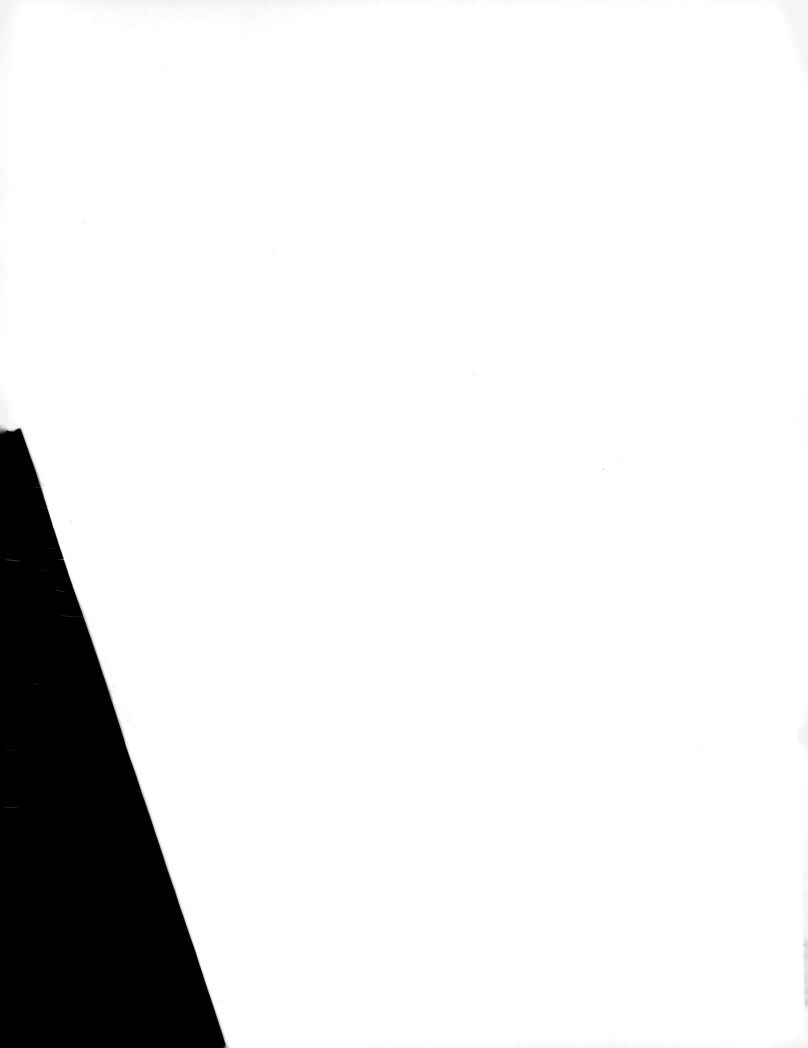

# Assessing and Treating Dysphagia

A Lifespan Perspective

**Debra M. Suiter, PhD, CCC-SLP, BCS-S, F-ASHA**
Director, Voice and Swallow Clinic
Professor
Department of Communication Sciences and Disorders
University of Kentucky
Lexington, Kentucky

**Memorie M. Gosa, PhD, CCC-SLP, BCS-S**
Associate Professor, Speech-Language Pathologist
Department of Communicative Disorders
The University of Alabama
Neonatal Intensive Care Unit
Druid City Hospital
Tuscaloosa, Alabama

201 illustrations

Thieme
New York • Stuttgart • Delhi • Rio de Janeiro

Executive Editor: Tim Hiscock
Managing Editor: Elizabeth Palumbo
Editorial Assistant: Keith Palumbo
Director, Editorial Services: Mary Jo Casey
Production Editor: Kenny Chumbley
International Production Director: Andreas Schabert
Editorial Director: Sue Hodgson
International Marketing Director: Fiona Henderson
International Sales Director: Louisa Turrell
Director of Institutional Sales: Adam Bernacki
Senior Vice President and Chief Operating Officer: Sarah Vanderbilt
President: Brian D. Scanlan

**Library of Congress Cataloging-in-Publication Data**

Names: Suiter, Debra M., editor. | Gosa, Memorie M., editor.

Title: Assessing and treating dysphagia : a lifespan perspective / [edited by] Debra M. Suiter, Memorie M. Gosa.

Description: New York : Thieme, [2019] | Includes bibliographical references.

Identifiers: LCCN 2019007265| ISBN 9781626232143 (hardcover : alk. paper) | ISBN 9781626232150 (e-book)

Subjects: | MESH: Deglutition Disorders--diagnosis | Deglutition Disorders--therapy

Classification: LCC RC815.2 | NLM WI 258 | DDC 616.3/23--dc23

LC record available at https://lccn.loc.gov/2019007265

**Important note:** Medicine is an ever-changing science undergoing continual development. Research and clinical experience are con- tin- ually expanding our knowledge, in particular our knowledge of proper treatment and drug therapy. Insofar as this book mentions any dosage or application, readers may rest assured that the authors, editors, and publishers have made every effort to ensure that such references are in accordance with **the state of knowledge at the time of production of the book**.

Nevertheless, this does not involve, imply, or express any guarantee or responsibility on the part of the publishers in respect to any dosage instructions and forms of applications stated in the book. **Every user is requested to examine carefully** the manufacturers' leaflets accompanying each drug and to check, if necessary in consultation with a physician or specialist, whether the dosage schedules mentioned therein or the contraindications stated by the manufacturers differ from the statements made in the present book. Such examination is particularly important with drugs that are either rarely used or have been newly released on the market. Every dosage schedule or every form of application used is entirely at the user's own risk and responsibility. The authors and publishers request every user to report to the publishers any discrepancies or inaccuracies noticed. If errors in this work are found after publication, errata will be posted at www.thieme.com on the product description page.

Some of the product names, patents, and registered designs referred to in this book are in fact registered trademarks or proprietary names even though specific reference to this fact is not always made in the text. Therefore, the appearance of a name without designation as proprietary is not to be construed as a representation by the publisher that it is in the public domain.

© 2019 Thieme Medical Publishers, Inc.
Thieme Publishers New York
333 Seventh Avenue, New York, NY 10001 USA
+1 800 782 3488, customerservice@thieme.com

Thieme Publishers Stuttgart
Rüdigerstrasse 14, 70469 Stuttgart, Germany
+49 [0]711 8931 421, customerservice@thieme.de

Thieme Publishers Delhi
A-12, Second Floor, Sector-2, Noida-201301
Uttar Pradesh, India
+91 120 45 566 00, customerservice@thieme.in

Thieme Publishers Rio de Janeiro, Thieme Publicações Ltda.
Edifício Rodolpho de Paoli, 25º andar
Av. Nilo Peçanha, 50 – Sala 2508
Rio de Janeiro 20020-906, Brasil
+55 21 3172 2297

Cover design: Thieme Publishing Group
Typesetting by Prairie Papers

Printed in the United States of America by King Printing Co., Inc.

ISBN 978-1-62623-214-3

Also available as an e-book:
eISBN 978-1-62623-215-0

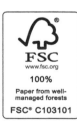

FSC
www.fsc.org
100%
Paper from well-managed forests
FSC® C103101

# Dedication

To Steve Leder who taught me to question everything and never accept anything less than the best for the patients we serve.

A thank you to my husband, Steve, and daughter, Lauren, for their unwavering support and patience as we worked on this book.

And, thank you to my patients and students throughout the years for teaching me how to be a better clinician and educator.

*Debra M. Suiter*

To my children, Tucker and Sam. You changed everything about me and continue to have a profound influence on the way I approach feeding and swallowing difficulties in pediatric populations.

To my husband, Joe, and my parents, Bill and Sharon Mintz. You all have been a source of tremendous support and encouragement throughout my education and career. Thank you for loving me, believing in me, and pushing me outside of my comfort zone to achieve things I did not always know were possible.

To the infants and children with feeding and swallowing difficulties and their families, who inspire me every day to strive for advances in this area.

*Memorie M. Gosa*

# Contents

# Foreword

A reader often measures the purchase of a book by looking at the collective content, contributors, and quality of direction offered in a text. Many believe a good book will contain enough wisdom to outlast changes in technology or shifts in conventional wisdom. Sometimes this is true. The scope of study in the area of swallowing disorders is vast, and clinicians perceive a constant need for more instruction and shepherding as clinical conventions are challenged and timeworn information is supplanted by new ideas.

But replacing the old with the new occurs slowly, and the increments of change can only be achieved through the protracted process of replication and, sometimes, origination, in both the clinic and the lab. The process is often so slow that changes go unnoticed. There are rare moments when there is a union of time, place, and acquaintance that only those most sensitive to perturbations in their field realize. There are rarer moments when these sensitive souls recognize the opportunity to express the refinement. This book, written by my friends and colleagues Debra Suiter and Memorie Gosa, is an example of such a realization. They perceived and took advantage of the intersection of knowledge and favorable conditions, gathered the right experts at the right time, and expressed a state of change that will be meaningful to clinician, researcher, instructor, and student.

I firmly believe that the clinic always informs research. Less often the reverse is true; researchers who are cloistered in a lab will find it difficult to develop the insight necessary to ask important questions and create a construct for answering them that can be translated into clinical practice. Dr. Suiter and Dr. Gosa are both consummate clinician-scientists who have successfully straddled both worlds. Both have decades of service to patients and many peer-reviewed manuscripts from their labs. They recognize good clinical practice and good data. The proof is in this book. The difficulty of editing a book with multiple authors is to create a singular and seamless "voice" for the reader. The authors of the contributed chapters are numerous and bring a wide-range of both clinical and technical expertise to each of the areas covered. My joy as I read the assembled work was that I was not encumbered to slog through a technical review of measurement and analysis but was instead offered a nuanced and helpful treatment in each chapter. The range of topics is also impressive. Along with new and technically advanced information related to videofluoroscopy, laryngoscopy, and manometrics, this book includes essential advice regarding counseling and the shepherding of patients and family at the end of life.

The reader will find that Debra and Memorie have identified and convinced leaders in the field, who are at the height of their command in their area of specialization, to give both exacting and useful information. Many will continue to expand their expertise and innovation. Sadly, at least one author has left us in the time between the writing and publication. Dr. Steven Leder would be appropriately proud of his contribution to this book. He'd be even more proud of the entirety of the creations that accompany it, especially of his colleague Debra Suiter who, with Memorie Gosa, produced this excellent work. There are no weaknesses here. Each chapter shines, and I believe each author has produced their very best work.

George Herbert (1593–1633) said, "The best mirror is an old friend." I have watched both Debra and Memorie work together for years, and I know they are old friends. When each looks in the mirror, she sees a productive scientist, a careful and caring clinician, and now, a very successful author of an excellent book. I am proud to know them both.

*Joseph Murray, PhD, CCC-SLP*
*Chief, Audiology/Speech Pathology Service*
*VA Ann Arbor Healthcare System*
*Ann Arbor, Michigan*

# Preface

This book is the culmination of an academic and clinical partnership between two clinician-researchers who practice across the lifespan. Throughout our careers, we have drawn information from experts in the field of dysphagia to inform our clinical practice and to transfer knowledge about the complexities of dysphagia to students and colleagues. Now, this book represents a referenced, accessible, and tangible culmination of those efforts.

The chapters are intentionally arranged to integrate swallowing concepts that are relevant across the human lifespan, and each chapter is authored by a respected expert in the area of interest. Unique to this text is a section on ethical and multicultural considerations for dysphagia practice. As such, this up-to-date reference represents a complete source of evidence-based practice information that will benefit students and novice and seasoned clinicians.

It is our hope that you, our readers, will find this book useful in every phase of your career as you strive to provide the best possible care for people with dysphagia.

*Debra M. Suiter*
*Memorie M. Gosa*

# Contributors

**Saima Aftab, MD**
Director
Fetal Care Center
Medical Director
Victor Center
Miami, Florida

**Paras M. Bhattarai, MD, MBA**
Assistant Professor and Director, Pediatric Stroke Program
Department of Pediatrics, Division of Pediatric Neurology
University of Tennessee Health Science Center
Le Bonheur Children's Hospital
Memphis, Tennessee

**Susan Brady, DHEd, MS, CCC-SLP, BCS-S**
Director of Quality and Research
Department of Quality, Outcomes, Research, and Education
Marianjoy Rehabilitation Hospital, Northwestern Medicine
Wheaton, Illinois

**Martin B. Brodsky, PhD, ScM, CCC-SLP, F-ASHA**
Associate Professor
Department of Physical Medicine and Rehabilitation
Johns Hopkins University
Baltimore, Maryland

**Giselle Carnaby, MPH, PhD, CCC=SLP, FASHA**
Professor
Internal Medicine and Communication Sciences and
  Disorders
University of Central Florida
Orlando, Florida

**Mary L. Casper, MA, CCC-SLP, FNAP**
Corporate Rehabilitation Consultant
Rehabilitation Department
HCR ManorCare
Rockville, Maryland

**Edgar Chambers IV, PhD**
University Distinguished Professor
Center for Sensory Analysis and Consumer Behavior
Kansas State University
Manhattan, Kansas

**Kelly Green Corkins, MS, RD, CSP, LDN, CNSC**
Pediatric Clinical Dietitian III
LeBonheur Children's Hospital
Memphis, Tennessee

**Mark R. Corkins, MD, FAAP**
Professor of Pediatrics
University of Tennessee Health Science Center
Division Chief
Pediatric Gastroenterology
LeBonheur Children's Hospital
Memphis, Tennessee

**Scott Dailey, PhD, CCC-SLP**
Speech-Language Pathologist, Adjunct Assistant Professor
Department of Otolaryngology–Head and Neck Surgery
University of Iowa Hospitals and Clinics
Iowa City, Iowa

**Amy L. Delaney, PhD, CCC-SLP**
Assistant Professor
Department of Speech Pathology and Audiology
Marquette University
Milwaukee, Wisconsin

**Pamela Dodrill, PhD, CCC-SLP**
Clinical Specialist
Feeding and Developmental Therapy Team
Neonatal Intensive Care Unit
Brigham and Women's Hospital
Boston, Massachusetts

**Caryn Easterling, PhD CCC ASHA Fellow**
Adjunct Faculty
Department of Communication Sciences and Disorders
University of Wisconsin-Milwaukee
Milwaukee, Wisconsin

**Jane Mertz Garcia, PhD**
Professor
Department of Communication Sciences and Disorders
Kansas State University
Manhattan, Kansas

**Memorie M. Gosa, PhD, CCC-SLP, BCS-S**
Associate Professor, Speech-Language Pathologist
Department of Communicative Disorders
The University of Alabama
Neonatal Intensive Care Unit
Druid City Hospital
Tuscaloosa, Alabama

**Melanie P. Hiorns, MBBS, FRCR, FRCP**
Consultant, Paediatric Radiologist
Radiology Department
Institution Great Ormond Street Hospital for Children
London, United Kingdom

**Sudarshan R. Jadcherla, MD, FRCPI, DCH**
Professor and Associate Division Chief, Academics
Department of Pediatrics
Nationwide Children's Hospital
The Ohio State University College of Medicine
Columbus, Ohio

**Jason Nathaniel Johnson, MD, MHS**
Director, Cardiac MRI
Assistant Professor of Pediatrics and Radiology
University of Tennessee Health Sciences Center
LeBonheur Children's Hospital
Memphis, Tennessee

**Molly A. Knigge, MS**
Senior Speech Pathologist
Department of Surgery, Division of Otolaryngology
University of Wisconsin–Madison
Madison, Wisconsin

**Steven B. Leder, PhD, CCC-SLP (deceased)**
Professor
Department of Surgery
Section of Otolaryngology
Yale University School of Medicine
New Haven, Connecticut

**Paula Leslie, PhD, MA (Bioethics), FRCSLT, CCC-SLP**
Senior Lecturer
School of Health Sciences
Faculty of Health and Wellbeing
University of Central Lancashire
Lancashire, United Kingdom

**Georgia A. Malandraki, PhD, CCC-SLP, BCS-S**
Associate Professor
Department of Speech, Language, and Hearing Sciences
Purdue University
West Lafayette, Indiana

**Jaime Bauer Malandraki, MS, CCC-SLP, BCS-S**
Clinical Assistant Professor
Department of Speech, Language and Hearing Sciences
West Lafayette, Indiana

**Claire Kane Miller, PhD, MHA**
Program Director
Aerodigestive and Esophageal Center
Interdisciplinary Feeding Team
Division of Speech-Language Pathology
Cincinnati Children's Hospital Medical Center
Cincinnati, Ohio

**William G. Pearson Jr., PhD**
Associate Professor
Department of Cellular Biology and Anatomy
Medical College of Georgia
Augusta University
Augusta, Georgia

**Emily K. Plowman, PhD, CCC-SLP**
Associate Professor
Departments of Communication Sciences and Disorders
    and Neurology
Co-Director, Swallowing Systems Core
Clinical Director, Center for Respiratory Rehabilitation
    and Research
University of Florida
Gainesville, Florida

**Luis F. Riquelme, PhD, CCC-SLP, BCS-S**
Associate Professor, Director
Department of Speech-Language Pathology,
    School of Health Sciences and Practice
New York Medical College
Valhalla, New York
Center for Swallowing and Speech-Language Pathology
New York-Presbyterian Brooklyn Methodist Hospital
Brooklyn, New York

**Erin Sundseth Ross, PhD, CCC-SLP**
Developmental Therapist, Speech/Language Pathologist
Physical Medicine and Rehabilitation
Rose Medical Center
Denver, Colorado

**Martina Ryan, LRSLT, MRSLT**
Specialist, Speech and Language Therapist
Department of Speech and Language Therapy
Great Ormond Street Hospital
London, United Kingdom

**Reza Shaker, MD**
Senior Associate Dean, Chief, Professor
Division of Gastroenterology
Director
Digestive Disease Center
Clinical and Translational Research
Medical College of Wisconsin
Milwaukee, Wisconsin

**Pamela A. Smith, PhD, CCC-SLP**
Professor of Speech Pathology
Department of Communication Sciences and Disorders
Bloomsburg University
Bloomsburg, Pennsylvania

**Heather M. Starmer, MA, CCC-SLP, BCS-S**
Director, Head and Neck Speech and Swallowing
  Rehabilitation
Department of Otolaryngology–Head and Neck Surgery
Stanford University
Palo Alto, California

**Catriona M. Steele, PhD, S-LP(C), CCC-SLP, BCS-S**
Senior Scientist
Swallowing Rehabilitation Research Laboratory
Toronto Rehabilitation Institute–University Health
  Network
Toronto, Ontario, Canada

**Debra M. Suiter, PhD, CCC-SLP, BCS-S, F-ASHA**
Director, Voice & Swallow Clinic
Professor
Department of Communication Sciences & Disorders
University of Kentucky
Lexington, Kentucky

**Nancy B. Swigert, MA, CCC-SLP, BCS-S**
President
Swigert & Associates, Inc.
Biltmore Lake, North Carolina

**Lauren Tabor, MS, CCC-SLP**
Swallowing Systems Core
University of Florida
Gainesville, Florida

**Susan L. Thibeault, PhD, CCC-SLP**
Professor, Diane M. Bless Endowed Chair
Department of Surgery
University of Wisconsin–Madison
Madison, Wisconsin

**Kay A. Toomey, PhD**
President, Toomey & Associates, Inc.
Clinical Supervisor, The Feeding Clinic @ STAR
Developer, SOS Approach to Feeding program
Pediatric Psychologist
Denver, Colorado

**James D. Tutor, MD**
Professor of Pediatrics
Program in Pediatric Pulmonary Medicine
University of Tennessee Health Science Center
Le Bonheur Children's Hospital
Memphis, Tennessee

**Heather L. Warner, PhD, CCC-SLP**
Assistant Professor
Department of Communication Disorders
Southern Connecticut State University
New Haven, Connecticut

**Tammy Wigginton, MS, CCC-SLP, BCS-S**
Speech Language Pathologist
University of Kentucky Voice and Swallow Clinic
Lexington, Kentucky

**Jay Paul Willging, MD**
Professor
Department of Otolaryngology–Head and Neck Surgery
University of Cincinnati College of Medicine
Cincinnati Children's Hospital Medical Center
Cincinnati, Ohio

# 1 Introduction

*Debra M. Suiter and Memorie M. Gosa*

## Summary

This book is a comprehensive, yet accessible, volume of information on dysphagia and its many manifestations across the lifespan. It is written for graduate-level students, practicing clinicians currently working with individuals with swallowing disorders, and practicing clinicians wishing to transition to working with individuals with swallowing disorders. Experts in their respective areas provide the latest, most evidence-based information available on swallowing disorders, including their assessment and treatment.

## *Keywords*

dysphagia, deglutition, penetration, aspiration, mastication, bolus

---

### *Learning Objectives*

In order to understand swallowing disorders, it is important to first understand the following terms.

- **Dysphagia** is the medical term for swallowing disorders. As Dr. Jerilyn Logemann, a pioneer in the field of dysphagia assessment and treatment, described it, dysphagia is "any difficulty in moving food from the mouth to the stomach."
- **Deglutition** is the medical term for swallowing.
- **Penetration** is the entrance of anything ingested by mouth, secretions (saliva or mucus), or refluxed or regurgitated stomach contents into the laryngeal vestibule, which is bounded superiorly by the epiglottis, laterally by the aryepiglottic folds, and inferiorly by the true vocal folds. The term *penetration* indicates that material has entered the laryngeal vestibule but has not spilled below the level of the true vocal folds.
- **Aspiration** is the entrance of anything ingested by mouth, secretions (saliva or mucus), or refluxed or regurgitated stomach contents into the laryngeal vestibule and below the level of the true vocal folds.
- **Mastication** is the medical term for chewing.
- **Bolus** is a cohesive mass of food or liquid to be swallowed.

Additional terms specific to dysphagia in various settings and across various patient populations are defined in each chapter of this book.

---

## 1.1 Introduction to Swallowing Disorders

Each chapter begins with an introduction to its topic, a summary of what will be discussed, and a list of learning objectives. At the end of each chapter, the reader is asked a number of review questions to facilitate retention of the material. We hope our readers will find this approach to be beneficial.

This is not a "how-to" manual by design. Instead of "if you see this, do this," this text was designed to prepare current and future clinicians to assess and treat patients with dysphagia by equipping them with the underlying knowledge necessary to facilitate safe oral intake whenever possible. The text begins with foundational knowledge on the anatomy and physiology of typical swallowing across the life span. These chapters are purposefully dense; they are meant to provide the reader with a complete understanding of what is known about typical swallowing across the life span. This sets the stage for clinicians to apply the knowledge when evaluating swallowing in populations with various disorders that are known to impact swallowing function. Once readers understand how structure and physiology work together to create a typical, safe swallow, they can conceptualize how disorders that impact normal structure or function will impact swallowing.

The book transitions to chapters on assessment and again provides foundational knowledge for these concepts throughout the life span. The knowledge from these chapters should guide readers as they delve into population-specific chapters later in the book and apply the concepts gleaned from the assessment chapters to populations of interest.

From assessment, the book moves on to comprehensive chapters on treatment for individuals with dysphagia. Chapters 8 to 10 provide the fundamental concepts that underlie all treatment, regardless of specific etiology. Again, readers will apply these foundational concepts as they evaluate treatment-specific options in each of the population chapters. Readers are then ready to examine population-specific information about dysphagia in conditions that affect individuals across the life span, beginning with prematurity and ending with pulmonary disease.

Finally, readers will have the opportunity to evaluate the knowledge gained in this text in the context of biomedical ethical considerations. At that point, it is our hope that clinicians (future and currently practicing) have the knowledge needed to accurately diagnose and treat dysphagia across populations and diagnoses, which is more than could be accomplished with a simple "how-to" manual. Individuals with dysphagia deserve no less than a competent clinician equipped with the knowledge necessary to help them reach their specific goals related to feeding and swallowing. All those who contributed to this text invested the necessary time and energy to create this type of resource out of a desire to provide the best care possible to patients with dysphagia. We hope it will become a valuable resource to all readers.

## 1.2 Scope of the Problem

Human beings begin life taking all nutrition and hydration in liquid form, from either the breast or the bottle, consuming breast milk or formula. In rapid order, infants transition from a full liquid diet to a diet of varied textures and consistencies, typically by age 2. As infants learn to eat a variety of foods, there will be periods of increased coughing and gagging that resolve as the oral–motor patterns to support mastication of increasing textures are mastered. As infants mature into childhood, adolescence, and adulthood they will most likely continue to experience transient difficulty with swallowing.

Most people can relate to coughing on a piece of dry, crumbly food, such as cornbread or tortilla chips, or experiencing the feeling of something "going down the wrong tube." During times of illness, people experience painful swallowing due to a sore throat and choose to avoid certain foods or liquids that exacerbate the pain. As people age, they may have difficulty swallowing large pills and will need to find ways to facilitate safe swallowing. In most instances, these encounters with swallowing difficulty are transient and do not have lasting negative effects on a person's health or well-being. However, for some individuals, difficulty swallowing is an ongoing issue that can have a significant impact on health and quality of life, forcing them into scenarios that seem out of their control.

Swallowing disorders can occur at any age, from birth to old age. Dysphagia can have a variety of causes, including prematurity. It can be neurogenic, resulting from a stroke, brain injury, Parkinson's disease, or amyotrophic lateral sclerosis (Lou Gehrig's disease). It can arise from structural abnormalities, such as craniofacial disorders, head and neck tumors, narrowing of the esophagus, or trauma to the head and neck, or from systemic diseases such as pulmonary disease. Chapters 11 through 22 of this book provide relevant information on dysphagia resulting from specific etiologies, including diagnostic and treatment consideration of the specific etiology, not just information specific to dysphagia in this population.

Dysphagia occurs in approximately 1 in 25 adults per year,[1] and dysphagia occurs in 9 in 1,000 children between the ages of 3 and 17 years.[2] Dysphagia is more prevalent in some developmental and disease-specific pediatric populations, such as those with congenital heart disease and syndromes with craniofacial disorders, but accurate information on incidence and prevalence is difficult to discern due to various definitions and diagnostic modalities. Dysphagia is most common in older adults.[1,3,4] In a large acute care hospital, dysphagia referral rates doubled between the years 2000 and 2007, and over 70% of those referrals were for adults 60 years of age or older, with 42% of those referrals being for adults over the age of 80 years.[4] The prevalence of dysphagia in community-dwelling adults over the age of 50 is estimated to be somewhere between 15 and 22%,[5,6] and in skilled nursing facilities the prevalence rises to over 60%.[7]

## 1.3  Consequences of Dysphagia

Dysphagia can have devastating consequences for an individual's health. Malnutrition and dehydration often occur in individuals with swallowing disorders. An individual who coughs frequently when attempting to eat or drink, or who has significant difficulty getting food or liquid to clear, may avoid those foods and liquids and ultimately limit the overall intake of food and liquid.

Malnutrition can lead to additional health consequences, including a weakened immune system, which increases infection

risk, results in poor wound healing, and leads to muscle weakness, all of which can increase the risk of falls or other injuries. Infants and children do not have the nutritional reserves to withstand prolonged periods of dehydration and malnutrition, and these can lead to significant morbidity and mortality in pediatric populations. Therefore, dysphagia must be diagnosed accurately and treated effectively to avoid these undesirable consequences.

In addition to malnutrition and dehydration, dysphagia can also result in pulmonary complications, including aspiration pneumonia. Aspiration pneumonia is demonstrated by radiographic evidence of infiltrates in the lungs of individuals known to be at risk for dysphagia.[8,9] Aspiration pneumonia is caused when bacteria that normally reside in the oropharynx or nasopharynx enter the lungs. According to the Agency for Health Care Policy and Research (AHCPR), approximately one-third of individuals with dysphagia develop aspiration pneumonia, and 60,000 individuals die each year from complications related to aspiration pneumonia.[1,10] The 30-day mortality rate from aspiration pneumonia is 21% overall, with a higher percentage (29.7%) for health care–associated aspiration pneumonia.[11]

Although aspiration pneumonia occurs more frequently in adults, it can occur at any point across the life span. Aspiration is also recognized as a significant source of respiratory morbidity in pediatric patients because it has potential to cause permanent damage to developing lungs.[12]

In addition to impacting an individual's health adversely, dysphagia can also significantly impact quality of life. So many special moments in a person's life are celebrated and acknowledged in the context of eating and drinking. Birthdays are celebrated with cake, weddings are toasted with champagne, holidays are celebrated around the dinner table with friends and family, families are comforted by friends bringing food after the death of a loved one. Eating and drinking are a part of everyday life. An individual who is experiencing dysphagia may not be able to participate in these activities and may be able only to watch while others take part. Inability to participate in these types of activities can lead to social isolation, anxiety, and depression. Sometimes, even taking a small amount of food or liquid by mouth can lead to coughing or the need to regurgitate food or liquid and may become too embarrassing for a person to participate in situations that involve any eating and drinking. Many individuals with dysphagia report avoiding certain activities, such as eating out in a restaurant, because they do not wish to draw embarrassing attention.

Parents of children with dysphagia have to be hypervigilant and often have to restrict their child's involvement in typical social activities, such as school events, play dates with friends, and birthday parties. In a survey of individuals with dysphagia, clinical depression was found in 7% of respondents, and 20% of respondents reported experiencing anxiety related to their dysphagia.[13] Hewetson and Singh[14] reported on the experience of mothers of children with dysphagia and found that mothers describe the experience as two intertwined journeys: one of deconstruction, where their previous expectations of motherhood are lost, and one of reconstruction, where they learn to function in the reality of having a child with dysphagia. The authors emphasize the need for health care professionals to incorporate the parent's experience into true family-focused interventions.

## 1.4 The Dysphagia Team

The dysphagia team comprises individuals from a number of health care specialties. These include speech-language pathology, nursing, nutrition, medicine, psychology, allied health professions (e.g., occupational therapy or physical therapy), and respiratory therapy. This list is not exhaustive, and, depending on the patient's needs, other health care professionals may serve as members of the dysphagia team. Members of the team work together to ensure that all the individual's dysphagia-related needs are met. For instance, physical therapists are often involved with individuals who have dysphagia across the life span to determine optimal positioning and develop seating systems for head and neck supports. Occupational therapists may identify utensils or plates that facilitate the individual's ability to self-feed; again this is seen across the life span. Speech-language pathologists (SLPs) work closely with dietitians to ensure that individuals with dysphagia are meeting their nutrition and hydration needs and doing so safely. Psychologists may address the negative social consequences individuals with swallowing disorders experience.

SLPs often take the lead role in caring for individuals with dysphagia. This is because SLPs receive extensive training in the anatomy and physiology of the upper aerodigestive tract, including the oral, pharyngeal, and cervical esophageal regions that are involved in swallowing. The SLP is a primary professional involved in assessment and management of individuals with dysphagia and is responsible for the following:

- Performing a clinical swallowing and feeding evaluation
- Performing an instrumental assessment of swallowing function with medical professionals as appropriate
- Identifying normal and abnormal swallowing anatomy and physiology
- Identifying signs of possible or potential disorders in upper aerodigestive tract swallowing and making referrals to appropriate medical personnel
- Making decisions about management of swallowing and feeding disorders
- Developing treatment plans
- Providing treatment for swallowing and feeding disorders, documenting progress, and determining appropriate dismissal criteria
- Providing teaching and counseling to individuals and their families
- Educating other professionals on the needs of individuals with swallowing and feeding disorders and the SLP's role in the diagnosis and management of swallowing and feeding disorders
- Serving as an integral part of a team as appropriate
- Advocating for services for individuals with swallowing and feeding disorders
- Advancing the knowledge base through research activities[15]

Because of the negative health consequences of unrecognized or improperly treated dysphagia, it is imperative that SLPs who wish to work with individuals with swallowing disorders have proper training and knowledge to do so. As with other areas of clinical practice, this is required by the American Speech-Language-Hearing Association Code of Ethics.[16]

## 1.5 Assessment and Treatment for Dysphagia

Proper management of individuals with dysphagia begins with accurate assessment. Assessment can include screening, clinical swallow evaluation, or instrumental assessment, such as videofluoroscopy (X-ray), endoscopy, or manometry. The purpose of each of these assessments, optimal means of completing them, and indications/contraindications for each type of examination are discussed in Chapters 4 to 10.

Dysphagia is often a treatable condition. As already described, SLPs work closely with other health care professionals to determine an appropriate course of treatment. Treatments may include direct, rehabilitative treatments (e.g., active exercises to strengthen the structures involved in swallowing); indirect, compensatory treatments (e.g., suggestions for optimal posture for swallowing); or diet modifications (e.g., altering the texture of the individual's food or liquid). In some cases, when treatment outcomes are not successful, or are progressing more slowly than anticipated, an alternative means of nutrition is recommended. Treatments for dysphagia are discussed at length in Chapters 11 to 13 of this book. Additionally, treatment for dysphagia related to specific etiologies is discussed in Chapters 14 to 25.

## 1.6 Conclusion

Dysphagia is common in both adults and children. Its consequences can be devastating and isolating. It is our hope that the remainder of this book will serve to educate and prepare current and future clinicians who wish to work with individuals with swallowing disorders.

## References

[1] Bhattacharyya N. The prevalence of dysphagia among adults in the United States. *Head Neck Surg* 2014;*151*(5):765–769

[2] Bhattacharyya N. The prevalence of pediatric voice and swallowing problems in the United States. *Laryngoscope* 2015;*125*(3):746–750

[3] Baine WB, Yu W, Summe JP. Epidemiologic trends in the hospitalization of elderly Medicare patients for pneumonia, 1991-1998. *Am J Public Health* 2001;*91*(7):1121–1123

[4] Leder SB, Suiter DM. An epidemiologic study on aging and dysphagia in the acute care hospitalized population: 2000-2007. *Gerontology* 2009;*55*(6):714–718

[5] Aslam M, Vaezi MF. Dysphagia in the elderly. *Gastroenterol Hepatol (N Y)* 2013;*9*(12):784–795

[6] Barczi SR, Sullivan PA, Robbins J. How should dysphagia care of older adults differ? Establishing optimal practice patterns. *Semin Speech Lang* 2000;*21*(4):347–361

[7] Steele CM, Greenwood C, Ens I, Robertson C, Seidman-Carlson R. Mealtime difficulties in a home for the aged: not just dysphagia. *Dysphagia* 1997;*12*(1):43–50, discussion 51

[8] Marik PE, Kaplan D. Aspiration pneumonia and dysphagia in the elderly. *Chest* 2003;*124*(1):328–336

[9] Marik PE. Aspiration pneumonitis and aspiration pneumonia. *N Engl J Med* 2001;*344*(9):665–671

[10] Group EHTA; ECRI Health Technology Assessment Group. Diagnosis and treatment of swallowing disorders (dysphagia) in acute-care stroke patients. *Evid Rep Technol Assess (Summ)* 1999; (8):1–6

[11] Lanspa MJ, Jones BE, Brown SM, Dean NC. Mortality, morbidity, and disease severity of patients with aspiration pneumonia. *J Hosp Med* 2013;8(2):83–90

[12] Tutor JD, Gosa MM. Dysphagia and aspiration in children. *Pediatr Pulmonol* 2012;47(4):321–337

[13] Eslick GD, Talley NJ. Dysphagia: epidemiology, risk factors and impact on quality of life—a population-based study. *Aliment Pharmacol Ther* 2008;27(10):971–979

[14] Hewetson R, Singh S. The lived experience of mothers of children with chronic feeding and/or swallowing difficulties. *Dysphagia* 2009;24(3):322–332

[15] American Speech-Language-Hearing Association. Roles of speech-language pathologists in swallowing and feeding disorders: Technical report. 200

[16] American Speech-Language-Hearing Association. Code of ethics. 2016. www.asha.org/policy/

# 2 Anatomy of Swallowing

*William G. Pearson Jr. and Memorie M. Gosa*

## Summary

Thirty-plus muscles under the control of five cranial nerves and several spinal nerves convert a respiratory channel into a digestive tract and back within 500 milliseconds. To understand what goes wrong with swallowing, a master clinician must have a working knowledge of normal structure relevant to swallowing function. This chapter describes in some detail the oral cavity and pharynx in relationship to the skeleton. The text then discusses functional groups of neuromuscular structures that underlie the various physiological elements of swallowing, including ingestion, bolus formation, oral transport of the bolus, and pharyngeal conversion. Developmental differences in children and adults are discussed followed by the anatomy relevant to airway protection, salivation, neurobiology of swallowing, the esophagus, and development of the upper aerodigestive tract. Compromise of these structures, their function, or their development can lead to swallowing impairment. A strong knowledge of the functional anatomy of swallowing leads to effective understanding of swallowing function, impairment, and rehabilitation throughout the life span

## Keywords

oral cavity, pharynx, ingestion, bolus formation, oral transport of the bolus, pharyngeal conversion

## Learning Objectives
- List the surface features of the oral cavity and pharynx.
- Identify the muscles of the face, oral cavity, and pharynx that contribute to safe and effective swallowing.
- Explain the concept of a muscular hydrostat as it applies to the tongue.
- Identify the muscles underlying pharyngeal conversion.
- Describe the differences between the anatomical features for swallowing in the adult and infant.
- Describe the embryological development of the oral and pharyngeal cavities.

## 2.1 Introduction

The study of anatomy and physiology can be fascinating. Unfortunately, just reading the descriptions of anatomy and physiology can be tedious. If the reader becomes bogged down in the details of this anatomy chapter, reading Chapter 3 first, on physiology, may help. Once the function of the swallowing apparatus is understood, curiosity can motivate the study of the structures underlying function. As noted, the neuromuscular elements of anatomy in this chapter are organized by function. Because these structures serve multiple functions, some redundancy should be expected.

Students should have a basic understanding of human anatomy and physiology from their undergraduate coursework, ideally from a complete human anatomy and physiology class with lab. If students did not complete a comprehensive human anatomy and physiology course, then they are encouraged to obtain a human anatomy and physiology textbook and medical dictionary to read along with these chapters as needed. So often in the study of speech-language pathology, students are taught to consider just the overlaid functions pertinent to the field; however, to truly grasp the complexities of dysphagia, students need to consider the human body and its biological functions as a whole. It is suggested that, in addition to reading the chapters here, students also participate in a simultaneous lab experience, if possible. If a live lab experience is not available, students may consider one of many virtual anatomy software programs to augment reading. Additionally, students should read these chapters in an active, purposeful way. Use every means available to try to visualize the anatomy during the swallowing sequence. The point of studying anatomy is not memorizing lists of structures, but gaining a working knowledge of the **morphology** that underlies function so that you might effectively rehabilitate swallowing impairment and educate your patients and other clinicians concerning sources of swallowing dysfunction. Speech-language pathologists working in a medical setting are expected to be the experts on the anatomy and physiology of swallowing.

## 2.2 Surface Anatomy of the Oral Cavity

The oral cavity includes lips, cheeks, hard and soft palate, tongue, and teeth. The lips and teeth are at the anterior boundary of the oral cavity, with the teeth and cheeks forming the lateral boundary. The hard and soft palate form the superior boundary of the oral cavity, with the uvula hanging midline at the posterior edge of the soft palate. Faucial pillars, formed by the palatoglossal and palatopharyngeal folds, are found at the lateral posterior boundary of the oral cavity. On the surface of the tongue various types of papillae (filiform, foliate, and vallate) can be found that house many taste receptors. **Epithelium** is moistened by saliva, produced by salivary glands that line the oral cavity. In the **mucosa** of the floor of the mouth are found openings for the submandibular and sublingual glands, whereas the openings of the parotid glands are found between the cheeks and upper molars (**Fig. 2.1**). The entire oral cavity is innervated with somatosensory neurons that provide information about the temperature, volume, consistency, and position of a bolus that is critical to effective swallowing.

## Clinical Note
- The lips, tongue, and soft palate are focal structures visualized in a videofluoroscopic study to assess the oral phase of swallowing.

## 2.3 Surface Anatomy of the Pharynx

The pharynx is the crossroads for the passage of food and oxygen into the human body. Historically it has been called a quadrivium, which in Latin is transliterated as "the place where four roads meet." The pharynx incorporates four portals to other conduits, including the oral cavity, nasal cavity, trachea, and esophagus.[1] The pharynx is connected to and integrates with multiple skeletal elements, including bones and cartilage. The inner surface of the muscular pharynx is covered with a tough sheet of deep **fascia** called the pharyngobasilar fascia, a membrane that is lined with a continuous layer of mucosa. This mucosal lining drapes over the entire inner surface of the pharynx, including muscles, bone, and cartilage. This mucosal draping creates named spaces and folds. The pharynx can be divided into three sections: nasopharynx, oropharynx, and laryngopharynx. The laryngopharynx is more often clinically referred to as the hypopharynx. A bolus passes from the oral cavity through the oropharynx and hypopharynx to the esophagus (**Fig. 2.2**).

The spaces most relevant to swallowing in the pharynx are the **valleculae** and the **piriform recesses,** or **sinuses.** The valleculae, or "little valleys," lie between the median and lateral glossoepiglottic folds and become a potential reservoir for pharyngeal residue. The other common sites for residue are the piriform recesses, spaces lateral to the larynx created by the muscosa draping from the laryngeal inlet to the muscular pharyngeal wall on either side. When the pharynx is relaxed, residue can pool in either piriform recess on the side of the upper esophageal sphincter (**Fig. 2.3**).

Additional folds are formed by structures that lie within each fold. The median glossoepiglottic fold is formed by mucosa draping over the glossoepiglottic ligament. The aryepiglottic folds border the **laryngeal vestibule** and contain small variable muscle fascicles. The palatoglossal fold and palatopharyngeal folds, formed by muscles with the same name, descend from the palate on either side of the palatine **tonsil** and are referred to as the anterior and posterior faucial pillar, respectively. The salpingopharyngeal fold forms around the salpingopharyngeal muscle, beginning at the opening of the auditory tube in the nasopharynx and extending inferiorly into the hypopharynx on the lateral pharyngeal walls (**Fig. 2.4**).

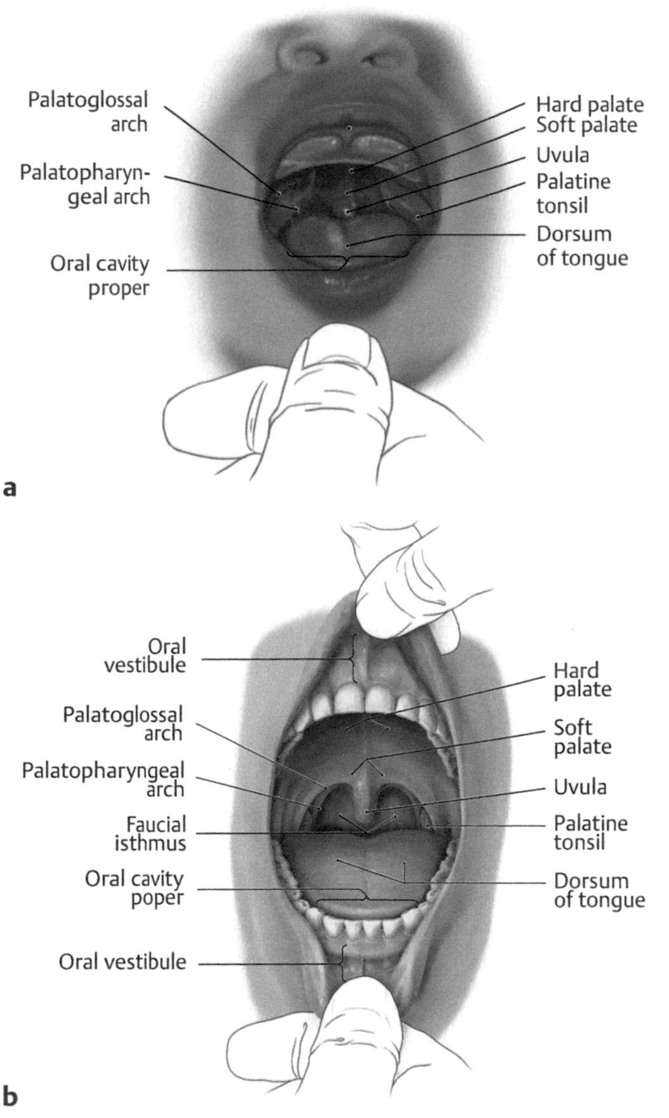

Palatoglossal arch

Palatopharyn-geal arch

Oral cavity proper

Hard palate
Soft palate

Uvula

Palatine tonsil

Dorsum of tongue

**a**

Oral vestibule

Palatoglossal arch

Palatopharyngeal arch

Faucial isthmus

Oral cavity poper

Oral vestibule

Hard palate

Soft palate

Uvula

Palatine tonsil

Dorsum of tongue

**b**

Fig. 2.1 **(a)** Infant and **(b)** adult oral cavity with structures labeled. **(b)** From Gilroy AM, MacPherson BR. *Atlas of Anatomy.* 3rd ed. New York, NY: Thieme, 2016.

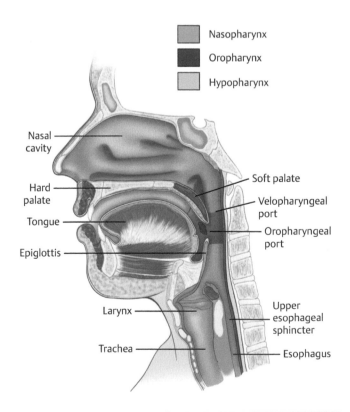

Nasopharynx

Oropharynx

Hypopharynx

Nasal cavity

Hard palate

Tongue

Epiglottis

Soft palate

Velopharyngeal port

Oropharyngeal port

Larynx

Trachea

Upper esophageal sphincter

Esophagus

Fig. 2.2 Regions of the pharynx, sagittal view.

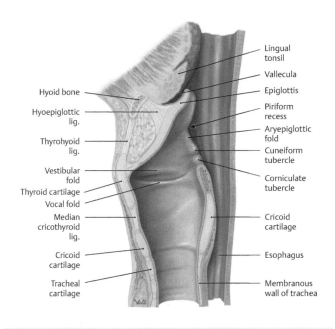

Lingual tonsil
Vallecula
Epiglottis
Piriform recess
Aryepiglottic fold
Cuneiform tubercle
Corniculate tubercle
Cricoid cartilage
Esophagus
Membranous wall of trachea

Hyoid bone
Hyoepiglottic lig.
Thyrohyoid lig.
Vestibular fold
Thyroid cartilage
Vocal fold
Median cricothyroid lig.
Cricoid cartilage
Tracheal cartilage

**Fig. 2.3** Valleculae and piriform recesses. From Gilroy AM, MacPherson BR. *Atlas of Anatomy*. 3rd ed. New York, NY: Thieme, 2016.

The pharynx is subdivided anatomically, and its regions are named after their adjacent apertures. The nasopharynx, opening into the **choanae** of the nasal cavity, is closed inferiorly by the soft palate or velum and is bordered posteriorly and laterally by the pharyngeal walls. The boundaries of the oropharynx are marked by the oropharyngeal isthmus anteriorly, the velum (soft palate) superiorly, the epiglottis inferiorly, and the pharyngeal walls posteriorly and laterally. The epiglottis, laryngeal vestibule, esophagus, and pharyngeal walls, including the piriform recesses, border the hypopharynx.

Recognizable features of the oropharynx and hypopharynx include the soft palate, uvula, faucial pillars, palatine tonsils, laryngeal vestibule, upper esophageal sphincter, valleculae, and piriform recess. Features of the nasopharynx are oriented around the opening to the auditory or **pharyngotympanic tube**. The tubal tonsils are located on mucosa covering the opening of the auditory tube, whereas the pharyngeal tonsils, also called the adenoids, are located posterior to the opening of the auditory tube. Enlarged adenoids can block both the nasal cavity and the auditory tube, leading to mouth breathing and problems in craniofacial development in children.[2] The palatine tonsils, often called the tonsils, are located inferior to the palate between the faucial pillars. All of these tonsils form a ring of

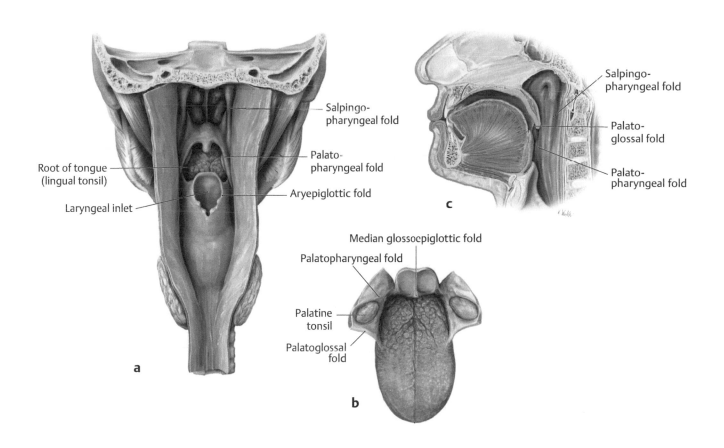

Salpingo-pharyngeal fold
Palato-pharyngeal fold
Aryepiglottic fold

Root of tongue (lingual tonsil)
Laryngeal inlet

a

Salpingo-pharyngeal fold
Palato-glossal fold
Palato-pharyngeal fold

c

Median glossoepiglottic fold
Palatopharyngeal fold
Palatine tonsil
Palatoglossal fold

b

**Fig. 2.4** Pharyngeal folds. From Gilroy AM, MacPherson BR. *Atlas of Anatomy*. 3rd ed. New York, NY: Thieme, 2016.

lymphoid tissue (Waldeyer's ring) surrounding the oral and nasal cavity portals to the pharynx, serving to protect the body from exogenous material. Severe inflammation of tonsils makes swallowing painful and difficult (**Fig. 2.5**). The pharynx does not have the same degree of somatosensory innervation as the oral cavity; however, the mucosa covering the faucial arches, opening of the larynx, and laryngeal vestibule is densely innervated.

## Clinical Note

Competent fiberoptic endoscopic evaluation of swallowing (FEES) requires recognition of the features and function of the nasopharynx, oropharynx, and hypopharynx.

## 2.4  Osteology of the Upper Digestive Tract

The **proximal** openings of the pharynx into the oral and nasal cavity are connected to bones of the **viscerocranium** and **cranial base**, whereas the distal openings into the trachea and esophagus connect to the **hyolaryngeal complex**. The oral cavity encompasses the mandible, the maxilla, the teeth, and the palatine bone, from which the soft palate extends posteriorly. Teeth are housed within the **alveolar processes of the maxilla and mandible**. Deciduous teeth emerge at approximately 7 months of age and are replaced by permanent teeth, typically by adolescence. The medial pterygoid plates serve as an attachment site for the superior end of the pharynx leading into the nasal cavity. The pharyngeal **tubercle** of the occipital bone, the styloid process and mastoid process of the temporal bone, and other surfaces of the temporal and

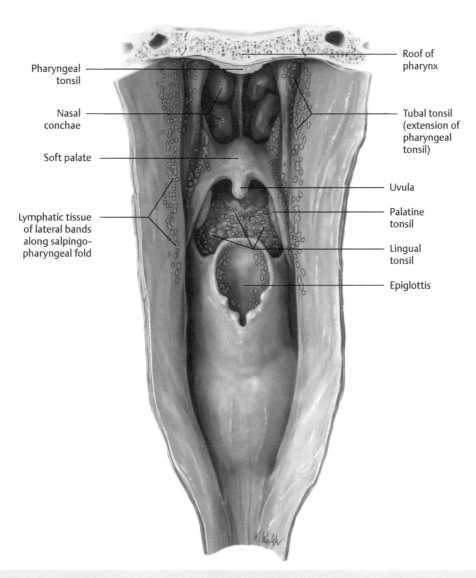

**Fig. 2.5** Tonsils. From Gilroy AM, MacPherson BR. *Atlas of Anatomy.* 3rd ed. New York, NY: Thieme, 2016.

sphenoid bones are all important cranial base attachment sites for muscles underlying mastication and swallowing (**Fig. 2.6**).

The hyolaryngeal complex is composed of the hyoid bone, laryngeal cartilages, and associated structures. The laryngeal skeleton is composed primarily of five cartilages, including the thyroid, cricoid, paired arytenoids, and epiglottis. Ligaments attach the epiglottis to the hyoid and thyroid cartilage. Of the laryngeal cartilages, the thyroid and cricoid cartilages serve as important attachment sites for the inferior pharyngeal constrictor muscle connecting the pharynx and esophagus.

Dense ligaments tether the thyroid cartilage to the hyoid (called the thyrohyoid membrane), and the cricoid to the thyroid cartilages (called the cricothyroid ligament) (**Fig. 2.7**). The valve function of the larynx primarily involves the arytenoid, cricoid, and thyroid cartilages. Muscles anchoring the hyoid inferiorly attach to the posterior facet of the sternum and scapula (**Fig. 2.8**). In sum, the osteology directly relevant to the functional

swallowing apparatus includes the mandible, the hard palate (maxilla and palatine bones), the medial pterygoid plates of the sphenoid, the styloid and mastoid process of the temporal bone, the temporomandibular joint, the hyoid and laryngeal cartilages (thyroid, cricoid, arytenoid, and epiglottis), and the sternum and scapulae.

The larynx is a visible structure in the anterior portion of the neck. It is located in the most inferior portion of the pharynx, the hypopharynx or laryngopharynx. The vocal folds and the muscles that accomplish movement of and within this organ are attached to these cartilages. The laryngeal cartilages form a series of synovial joints: the cricothyroid joint and the cricoarytenoid joints. The cricothyroid joint allows the cricoid cartilage to rotate around the thyroid cartilage, which shortens or lengthens the vocal folds. Movement at the cricoarytenoid joints allows for the vocal folds sliding toward or away from each other. Also, the cricoarytenoid joint allows for anterior tilting of the vocal folds (**Fig. 2.9**).

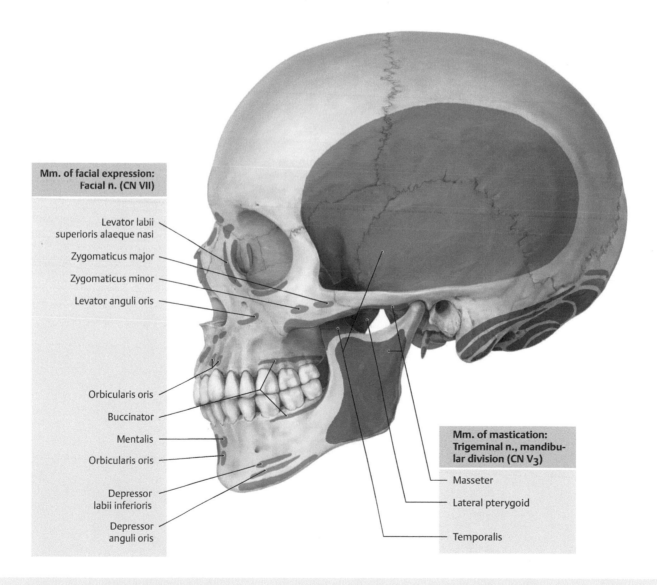

Fig. 2.6 Bony support of the face and oral cavity. From Gilroy AM, MacPherson BR. *Atlas of Anatomy.* 3rd ed. New York, NY: Thieme, 2016.

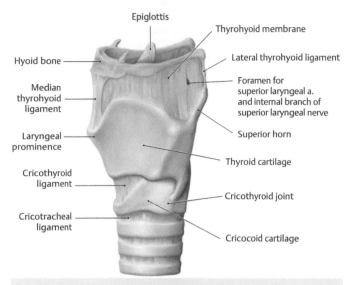

Fig. 2.7 Hyolaryngeal complex, lateral view. From Gilroy AM, MacPherson BR. *Atlas of Anatomy.* 3rd ed. New York, NY: Thieme, 2016.

Other elements of the skeleton are indirectly relevant to swallowing and are important to dysphagia management. The cervical vertebrae, atlantoaxial joint, and atlantooccipital joint all lie within the **prevertebral compartment of the neck**. Muscles and bones in this compartment are primarily concerned with the position of the head and neck. Flexing and extending the head and neck or turning the head from one side to another changes the morphology of the pharynx and may add mechanical advantage to swallowing musculature.[3]

## Clinical Note

It is important to differentiate the actions and functions of the skeletal elements of the swallowing apparatus from those of the vertebrae. Although the hyoid appears to be related to the vertebrae, movement of the hyoid should be evaluated in relationship to the mandible to which it is attached, and not the vertebrae, to which it is not attached.

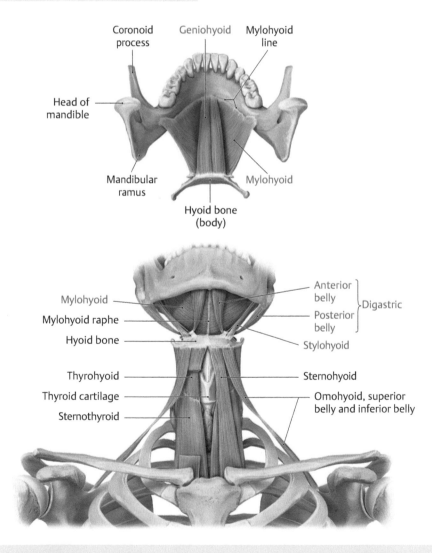

Fig. 2.8 Supra- and infrahyoid musculature. From Gilroy AM, MacPherson BR. *Atlas of Anatomy.* 3rd ed. New York, NY: Thieme, 2016.

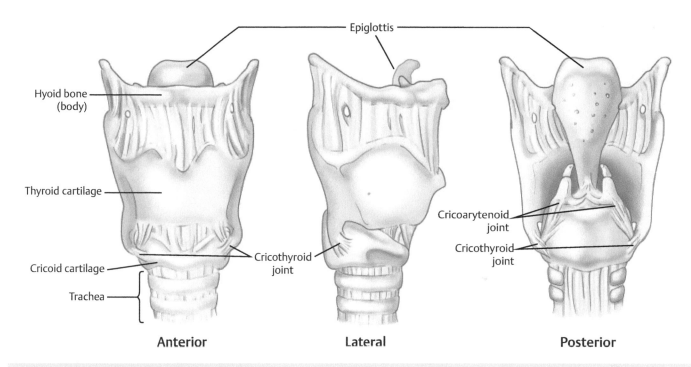

Fig. 2.9 Laryngeal skeleton.

### 2.4.1 Importance in Infants

When an infant is born, assuming no deviations in typical embryological and fetal development, it has an intact oral cavity with functioning articulators. The intactness of this space and its articulators make nipple feeding possible. At birth, the muscular system of the orofacial anatomy is one of the most developed muscular systems in the infant's body. This maturity gives the infant the capacity for suckling, sucking, and swallowing at birth.[4] However, it is not just the feeding dynamic that place demands on the infant's oral cavity. The major functions of the oral cavity, pharynx, and larynx are summarized into the following categories in order of importance: positional, respiratory, and feeding.[5] To understand the positional importance that maintains airway patency, consider the contributions of the infant's skull, specifically the region of the basicranium.

The basicranium is the underside of the skull (not including the hard palate). It forms the base of the calvarium (braincase) and posterior portion of the pharynx (**Fig. 2.6**). At birth, the basicranium shows a general flatness with no marked angulation, which is significantly different than the sharp angle seen in the adult basicranium.[6] The lack of angulation in the infant basicranium is desirable for maintaining patency in the pharynx for respiration; however, it limits the verbalization potential for the infant by shortening the vocal tract.[7] There is rapid change to the head and neck regions, due in large part to the rapid growth of the brain, during the first several years of life. This results in visible changes to the basicranium.[8]

The infant depends on the patency of the pharynx to facilitate respiration, making it a vital area for survival. However, it is infants' oral cavity that allows them to communicate their awareness of the world around them and its ever-changing stimuli.[9] The bones of the oral cavity and the subsequent shape of that cavity are influenced by the strong forces applied by the muscles surrounding this region.

### Clinical Note

The forces generated by the tongue heavily influence the shape of the hard palate. A high-arched palate may be a developmental feature, or it can be caused by chronic thumb-sucking. This condition may contribute to a narrow airway and influence disordered breathing during sleep.

## 2.5 Muscles Underlying Ingestion and Bolus Formation

Muscles underlying ingestion and bolus formation include facial muscles, muscles of mastication, and muscles of the tongue. These muscle groups work in concert to receive food or liquid into the oral cavity and to form a bolus in preparation for bolus transport.

## 2.5.1 Facial Musculature Relevant to Feeding

Muscles of the circumoral region
- Orbicularis oris
- Buccinator
- Levator labii superioris
- Depressor labii inferioris
- Levator anguli oris
- Depressor anguli oris
- Mentalis
- Zygomaticus major
- Zygomaticus minor

Feeding begins with muscles of the face (**Fig. 2.10**). The orbicularis oris lies deep to the lips in the superficial fascia of the face and is positioned by several muscles that converge on the lateral angle of the mouth, creating a mass called the **modiolus**. This sphincter closes the mouth and helps contain a bolus within the oral cavity along with the buccinator, the muscular lining of the cheeks. The buccinator connects with the orbicularis oris anteriorly and the superior pharyngeal constrictor posteriorly. All facial muscles are innervated by the facial nerve (CN VII).

## Clinical Note

Patients with a Bell's palsy affecting CN VII may present with difficulty ingesting or retaining a bolus in the oral cavity.

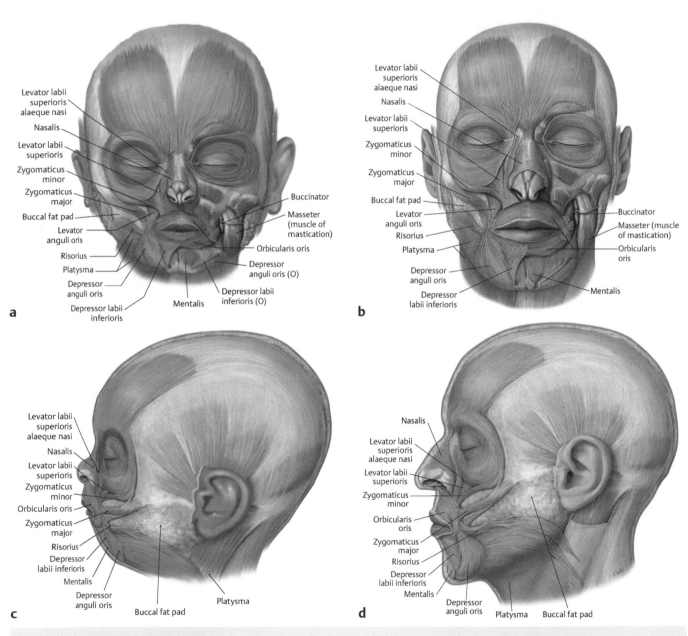

**Fig. 2.10** (**a,c**) Infant face and (**b,d**) adult face.

## 2.5.2 Muscles of Mastication

- Masseter
- Temporalis
- Medial pterygoid
- Lateral pterygoid
- Anterior digastric
- Mylohyoid

Mastication includes muscles that open and close the jaw (**Fig. 2.11**). Jaw closers include the masseter and medial pterygoid, which form the "V-sling" muscles. The bottom of the "V" is made up of the distal attachments of each muscle meeting at the superficial and deep surface of the mandibular angle, respectively. The proximal attachment site of the masseter is located at the zygomatic arch, whereas the medial surface of the lateral pterygoid plate is the proximal attachment of the medial pterygoid, completing the **V**-shaped sling. The temporalis, a powerful jaw-closer, has broad attachments on the flat bones of the skull in the temporal fossa. Muscle fibers converge as they descend deep to the zygomatic arch and form a tendon inserting on the coronoid process of the mandible. These three muscles and the lateral pterygoid muscle discussed below are known as muscles of mastication, and all are innervated by the mandibular nerve, the third division of the trigeminal nerve (CN V$_3$).

Jaw openers include the lateral pterygoid and **suprahyoid muscles**. The lateral pterygoid muscle arises from the lateral surface of the lateral pterygoid plate and inserts both postero-laterally on the anterior surface of the neck of the mandible and on the articular disk of the temporomandibular joint. Suprahyoid muscles, including the digastric, mylohyoid, geniohyoid, and stylohyoid, form a muscular sling attached to the inner surface of the body of the mandible anteriorly (**Fig. 2.8**), the cranial base posteriorly, and the hyoid in the middle. Together, these muscles have the mechanical advantage to open the jaw.[10] The mandibular branch of the trigeminal nerve innervates the mylohyoid and anterior digastric, the facial nerve the posterior digastric and stylohyoid, and the C1 spinal nerve the geniohyoid. Although all of these muscles are positioned to open the jaw, the lateral pterygoid is the primary jaw opener under normal conditions. The suprahyoid muscles have other important functions, including supporting the actions of the tongue in the oral cavity. The

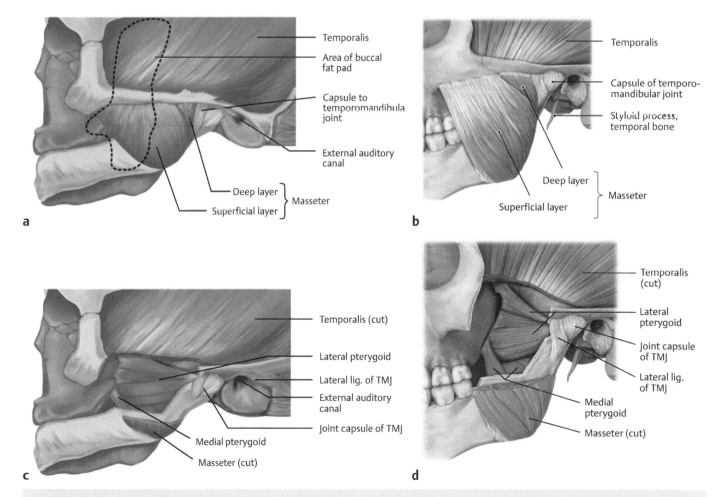

Fig. 2.11 (**a,c**) Infant and (**b,d**) adult muscles of mastication. (**b,d**) From Gilroy AM, MacPherson BR. *Atlas of Anatomy*. 3rd ed. New York, NY: Thieme, 2016.

mylohyoid, geniohyoid, and anterior digastric muscles as a group are referred to as the floor of the mouth or **submental muscles** in reference to the mental protuberance of the mandible.

### 2.5.3 Tongue

The tongue is a muscular hydrostat with intrinsic muscles oriented in longitudinal, vertical, and transverse planes, allowing for multiple degrees of freedom[11] (**Fig. 2.12**). The potential combinations of muscular contraction are enormous, allowing the tongue to move and manipulate various food types around the oral cavity. The superior and inferior longitudinal muscles course through the long axis of the tongue. The transversus and verticalis muscles are interwoven throughout the body of the tongue. The intrinsic muscles largely control the shape of the tongue, while the position of the tongue in the oral cavity is controlled directly by the extrinsic muscles and indirectly by the suprahyoid muscles and muscles of mastication.

The genioglossus, palatoglossus, styloglossus, and hyoglossus reposition the tongue in the oral cavity. These extrinsic muscles of the tongue are named for their respective attachments: anteriorly to the **genial tubercle of the mandible**, superiorly to the palate, posteriorly to the styloid process, and inferiorly to the hyoid. The extrinsic muscles of the tongue insert into the substance of tongue via muscle fibers interwoven with intrinsic tongue muscles and therefore highly influence tongue shape, especially the geniohyoid.

Tongue muscles are often classified functionally as protruders or retruders.[12] The genioglossus, transversus, and verticalis primarily protrude the tongue, whereas the hyoglossus, styloglossus, and longitudinal muscles primarily retrude the tongue.

The suprahyoid muscles (**Fig. 2.8**) and muscles of mastication (**Fig. 2.11**) support the posture of the tongue in the oral cavity. The floor of mouth muscles are especially involved in mastication to support the tongue during bolus formation. The submental muscles stiffen to support the tongue pressing against the palate, for example. Additionally, the posture of the tongue is influenced by the posture of the jaw. Coordination of tongue movements, facial muscles, muscles of mastication, and floor of mouth muscles involve central pattern generators in the brainstem, coordinating motor nuclei of cranial nerves V, VII, and XII.[13]

### Clinical Note

The location of these central pattern generators explains why a brainstem stroke (also called a bulbar stroke) is so devastating for swallowing.

## 2.6  Muscles Underlying Oral Transport

Bolus transport through the oral cavity involves the tongue accommodating the bolus and moving it toward the pharynx, and concludes with forceful tongue base retraction. The facial muscles (**Fig. 2.10**) contain the bolus by keeping the mouth closed or fixed around a cup or straw. The muscles of mastication (**Fig. 2.11**) keep the jaw fixed, and the submental muscles support the effort of the tongue. Anterior fibers of the genioglossus and the verticalis accommodate the bolus. A wavelike motion formed by serial contraction of the genioglossus from anterior to posterior with the intrinsic muscles of the tongue rolls the bolus through the oral cavity.[14] The tongue base, pulled like a piston by the hyoglossus and styloglossus, drives the bolus into the hypopharynx. These muscles are innervated by cranial nerve XII (hypoglossal nerve).

### Clinical Note

Recent evidence suggests that intentional bracing of the tongue tip against the upper alveolar ridge and hard palate facilitates tongue wave motion and increases pharyngeal pressure.[15]

## 2.7  Muscles Underlying Pharyngeal Conversion

The most complicated phase of swallowing is the pharyngeal phase. The key contractile elements are a series of muscular slings that insert on bones, cartilages, other muscles, or fascia. It would be misleading to think of each muscle as acting independently. These sling muscles function cooperatively and are often bound together by deep fascia, so that muscles function less like ropes pulling on a structure and more like two ends of a hammock that surround and displace a structure. These muscular slings function to seal off openings and help transform the morphology of the pharynx.

### 2.7.1 Muscles of the Soft Palate

The tensor veli palatini (innervated by the mandibular branch of the trigeminal nerve [CN V$_3$]) originates in the **fossa** between the pterygoid plates and uses the pterygoid hamulus as a pulley to stiffen the palatine **aponeuroses** embedded in the soft palate (**Fig. 2.13**). The levator veli palatini attaches to the cranial base near the carotid canal and the auditory tube on the temporal bone. It passes over the edge of the superior pharyngeal constrictor and into the soft palate to form a sling of muscle within the substance of the soft palate. These muscle fibers attach to the palatine aponeuroses and associate with the musculus uvulae (innervated by the pharyngeal branch of the vagus nerve [CN X]), the only intrinsic muscle of the soft palate, which attaches to the posterior nasal spine. The primary function of the levator veli palatini in swallowing is to seal the velopharyngeal port.[16] Secondarily, this muscle anchors and leverages the proximal attachments of the palatopharyngeus (innervated by the pharyngeal branch of the vagus nerve [CN X]) and therefore indirectly contributes to important functions of swallowing other than the closure of the soft palate.[17]

### Clinical Note

Surgical procedures that are designed to address obstructive sleep apnea may inadvertently cause swallowing impairment if these muscles or nerves are compromised.

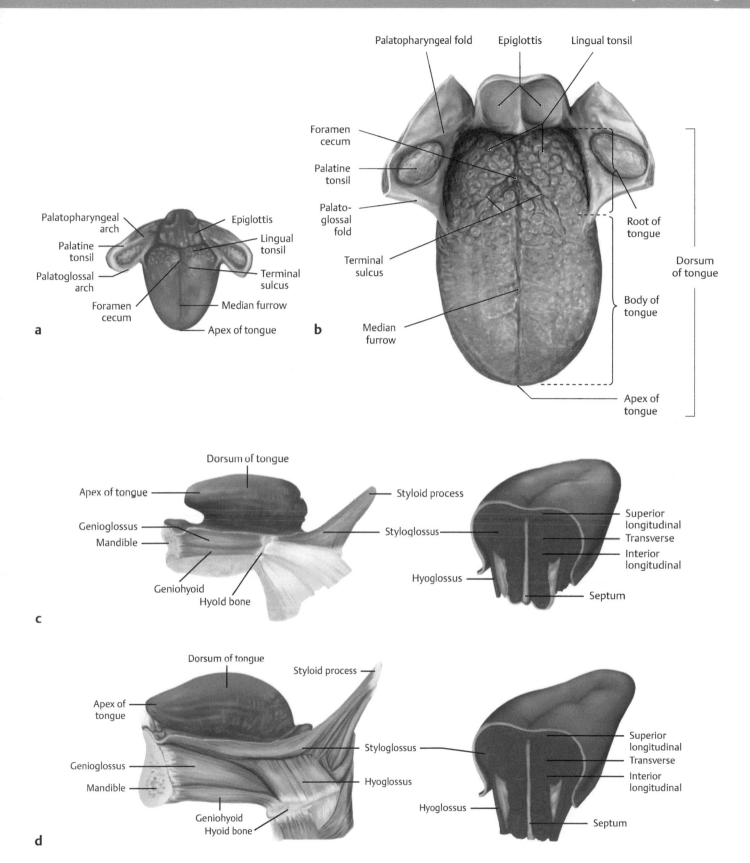

**Fig. 2.12** (**a,c**) Infant and (**b,d**) adult tongue muscles (intrinsic and extrinsic). (**b,d**) From Gilroy AM, MacPherson BR. *Atlas of Anatomy*. 3rd ed. New York, NY: Thieme, 2016.

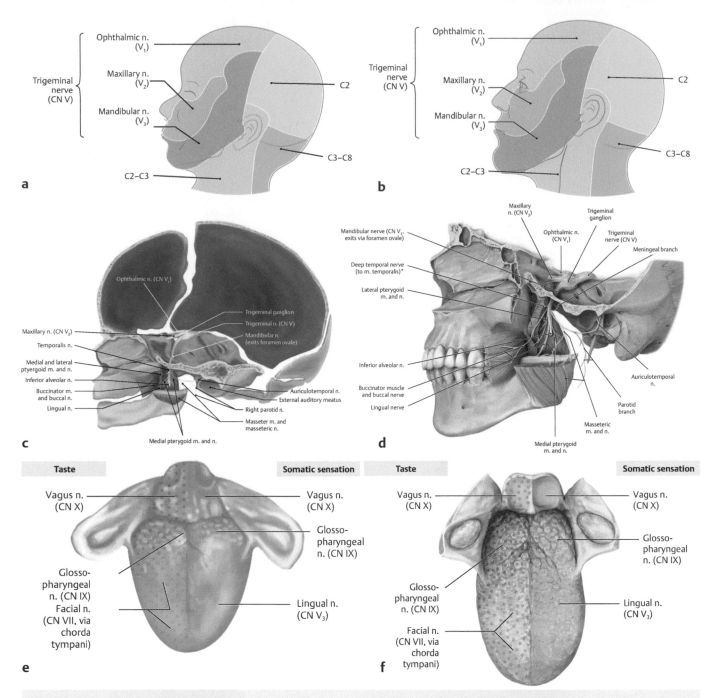

**Fig. 2.13** Sensory and motor innervation of the face and oral cavity in (**a,c,e**) infants and (**b,d,f**) adults. From Gilroy AM, MacPherson BR. *Atlas of Anatomy.* 3rd ed. New York, NY: Thieme, 2016.

## 2.7.2 Extrinsic Tongue Muscles

The tongue itself is slung in the oral cavity by the genioglossus anteriorly and the styloglossus posteriorly. The hyoglossus attaches to the greater horn of the hyoid and rises through the lateral walls of the tongue. The styloglossus attaches to the styloid process and inserts into the lateral tongue, embracing the fibers of the hyoglossus. These two muscles contract and together pull the tongue base posteriorly in tongue base retraction.[18] The palatoglossus is positioned to suspend the tongue; however, this little muscle approximates the palate to the tongue base, helping to seal the oropharyngeal isthmus during pharyngeal conversion. The palatoglossus muscles receive innervation from the vagus nerve (CN X); all other tongue muscles are innervated by the hypoglossal nerve (CN XII) (**Fig. 2.12**).

### 2.7.3 Two-Sling Mechanism of Hyolaryngeal Elevation

Elevation of the hyolaryngeal complex (**Fig. 2.7**) contributes to the inversion of the epiglottis, helps stretch open a relaxed upper esophageal sphincter, and relocates the airway from the pathway of the bolus. The hyolaryngeal complex comprises the hyoid, larynx, and associated structures, including the cricopharyngeus muscle, which forms the upper esophageal sphincter. Underlying hyolaryngeal elevation is an anterior sling, formed by the suprahyoid muscles (**Fig. 2.8**), and a posterior sling, formed by the long pharyngeal muscles (see Chapter 3, **Fig. 3.14**).[19]

The suprahyoid muscles (mylohyoid, geniohyoid, stylohyoid, and digastric) have proximal attachments to the mandible anteriorly and to the cranial base posteriorly, as discussed earlier. The distal insertions of the suprahyoid muscles exert force principally on the body of the hyoid and therefore function together as the anterior sling to displace the hyoid in an anterosuperior direction. Furthermore, these muscles are connected to one another through dense fascia deep in the floor of the mouth. This sling functions via the thyrohyoid membrane and muscle to advance the hyoid and the larynx and to support tongue function in the oral cavity. These muscles function collectively to displace the hyoid along a somewhat triangular path, which indicates that different muscles are exerting a pulling force on the hyoid at differing times. The digastric muscles work together to elevate the hyoid but more or less cancel each other out in the anterior-posterior direction. The mylohyoid has the greatest mechanical advantage for hyoid elevation, and the geniohyoid has the greatest mechanical advantage for anterior advancement of the hyoid.[20]

The long pharyngeal muscles, including the stylopharyngeus, salpingopharyngeus, and palatopharyngeus, constitute the posterior muscular sling. The stylopharyngeus is attached to the styloid process superiorly. This muscle passes between the superior and middle pharyngeal constrictor and inserts on the posterior edge of the thyroid cartilage, in addition to other structures, including the lateral pharyngeal wall.[21] The palatopharyngeus attaches superiorly into the palatine aponeuroses and muscles of the velum.[17] It broadens and descends, filling the lateral walls of the pharynx, and often inserts on the thyroid cartilage as well. As noted previously, this muscle is elevated and stabilized by the actions of the levator veli palatini. The palatopharyngeus forms the substance of the palatopharyngeal fold, which is the posterior faucial pillar of the pharynx. The diminutive proximal portion of the salpingopharyngeus attaches to the auditory tube and blends inferiorly with the stylopharyngeus and palatopharyngeus in the lateral walls of the pharynx.

The long pharyngeal muscles essentially crisscross for mechanical advantage. The palatopharyngeus begins inside the pharynx in a slightly anterior and medial position, whereas the stylopharyngeus begins in a slightly posterolateral position outside the pharynx. They cross at the level of the hyoid such that the stylopharyngeus inserts anteriorly on the larynx and the palatopharyngeus on the pharynx. Taken together, they both contribute to laryngeal elevation and pharyngeal shortening. The stylopharyngeus has more connections to and primarily elevates the larynx, whereas the palatopharyngeus has more attachments to and primarily shortens the pharynx. All pharyngeal muscles are innervated by CN X, except the stylopharyngeus, which is innervated by the glossopharyngeal nerve (CN IX).

## Clinical Note

Long pharyngeal muscles, critical to laryngeal elevation and airway protection, may be damaged in radiation treatment of head and neck cancer, thereby compromising airway protection.

### 2.7.4 Infrahyoid Muscles Help Stabilize the Larynx

The infrahyoid muscles oppose the suprahyoid and long pharyngeal muscles. Together these muscles raise and lower the larynx within the pharynx and are critical in stabilizing the laryngeal skeleton so that the delicate functions of the intrinsic laryngeal musculature can be achieved.[22] Four pairs of muscles anchor the hyoid and thyroid inferiorly, including the thyrohyoid, sternothyroid, sternohyoid, and omohyoid. Together they form two layers and are referred to as the infrahyoid, or strap, muscles (**Fig. 2.8**). The thyrohyoid, an intrinsic muscle of the hyolaryngeal complex, is structurally positioned to assist in approximating the thyroid cartilage and hyoid. The sternothyroid lowers the larynx, whereas the sternohyoid lowers the hyoid. The omohyoid exerts downward pressure on the hyoid. All but the thyrohyoid are innervated by C2–C4 from the **ansa cervicalis**. A C1 spinal nerve coursing with the hypoglossal nerve innervates the thyrohyoid muscle.

### 2.7.5 Muscles of the Larynx

Intrinsic and extrinsic muscles are necessary for movement of and within the larynx. The intrinsic muscles are responsible for abduction (posterior cricoarytenoid), adduction (lateral cricoarytenoid and interarytenoids, transverse and oblique arytenoid muscles), and changing tension (cricothyroid and internal thyroarytenoid) of the true vocal folds.

The thyroarytenoid, lateral cricoarytenoid, and interarytenoid are important for adducting the vocal folds and protecting the airway. All of the intrinsic laryngeal muscles are composed of skeletal muscle fibers. There is greater variability in muscle fiber diameter in laryngeal muscles than in other skeletal muscle fibers. Many laryngeal motor units have multiple neural innervations for the multiple functions of the larynx (**Fig. 2.13; Table 2.1**).[23,24,25]

#### Differences in Infant and Adult Oral Cavity

There are definite differences in the oral cavity of the infant as compared to the oral cavity of the adult, which should be apparent to the reader after review of the foregoing illustrations. The infant's oral cavity is relatively small in size secondary to the small size and placement of the mandible (there is slight retrusion of the mandible at birth). Additionally, the infant has sucking/buccal pads in the oral cavity that are resorbed with growth and maturation and not present in the older child or adult. Additionally, it is important to note that the infant tongue is relatively large, taking up most of the space in the oral cavity,

**Table 2.1** Sensory and motor innervation of the face and oral cavity

| Anatomical region | Cranial nerve innervations |
| --- | --- |
| Face | V—Trigeminal: all sensory innervation to face<br>VII—Facial: motor innervation to muscles of facial expression |
| Craniomandibular Muscles | V—Trigeminal: motor innervation to muscles responsible for chewing |
| Oral cavity | V—Trigeminal: all sensory innervation to oral cavity |
| Salivary glands | IX—Glossopharyngeal: parotid gland<br>VII—Facial: sublingual and submandibular glands |
| Tongue | V—Trigeminal: sensory innervation to the anterior 2/3 of the tongue<br>VII—Facial: taste to anterior 2/3 of the tongue<br>IX—Glossopharyngeal: taste to posterior 1/3 of tongue and faucial pillars<br>X—Vagus (superior laryngeal nerve): taste to small posterior portion of base of tongue and valleculae<br>XII—Hypoglossal: motor innervation to intrinsic and extrinsic muscles |
| Velum | V—Trigeminal: innervates tensor veli palatini, responsible for dilation of auditory tubes<br>X—Vagus: innervates four paired muscles of soft palate, responsible for velar movement |

and it is housed entirely in the oral cavity (blade and root). The normal infant also has a relatively large head with shorter neck as compared to the adult head and neck regions.[4,5,26,27,28,29,30]

All the anatomical features reviewed thus far combined with a series of primitive reflexes present at birth (**Table 2.2**) enable the infant to successfully complete bolus ingestion, manipulation, and transfer for intake of adequate nutrition.

## 2.8 Differences between the Mature and Pediatric Larynx

There are well-known differences between the mature larynx of the adult and the newborn larynx.[31,32] The larynx itself is seated higher in the pharynx as compared to adult larynges. The pediatric larynx lies between the first and third cervical vertebrae in infants and young children. The posterior border of the cricoid cartilage is found between the sixth and seventh cervical vertebrae in the mature larynx.[31] The epiglottis may make direct contact with the soft palate in some cases due to the high laryngeal positioning, particularly in newborns. The epiglottis also has more direct contact with the base of the tongue in infants and children.[31,33]

**Table 2.2** Infant reflexes with age of appearance and diminishing

| Reflex | Age of appearance in weeks (gestational age) | Age of diminishing in months (chronological age) |
| --- | --- | --- |
| Suckling | 11–15 | 5–6 |
| Gag | 26–27 | 6–12 |
| Phasic bite | 28 | 9–12 |
| Rooting | 32 | 3 |
| Tongue protrusion | 38–40 | 6 |
| Tongue lateralization | 40 | 6 |

## 2.9 Laryngeal Descent

Infants are preferential nasal breathers until approximately 4 to 6 months of age, when there is notable initiation of oral breathing. This transition from preferential nasal breathing coincides with the maturational descent of the larynx and the subsequent lowering of the tip of the epiglottis from C2–C3 to that of the adult position.[33,34]

## Clinical Note

Initiation of the laryngeal descent and the initiation of oral respiration represents a reorganization in respiratory functioning and interestingly coincides with the height of risk for sudden infant death syndrome (SIDS), which occurs from 3 to 5 months of age (**Fig. 2.14**).[33,34]

## 2.10 Maturation of Laryngeal Reflexes

There are multiple upper airway reflexes designed to protect the lower airway from foreign-body invasion. Examples of upper airway reflexive responses include sneezing, apnea, swallowing, laryngeal closure, coughing, expiration, and negative pressure reflex.[37] Specifically, a group of reflexes common in the newborn, known as the laryngeal chemoreflexes, include startle, rapid swallowing, laryngeal constriction, apnea, hypertension, and bradycardia. These responses are initiated with activation of receptors in the interarytenoid space. With maturation, rapid swallowing and apnea commonly seen with aspiration in infancy become less prominent and are replaced with cough and, less commonly, laryngeal constriction. This reflexive shift is related to maturational changes of central neural processing rather than changes to the laryngeal chemoreceptors.[37,38]

## 2.11 Mechanisms of Airway Protection

The aerodigestive tract represents a crossroads for the passage of food and oxygen into the human body. Both are necessary for survival, and both mediums cross through the pharynx on the way to their final destinations. The larynx lies in the most inferior region of the pharynx, the hypopharynx, and serves many functions. It is responsible for lower airway protection, vocalization, and respiration. The larynx, like the rest of the upper aerodigestive tract, is complete in terms of form at birth but undergoes rapid evolution throughout the life span to allow for increasing levels of function as maturity demands.[39,40]

Important to the surveillance of the laryngeal vestibule is the internal branch of the superior laryngeal nerve (CN X).[41] This nerve elicits a swallow or a cough response to protect the airway from obstruction. During laryngeal elevation, the thyroarytenoid, forming the substance of the vocal folds, approximates the arytenoids toward the petiole of the epiglottis. The epiglottis is suspended over the opening of the airway and is attached to the larynx, hyoid, and tongue by a series of ligaments located in the

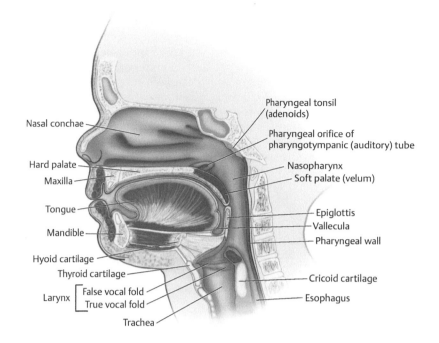

Pharyngeal tonsil (adenoids)

Pharyngeal orifice of pharyngotympanic (auditory) tube

Nasal conchae

Hard palate

Maxilla

Nasopharynx

Soft palate (velum)

Tongue

Mandible

Epiglottis

Vallecula

Pharyngeal wall

Hyoid cartilage

Thyroid cartilage

Cricoid cartilage

Larynx — False vocal fold / True vocal fold

Esophagus

Trachea

a

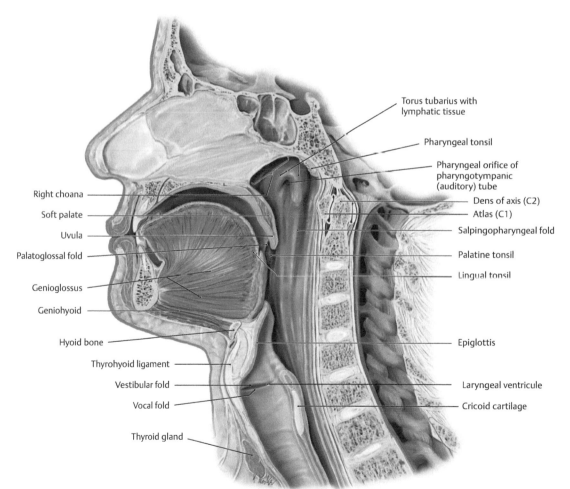

Torus tubarius with lymphatic tissue

Pharyngeal tonsil

Pharyngeal orifice of pharyngotympanic (auditory) tube

Right choana

Soft palate

Uvula

Palatoglossal fold

Genioglossus

Geniohyoid

Dens of axis (C2)

Atlas (C1)

Salpingopharyngeal fold

Palatine tonsil

Lingual tonsil

Hyoid bone

Thyrohyoid ligament

Vestibular fold

Vocal fold

Thyroid gland

Epiglottis

Laryngeal ventricule

Cricoid cartilage

b

**Fig. 2.14** Comparison of laryngeal position in (**a**) infants and (**b**) adults. (**b**) From Gilroy AM, MacPherson BR. *Atlas of Anatomy.* 3rd ed. New York, NY: Thieme, 2016.

midline of the epiglottis, including the thyroepiglottic ligament, median hyoepiglottic ligament, and glossoepiglottic ligament. The lateral hyoepiglottic ligaments are variable, but they help keep the epiglottis in position when present. The epiglottis is encased by the quadrangular membrane, which forms the aryepiglottic fold laterally. Small wisps of contractile tissue, including the thyroepiglottis and aryepiglottis, are found within the aryepiglottic fold. Despite the actions of these tiny muscles, epiglottic inversion is a largely passive event that occurs as muscular slings retract the tongue base and elevate the larynx.[42] The final measure of airway protection is the adduction of the vocal folds by the lateral cricoarytenoid and transverse and oblique arytenoid muscles.[43]

## Clinical Note

Impairment of sensory neurons protecting the airway may contribute to aspiration of a bolus into the trachea.

## 2.12 Salivary Glands

Two sets of salivary glands (see Chapter 3, **Fig. 3.4**) are important for swallowing.[44] Xerostomia (dry mouth) is a contributing factor to dysphagia. The superior salivatory nucleus, associated with CN VII, controls the two pairs of salivary glands that open into the floor of the mouth. The submandibular gland is located superficial to the mylohyoid under the angle of the mandible. The duct wraps around the posterior edge of the mylohyoid and runs forward into the floor of the mouth, where it ends at the sublingual papilla on both sides of the frenulum. The sublingual gland surrounds the submandibular duct in the oral cavity and has numerous openings into the epithelial lining of the floor of the mouth. The parotid gland is situated on the ramus of the mandible, with a portion of the gland wrapping around the back edge of the ramus. The parotid duct leaves the gland anteriorly, crosses over the masseter, and dives through the buccinator to empty saliva behind a mucosal fold lateral to the upper molars. Visceromotor signals to the parotid originate in the inferior salivatory nucleus, associated with CN IX. This brainstem nucleus also provides innervation to scattered glands throughout the oropharynx via the pharyngeal branches of CN X.

## Clinical Note

A common sequela of radiation treatment of head and neck cancer is xerostomia resulting from damage to the salivary glands or the nerve innervating the salivary glands.

## 2.12.1 Neurobiology of Swallowing

Developmentally, motor innervation of the tongue and the remaining muscles relevant to swallowing arises from different locations. The hypoglossal nerve and the tongue are derived from occipital **somites**. Nearly every other muscle was formed from the **pharyngeal arches**. The tongue therefore functions semi-independently. When the tongue propels a bolus into the hypopharynx, the internal superior laryngeal nerve triggers the

central pattern generators (CPGs) in the brainstem. These CPGs begin with the "leading complex," firing pharyngeal arch–derivative nerve and muscle, including submental muscles innervated by CN V$_3$. The nuclei for CN V$_3$, VII, IX, and X are organized sequentially from superior to inferior in the lateral pons and medulla. A cascade of signals produces a wave of depolarization in these pharyngeal arch derivatives, facilitating the movement of the bolus from the oral cavity through the pharynx.

Taste, temperature, proprioception, and tactile sensory receptors in the oral cavity provide information to the cortex that modifies the rhythmic pattern of each swallowing episode from the start of oral transport through the completion of pharyngeal clearance. Corticobulbar tracts modulate the brainstem CPG, which coordinates the motor unit recruitment of muscles that are under the control of five cranial nerves (CN V, VII, IX, X, XII) and five spinal nerves (C1–C5). Other functions regulated by the brainstem important to pharyngeal swallowing include respiratory cessation and salivary flow. Together these peripheral and central pathways monitor, modulate, and synchronize the complex physiological process known as deglutition.

## Clinical Note

Neurogenic dysphagias have multiple presentations and prognoses depending on the structures of the peripheral and central nervous system that are affected.

## 2.12.2 Esophagus

The esophagus is a muscular tube that is continuous with the pharynx. It is attached to the cricoid cartilage by the cricopharyngeus. The esophagus is composed of skeletal and smooth muscle that is innervated by a plexus of autonomic nerves, including the vagus nerve. Muscle fibers are oriented in circumferential and longitudinal directions, allowing the esophagus to push a bolus through the tube and shorten the tube around the bolus. The longitudinal fibers are external to the circumferential fibers. The esophagus passes through the esophageal hiatus of the respiratory diaphragm at the T10 vertebral level. The right crus of the diaphragm wraps around the esophagus and forms the lower esophageal sphincter.

## 2.12.3 Development

There is evidence from ultrasound examination that human fetuses begin swallowing as early as 12 weeks' gestational age.[29] The development of the oral cavity begins approximately 3 weeks after conception, when three germ layers (group of cells or primary tissue layers) are present: the ectoderm, the mesoderm, and the endoderm. The skin and nervous system arise from the ectoderm. The connective tissue and blood vessels arise from the middle layer, the mesoderm. From the endoderm, the digestive and respiratory systems will develop. Beginning in the fourth week after conception, the pharyngeal arches develop from these primitive germ layers.[45] Pharyngeal arches are separated from each other by apparent branchial grooves or clefts. Most of the anatomy important to swallowing, except for the tongue, is derived from five pharyngeal arches (**Fig. 2.15**).[46,47]

Within the first arch, the mylohyoid and anterior belly of the digastric develop, in addition to the muscles of mastication. The mylohyoid and anterior digastric are important for jaw opening but are also considered part of the leading complex, or the muscles that displace the hyoid as the initiating movement in pharyngeal swallowing. The third division of the trigeminal nerve innervates arch 1 muscles. The stylohyoid, posterior digastric, and muscles of the face are arch 2 derivatives and are innervated by the facial nerve (CN VII). The stylohyoid and posterior digastric muscles displace the hyoid. Two facial muscles in particular (the orbicularis oris surrounding the lips and the buccinator, which manipulates the cheeks) are important for ingestion and bolus formation. The stylopharyngeus, the lower portion of the hyoid body, and the greater horns of the hyoid are derived from pharyngeal arch 3. The stylopharyngeus is innervated by the glossopharyngeal nerve (CN IX). The laryngeal cartilages and muscles manipulating the soft palate, pharynx, and larynx are derived from the fourth and sixth pharyngeal arches. Pharyngeal branches of the vagus nerve (CN X) innervate arch 4 muscles, including the levator veli palatini and all pharyngeal muscles except the stylopharyngeus, whereas the recurrent laryngeal nerve (CN X) innervates muscles from the sixth pharyngeal arch. The fifth arch does not develop in humans.

The mucosa lining the conduit formed by these arches is innervated by these same nerves, most importantly, CN V in the oral cavity and CN IX and X in the pharynx and larynx, respectively.

Occipital somites migrate into the pharynx to develop the tongue under the control of the hypoglossal nerve (CN XII), a motor-only nerve. Somatosensory receptors in the anterior two-thirds of the tongue send signals through the mandibular division of the trigeminal nerve (CN $V_3$). Taste in this same region follows the trigeminal nerve but is ultimately a sensory function of CN VII. Taste and somatosensory sensation in the posterior one-third of the tongue are mediated by CN IX. CN VII provides visceromotor innervation to the submandibular and sublingual glands, CN IX to the parotid glands, and CN X to mucosal glands scattered throughout the pharynx. The pharyngeal arch structures and tongue develop in synchrony with the mandible and skull to form overlapping respiratory, digestive, and vocal tracts.

## Clinical Note

Children born with orofacial clefts may have early difficulty with feeding/swallowing secondary to the cleft impacting their ability to generate suction in the oral cavity for transfer of liquid from the bottle or the breast. There are many specialized bottle/nipple systems on the market to help the infant compensate for the anatomical defect and successfully feed by mouth. See Chapter 14 for a discussion of swallowing and feeding disorders associated with orofacial clefts.

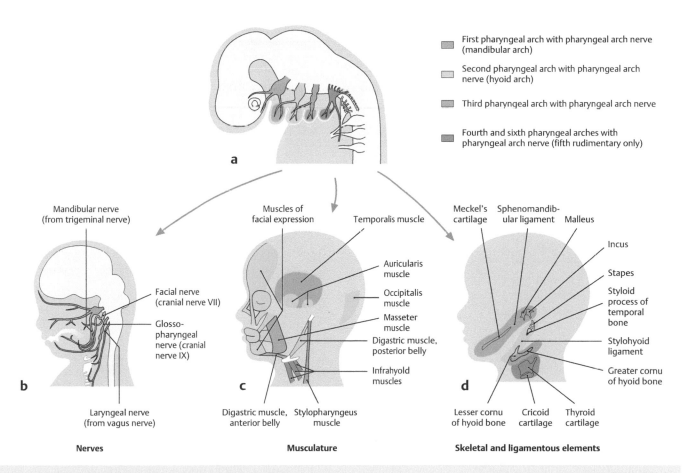

First pharyngeal arch with pharyngeal arch nerve (mandibular arch)

Second pharyngeal arch with pharyngeal arch nerve (hyoid arch)

Third pharyngeal arch with pharyngeal arch nerve

Fourth and sixth pharyngeal arches with pharyngeal arch nerve (fifth rudimentary only)

**Nerves**

Mandibular nerve (from trigeminal nerve)

Facial nerve (cranial nerve VII)

Glosso-pharyngeal nerve (cranial nerve IX)

Laryngeal nerve (from vagus nerve)

**Musculature**

Muscles of facial expression

Temporalis muscle

Auricularis muscle

Occipitalis muscle

Masseter muscle

Digastric muscle, posterior belly

Infrahyoid muscles

Digastric muscle, anterior belly

Stylopharyngeus muscle

**Skeletal and ligamentous elements**

Meckel's cartilage

Sphenomandibular ligament

Malleus

Incus

Stapes

Styloid process of temporal bone

Stylohyoid ligament

Greater cornu of hyoid bone

Lesser cornu of hyoid bone

Cricoid cartilage

Thyroid cartilage

Fig. 2.15 Comparison of laryngeal position in infants and adults.

## 2.13 Questions

**1.** The laryngeal skeleton is composed of all of the following except:

A. Thyroid
B. Paired arytenoids
C. Cricoid
D. Hyoid bone
E. Epiglottis

**2.** Which infrahyoid muscle is structurally positioned to assist in approximating the thyroid cartilage and hyoid?

A. Thyrohyoid
B. Sternothyroid
C. Sternohyoid
D. Omohyoid
E. Mylohyoid

**3.** Which two muscles are primarily responsible for tongue base retraction?

A. Genioglossus and styloglossus
B. Genioglossus and hyoglossus
C. Palatoglossus and genioglossus
D. Styloglossus and hyoglossus
E. Palatoglossus and styloglossus

**4.** Which muscle of the soft palate is primarily responsible for sealing the velopharyngeal port during swallowing?

A. Tensor veli palatini
B. Levator veli palatini
C. Musculus uvulae
D. Palatoglossus
E. Palatopharyngeus

**5.** Which salivary glands are most important for swallowing due to their secretion to the floor of the mouth?

A. Parotid and sublingual
B. Thyroid and submandibular
C. Sublingual and thyroid
D. Parotid and submandibular
E. Submandibular and sublingual

## 2.14 Answers and Explanations

**1. Correct: hyoid bone (D).**
The hyoid bone is part of the hyolaryngeal framework, but it is not part of the laryngeal skeleton. The laryngeal skeleton is composed primarily of five cartilages, including the thyroid (**A**), paired arytenoids (**B**), cricoid (**C**), and epiglottis (**E**).

**2. Correct: thyrohyoid (A).**
The thyrohyoid, an intrinsic muscle of the hyolaryngeal complex, is structurally positioned to assist in approximating the thyroid cartilage and hyoid due to its origin on the thyroid cartilage and its insertion in the hyoid bone.

The sternothyroid (**B**), sternohyoid (**C**), and omohyoid (**D**) are all infrahyoid muscles that anchor the hyoid and thyroid inferiorly. The mylohyoid (**E**) is a suprahyoid muscle. None of these muscles is structurally positioned to assist in approximating the thyroid cartilage to the hyoid bone as the thyrohyoid is.

**3. Correct: styloglossus and hyoglossus (D).**
The hyoglossus attaches to the greater horn of the hyoid and rises through the lateral walls of the tongue. The styloglossus attaches to the styloid process and inserts into the lateral tongue, embracing the fibers of the hyoglossus. These two muscles contract and together pull the tongue base posteriorly in tongue base retraction.

The tongue itself is slung in the oral cavity by the genioglossus anteriorly and the styloglossus posteriorly. The palatoglossus is positioned to suspend the tongue; however, this little muscle approximates the palate to the tongue base, thereby helping to seal the oropharyngeal isthmus during pharyngeal conversion.

**4. Correct: levator veli palatini (B).**
The levator veli palatini attaches to the cranial base near the carotid canal and the auditory tube on the temporal bone. It passes over the edge of the superior pharyngeal constrictor and into the soft palate to form a sling of muscle within the substance of the soft palate. The primary function of the levator veli palatini in swallowing is to seal the velopharyngeal port.

The tensor veli palatini (**A**) originates in the fossa between the pterygoid plates and utilizes the pterygoid hamulus as a pulley to stiffen the palatine aponeuroses embedded in the soft palate. The muscle fibers of the levator veli palatini attach to the palatine aponeuroses and associate with the musculus uvulae (**C**). The levator veli palatini muscle anchors and leverages the proximal attachments of the palatopharyngeus (**E**) and therefore indirectly contributes to important functions of swallowing other than the closure of the soft palate. The palatopharyngeus functions to shorten the pharynx and indirectly aids laryngeal elevation.

**5. Correct: submandibular and sublingual salivary glands (E).**
The sublingual and submandibular salivary glands are the two sets of salivary glands most important for swallowing. The superior salivatory nucleus associated with CN VII controls the two pairs of salivary glands that open into the floor of the mouth. The parotid gland is situated on the ramus of the mandible, with a portion of the gland wrapping around the back edge of the ramus. The parotid duct leaves the gland anteriorly, crosses over the masseter, and dives through the buccinator to empty saliva behind a mucosal fold lateral to the upper molars. The thyroid gland is not a salivary gland, and it does not have a duct. Instead, the thyroid gland secretes hormones in the body to regulate metabolic rate.

# References

[1] Shaw SM, Martino R. The normal swallow: muscular and neurophysiological control. *Otolaryngol Clin North Am* 2013;46(6):937–956

[2] Linder-Aronson S. Adenoids. Their effect on mode of breathing and nasal airflow and their relationship to characteristics of the facial skeleton and the dentition. A biometric, rhino-manometric and cephalometro-radiographic study on children with and without adenoids. *Acta Otolaryngol Suppl* 1970;265:1–132

[3] Ekberg O. Posture of the head and pharyngeal swallowing. *Acta Radiol Diagn (Stockh)* 1986;27(6):691–696

[4] Kent RD, Vorperian HK. Development of the Craniofacial-Oral-Laryngeal Anatomy. San Diego, CA: Singular Publishing Group; 1995

[5] Bosma JF. Anatomic and physiologic development of the speech apparatus. In: Tower DB, ed. The Nervous System. Vol 3. New York: Raven; 1975:469–481

[6] Laitman JT, Crelin ES. Postnatal development of the basicranium and vocal tract region in man. Paper presented at: Symposium on Development of the Basicranium 1976

[7] Crelin ES. The skulls of our ancestors: implications regarding speech, language, and conceptual thought evolution. *J Voice* 1989;3(1):18–23

[8] Holzman RS. Anatomy and embryology of the pediatric airway. *Anesthesiol Clin North Am* 1998;16(4):707–727

[9] Bosma JF, Showacre J. Symposium on Development of Upper Respiratory Anatomy and Function: Implications for Sudden Infant Death Syndrome. Baltimore, MD: National Institutes of Health; 1975

[10] Van Eijden TM, Korfage JA, Brugman P. Architecture of the human jaw-closing and jaw-opening muscles. *Anat Rec* 1997;248(3):464–474

[11] Gilbert RJ, Napadow VJ, Gaige TA, Wedeen VJ. Anatomical basis of lingual hydrostatic deformation. *J Exp Biol* 2007;210(Pt 23):4069–4082

[12] Sawczuk A, Mosier KM. Neural control of tongue movement with respect to respiration and swallowing. *Crit Rev Oral Biol Med* 2001;12(1):18–37

[13] Jean A. Brain stem control of swallowing: neuronal network and cellular mechanisms. *Physiol Rev* 2001;81(2):929–969

[14] Felton SM, Gaige TA, Reese TG, Wedeen VJ, Gilbert RJ. Mechanical basis for lingual deformation during the propulsive phase of swallowing as determined by phase-contrast magnetic resonance imaging. *J Appl Physiol (1985)* 2007;103(1):255–265

[15] Huckabee ML, Steele CM. An analysis of lingual contribution to submental surface electromyographic measures and pharyngeal pressure during effortful swallow. *Arch Phys Med Rehabil* 2006;87(8):1067–1072

[16] Kogo M, Hamaguchi M, Matsuya T. Observation of velopharyngeal closure patterns following isolated stimulation of levator veli palatini and pharyngeal constrictor muscles. *Cleft Palate Craniofac J* 1996;33(4):273–276

[17] Okuda S, Abe S, Kim H-J, et al. Morphologic characteristics of palatopharyngeal muscle. *Dysphagia* 2008;23(3):258–266

[18] Gassert RB, Pearson WG. Evaluating muscles underlying tongue base retraction in deglutition using muscular functional magnetic resonance imaging (mfMRI). *Magn Reson Imaging* 2015

[19] Pearson WG Jr, Langmore SE, Yu LB, Zumwalt AC. Structural analysis of muscles elevating the hyolaryngeal complex. *Dysphagia* 2012;27(4):445–451

[20] Pearson WG Jr, Langmore SE, Zumwalt AC. Evaluating the structural properties of suprahyoid muscles and their potential for moving the hyoid. *Dysphagia* 2011;26(4):345–351

[21] Meng H, Murakami G, Suzuki D, Miyamoto S. Anatomical variations in stylopharyngeus muscle insertions suggest interindividual and left/right differences in pharyngeal clearance function of elderly patients: a cadaveric study. *Dysphagia* 2008;23(3):251–257

[22] Loucks TMJ, Poletto CJ, Saxon KG, Ludlow CL. Laryngeal muscle responses to mechanical displacement of the thyroid cartilage in humans. *J Appl Physiol (1985)* 2005;99(3):922–930

[23] Orlikoff RF, J.C. Structure and function of the larynx. In: Lass NJ, ed. Principles of Experimental Phonetics. St. Louis, MO: Mosby; 1996:112–180

[24] Pretterklieber ML. Functional Anatomy of the Human. *Eur Surg* 2003;35(5):250–258

[25] Sataloff RT, Heman-Ackah YD, Hawkshaw MJ. Clinical anatomy and physiology of the voice. *Otolaryngol Clin North Am* 2007;40(5):909–929, v

[26] Crelin ES. Functional Anatomy of the Newborn. New Haven, CT: Yale University Press; 1973

[27] Carr RJ, Beebe DS, Belani KG. The difficult pediatric airway. Seminars in Anesthesia. *Perioperative Medicine and Pain.* 2001;20(3):219–227

[28] Newman LA. Anatomy and physiology of the infant swallow. SIG 13 Perspectives on Swallowing and Swallowing Disorders. *Dysphagia* 2001;10:3–4

[29] Cichero JAY. Swallowing from infancy to old age. In: Cichero JAY, Murdoch B, eds. Dysphagia: Foundation, Theory and Practice. West Sussex, England: John Wiley & Sons; 2006:26–46

[30] Matsuo K, Palmer JB. Anatomy and physiology of feeding and swallowing: normal and abnormal. *Phys Med Rehabil Clin N Am* 2008;19(4):691–707, vii

[31] Kahane JC. Postnatal development and aging of the human larynx. Semin Speech Lang 1983:189–203

[32] Klock LE. The growth and development of the human larynx from birth to adolescence. University of Washington School of Medicine; 1968

[33] Soloff H. The epiglottis in infants and adults: A study of linear measurements and the relationship between measurements in infant and adult groups. 1984.

[34] Sasaki CT, Levine PA, Laitman JT, Crelin ES Jr. Postnatal descent of the epiglottis in man. A preliminary report. *Arch Otolaryngol* 1977;103(3):169–171

[35] Schwartz DS, Keller MS. Maturational descent of the epiglottis. *Arch Otolaryngol Head Neck Surg* 1997;123(6):627–628

[36] Nishino T. Physiological and pathophysiological implications of upper airway reflexes in humans. *Jpn J Physiol* 2000;50(1):3–14

[37] Thach BT. Maturation and transformation of reflexes that protect the laryngeal airway from liquid aspiration from fetal to adult life. *Am J Med* 2001;111(Suppl 8A):69S–77S

[38] Thach BT. Maturation of cough and other reflexes that protect the fetal and neonatal airway. *Pulm Pharmacol Ther* 2007;20(4):365–370

[39] Laitman JT, Reidenberg JS. Specializations of the human upper respiratory and upper digestive systems as seen through comparative and developmental anatomy. *Dysphagia* 1993;8(4):318–325

[40] Polgar G, Weng TR. The functional development of the respiratory system from the period of gestation to adulthood. *Am Rev Respir Dis* 1979;120(3):625–695

[41] Mu L, Sanders I. Sensory nerve supply of the human oro- and laryngopharynx: a preliminary study. *Anat Rec* 2000;258(4):406–420

[42] Pearson WG, Taylor BK, Blair J, Martin-Harris B. Computational analysis of swallowing mechanics underlying impaired epiglottic inversion. *Laryngoscope* 2015

[43] McCulloch TM, Van Daele D, Ciucci MR. Otolaryngology head and neck surgery: an integrative view of the larynx. *Head Neck* 2011;33(Suppl 1):S46–S53

[44] Hughes PJ, Scott PM, Kew J, et al. Dysphagia in treated nasopharyngeal cancer. *Head Neck* 2000;22(4):393–397

[45] Graney DO, Sie KCY. Developmental anatomy. In: Cummings CW, ed. Otolaryngology-Head & Neck Surgery: Pediatric Otolaryngology. St. Louis, MO: Mosby; 1998:11–24

[46] Crelin ES. Development of the vocal tract. In: The Human Vocal Tract: Anatomy, Function, Development, and Evolution. New York, NY: Vantage Press; 1987:42–128

[47] German RZ, Palmer FB. Anatomy and development of oral cavity and pharynx. GI Motility Online. 2006

# 3 Physiology of Swallowing

*William G. Pearson Jr. and Memorie M. Gosa*

## Summary

Drinking and eating provide the necessary nutrition for human growth and development; however, feeding provides more in the human experience than mere nutrition. Although technical interventions, such as a percutaneous endoscopic gastronomy tube, can provide nutrition to the human body and prevent prandial aspiration, such methods prohibit the social and spiritual benefits derived from sharing food and drink together. Special events, milestones, and occasions worth celebrating through a person's lifetime involve eating and drinking. So then, to fully participate in the human experience, one must be able to swallow safely.

## Keywords

suckling, sucking, taste, flavor, chemestesis, muscular hydrostat

### Learning Objectives
- Describe the differences between suckling and sucking.
- List the components of ingestion.
- Compare and contrast the concepts of taste, flavor, and chemesthesis.
- Explain the concept of "muscular hydrostat" and describe its function in the human body.
- List the components of pharyngeal conversion.

## 3.1 Introduction

Complicating swallowing is the seemingly vulnerable overlapping design of the upper respiratory tract, upper digestive tract, and vocal tract (**Fig. 3.1**). Enjoying a meal with others becomes problematic when human goals of eating and drinking, dialogue, and the basic need for oxygen compete with each other. Deglutition (swallowing) is the complicated process that enables food and air to find their proper passage through the various spaces of the upper aerodigestive tract. Airway protection and efficient transport of the bolus are the twin goals of effective swallowing.

Deglutition is often divided into stages including oral preparatory, oral transit, pharyngeal, and esophageal stages.[1,2] This chapter similarly describes stages of the swallowing process as ingestion, bolus formation, oral transport of the bolus, and conversion of the **pharynx** followed by the esophageal transport of the bolus to the stomach. Within each swallowing stage there are specific elements that ensure the overall adequacy and efficiency of the swallowing process. Although this chapter attempts to describe "normal" functional elements of swallowing physiology, with specific emphasis on the differences across the life span, be aware that swallowing is variable. The swallowing apparatus is adaptable to various conditions, developmental stages, and even injury.

As discussed in the anatomy chapter, the study of anatomy and physiology is fascinating, but reading the descriptions of physiology alone can be cumbersome. Other resources, such as animations, dynamic models of swallowing, or clinical diagnostic imaging of functional swallowing, are especially helpful for visualizing the various elements that constitute swallowing physiology. This will be especially helpful when you consider how the loss of one element of swallowing may be compensated for by another element to achieve safe and efficient swallowing. It is critical that speech-language pathologists working in medical settings gain expert knowledge of swallowing physiology, because the patient care team will depend on this knowledge to interpret findings and manage care.

## 3.2 Feeding Begins with Ingestion and Bolus Formation

In infancy, ingestion involves the transfer of bolus material from either the breast or the bottle by suckling and eventually sucking. Both suckling and sucking require the creation of

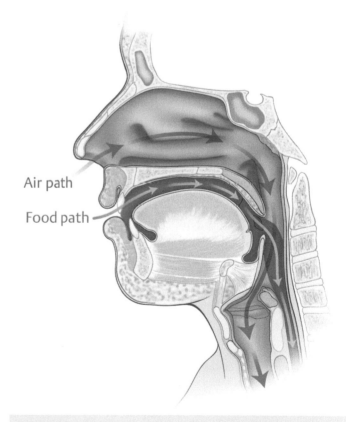

Air path

Food path

**Fig. 3.1** Overlapping functions of the upper respiratory tract.

lowered pressure within the oral cavity to draw fluid from its source into the mouth. The two processes can be differentiated by their primary oral motor characteristics. Suckling is a reflexive response that is present in healthy, full-term infants and is characterized by the following: loose upper and lower lip approximation around the nipple; effective intraoral seal achieved by tongue to hard palate compressing the nipple, with stabilization of the nipple achieved by bilateral fat pads and the alveolar ridge; and wide **mandibular excursions** with tongue blade movements characterized by protrusion and retrusion. The mandibular excursions and movement of the tongue increase the volume of the oral cavity, lowering the pressure within it, and effectively draw the fluid from its source (breast or bottle) into the mouth. In suckling the infant is expected to achieve suckle to swallow to respiration coordination in a 1:1:1 ratio. That is, the infant should demonstrate one suckle, one swallow, and one breathe per second. Suckling for nutritional intake (nutritive suckling), because it is reflexive, is automatic and involuntary. It occurs when the infant perceives sufficient sensory stimuli within the oral cavity to activate the reflex.[3,4]

Sucking is the more mature, learned pattern for nipple feeding. Sucking is the result of cortical maturation and depends on the infant having nipple feeding experience that then results in learned nipple feeding behavior. Sucking is not purely reflexive and therefore does not necessarily occur automatically with sensory stimulation to the oral cavity. An infant who is experiencing pain or discomfort may not suck despite sufficient oral stimulation from a nipple source. Sucking typically replaces suckling after 5 months of age and differs from its predecessor in the following ways: lips are tightly approximated around the nipple, looser approximation of the tongue to the hard palate, graded/focused mandibular movements, and tongue movements characterized by elevation and depression as opposed to protrusion and retrusion. In sucking, the tongue and mandible are again responsible for increasing the volume of the oral cavity, although through different planes of movement, which lowers the intraoral pressure and draws the fluid into the mouth. Sucking has more variation within its expected ratios for swallowing and breathing. It is acceptable for a healthy infant without dysphagia to use two or even three sucks per one swallow and one breath when sucking, as opposed to the previous ratio of 1:1:1 for suckling. Both patterns are effective for ingestion of fluids during infancy, and sucking continues to evolve during development to allow for eventual open cup drinking and straw drinking when there is sufficient neurologic and physical maturation to allow for these more advanced methods of fluid ingestion.[4,5,6,7,8,9,10]

## Clinical Note

Infants and children may have congenital or acquired dysphagia resulting from a number of different conditions. Similarly, the dysphagia may be transient or chronic depending on the causal factor. The most commonly reported conditions in pediatric populations with dysphagia include cerebral palsy, acquired/traumatic brain injury, craniofacial malformations, airway malformations, cardiac disease, gastrointestinal disorders, and infants born prematurely.

For most, feeding follows a predictable, developmental progression driven by physical and neurologic maturation. Newborn infants, as reviewed earlier, receive all their nutrition from nipple feedings for the first 4 to 6 months of life. At around 4 to 6 months of age, some form of spoon-feeding is typically introduced as the infant demonstrates greater head and neck control to allow for sitting with external trunk support. Initially, infants suck on pureed textures offered to them from the spoon until they learn, through repeated experiences, to close their lips around the spoon and use their upper lip to assist in removing the pureed or semisolid material from the spoon. At 5 to 6 months of age, infants have the ability to use a primitive, reflexive munching pattern on more solid textures that have the ability to melt when they come into contact with saliva. A more mature biting pattern, necessary to consume solids that do not have the property of melting, requires infants to close their lips around the utensil or food substance, use their incisors (if necessary) to bite, use their molar surfaces to chew, use their tongue to move the bolus laterally within the oral cavity for further manipulation before gathering the bolus on the midblade of the tongue for initiation of bolus transport to the pharynx. In general, feeding development can be summarized into five distinct stages: (1) nipple feeding, (2) spoon-feeding, (3) chewing, (4) self-feeding, and (5) managing a cup.[11,12,13] Each stage of feeding development depends on the physical growth and maturation of the infant. While all the individual components for successful nutritional intake are in place by 2 years of age, they continue to be refined throughout childhood until they reach the familiar patterns of adult feeding skills.

As the human diet expands during growth and maturation, ingestion depends on the characteristics of the food source. The strategy for consuming liquids varies with the consistency and delivery method, whether it is via spoon, straw, or cup. Semisolids and eventually solids can be introduced to the oral cavity with help of fingers or a utensil, or by biting away a piece of foodstuff. Strategies such as biting food or sucking liquid from a straw by creating negative pressure both require **occlusion**. Muscular control of the lips surrounding the vestibule of the oral cavity is important for bolus containment during biting and chewing.

## Clinical Note

Peripheral or central lesions of the facial nerve (CN VII), known as a Bell's palsy, can result from a common cold and may present with oral dysphagia.

Bolus formation follows ingestion of fluid and food substances, serving both as preparation for the transport of the material and as the initiation of digestion. **Mastication** increases the surface area of food while partitioning food into a bolus of manageable size and consistency for swallowing. Chewing is both voluntary and rhythmic and is driven by brainstem **central pattern generators** (**Fig. 3.2**) that manage the **lower motor neurons** controlling muscles that open and close the jaw in response to the sensory stimuli. These rhythmic generators in the brainstem receive constant information from the teeth, muscles of mastication, and tongue to allow food to be reduced and swept around the oral cavity while

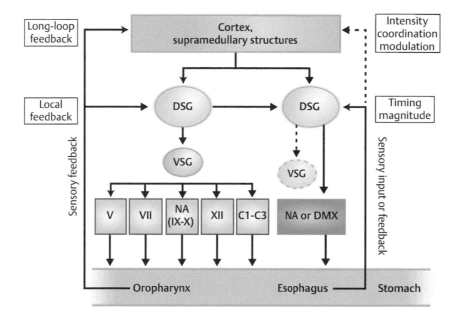

DSG = Dorsal swallowing group
VSG = Ventral swallowing group
NA = Nucleus ambiguus
DMX = Dorsal motor nucleus of X

**Fig. 3.2** Diagram of brainstem swallowing center.

protecting the tongue. Surrounding this process are **mucosa**-lined muscles of the cheeks and lips that contain the bolus in the oral cavity and provide sensory feedback to the cortex.

**Taste** plays an important role in swallowing and nutrition. Taste receptors are matched with the nutritional needs of the body and provide protection through an **emetic reflex** with projections to the **area postrema** in the **medulla** that induce vomiting in response to noxious **tastants**. Multiple taste receptors are located within taste buds on the tongue, and some are found in epiglottic mucosa. These receptors trigger taste-salivatory reflexes mediated by the **autonomic nervous system** (**Fig. 3.3**) to release saliva into the oral cavity. Saliva provides enzymes that begin to extract nutrients for eventual reuptake in the small bowel, and it lubricates the bolus and mucosa lining the oral and pharyngeal cavities.

Taste sensation is received within the **solitary nucleus** of the medulla and projects from there to many areas of the brain, including cognitive and hedonic pathways. Some sensory stimuli, such as capsaicin or menthol, often confused with taste, are mediated by pain receptors in the trigeminal system and are properly distinguished as **chemesthesis**. **Taste** perception is also confused with **flavor**, which is a perception influenced by smell, taste, temperature, chemesthesis, and even hormones. Experience with taste shows us that tastants elicit differences in swallowing mechanics. A bitter-tasting cough syrup may induce a rapid swallow, whereas a favorite dish or dessert may slow down the entire feeding sequence.

## Clinical Note

The use of various tastants and stimulants as possible neurorehabilitative treatments for dysphagia is under ongoing investigation.

Flavor perception develops and functions in utero. A fetus can distinguish flavors, and the amniotic fluid contains a wide range of nutrients and flavors, dependent upon the mother's diet. Infants show preference for previously experienced flavors.[14] Infants also show affective reactions to taste: Sweet/Umami elicits rhythmic tongue protrusion, lip smacking, and elevation of the corners of the mouth; Bitter elicits a gape, nose wrinkling, flailing of the arms, and a frown; Sour elicits a pursing of the lips, and with less extent gaping, nose wrinkling, head shaking, flailing of the arms, and frowning; Salty elicits a neutral response in newborns (taste recognition for salty doesn't emerge until approximately 4 months of age).[15] The senses of both taste and smell continue to develop after birth, and developmentally, taste and smell are major determinants of what children will eat.[14] Eventual food preference is a function of exposure within hypothesized critical periods for infant acceptance of increasing flavor and texture. Infants from 3 to 4 months of age are more willing to try new tastes of food, which happens to coincide with their physical development to support spoon-feeding. During the later half of the first year of

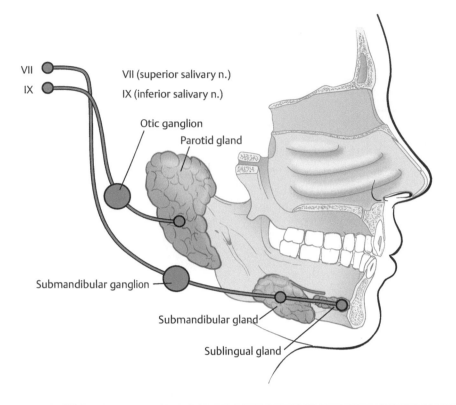

VII
IX

VII (superior salivary n.)
IX (inferior salivary n.)

Otic ganglion
Parotid gland

Submandibular ganglion

Submandibular gland

Sublingual gland

**Fig. 3.3** Salivary glands and innervation.

life to the second year of life, their willingness to try new foods decreases until the developmental stage of food neophobia becomes prominent.[16,17] Food neophobia peaks between 2 and 6 years of age and represents a predictable developmental stage when children display a reluctance to eat and avoidance of new foods.[17] In typically developing children, food neophobia is overcome, and diets continue to expand through repeated exposure to new foods (sometimes up to 15 exposures to a new food are necessary before acceptance).[18]

Sensory integration is the neurologic process of organizing the sensory information we receive from the environment in all aspects of human functioning. It is particularly relevant to eating because eating is one of the most sensory-rich activities available in the human experience. When sensory information is received and processed appropriately within the central nervous system, humans predictably respond with expected actions and behaviors. This can be witnessed during the process of eating and swallowing in individuals without dysphagia at every meal and snack opportunity. The processes of sensory modulation, inhibition, habituation, and facilitation enable the typically functioning person to subconsciously consume adequate volumes of nutrition without swallowing impairment. *Sensory integration dysfunction* is a general term that refers to the inability to process some information received through the senses. It may result in the inability to appropriately respond to some sensory stimuli affecting the individual's actions and behavior.

## Clinical Note

Sensory integration dysfunction has been implicated in some forms of oral dysphagia, particularly in pediatric patients.[4,19,20]

## 3.3 Oral Transport Initiates Swallowing

Bolus formation varies in time depending on the type of bolus and the competing hedonic and cognitive goals of the individual. In the well-controlled environment of the fluoroscopy suite, the bolus formation concludes when the bolus is gathered behind the teeth in the anterior chamber of the mouth. However, at times, a solid food bolus is parceled to the anterior chamber and the posterior surface of the tongue with the more caudal parcel ready for transport into the pharynx. Oral transport commences when the tongue accommodates the bolus and moves it through the oral cavity, and it concludes when the bolus is propelled into the hypopharynx through a wavelike movement of the tongue. Bolus transport is voluntary in the mature feeder and therefore under cortical control.

## Clinical Note

Stroke patients may exhibit tongue pumping preceding oral transport, indicating a disruption of upper motor neuron pathways.

The tongue is a **muscular hydrostat** that is deformed by intrinsic muscles oriented longitudinally and in the perpendicular plane, vertically and horizontally (**Fig. 3.4**).[21,22] Extrinsic muscles attaching the tongue to the mandible, hyoid, cranial base, and palate are interwoven into the intrinsic muscles (**Fig. 3.5**). Notably, the genioglossus spreads out like a handheld folding fan with the apex (tip) attached to the mandible. This muscle, in conjunction with the intrinsic muscle, creates a wave that pushes the bolus up against the palate and then propels the bolus into the hypopharynx as the tongue base is retracted against the **oropharyngeal isthmus**. As the bolus enters the **hypopharynx** (**Fig. 3.6**), swallowing moves from voluntary to involuntary control as the central pattern generator in the brainstem for pharyngeal swallowing is triggered

and a sequence of biomechanical events transforms a respiratory conduit into a digestive tract in less than 500 milliseconds.[23]

Recall from earlier discussion that an infant must be able to extract liquid from the bottle or the breast through suckling or sucking to successfully complete the oral preparatory phase. The tongue is primarily responsible for this action, and, depending on the number of suckles or sucks used to extract bolus material, the infant may need to collect small volumes of liquid bolus within the oral cavity until it is of a sufficient volume to trigger a swallow. Liquid bolus material may be collected between the tongue and soft palate, on the posterior portion of the tongue, or in the **valleculae—** due to the anatomical configuration of the oral cavity in infancy.[24] Unlike the swallow seen in a mature feeder, the swallow in an infant does not have distinct oral preparatory and transit phases. The continuous anterior to posterior wavelike motion of the tongue visible during suckling and sucking is responsible for the seamless transition between oral preparatory and deglution phases during nipple feeding. The wavelike component of suckling or sucking occurs in the medial portion of the tongue. As the wave progresses posteriorly, it applies both negative and positive pressure on the nipple, assisting in the transference of the bolus to the pharynx.[25]

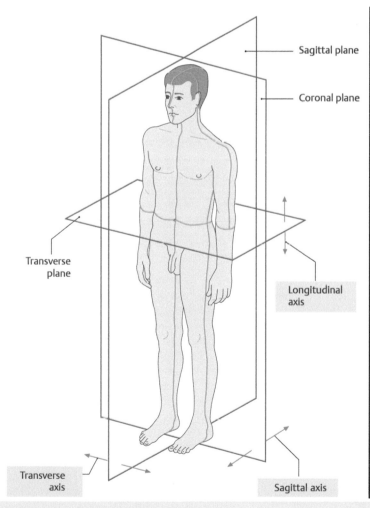

| Upper body (head, neck, and trunk | | |
|---|---|---|
| Term | Explanation | |
| Cranial | Pertaining to, or located toward, the head | |
| Caudal | Pertaining to, or located toward, the tail | |
| Anterior | Pertaining to, or located toward, the front synonym: Ventral (used for all animals) | |
| Posterior | Pertaining to, or located toward the back synonym: Dorsal (used for all animals) | |
| Superior | UPper or above | |
| Inferiot | Lower or below | |
| Axial | Pertaining to the axis of a structure | |
| Transverse | Situated at right angles to the long axis of a structure | |
| Longitudinal | Parallel to the long axis of a structure | |
| Horizontal | Parallel to the plane or the horizon | |
| Vertical | Perpendicular to the plane or the horizon | |
| Medial | Toward the median plane | |
| Lateral | Away from the median pane (toward the side) | |
| Median | Situated in the median plane or midline | |
| Peripheral | Situated away from the surface | |
| Superficial | Situated near the surface | |
| Deep | Situated deep beneath the surface | |
| External | Outer or lateral | |
| Internal | Inner or medial | |
| Apical | Pertaining to the top or apex | |
| Basal | pertaining to the bottom or base | |
| Sagittal | Situated parallel to the sagittal suture | |
| Coronal | Situated parallel to the coronal suture (pertaining to the crown of the head) | |
| Limbs | | |
| Term | Explanation | |
| Proximal | Close to, or toward, the trunk, or toward the point of origin | |
| Distal | Away from the trunk (toward the end of the limb), or away from the point of origin | |
| Radial | Pertaining to the radius of the lateral side of the forearm | |
| Ulnar | Pertaining to the ulna or the medial side of the forearm | |
| Tibial | Pertaining to the tibia or the medial side of the leg | |
| Fibular | Pertaining to the fibula or the lateral side of the leg | |
| Palmar (volar) | Pertaining to the palm of the hand | |
| Planar | Pertaining to the sale of the foot | |
| Dorsal | Pertaining to the back of the hand or top of the foot | |

**Fig. 3.4** Anatomical planes and terms.

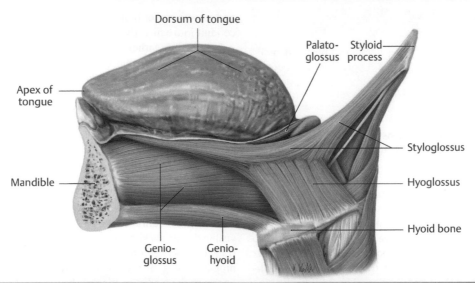

| Innervation of the tongue | | |
|---|---|---|
| **Nerve** | **Nerve Fibers** | **Distribution** |
| Lingual nerve (CN V$_3$) | General sensory | Anterior two thirds or the tongue |
| Chorda tympani (CN VII) | Taste | Anterior two thirds or the tongue |
| Glossopharyngeal nerve (CN IX) | General sensory and taste | Posterior third of the tongue |
| Vagus nerve (CN X) | General sensory and taste | Scattered taste buds at the tongue's base |
| Hypoglossal nerve (CN XII) | Somatic motor | Muscles of the tongue, except the palatoglossus, which is innervated by the vagus nerve (CN X) |

**Fig. 3.5** Muscles of the tongue and innervation of the tongue.

Operating in the background of oral transport is the respiratory swallow cycle. Respiration is driven by the body's need to supply oxygen for necessary metabolic functions and to remove carbon dioxide from the body to prevent toxicity. This is mostly an involuntary process involving the respiratory center of the central nervous system, housed in the medulla. The respiratory center responds to neural, chemical, and hormonal signals to regulate breathing by adjusting the rate and depth of inhalation and exhalation. In healthy individuals, it is usually the elevated presence of carbon dioxide detected by chemoreceptors in the blood that signals the respiratory center to breathe.[26] As the voluntary action of initiating swallowing occurs in the mature feeder, the brainstem signals respiratory inhibition. There is sufficient evidence in the literature to support that swallowing occurs optimally at mid to low expiratory volumes.[27] Inspiration immediately following a swallow may lead to aspiration of residue. Conversely, swallowing at a full lung volume preceding expiration introduces the problem of compensating for the downward pull of negative pressure generated by the decent of the respiratory diaphragm.[28] Respiratory cessation at mid to low volume benefits from residual exhale to oppose aspiration without necessitating the swallowing apparatus to work against the negative pressure of full lung volume.

## Clinical Note

The uncoupling of swallowing and respiratory control resulting from stroke or cancer treatment can lead to swallowing difficulty.

Infants are required to utilize a sophisticated, highly coordinated process of suckling/sucking, swallowing, and respiration to safely consume enough calories to support their rapid growth and development. It was previously thought that infants could breathe and swallow simultaneously.[29] Current understanding of infant swallow physiology includes the recognition of a brief swallow apnea.[30,31,32,33] In limited research of 10 infants followed longitudinally during the first year of life, researchers discovered that the majority of infants followed a nutritive swallow with expiration regardless of postgestational age, like the pattern of swallow and respiration generally reported for adults.[33]

Infants are preferential nasal breathers, and their coordination for suckle or suck/swallow/breath sequencing is typically described as follows: (1) inhalation through the nose, (2) suckle/suck with simultaneous transition to expiration, (3) swallow (with cessation of expiration due to complete closure of the

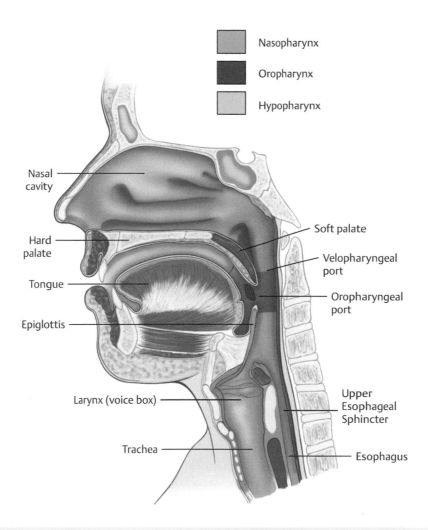

Nasopharynx

Oropharynx

Hypopharynx

Nasal cavity

Hard palate

Tongue

Epiglottis

Larynx (voice box)

Trachea

Soft palate

Velopharyngeal port

Oropharyngeal port

Upper Esophageal Sphincter

Esophagus

**Fig. 3.6** Regions of the pharynx and valves.

larynx), (4) finish expiratory phase of respiration.[34] A minimal period of airway closure with complete cessation of respiratory flow (mean of 530 milliseconds) has been reported.[35] A mature, coordinated suck, swallow, breathe pattern is typically present in healthy infants by 37 weeks postmenstrual age.[32,36] Whereas suck and swallow rhythms mature at ~ 37 weeks postmenstrual age, the stability of respiration and swallow cycles matures at a later time.[37]

## Clinical Note

Research to understand the dynamic relationships between suckling/sucking and swallowing is ongoing. Physiological research helps the clinician understand the relationship between suckling/sucking and swallowing in the healthy infant who can successfully feed and helps guide interventions in the infant with dysphagia.

## 3.4  Pharyngeal Conversion

As the bolus is propelled into the pharynx, conversion of the pharynx from the respiratory to the digestive tract is well under way. The pharynx is a **fibromuscular** tube lined with **membranous fascia** and mucosa. This pharyngeal tube has four openings that can each be closed or sealed off, namely, the oropharyngeal port, the velopharyngeal port, the larynx, and the upper esophageal sphincter (often called the pharyngeal esophageal segment). During normal respiration the portals to the oral and nasal cavity and trachea are open while the portal into the esophagus is closed. During oropharyngeal swallowing the three opened portals are closed and the portal to the esophagus is relaxed and stretched open. Simultaneous with the closing and opening of portals the configuration of the pharynx is changed, drastically reducing pharyngeal volume. As readers will recall from study of **Boyle's law**, as volume decreases, pressure increases. The propulsive force of the tongue base behind the bolus now benefits from this pressurized chamber adding increased force behind the bolus as it gains momentum passing through the upper esophageal sphincter.[38] Pharyngeal clearance is completed by a stripping wave of the pharynx, and in the typical swallow there is no perceivable residual material left in the pharynx after the swallow.

Safe and efficient swallowing depends on the proper function of each of the four portals of the pharynx. Each portal will now be discussed in turn followed by the changes in the pharynx.

As respiration is inhibited during swallowing, so is the tonic contraction of the **cricopharyngeus muscle**. This distal portion of the inferior (**Fig. 3.7**) pharyngeal constrictor is attached to the cricoid and connects the esophagus to the pharynx. The tonic contraction of this muscle creates a high-pressure zone called the upper esophageal sphincter or the pharyngeal esophageal segment.[39,40] This high-pressure zone varies in length and may also include the more superior portion of the inferior pharyngeal constrictor, called the **thyropharyngeus**, attaching to the thyroid cartilage. Tonic contraction is inhibited during pharyngeal conversion, allowing for the relaxation and opening of the upper esophageal sphincter as the pharynx is reconfigured and the bolus is pushed into the esophagus. As the bolus tail passes through this segment, phasic contraction of the cricopharyngeus helps push the bolus into the esophagus, followed by the resting state tonic activity of the cricopharyngeus.

The velum, or soft palate, hangs off the back edge of the hard palate. Closure of the soft palate occurs simultaneously with oral transport and is rarely compromised. When velopharyngeal port closure is compromised, swallowing impairment is certain. The levator veli palatini (**Fig. 3.9**) extends into the substance of the soft palate to form a sling to close this portal. The apparent result seen in a fiberoptic endoscopic examination of swallowing is that the soft palate is bunched together against the pharyngeal walls sealing off the velopharyngeal port (**Fig. 3.10**).[42]

The propulsive action of the tongue in oral transport propels the bolus into the hypopharynx and closes the oral cavity portal. The oropharyngeal portal is sealed off as the tongue base is retracted and the pharyngeal isthmus is pulled toward the tongue base by the palatoglossus.

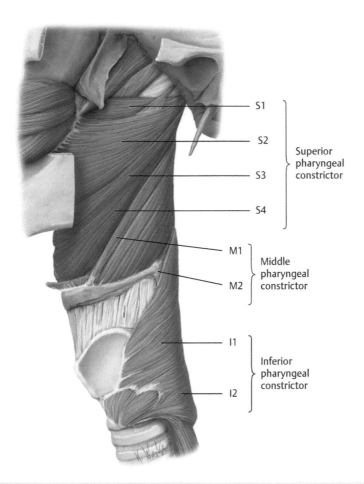

**Fig. 3.7** Pharyngeal constrictor muscles 12, cricopharyngeus.

There are multiple functions that close off the larynx and protect the airway. The laryngeal inlet is highly innervated and under constant surveillance in wakefulness or sleeping (**Fig. 3.11**).[43] As a bolus nears the laryngeal inlet, pharyngeal swallowing is triggered. The hyoid bursts toward the mandible, pulling the larynx along with it. As the larynx is elevated, and the base of the tongue retracts, the arytenoids tilt toward the base of the epiglottis as it closes over the larynx. Two epiglottic movements can be observed in epiglottic inversion: one movement to horizontal and the next to full inversion to shield the airway from the bolus. Laryngeal elevation and tongue base retraction underlie both movements.[44] Finally, vocal fold adduction provides the last measure of protection for the airway.

## Clinical Note

In a fiberoptic endoscopic examination of swallowing, the arytenoids can be seen approximating toward the epiglottis to narrow the laryngeal inlet before the bolus arrives on the scene.[45]

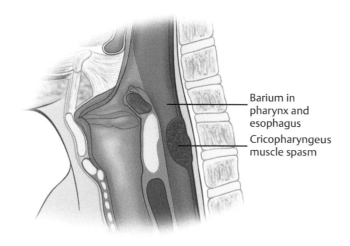

Barium in pharynx and esophagus

Cricopharyngeus muscle spasm

**Fig. 3.8** Cricopharyngeal bar as seen on videofluoroscopy.

Concurrent with the opening and closing of these portals to redirect the bolus, the morphology of the pharynx is reconfigured to accomplish several physiological objectives. The larynx is relocated under the retracting tongue base away from of the trajectory of the oncoming bolus. The pharynx is shortened and is pulled up to engulf the head of the bolus.[46] Finally the volume of the pharynx is compressed by shortening the pharynx, but also by the radial compression of the pharynx to increase pressure pushing the bolus through the upper esophageal sphincter. The relocation of the larynx and shortening of the pharynx are accomplished through a series of muscular slings that suspend the swallowing apparatus.[47] The muscular slings in the pharynx, referred to as the long pharyngeal muscles (**Fig. 3.12**), are fatigue-resistant and shorten the pharynx. Fast-twitch pharyngeal constrictor muscles wrap these longitudinally oriented muscles and radially collapse the pharynx from superior to inferior, producing what is referred to as the pharyngeal stripping wave, which in normal conditions ensures pharyngeal clearance.[48]

## Clinical Note

Radiation treatment of head and neck cancer can lead to muscle fibrosis, which greatly reduces muscle function and is a common cause of dysphagia. Swallowing exercises before and during radiation treatment have been shown to help patients retain swallowing function.[49]

After the bolus head passes through the upper esophageal sphincter and the stripping wave of the pharynx pushes the bolus into the esophagus, the pharynx reverts to a respiratory tract. When the portal to the esophagus closes, all muscular slings that underlie closure of the oropharyngeal port, velopharyngeal port, and airway relax and open these portals. Respiration optimally resumes at a midexhalation.[50]

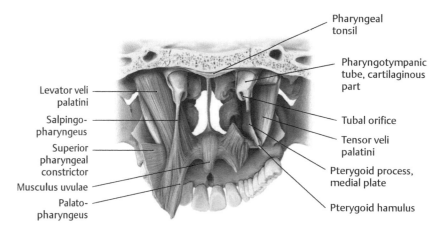

Pharyngeal tonsil

Pharyngotympanic tube, cartilaginous part

Levator veli palatini

Salpingo-pharyngeus

Superior pharyngeal constrictor

Musculus uvulae

Palato-pharyngeus

Tubal orifice

Tensor veli palatini

Pterygoid process, medial plate

Pterygoid hamulus

**Fig. 3.9** Muscles of the velopharyngeal sling.

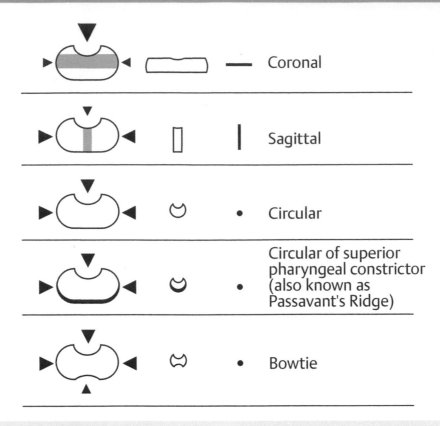

| | | | |
|---|---|---|---|
| | ▬ | — | Coronal |
| | ▯ | \| | Sagittal |
| | ☾ | • | Circular |
| | ☽ | • | Circular of superior pharyngeal constrictor (also known as Passavant's Ridge) |
| | ⧖ | • | Bowtie |

**Fig. 3.10** Patterns of velopharyngeal closure.

The pharyngeal stage of the infant swallow is similar to that of the adult swallow. A notable difference, however, is the frequency with which the infant swallow occurs. Infants swallow more frequently and with greater speed than their adult counterparts, due in part to the smaller volume of fluid extracted with each suckle/suck, reduced space within the oral cavity, and the reduced pharyngeal length present in infants as compared to adults.[51] There is also some question about the presence of epiglottic retroflexion over the laryngeal inlet during the infant swallow.[52,53]

In infants, the epiglottis may be omega shaped, more pliant and soft, and has been seen to make direct contact with the soft palate (in some cases) due to the high laryngeal positioning found in infants. The epiglottis also has more direct contact with the base of the tongue in infants and children, again due to the superior positioning of the larynx in the pharynx.[54,55] The thyroid cartilage and hyoid bone are in closer approximation at rest in the infant than in the adult.[56] These anatomical and positional differences between the infant and adult larynx may explain the lack of epiglottic tilting reported by some authors.[52,53] Rommel first reported that infants and children do not show consistent epiglottic tilting until after 5 years of age.[52] Rommel proposed that the anterior movement of the arytenoids was sufficient for laryngeal closure in the smaller laryngeal vestibule found in infants and younger children. Additionally, she proposed that epiglottic tilting might represent a maturational factor that changes with laryngeal and pharyngeal growth.[52]

## 3.5 Timing of Pharyngeal Conversion

The timing of events underlying pharyngeal conversion, although variable, is critically important for airway protection and swallowing efficiency.[57] If the bolus arrives at the laryngeal inlet before this portal is relocated, protected, and sealed, then aspiration is inevitable. If the larynx is sealed by vocal cord closure but is not sufficiently protected by epiglottic inversion or arytenoid-to-epiglottis approximation (as described by Rommel[52]), or relocated by hyolaryngeal excursion (as happens in the adult swallow), then penetration of the bolus into the laryngeal inlet is likely. Both penetration and aspiration threaten swallowing safety.

Swallowing efficiency is observed when the bolus is cleared from the pharynx.[58] If the momentum of the bolus propelled into the pharynx by the tongue is not followed by both the application of compressive forces to the bolus by the conversion of the pharynx and the efficient opening of the upper esophageal sphincter, then residue in the pharynx is likely. Residue is most often found in valleculae or the piriform recess, but it can be located on the pharyngeal walls or tongue. Residue in the valleculae is most likely to indicate inadequate tongue base retraction, laryngeal elevation, epiglottic inversion, or pharyngeal squeeze during the adult swallow, resulting in some portion of the bolus being retained in that space. In contrast, infants participating in nipple feeding typically have small-volume residue in the valleculae after the swallow due to the more caudal positioning of the infant larynx. The infant laryngeal position at rest resembles the laryngeal position of the

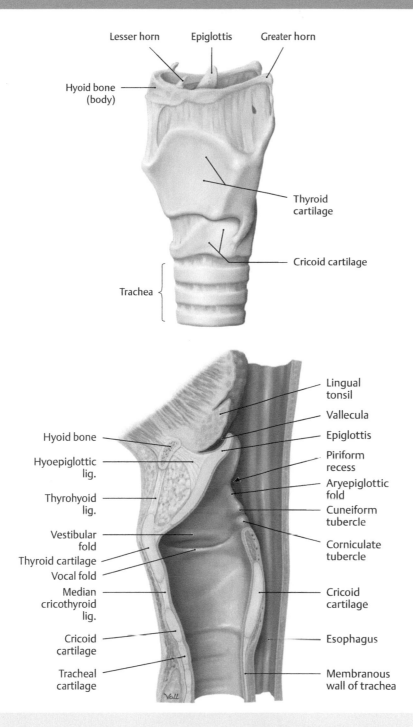

Lesser horn   Epiglottis   Greater horn

Hyoid bone
(body)

Thyroid
cartilage

Cricoid cartilage

Trachea

a

Lingual
tonsil

Vallecula

Hyoid bone

Epiglottis

Hyoepiglottic
lig.

Piriform
recess

Thyrohyoid
lig.

Aryepiglottic
fold

Vestibular
fold

Cuneiform
tubercle

Thyroid cartilage

Corniculate
tubercle

Vocal fold

Median
cricothyroid
lig.

Cricoid
cartilage

Cricoid
cartilage

Esophagus

Tracheal
cartilage

Membranous
wall of trachea

b

**Fig. 3.11** Larynx.

adult at the height of the pharyngeal swallow.[51,59] Residue in the piriform sinuses is multifactorial, though incidence is likely with ineffective opening of the upper esophageal sphincter in both populations. Pathological residue increases the risk of penetration–aspiration events. Residue in the piriform sinuses indicates impaired swallowing physiology in both populations, and residue in the valleculae is indicative of impaired swallowing physiology in those with mature swallowing function.

It is generally accepted that the internal superior laryngeal nerve is the afferent trigger for involuntary swallowing.[60] These axons belong to the vagus nerve (CN X) and populate the mucosa within and surrounding the laryngeal inlet. When stimulated in animal models, this nerve initiates the cascade of events synchronizing over 20 muscles under the control of five cranial nerves and several spinal nerves to move the bolus from the oral cavity and through the pharynx and esophagus. Swallowing centers in the brainstem coordinate with

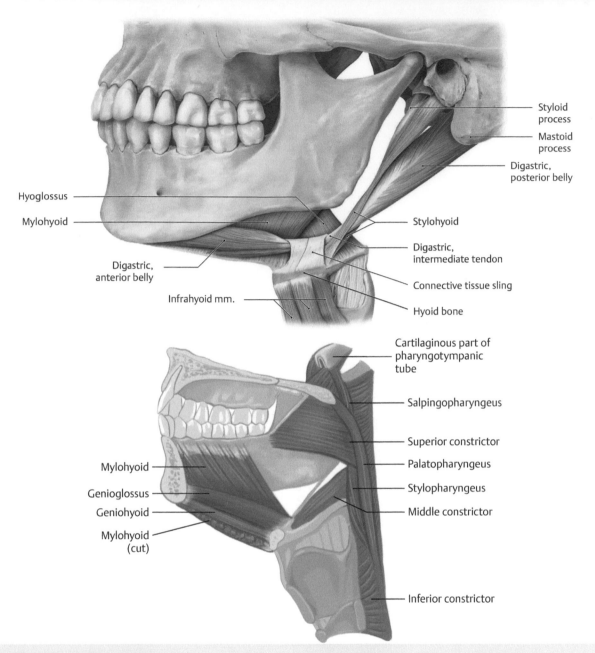

**Fig. 3.12** Pharyngeal muscles and slings

masticatory and respiratory centers to time deglutition effectively.[61] In normal physiological swallowing, sensory assessment of bolus consistency in the oral cavity allows for motor planning and cortical drive to modulate the timing and intensity of pharyngeal swallowing.

## Clinical Note

Lesions to the cortex may impair swallowing efficiency and safety, which can be recovered with rehabilitation, whereas a brainstem stroke or malformation involving the central pattern generators will have a prolonged deleterious impact on swallowing function. A more detailed outline of neurologic control of swallowing function is provided at the conclusion of this chapter in **Appendix 3.1**.

## 3.6 Esophageal Phase of Swallowing

The esophagus is a muscular tube composed of striated and smooth muscle. The upper and lower esophageal sphincters are created by continuous contraction of muscles that relax during swallowing but otherwise function to keep acidic digestive juices in their proper place. Due to neurologic immaturity, there are transient relaxations of the esophageal sphincters in infants that result in nonpathological, developmental, gastroesophageal reflux that typically resolves by 1 year of age with physical and neurologic maturation. Reflux is a common comorbidity of incompetent sphincters in both populations. Muscles in the esophagus are arranged in longitudinal and circumferential patterns, allowing for peristaltic waves of contraction to move the bolus forward. The primary peristalsis of the esophagus is a continuation of the peristaltic stripping wave of the pharynx that descends to the lower esophageal sphincter. The esophagus has a rich network of sensory nerves that give feedback to smooth muscle through local circuits. If a bolus gets stuck in transit, local stretch receptors induce a secondary peristalsis to push the bolus along. Problems with the esophageal phase of swallowing may include retention of the bolus in the esophagus, retrograde flow of the bolus through the upper esophageal sphincter, or complete retention of the bolus without any clearance.

## Clinical Note

Gastroesophageal reflex disease, or GERD, is a chronic condition of the lower esophageal sphincter allowing stomach acid back into the esophagus and is commonly exacerbated by being in a supine position during sleep.

Deglutition is a complex physiological process that integrates multiple functions to meet nutritional and eventual hedonic needs of the organism. The pharynx is at the crossroads of medical specialties, including otolaryngology, neurology, gastroenterology, pulmonology, and physical and rehabilitative medicine. It is imperative that speech-language pathology clinicians possess a comprehensive understanding of function and structure underlying deglutition to enable the health care team to best serve each individual patient.

## 3.7 Questions

1. Incidence of residue in the piriform sinuses is likely in both populations (infants and adults) when which physiological correlate is observed?

A. Delayed oral transit
B. Delayed pharyngeal transit
C. Ineffective velopharyngeal closure
D. Ineffective opening of the upper esophageal sphincter
E. Ineffective base of tongue to posterior pharyngeal wall contact

2. Which extrinsic muscle of the tongue, in conjunction with the intrinsic muscles of the tongue, contributes most notably to the transport of the bolus through the oral cavity?

A. Hyoglossus
B. Styloglossus
C. Genioglossus
D. Palatoglossus
E. Inferior longitudinal

3. In infants, there are notable differences in the form and function of the epiglottis that include all of the following except:

A. Epiglottis may be omega shaped
B. Epiglottis may be more pliant and soft
C. Epiglottis may make direct contact with the soft palate

D. Epiglottis has more direct contact with the base of the tongue
E. Epiglottis is noted to have a greater degree of retroflexion during the swallow

4. There is sufficient evidence in the literature to support that swallowing optimally occurs during which phase of the respiratory cycle?

A. Early expiratory phase
B. Mid to late expiratory phase
C. Early inspiratory phase
D. Mid inspiratory phase
E. In between expiration and inspiration

5. During pharyngeal swallowing, pharyngeal shortening compressing the bolus is primarily achieved by action of which of the following muscles?

A. Long pharyngeal muscles
B. Pharyngeal constrictors
C. Cricopharyngeus
D. Hyolaryngeal complex

## 3.8 Answers and Explanations

1. **Correct: ineffective opening of the upper esophageal sphincter (D).**
   Residue in the piriform sinuses is multifactorial, though incidence is likely with ineffective opening of the upper esophageal sphincter in both populations. Delayed oral or pharyngeal transit (**A, B**) is likely to increase the incidence of laryngeal penetration or aspiration, but it is not correlated with increases in piriform sinus residue. Ineffective velopharyngeal closure (**C**) is likely to result in nasopharyngeal backflow, and ineffective base of tongue to posterior pharyngeal wall contact (**E**) is likely to result in increased incidence of residue in the valleculae.

2. **Correct: genioglossus (C).**
   The genioglossus muscle spreads out like a handheld folding fan with the apex (tip) attached to the mandible and, in conjunction with the intrinsic lingual muscle, creates a wave that pushes the bolus up against the palate and then propels the bolus into the hypopharynx as the tongue base is retracted against the oropharyngeal isthmus.
   The hyoglossus (**A**), styloglossus (**B**), and palatoglossus (**D**) are also extrinsic muscles of the tongue; however, they are not primary contributors to the oral transit stage of swallowing. The inferior longitudinal muscle (**E**) is an intrinsic tongue muscle.

3. **Correct: the epiglottis is noted to have a greater degree of retroflexion during the swallow (E).**
   Due to documented differences in the epiglottic shape and positioning in the infant, there is currently thought to be a lack of epiglottic retroflexion. Rommel[52] first reported that infants and children do not show consistent epiglottic

tilting until after 5 years of age. Rommel proposed that the anterior movement of the arytenoids was sufficient for laryngeal closure in the smaller laryngeal vestibule found in infants and younger children. Additionally, she proposed that epiglottic tilting might represent a maturational factor that changes with laryngeal and pharyngeal growth.[52]

In infants, the epiglottis may be omega shaped (**A**), more pliant and soft (**B**), and has been seen to make direct contact with the soft palate (**C**) (in some cases) due to the high laryngeal positioning found in infants. The epiglottis also has more direct contact with the base of tongue (**D**) in infants and children, again due to the superior positioning of the larynx in the pharynx.[54,55] The thyroid and hyoid cartilages are in closer approximation at rest in the infant than in the adult.[56]

4. **Correct: mid to late expiratory phase (B).**
There is sufficient evidence in the literature to support that swallowing occurs optimally at mid to low expiratory volumes.[27] Respiratory cessations at mid to low volume benefit from residual exhale to oppose aspiration without necessitating the swallowing apparatus to work against the negative pressure of full lung volume. Inspiration immediately following a swallow (as would occur with swallow happening between the expiratory and inspiratory phases) may lead to aspiration of residue. Conversely, swallowing at a full lung volume preceding expiration introduces the problem of compensating for the downward pull of negative pressure generated by the descent of the respiratory diaphragm.[28]

5. **Correct: the long pharyngeal muscles (A).**
The relocation of the larynx and shortening of the pharynx are accomplished through a series of muscular slings that suspend the swallowing apparatus.[47] The muscular slings in the pharynx, referred to as the long pharyngeal muscles, are fatigue-resistant and shorten the pharynx.

The fast-twitch pharyngeal constrictor muscles (**B**) wrap these longitudinally oriented muscles and radially collapse the pharynx from superior to inferior, producing what is referred to as the pharyngeal stripping wave, which in normal conditions ensures pharyngeal clearance.[48] The cricopharyngeus (**C**) is the tonically contracted muscle of the upper esophageal sphincter. The palatopharyngeus assists in approximating the velum and pharynx. The hyolaryngeal complex (**D**) is made of the hyoid bone and the larynx and is acted upon by various muscles to accomplish hyolaryngeal excursion during the swallow.

# Appendix 3.1 Outline of Neurologic Influence and Control for Swallowing[62,63,64,65]

## Basic Sequence of Neural Events

1. Before the bolus enters the mouth, the individual recognizes the bolus (through sight and smell); this is registered by the cortical structures, which prepare the swallowing system for that particular bolus.

2. The bolus enters the oral cavity and is sensed by the peripheral nerves, which send sensory (afferent) information to the nucleus tractus solitarii (NTS) in the brainstem swallowing center. The brainstem communicates with the cortical structures to ultimately determine the precise physiological nature of the swallow.

3. The reflexive swallow is triggered by sensory stimulation (i.e., bolus contact on the faucial arches, tonsils, soft palate, posterior pharyngeal wall, and deep muscle receptors in the base of the tongue).

4. The NTS (where all the sensory information accumulates) in the brainstem swallowing center instructs the cranial nerve motor nuclei to execute motoric responses.

Afferent information on taste and general sensation associated with deglutition:

- Cranial nerve (CN) V trigeminal, VII facial, IX glossopharyngeal, X vagus

Efferent control of oral and pharyngeal phases of the swallow:

- CN V trigeminal, VII facial, IX glossopharyngeal, X vagus, and XII hypoglossal

Division of cranial nerve innervation by swallowing phase:

## Oral Phase

- Sensation:
  - CN V—trigeminal
  - Maxillary branch
    - Mucous membranes of the nasopharynx
    - Hard and soft palates
    - Upper teeth
    - Tonsils
  - Mandibular branch
    - Mucous membranes of anterior two-thirds of tongue
    - Cheek
    - Floor of mouth
    - Lower teeth
    - Gums
    - Skin of lower lip and jaw
    - Temporomandibular joint
  - CN VII—facial
    - Conveys taste sensation from anterior two-thirds of tongue
  - CN IX—glossopharyngeal
    - Taste sensation from posterior third of tongue
    - Touch, pain, and thermal sensation from mucous membrane of oropharynx, palatine tonsils, faucial pillars, and posterior third of tongue
- Motor
  - CN V—trigeminal, mandibular branch

- Muscles of mastication (temporalis, masseter, medial pterygoid, lateral pterygoid)
  - CN VII—facial
    - Mimetic muscles including orbicularis oris and buccinator
    - Visceromotor neurons originating in the facial nerve supply submandibular and sublingual glands
  - CN IX—glossopharyngeal
    - Visceromotor neurons originating in the glossopharyngeal nerve supply parotid glands
  - CN X—vagus
    - Visceromotor neurons originating in the glossopharyngeal nerve supply mucus glands scattered throughout the pharynx
  - CN XII—hypoglossal
    - Controls the intrinsic muscles of the tongue and genioglossus that underlie bolus transport

## Pharyngeal Phase

- Sensation:
  - CN IX—glossopharyngeal
    - Transmits visceral sensation from posterior tongue and faucial pillars
  - CN X—vagus
    - Pharyngeal branches of the vagus transmit visceral sensation from the pharynx
    - Internal branch of superior laryngeal nerve (SLN) conveys general sensation from mucosa of laryngopharynx, epiglottis, laryngeal mucosa above vocal folds, joint receptors in larynx, and small area on posterior tongue
    - Recurrent laryngeal nerve (RLN) conveys general sensation from mucosa below vocal folds and mucosa of esophagus
- Motor (in sequence of events)
  - CN V—trigeminal, mandibular branch
    - Mylohyoid
    - Anterior belly of the digastric muscle
    - Tensor veli palatini
  - CN VII—facial
    - Posterior belly of the digastric muscle
    - Stylohyoid
  - CN IX—glossopharyngeal
    - Stylopharyngeus
  - CN X—vagus
    - Levator veli palatini
    - Palatoglossus
    - Palatopharyngeus and salpingopharyngeus
    - Laryngeal muscles that close the larynx
    - Pharyngeal constrictor muscles
  - CN XII—hypoglossal
    - Controls the intrinsic muscles of the tongue and the hyoglossus and styloglossus that underlie tongue base retraction

- C1 spinal nerve (branches that travel with CN XII)
  - Geniohyoid
  - Thyrohyoid
- C2–C4 (ansa cervicalis)
  - Omohyoid
  - Sternohyoid
  - Sternothyroid

## Esophageal Phase

- CN X provides the parasympathetic innervation to the whole esophagus
  - Pharyngeal branches innervate the pharyngoesophageal segment
  - Recurrent laryngeal nerves innervate the cervical part
  - Upper thoracic esophagus is innervated by recurrent laryngeal nerves and the primary branches of the vagus nerve

## Brainstem Swallowing Center

- The brainstem has primitive control of coordination of sequential muscle activity
- The brainstem swallowing center is in the medulla
- The swallowing center initiates and coordinates the muscles involved in swallowing
- Neurons in the brainstem involved in swallowing are within and around the NTS and in and around the Nucleus Ambiguus (NA)
- Swallowing control is bilateral
- Stimulation of motor nuclei in the brainstem only, stimulates muscle contraction and does not initiate the swallowing sequence
- The interneurons of the brainstem are essential to the coordination of pharyngeal and esophageal muscle activity

## Central Organization of Swallowing

- Three regions of the cortex are important to chewing and swallowing:

  1. Premotor cortex
  2. Precentral gyrus (i.e., primary motor cortex)
  3. Anterior insula

- The inferior and posterior regions of the primary motor cortex and regions of the supplementary cortex must remain intact for normal swallowing
- The lower precentral and posterior inferior frontal gyri are involved in the oral phase of swallowing
- The anterior inferior and middle frontal gyri are involved in the pharyngeal and esophageal phases of swallowing
- Individuals show hemispheric dominance for swallowing; as with language, most are left hemisphere dominant for initiating swallowing

# References

[1] Matsuo K, Palmer JB. Anatomy and physiology of feeding and swallowing: normal and abnormal. *Phys Med Rehabil Clin N Am* 2008;*19*(4):691–707, vii

[2] Hiiemae KM, Palmer JB. Food transport and bolus formation during complete feeding sequences on foods of different initial consistency. *Dysphagia* 1999;*14*(1):31–42

[3] Wolff PH. The serial organization of sucking in the young infant. *Pediatrics* 1968;*42*(6):943–956

[4] Morris SE, Klein MD. *Normal development of feeding skills.* In: Morris SE, Klein MD, eds. Pre-feeding Skills, Second Edition: A Comprehensive Resource for Mealtime Development. Austin, TX: Pro-Ed; 2000:59–95

[5] Colley JR, Creamer B. Sucking and swallowing in infants. *BMJ* 1958;*2*(5093):422–423

[6] Gewolb IH, Bosma JF, Reynolds EW, Vice FL. Integration of suck and swallow rhythms during feeding in preterm infants with and without bronchopulmonary dysplasia. *Dev Med Child Neurol* 2003;*45*(5):344–348

[7] Lau C, Alagugurusamy R, Schanler RJ, Smith EO, Shulman RJ. Characterization of the developmental stages of sucking in preterm infants during bottle feeding. *Acta Paediatr* 2000;*89*(7):846–852

[8] Lau C, Hurst N. Oral feeding in infants. *Curr Probl Pediatr* 1999;*29*(4):105–124

[9] Medoff-Cooper B, Bilker WB, Kaplan JM. Suckling behavior as a function of gestational age: A cross-sectional study. *Infant Behav Dev* 2001;*24*(1):83–94

[10] Steeve RW, Moore CA, Green JR, Reilly KJ, Ruark McMurtrey J. Babbling, chewing, and sucking: oromandibular coordination at 9 months. *J Speech Lang Hear Res* 2008;*51*(6):1390–1404

[11] Evans SM, Klein MD. *Pre-feeding Skills, Second Edition: A Comprehensive Resource for Mealtime Development.* Austin, TX: Pro-Ed; 2000

[12] Gisel EG. Effect of food texture on the development of chewing of children between six months and two years of age. *Dev Med Child Neurol* 1991;*33*(1):69–79

[13] Hall KD. *Core Knowledge: Pediatric Dysphagia Resource Guide.* Stamford, CT: Cengage Learning; 2000:1–40

[14] Ventura AK, Mennella JA. Innate and learned preferences for sweet taste during childhood. *Curr Opin Clin Nutr Metab Care* 2011;*14*(4):379–384

[15] Steiner JE. The gustofacial response: observation on normal and anencephalic newborn infants. *Symp Oral Sens Percept* 1973; (4):254–278

[16] Mason SJ, Harris G, Blissett J. Tube feeding in infancy: implications for the development of normal eating and drinking skills. *Dysphagia* 2005;*20*(1):46–61

[17] Dovey TM, Staples PA, Gibson EL, Halford JC. Food neophobia and 'picky/fussy' eating in children: a review. *Appetite* 2008;*50*(2-3):181–193

[18] Nicklaus S. Development of food variety in children. *Appetite* 2009;*52*(1):253–255

[19] Arvedson JC, Brodsky L. *Anatomy, embryology, physiology, and normal development.* In: Arvedson JC, Brodsky L, eds. Pediatric Swallowing and Feeding: Assessment and Management. 2nd ed. Albany, NY: Singular Thomson Learning; 2002:13–79

[20] Lumb BM, Lovick TA. The rostral hypothalamus: an area for the integration of autonomic and sensory responsiveness. *J Neurophysiol* 1993;*70*(4):1570–1577

[21] Palmer PM, Jaffe DM, McCulloch TM, Finnegan EM, Van Daele DJ, Luschei ES. Quantitative contributions of the muscles of the tongue, floor-of-mouth, jaw, and velum to tongue-to-palate pressure generation. *J Speech Lang Hear Res* 2008;*51*(4):828–835

[22] Felton SM, Gaige TA, Reese TG, Wedeen VJ, Gilbert RJ. Mechanical basis for lingual deformation during the propulsive phase of swallowing as determined by phase-contrast magnetic resonance imaging. *J Appl Physiol (1985)* 2007;*103*(1):255–265

[23] Hiiemae KM, Palmer JB. Tongue movements in feeding and speech. *Crit Rev Oral Biol Med* 2003;*14*(6):413–429

[24] Bosma JF. Human infant oral function. In: Symposium on Oral Sensation and Perception. Springfield, IL: Charles C Thomas; 1967:98–110

[25] Bosma JF, Hepburn LG, Josell SD, Baker K. Ultrasound demonstration of tongue motions during suckle feeding. *Dev Med Child Neurol* 1990;*32*(3):223–229

[26] Bhatnagar SC. *Axial-Limbic Brain: Autonomic Nervous System, Limbic System, Hypothalamus, & Reticular Formation Neuroscience for the Study of Communicative Disorders.* 3th ed. Philadelphia, PA: Wolters Kluwer Lippincott Williams & Wilkins; 2008:353–398

[27] Martin-Harris B, McFarland D, Hill EG, et al. Respiratory-swallow training in patients with head and neck cancer. *Arch Phys Med Rehabil* 2015;*96*(5):885–893

[28] Tran TTA, Martin-Harris B, Pearson WG. Improvements from post respiratory-swallow phase training visualized in patient specific computational analysis of swallowing mechanics. *Comput Methods Biomech Biomed Eng Imaging Vis* 2016.

[29] Negus VE. The second stage of swallowing: simple mechanism of swallowing. *Acta Otolaryngol* 1948;*36*(1):78–82

[30] Thach BT, Menon A. Pulmonary protective mechanisms in human infants. *Am Rev Respir Dis* 1985;*131*(5, S5):S55–S58

[31] Wilson SL, Thach BT, Brouillette RT, Abu-Osba YK. Coordination of breathing and swallowing in human infants. *J Appl Physiol* 1981;*50*(4):851–858

[32] Bu'Lock F, Woolridge MW, Baum JD. Development of co-ordination of sucking, swallowing and breathing: ultrasound study of term and preterm infants. *Dev Med Child Neurol* 1990;*32*(8):669–678

[33] Kelly BN, Huckabee ML, Jones RD, Frampton CM. The first year of human life: coordinating respiration and nutritive swallowing. *Dysphagia* 2007;*22*(1):37–43

[34] Bamford O, Taciak V, Gewolb IH. The relationship between rhythmic swallowing and breathing during suckle feeding in term neonates. *Pediatr Res* 1992;*31*(6):619–624

[35] Koenig JS, Davies AM, Thach BT. Coordination of breathing, sucking, and swallowing during bottle feedings in human infants. *J Appl Physiol (1985)* 1990;*69*(5):1623–1629

[36] Hanlon MB, Tripp JH, Ellis RE, Flack FC, Selley WG, Shoesmith HJ. Deglutition apnoea as indicator of maturation of suckle feeding in bottle-fed preterm infants. *Dev Med Child Neurol* 1997;*39*(8):534–542

[37] Gewolb IH, Vice FL. Maturational changes in the rhythms, patterning, and coordination of respiration and swallow during feeding in preterm and term infants. *Dev Med Child Neurol* 2006;*48*(7):589–594

[38] McConnel FM. Analysis of pressure generation and bolus transit during pharyngeal swallowing. *Laryngoscope* 1988;*98*(1):71–78

[39] Kahrilas PJ, Dodds WJ, Dent J, Logemann JA, Shaker R. Upper esophageal sphincter function during deglutition. *Gastroenterology* 1988;*95*(1):52–62

[40] Sivarao DV, Goyal RK. Functional anatomy and physiology of the upper esophageal sphincter. *Am J Med* 2000;*108*(Suppl 4a):27S–37S

[41] Dantas RO, Cook IJ, Dodds WJ, Kern MK, Lang IM, Brasseur JG. Biomechanics of cricopharyngeal bars. *Gastroenterology* 1990;*99*(5):1269–1274

[42] Kogo M, Hamaguchi M, Matsuya T. Observation of velopharyngeal closure patterns following isolated stimulation of levator veli palatini and pharyngeal constrictor muscles. *Cleft Palate Craniofac J* 1996;*33*(4):273–276

[43] Mu L, Sanders I. Sensory nerve supply of the human oro- and laryngopharynx: a preliminary study. *Anat Rec* 2000;*258*(4):406–420

[44] Pearson WG, Taylor BK, Blair J, Martin-Harris B. Computational analysis of swallowing mechanics underlying impaired epiglottic inversion. *Laryngoscope* 201 6;*126*(8):1854–1858

[45] Langmore SE. *Endoscopic evaluation of oral and pharyngeal phases of swallowing.* GI Motility Online 2006

[46] Kahrilas PJ, Logemann JA, Lin S, Ergun GA. Pharyngeal clearance during swallowing: a combined manometric and videofluoroscopic study. *Gastroenterology* 1992;*103*(1):128–136

[47] Pearson WG Jr, Langmore SE, Yu LB, Zumwalt AC. Structural analysis of muscles elevating the hyolaryngeal complex. *Dysphagia* 2012;*27*(4):445–451

[48] Mu L, Sanders I. Neuromuscular specializations within human pharyngeal constrictor muscles. *Ann Otol Rhinol Laryngol* 2007;*116*(8):604–617

[49] Carnaby-Mann G, Crary MA, Schmalfuss I, Amdur R. "Pharyngocise": randomized controlled trial of preventative exercises to maintain muscle structure and swallowing function during head-and-neck chemoradiotherapy. *Int J Radiat Oncol Biol Phys* 2012;*83*(1):210–219

[50] Martin-Harris B, Brodsky MB, Michel Y, Ford CL, Walters B, Heffner J. Breathing and swallowing dynamics across the adult lifespan. *Arch Otolaryngol Head Neck Surg* 2005;*131*(9):762–770

[51] Newman LA, Cleveland RH, Blickman JG, Hillman RE, Jaramillo D. Videofluoroscopic analysis of the infant swallow. *Invest Radiol* 1991;*26*(10):870–873

[52] Rommel N. *Diagnosis of Oropharyngeal Disorders in Young Children: New Insights and Assessment with Manofluoroscopy.* Leuven, Belgium: University of Leuven; 2002

[53] Gosa MM, Suiter DM, Kahane JC. Videofluoroscopic analysis to determine the effects of thickened liquids on oropharyngeal swallowing function in infants with respiratory compromise. Oral Research Presentation presented at 22 Annual Dysphagia Research Society Meeting; March, 2014; Nashville, TN

[54] Kahane JC. Postnatal development and aging of the human larynx. *Semin Speech Lang* 1983:189–203

[55] Soloff H. The epiglottis in infants and adults: A study of linear measurements and the relationship between measurements in infant and adult groups. 1984.

[56] Sapienza CM, Ruddy BH, Baker S. Laryngeal structure and function in the pediatric larynx: clinical applications. *Lang Speech Hear Serv Sch* 2004;*35*(4):299–307

[57] Kendall KA, Leonard RJ, McKenzie SW. Sequence variability during hypopharyngeal bolus transit. *Dysphagia* 2003;*18*(2):85–91

[58] Eisenhuber E, Schima W, Schober E, et al. Videofluoroscopic assessment of patients with dysphagia: pharyngeal retention is a predictive factor for aspiration. *AJR Am J Roentgenol* 2002;*178*(2):393–398

[59] Ardran GM, Kemp FH. The mechanism of the larynx. II. The epiglottis and closure of the larynx. *Br J Radiol* 1967;*40*(473):372–389

[60] Jean A. Brain stem control of swallowing: neuronal network and cellular mechanisms. *Physiol Rev* 2001;*81*(2):929–969

[61] Mistry S, Hamdy S. Neural control of feeding and swallowing. *Phys Med Rehabil Clin N Am* 2008;*19*(4):709–728, vii–viii

[62] Miller AJ. Deglutition. *Physiol Rev* 1982;*62*(1):129–184

[63] Miller AJ. The neurobiology of swallowing and dysphagia. *Dev Disabil Res Rev* 2008;*14*(2):77–86

[64] Miller AJ. The search for the central swallowing pathway: the quest for clarity. *Dysphagia* 1993;*8*(3):185–194

[65] Steele CM, Miller AJ. Sensory input pathways and mechanisms in swallowing: a review. *Dysphagia* 2010;*25*(4):323–333

# 4 Adult Swallow Screening and Clinical Swallow Evaluation

*Debra M. Suiter and Heather L. Warner*

## Summary

The literature provides a plethora of swallow-screening options. The discerning clinician must make an informed decision about what screen is desired for use. Considerations are multifactorial. The clinician must first consider the quality of the research, ensuring adequate statistical evidence for clinical use, and methodology that is well substantiated by evidence from the literature. Other factors that must be taken into account include ease of administration, time of administration, and any necessary equipment to carry out the screen. The screen should provide the clinician with a clear pass/fail choice and explicitly state what action should be taken after completion of the screen.

The clinician should be cognizant that, as with any swallow test, a swallow screen provides only a snapshot-in-time of a patient's swallowing abilities and cannot guarantee continued swallowing success in the future. This is an inherent limitation of any swallow screen or dysphagia evaluation. Therefore, clinicians and caregivers must remain vigilant to signs of aspiration risk (e.g., coughing at mealtimes, febrile status, or signs/symptoms of upper respiratory infection), and use this information to recommend a formal swallowing evaluation.

## Keywords

deglutition, screening, evaluation, sensitivity, specificity, aspiration

---

### Learning Objectives

- Explain the difference between a swallow screening and a clinical swallow evaluation.
- Discuss the 3-ounce water swallow test and evidence supporting its use as a swallow screening tool.
- List at least three indications for a clinical swallow evaluation.
- Explain information that can be gathered during the chart review, case history, cognitive-linguistic assessment and oral mechanism examination and how this information contributes to the clinical swallow evaluation.
- Describe what clinicians should observe during the bolus administration portion of the clinical swallow evaluation.

---

## 4.1 Introduction

Accurate assessment of individuals with aspiration due to oropharyngeal dysphagia is critically important. Unrecognized dysphagia can lead to serious health consequences for our patients, including dehydration, malnutrition, aspiration pneumonia, and even death. The first steps toward making an accurate assessment of oropharyngeal dysphagia are noninstrumental tools, namely screening and the clinical swallow evaluation. Screening is a pass/fail process in which the clinician determines whether the patient is at risk for aspiration. If passed, no further intervention is recommended. If failed, however, further assessment, such as a clinical swallow evaluation or instrumental assessment, is necessary. The clinical swallow assessment provides the clinician with additional information about the patient, including the feasibility of taking an oral diet safely, treatment options, and whether the patient will be able to participate in an instrumental swallow evaluation. This chapter discusses the purposes of swallow screening and the clinical swallow evaluation and describes the specific information that can be gleaned from each.

## 4.2 Purpose of Screening

Accurate and timely evaluation of swallowing and aspiration risk is necessary to determine how to safely administer medications, maintain adequate nutrition and hydration for healing, and avoid deleterious sequelae of dysphagia, specifically aspiration pneumonia. It is widely accepted that the gold standards for instrumental dysphagia evaluation are videofluoroscopic swallow study (VFSS) and fiberoptic endoscopic evaluation of swallowing (FEES). However, it is not feasible to complete instrumental assessment with every patient who is at risk for aspiration. Although these tests have become more widely available, not all facilities have access to equipment and staffing needed to carry them out. Instrumental testing, while often necessary, is both time consuming and costly, and as a result, it is not prudent to expect that each patient with suspected dysphagia undergo an instrumental assessment. Therefore, noninstrumental swallowing screening for potential aspiration risk is a critical component of dysphagia management.

Swallow screening can help speech-language pathologists (SLPs) identify patients who are at risk for aspiration and in need of additional dysphagia assessment as well as patients who are at minimal risk for aspiration. Additionally, in the case of the 3-ounce water swallow screen, screening can also determine whether a patient is able to resume oral intake. If a patient passes the 3-ounce water swallow screen, a diet can be recommended without the need for additional testing.[1]

Swallow screening can also be used by other health care professionals to assist with appropriate referrals for swallowing assessment. In most institutions, speech-language pathology is a consult service and clinicians do not have independent direct access to each and every patient who could potentially benefit from a swallow screen. Other members of the health care team, specifically registered nurses (RNs), licensed independent practitioners, and physicians, are often responsible for identifying patients who are at risk for potential aspiration. The usual procedure is to rely on some form of screening process to determine the need for a referral. Unfortunately, these screening processes vary widely, are not standardized even within the same institution, and are usually not evidence based and therefore unsubstantiated by the literature.[2] It is critical that discerning clinicians and other health care professionals be aware of the literature available to them prior to choosing a swallowing screen to ensure that the screen has adequate statistical support to justify use.

## 4.3 Swallow Screening versus Swallow Evaluation

Swallow screening is defined by the American Speech-Language-Hearing Association (ASHA) as "a pass/fail procedure to identify individuals who require a comprehensive assessment of swallowing function or a referral for other professional and/or medical services."[3] A swallow screening should be simple, quick, and easy to administer, have defined pass/fail criteria, and accurately determine the presence or absence of aspiration risk. A swallow screening cannot determine pharyngeal and laryngeal anatomy and physiology or bolus flow characteristics; it can determine only the presence or absence of aspiration *risk*. Ideally, a swallow screening should have defined parameters for pass/fail criteria and should define what action the clinician should take based on the results of the screen.

An effective screen must be defined by more than methodology—it must also be defined statistically. A number of standard statistical measures are prevalent in the swallow screening literature. Sensitivity and specificity are often presented to assist clinicians in making a sound choice for use of a given screen. *Sensitivity* of a particular clinical sign (e.g., cough after swallow) for detecting a sign on criterion measure (aspiration on VFSS) is defined as the proportion of patients who have the sign (aspiration) who also have the clinical sign (cough after swallow). Sensitivity measures a test's ability to identify an individual with the disease as positive. Tests that are found to be highly sensitive indicate that there are few false-negative results; thus fewer cases of disease are missed.[4]

*Specificity* of a particular clinical sign (cough after swallow) is the proportion of patients who do not have the sign on the criterion measure (aspiration on VFSS) who also do not have the clinical sign (cough after swallow). Specificity measures a test's ability to identify an individual without the disease as negative. Tests that are found to be highly specific indicate fewer false-positive results and are able to help "rule in" the diagnosis.[4]

Ideally each screening tool should have equally high sensitivity and specificity, but this is often not the case. In the swallow screening literature, it is often found that screening procedures with higher sensitivities have lower specificities. That is, the screening tools that are successful at identifying those patients with a particular disorder often overidentify patients who do not have the disorder.[5] Although favorable from an identification perspective, the clinical implication of a low specificity is overreferral for further testing, withholding of oral feeds and medications, and unnecessary use of nasogastric feeding tubes.[6] These potential drawbacks must be considered when determining criteria for a statistically sound screening tool, and clinicians must determine their own ethically driven parameters for accuracy.

Although there is no consensus for a defined target parameter for sensitivity, Leder and Espinosa[6] suggested that an effective screening tool should have a sensitivity of 95% or greater. Clinically, this means that one would miss 5% or fewer patients who are aspirating. To give another example, a sensitivity of 85%

means that one could miss up to 15% of patients who are aspirating. It is critical that individuals that are using screening procedures understand the clinical meaning of the reported statistics associated with the screen being used.

## 4.4 Who Should Screen?

SLPs are the primary professionals responsible for swallowing assessment. Many clinicians use screening as part of their assessment process to determine the need for further assessment. In other words, if the patient fails the screen, an instrumental assessment (FEES or VFSS) is completed. Instrumental swallow assessments (VFSS and FEES) allow the SLP to define the anatomy of the swallow and identify characteristics such as bolus flow and swallow physiology. With this information, clinicians can definitively diagnose swallowing disorders as well as trial specific interventions, strategies, and modifications during the assessment. Additionally, with the use of instrumental assessment, dysphagia management is directly dependent upon the information obtained during the swallowing assessment, allowing clinicians to make informed decisions about their goals for intervention and care planning.

It is important to note that referrals from other health care professionals (e.g., nurses, physicians, licensed independent practitioners) often result from some form of screening process. The screen may be based on patient diagnosis, observation at mealtime, food trials, associated clinical signs, or the results of a formal swallow screening protocol. Additionally, RNs often conduct a swallow screening as part of their nursing practice. RNs are a logical first choice to provide assistance in implementing the screening process because they are the professionals who have the most direct, frequent, and continuous contact with patients. The issue remains that many of the screening protocols and criteria used are unsubstantiated by the literature.[2] Warner and colleagues[7] published a study that supports the RN's ability to effectively perform the Yale Swallow Protocol to detect aspiration risk. It is critical that SLPs and other health care professionals who are participating in the screening process use evidence from the literature to guide their practice so as not to leave patients vulnerable to non-evidence-based decision making.

## 4.5 Evidence-Based Screening

Swallow screening is a critical component of dysphagia management, especially in the acutely hospitalized patient. The literature provides a plethora of swallow screening options for the SLP. The discerning clinician, therefore, must make an informed decision about what screen is desired for use. A successful swallow screen should be simple to administer, cross-disciplinary, cost-effective, acceptable to patients, and able to identify the desired target in question.[8] The clinician must first consider the quality of the research, ensuring adequate statistical evidence for clinical use, and methodology that is well substantiated by evidence from the literature. Other factors that must be taken into account include ease of administration, time of administration, and necessary equipment to carry out the screen.

Unfortunately, swallow screening practice varies widely, and much is unsubstantiated by current research. McCullough et al[2] reported that only 56% of methods used for assessment had support from the literature. There is significant variability in the way screenings are conducted. The current literature does not provide a consensus on methodology, stimuli used, criteria for passing/failure, or variables that should be included as part of a screening tool for swallowing.

## 4.6 Critical Caveat: Silent Aspiration

Silent aspiration remains of critical importance in the discussion of swallowing screening. Silent aspiration occurs when material passes below the level of the true vocal folds without overt signs (e.g., coughing or choking) that can be detected solely by observation of the patient without visualization of the aspiration event. By this definition, silent aspiration would be undetected on all screening tools or clinical evaluations of swallowing. Leder et al[6] attributed the unreliability of clinical examinations to the high incidence of silent aspiration (i.e., 28–52% in patients referred for swallow testing). In theory, then, a clinician would have to consider that up to 50% of patients could be potentially missed via silent aspiration by any given screening tool.

In 2011, Leder and colleagues[9] published a study that contributed novel evidence that silent aspiration is volume dependent. In this study ($n$ = 4,102), results of the 3-ounce water swallow challenge were compared to FEES to demonstrate patients who were shown via FEES to be silent aspirators of smaller volumes (up to 5 mL) demonstrated overt signs of aspiration when they subsequently drank larger volumes (3 ounces or 90 mL). This finding helped to elucidate why particular swallowing screens had higher sensitivities and lent significant support for screening tools that include oral trials with larger volumes of liquid intake. Clinicians who are called upon to make an ethical determination about acceptable risk when evaluating swallowing must not only understand the validity of the tests they are using but also possess knowledge of the prevalence and characteristics of silent aspiration.

## 4.7 Screening Measures

Most, but not all, swallow screening tools use some form of a swallowing trial. There is, however, high variability in what boluses are administered. Swallowing trials may take the form of a water swallow test (WST) or a bolus swallow test (BST). WSTs are defined by swallow trials that involve water only and are generally identified using this nomenclature by the authors. BSTs are those that involve administration of multiple and alternative oral consistencies. Some screens are carried out using components of both WSTs and BSTs.

According to the literature, there is high variability in BSTs and WSTs. Volumes administered for the WSTs range from 3 milliliters (mL) to 100 mL with varying increments of 3, 5, 30, 60, 90, and 100 mL. BSTs vary by both consistency and volume. Consistencies offered include thin liquids, thickened liquids, puree, semisolids, and solid consistencies. Volumes of consistencies are also variable. Quantities range from 1 to 60 mL, with reported increments of 1, 3, 5, 10, 20, 50, and 60 mL.

Swallow screening tools often, though not always, include other measures that are purported to predict aspiration risk. Screens can include questionnaires, a medical history, subjective variables, oral mechanism evaluation, and other measures, such as pulse oximetry, and scores from scales such as the National Institutes of Health Stroke Severity Scale (NIHSS). Oral mechanism examination can include assessment of labial and lingual strength and range of motion, dentition status, and palatal range of motion. The category of subjective variables is arguably the most varied, including measures such as gag reflex, voluntary cough, dysphonia, dysarthria, secretion management, orientation, wet vocal quality, and command following.

The matrix of these measures is highly variable across screening tools. Logemann et al[5] used a total of 28 variables on their screening tool, 21 of which fall under the category of efforts not associated with swallowing, with the majority of those being subjective. In contrast, Smith Hammond et al[10] used sophisticated measurements of the voluntary cough alone to predict aspiration risk. Though these examples are outliers in terms of numbers of variables included, they demonstrate the wide range as well as the lack of standardization of the screening tools available to clinicians.

Another factor that should be considered when reviewing the literature on swallow screening is that many of the studies have been conducted using referred samples. This results in an inherent bias in these studies and in the literature because patients who are referred are more likely to screen positive for aspiration risk secondary to the fact that the referral process itself is in place to identify those patients that may require further dysphagia assessment. The factors that prompt a referral are varied and not standardized. Physicians, midlevel providers, and nurses can refer based on a variety of factors, including medical diagnosis or clinical judgment about level of arousal, mental status, observation of any clinical sign (e.g., wet vocal quality, difficulty managing secretions, facial droop), as well as other factors, such as a patient being postextubation. Although there is no official published standard on when a health care practitioner should refer for dysphagia assessment, the fact that the patients have been referred can potentially impact the results of studies with such samples and should be considered when one is reviewing the literature.

## 4.8 Swallow Screening

There is a plethora of swallow screenings presented in the literature. It is beyond the scope of this text to review all available screening options; however, a brief summary highlighting several frequently cited screening tools follows. The discerning clinician must review available information and take into account time and resources needed to administer, methodology of the study, as well as statistical support when determining best practice in swallow screening.

DePippo et al[11] were the first to report data on the 3-ounce WST. They investigated 44 patients with stroke and used VFSS as the measure by which to validate the 3-ounce WST. This screening tool required the patient to demonstrate uninterrupted drinking of 3 ounces of water without overt signs of aspiration. Failure criteria were inability to drink continuously, cough during or up to 1 minute after completion of the test, or a wet/hoarse voice quality postswallow. The authors reported the relationship between cough or wet/hoarse voice on the screen and aspiration on VFSS to have a sensitivity of 76% and specificity of 59%. Sensitivity and specificity of these same signs on the 3-ounce screen were revised to 94% and 26%, respectively, when considering the relationship between these signs and aspiration of greater than 10% of the bolus on VFSS. They went on to report that the relationship between these overt signs on the 3-ounce swallow and aspiration of thickened liquids or solids on VFSS was found to have a sensitivity of 94% and a specificity of 30%.

These data must be interpreted carefully. The sample size must be adequate to answer the question at hand, and statistics must be interpreted with caution. If the patient coughs on the 3-ounce screen, the clinician is most interested in what information this screen provides about overall aspiration risk. Caution must be taken when interpreting statistics of additional conditions reported, because clinical relevance must be determined. The clinician must determine the clinical utility of the information being reported—that is, information about thickened liquids, solids, or volume of aspirated material. The information reported still only leaves the clinician with one clinically relevant conclusion, that with a sensitivity of 76%, the 3-ounce WST will potentially miss 24% of patients who aspirate.

Daniels et al[12] used another form of WST combined with assessment of subjective clinical features to determine whether the screening tool could distinguish patients with mild dysphagia or normal swallowing from those with moderate to severe dysphagia. The screening tool consisted of a WST using 5, 10, and 20 mL volumes. The clinical signs included dysphonia, dysarthria, abnormal volitional cough, abnormal gag, cough following swallow, and voice change following swallow. Results of the screen were compared with VFSS. Subjects included 59 acute stroke patients. Results indicated that the presence of two out of six of these clinical features is able to distinguish dysphagia severity with a sensitivity of 92.3% and a specificity of 66.7%. To clarify, the presence of two out of these six features accurately predicted with 92.3% certainty which patients had moderate to severe dysphagia. It is important to note that, taken individually, the sensitivities and specificities of each of these clinical features were poor (sensitivity range of 30–76% and specificity range of 60–87%). Relative strengths of this screening tool included use of an instrumental assessment (VFSS) to corroborate severity of dysphagia, adequate statistical measurements, and report of both inter- and intrarater reliability. However, there were some methodological concerns, such as the length of time between screen and evaluation as well as a lack of power analysis to determine whether sample size was adequate. Although this is not a criticism of the study itself, clinicians should be cautioned that a sensitivity of 92% means that almost 10% of the time this screening tool is not going to be able to identify someone with a moderate to severe dysphagia.

Leder and Espinosa[6] published a study considering the "two out of six" clinical variables described by Daniels et al.[12] In this study they compared the clinical examination consisting of the same clinical factors: dysphonia, dysarthria, abnormal gag, abnormal volitional cough, cough following swallow, and voice change after swallow with FEES. Bolus trials consisted of single sips of water boluses via a straw. A rating of no aspiration risk was made if zero or one of the clinical identifiers was present, and a rating of aspiration risk was given if two or more of the clinical identifiers

were present. Results indicated that the water swallow screen had a sensitivity of 86% and a specificity of 30%. Leder and Espinosa[6] concluded that this clinical assessment underestimated aspiration risk in patients with aspiration and overestimated aspiration risk in patients who did not exhibit aspiration.

The Toronto Bedside Swallowing Screening Test (TOR-BSST) is a swallowing screen developed by Martino et al in 2009.[13] This screen was investigated using 311 stroke patients and consists of five items: voice before water swallow, lingual movement, pharyngeal sensation, water swallow, and voice after swallow. This screen was developed from the Kidd WST (50 mL). The exact procedure for the screen is provided to clinicians who attend the training course and become certified to administer the TOR-BSST. In the study, the results of the TOR-BSST were compared with VFSS. Martino et al report a sensitivity of 91.3%. Strengths of this study included reliability data provided and defined parameters for inclusion as well as the use of rating scales, such as the NIHSS, to define the patient population. In assessing results of this study, it is important to note that only 20% of the patients received VFSS for comparison to the TOR-BSST.

In 1999, Logemann et al published findings on a 28-item screening tool.[5] This screening procedure was compared with VFSS and contained screening items over five different categories: medical history, behavioral, gross motor, oral mechanism examination, and swallow trials (1 mL of thin liquid, puree, and one-fourth of a cookie). Ratings for bolus trials were safe and unsafe. Results indicated that the best single predictor of the presence of aspiration was a throat clear or cough during swallowing trials, with a sensitivity of 78% and a specificity of 58%.

Other studies have sought to use a single measure to detect aspiration. Ramsey et al[14] examined the utility of pulse oximetry to detect aspiration risk in 189 patients with stroke. The authors conducted what was described as a modified bedside swallow assessment (mBSA). Simultaneous VFSS and pulse oximetry was completed, and 5 and 75 mL of contrast were administered. Findings indicated a poor association between oxygen desaturation and aspiration status. Using VFSS as the criterion standard, sensitivity and specificity for detecting aspiration were 47% and 72%, respectively for mBSA, 33% and 62% for desaturation greater than 2%, and 13% and 95% for desaturation greater than 5%. Based on results of this study, we can conclude that pulse oximetry is not a good screening measure or indicator of aspiration risk.

In 2008, building on DePippo's prior research, Suiter and Leder published data on use of the 3-ounce WST in 3,000 hospitalized patients. Because of the limited of sample size in previous studies by DePippo, the goal of this study was to determine whether the 3-ounce WST could be generalized to a larger and more heterogeneous patient population. Additionally, they sought to determine whether recommendations for an oral diet could be made based on the result of the screen—a critical component of the literature that was also not addressed in prior studies. FEES was the reference test against which results of the 3-ounce water test were compared. Each participant first completed an FEES followed by administration of the 3-ounce WST. Participants were acutely hospitalized patients from 14 different diagnostic categories. Criteria for passing and failure were the same as in earlier studies; that is, the patient had to drink 3 ounces of water uninterrupted and without overt signs or symptoms of aspiration. Criteria for failure of the test included inability to drink the entire amount without stopping and/or coughing or choking during or immediately after completion. Findings were favorable and in support of generalization of the use of the 3-ounce water swallow screen in a heterogeneous population with a sensitivity for predicting aspiration of 96.5% and specificity of 48.7%. The 3-ounce WST was found to be an excellent predictor of aspiration risk in a heterogeneous population, potentially missing only 3.5% of patients.

As discussed by Suiter and Leder, the 3-ounce WST does not meet the strict criteria of an efficient screening tool because it does not have both high sensitivity and high specificity. The result of low specificity indicates that patients will be overreferred for further testing. That is, it unnecessarily restricts liquid intake for nearly half the people tested. Furthermore, approximately 70% of the individuals who failed the 3-ounce water test went on to tolerate some form of oral intake successfully based on FEES results.

Suiter and Leder[1] reported results for the test as a whole as well as statistics on each of the 14 diagnostic categories. Given the large sample size, each diagnostic category had meaningful statistical measures to guide clinicians on use of this screening tool in specific populations. The second question that Suiter and Leder[1] answered is of critical importance in clinical practice: What clinical information does one receive from the passing of a 3-ounce water swallow challenge? Based on the results of this study, clinicians can confidently recommend an oral diet based on the 3-ounce WST alone without the need for additional assessment. Statistical support indicates that sensitivity of the 3-ounce test for identifying individuals deemed safe for oral intake based on FEES is 96.4% and specificity is 46.4%. This study was the first published to provide information about diet recommendations that can be made based on the results of the 3-ounce WST. Importantly, this not only allows patients to resume earlier oral intake but also eliminates the need to use thickened liquids and reduces the potential risk associated with tube feeding while they await further assessment.

Although this study was largely methodologically sound and undoubtedly made significant contributions to the literature on swallowing screening, it came under criticism for lacking adequate reliability and rater blinding data. Several follow-up studies addressed these issues in the context of additional poststudy, blinded FEES testing resulting in 100% identification for tracheal aspiration,[15,16] and via a recent prospective double-blinded videofluoroscopic study confirmed the clinical usefulness and validity of the 3-ounce challenge for determining aspiration risk.[17]

There were several follow-up studies involving the 3-ounce water swallow screen. In 2009, Leder et al[18] published a study that supported the use of a brief cognitive screen in conjunction with assessment of swallowing. It was reported that the odds of liquid aspiration were 31% greater for patients not oriented to person, place, and time. Additionally, for patients who were unable to follow one-step commands, the odds of liquid aspiration, puree aspiration, and being deemed nil for oral diet were 57, 48, and 69% greater, respectively, than for patients who were able to do so. In 2011 and again in 2012, Leder and colleagues[19,20] reported more substantial evidence about diet recommendations based on the 3-ounce water swallow challenge. These studies, Leder et al 2011 (with $n = 75$ stroke patients)[19] and Leder et al 2012 ($n = 493$ intensive care and step-down unit patients),[20] investigated patients' ability to tolerate a recommended oral diet 24 hours following passing the 3-ounce water swallow screen. Results

indicated that diet recommendations were followed, and patients were tolerating recommended diets without overt signs or symptoms of aspiration with 100% success after 24 hours. A comparison study similarly supported the use of the 3-ounce swallow screen for making diet recommendations in 1,000 general hospitalized patients,[20] thereby expanding the use of this swallow screen protocol to virtually all hospitalized patients. An additional study indicated that the 3-ounce WST can be successfully used in the pediatric population with a sensitivity and specificity of predicting aspiration during FEES of 100% and 51.2%, respectfully.

The combined results of this series of studies on the 3-ounce water swallow screen offer compelling evidence in support of widespread use of this water swallow screening tool for detecting aspiration risk in the vast majority of hospitalized patients (**Table 4.1**).[21] The 3-ounce water swallow challenge protocol not only has one of the highest sensitivities reported; it is also validated against the criterion standards of FEES and VFSS and incorporates a large and heterogeneous population sample ($n = 3,000$) that far exceeds the breadth of subjects examined in previous studies. Perhaps most importantly, there is strong evidence that if a patient passes the 3-ounce screen, the clinician can confidently recommend an oral diet without need for further testing. These data support a significant shift in the way clinicians have used screening tools in the past. When taken collectively, there is significant empirical evidence supporting widespread use of this screening protocol.

**Table 4.1** Summary of the Yale Swallow Protocol

| Procedure | 1. Sit patient upright.<br>2. Ask patient to drink entire 3 oz. (90 mL) of water from a cup or through a straw in sequential swallows without stopping.<br>3. Assess patient for coughing, choking, or throat clearing during swallowing and immediately after drinking. |
|---|---|
| Criteria for Pass/Fail | Pass: Ability to drink 3 ounces of water sequentially without overt signs/symptoms of aspiration.<br>Fail: Inability to drink the entire amount sequentially or demonstration of coughing or choking during trial. |
| Interpretation: Pass | If patient passes and medically indicated, a diet can be ordered.<br>If patient is dentate (with teeth), order a modified or regular diet.<br>If patient is edentulous (without teeth), order a liquid and puree diet.<br>SLP can complete solid trials, or RN can consult speech-language pathologist to assist with diet recommendations if unclear secondary to oral mechanism findings. |
| Interpretation: Fail | If patient fails, keep nothing by mouth.<br>Instrumental dysphagia assessment (VFSS or FEES) required.<br>If patient improves clinically, may rescreen within 24 hours prior to placing consult for instrumental evaluation. |
| Defer screening if the following present | Patient is unable to remain alert for testing.<br>Existing percutaneous endoscopic gastrostomy (PEG) or abdominal feeding tube.<br>Head of bed restricted to less than 30 degrees.<br>Currently eating modified diet secondary to dysphagia.<br>Patient has a tracheotomy tube.<br>Nothing by mouth order per doctor. |

## 4.9 Clinical Swallow Evaluation

### Purpose

A clinical swallow evaluation (CSE), sometimes referred to as the bedside swallow evaluation, is often the first step in the assessment of an individual who is deemed to be at risk for dysphagia. According to ASHA,[22] the CSE allows the SLP to do as follows:

- Integrate information from interview/case history, review medical records, observations from physical exam
- Observe and assess integrity and function of structures of the upper airway and digestive tract
- Identify presence and observe the characteristics of a dysphagia based on clinical signs and symptoms
- Identify clinical signs/symptoms of esophageal dysphagia or gastroesophageal reflux
- Determine need for instrumental exam
- Determine whether patient is appropriate candidate for treatment and/or management
- Recommend route of nutritional management
- Recommend clinical interventions

The remainder of this chapter focuses on indications for a CSE, the suggested components of a CSE, the strengths and limitations of the CSE.

## 4.10 Indications for a Clinical Swallow Evaluation

Referral for a CSE may be based on a number of factors, including patient admitting diagnosis, physician concern regarding patient nutritional status, or patient complaints. When an SLP receives a referral for a CSE, it is important to understand what prompted the referral and what the referring provider's primary concern is regarding the patient.

Providers may make a referral for CSE based upon the patient's medical diagnosis. Medical diagnoses that are frequently associated with increased risk of oropharyngeal dysphagia include stroke;[23] neurodegenerative disease, such as Parkinson's disease,[24] amyotrophic lateral sclerosis,[24] or dementia;[25] and head and neck cancers.[26] Many medical facilities implement a policy whereby individuals with particular diagnoses, such as stroke, are automatically referred to speech-language pathology for a CSE.

In addition to medical diagnosis, physicians also consider the patient's nutritional status when deciding to recommend a CSE. Individuals who present with recent unintentional weight loss may be experiencing swallowing difficulty that leads them to avoid eating particular foods or drinking certain liquids. Avoidance of liquids can also result in dehydration, and patients who present with dehydration may thus be referred for a CSE.

Finally, it is often the patient's complaints that will prompt the physician to refer to a SLP for a CSE. Patients may complain of frequent coughing or choking during meals; feeling as if food or liquid gets stuck when they attempt to swallow; or prolonged meal times. They may also complain of pain associated with swallowing, odynophagia, or food or liquid coming out of their nose when they attempt to swallow. Any of these complaints may indicate an underlying swallowing problem and should result in referral for a CSE.

## 4.11 Components of the Clinical Swallow Evaluation

### 4.11.1 Chart Review

The first step in the evaluation actually takes place before the clinician meets the patient face to face. A thorough chart review will allow the SLP to obtain information that will aid in determining whether the patient is medically ready and appropriate for a swallow evaluation and assist the clinician in formulating a hypothesis regarding the nature of the patient's swallowing difficulty.

Typically, the chart review begins with a review of the patient's current and past medical history. We want to know who referred the patient. Was it a physician? Did the nurse or another health care professional have concerns regarding the patient's swallow safety? We also want to know what prompted the referral. Was the referral based on a patient failing a previously completed swallow screen? Did the patient or patient's family report issues swallowing? Does the patient's current diagnosis indicate an increased risk for dysphagia?

After reviewing the referral information, the next step is to review information regarding the patient's medical history. Often, a history and physical are available for review in the chart. These usually include information regarding the patient's admitting diagnosis (if the patient is an inpatient) and previous medical history. It is important to note any information in the patient's medical history that would indicate that the individual is at risk for dysphagia. This information may include a history of neurological disease, such as Parkinson's disease or amyotrophic lateral sclerosis, head and neck cancer, chronic obstructive pulmonary disease, or gastroesophageal reflux. If the patient has a history of frequent upper respiratory illness, the clinician should consider the possibility that this is related to chronic aspiration. McCullough and colleagues[27] found that presence of pneumonia or a history of pneumonia was highly predictive of aspiration risk. It is also important to review the patient's surgical history. Specifically, the SLP should pay particular attention to whether the patient has had any previous surgery to the head and neck, including tracheostomy placement or surgical resection of head and neck cancer. Surgeries can result in anatomical alterations that may, in turn, lead to changes in swallow physiology. A previous history of feeding tube placement may indicate a history of dysphagia or malnutrition.

In addition to the history and physical, it is important to review any imaging, such as chest X-rays, computed tomographic scans, or magnetic resonance imaging scans. Chest X-rays may reveal evidence of acute or chronic lung infection, which may be due to aspiration. The radiologist may note in the chest X-ray report the presence of infiltrates, foreign material in the lungs that should not be there. The location of infiltrates in the lungs depends on the patient's position, and aspiration can occur into any part of the lung, depending on the patient's position when aspiration occurs.

Patients who aspirate while in the recumbent positon will most commonly have infiltrates in the posterior segments of the upper lobes and the apical segments of the lower lobes.[28] Patients who aspirate when they are in an upright or semirecumbent position, are more likely to have infiltrates in the basal segments of the lower lobes.[28]

Results of neuroimaging, such as CT scans or MRI scans of the brain, can help the clinician formulate hypotheses regarding the nature of the patient's dysphagia. For instance, patients with right hemisphere stroke demonstrate different patterns of dysphagia than patients with left hemisphere stroke.[29,30,31,32] Specifically, patients with right hemisphere stroke have a higher incidence of dysphagia,[33] are more likely to demonstrate pharyngeal phase (vs. oral phase) dysphagia,[29,30] are more likely to aspirate, and have more severely impaired swallow function than patients with left hemisphere stroke.[32]

The chart review should also include a perusal of the patient's current medications and current lab values. Certain medications can adversely affect swallow function, either as a normal side effect of the drug or as a complication of the therapeutic action of the drug.[34,35] Medications that affect smooth or striated esophageal muscle function may cause dysphagia. Other medications may cause xerostomia (dry mouth) and interfere with oral transit of the bolus. Antipsychotic medications may cause involuntary movements of the face and tongue (tardive dyskinesia). Dysphagia resulting from a complication of the therapeutic action of a medication includes viral or fungal esophagitis in patients treated with immunosuppressive drugs or cancer therapeutic agents, or medications that can depress the central nervous system, such as benzodiazepines. Additionally, some medications, such as nonsteroidal anti-inflammatory drugs, can cause esophageal injury if they remain in the esophagus for a prolonged period of time.

A review of the patient's laboratory values can provide information regarding the patient's overall medical status and can reflect consequences of dysphagia. For instance, elevated white blood cell count indicates an active infectious process and may indicate presence of a bacterial infection, including aspiration pneumonia. Elevated blood urea nitrogen, albumin, or creatinine levels can be indicative of dehydration, whereas decreased albumin or blood urea nitrogen levels can be indicative of malnutrition.

Nurses' notes can provide valuable information to the SLP. If a patient is on an oral diet, nurses' notes will include information regarding the amount of intake. Decreased oral intake may indicate the patient is having difficulty swallowing. Nurses tend to spend the most one-on-one time with patients, and they are often the first to notice a patient is struggling to tolerate an oral diet or medications. Nurses are often the professionals who request a physician referral to the SLP for a dysphagia assessment. McCullough and colleagues determined that nurse report of a patient being at risk for dysphagia was highly predictive of aspiration noted during subsequent instrumental assessment of swallowing.[26]

Finally, the clinician may also wish to review the patient's advanced directives or living will if the patient has one. Enteral nutrition, or tube feeding, is considered to be a life-sustaining measure, and patients may indicate in their living will if they are willing to accept enteral nutrition and, if so, under what circumstances. This information, if known prior to the physical examination of swallow function, can cue the clinician as to what treatment options are available for the patient. If the patient does not wish to accept enteral nutrition under any circumstances, that information may be used to guide decision making regarding the need for instrumental assessment.

## 4.11.2 Case History

Following the chart review, the SLP should conduct a thorough case history. This can be obtained from the patient or other individuals, such as family members, significant others, or health care workers who have had the opportunity to observe and interact with the patient during attempts at oral feeding. Case history questions should be conducted using open-ended questions to avoid planting thoughts or suggestions the patient might not otherwise have regarding his or her current status. One of the purposes of the case history is to help the clinician formulate a hypothesis regarding what is wrong with the patient's swallow function. Is this is an oral phase issue or a pharyngeal phase issue? Is the patient describing symptoms more consistent with an esophageal dysphagia? The information gathered during the case history can be invaluable in determining the appropriate means of assessing swallowing function (e.g., fluoroscopy or endoscopy), and in determining whether other professionals (e.g., a gastroenterologist or a neurologist) should be consulted.

### Chief Complaint

Generally the first question to ask is what the patient's chief complaint is. Common complaints include coughing, choking or strangling with food or liquids, food or liquids sticking in the throat, difficulty chewing, or prolonged mealtimes. Patients may complain they feel as if they have a lump in their throat that never goes away, and they feel the need to swallow frequently. This is known as a globus sensation. Sometimes, patients will indicate that they have difficulty swallowing a particular food or liquid. Difficulty swallowing dry, crumbly foods, such as cornbread or tortilla chips, is a common complaint and may indicate difficulty with lingual control of the bolus or pharyngeal clearance. Patients may complain of difficulty swallowing liquids only. In this case, it is important to note whether there are specific liquids that are more difficult to swallow than others and whether the temperature of the liquid affects swallowing. Consumption of either very hot or very cold liquids can trigger esophageal spasms for some individuals. Knowing which foods or liquids are problematic for the patient can assist the clinician in forming a hypothesis regarding whether dysphagia is likely related to an oral phase or a pharyngeal phase issue. Additionally, patient complaints of feeling as if food sticks, difficulty swallowing solid foods (often breads or steak), or difficulty swallowing liquids of extreme temperatures (either hot or cold) only, may indicate an esophageal phase issue rather than an oropharyngeal swallowing difficulty.[36]

### History of Symptoms

Clinicians should also ask patients about the timeline of their dysphagia. How long have dysphagia symptoms been present? Did the patient experience any illness at the time dysphagia symptoms began? Do they vary depending upon time of day?

Were there other changes, such as alterations in vocal quality or speech intelligibility that accompanied onset of dysphagia? Have symptoms been stable, or have they gotten progressively better or worse? Knowing how long dysphagia symptoms have been present, the stability of the symptoms, and accompanying symptoms can point to the underlying etiology of swallowing difficulty and indicate the need for referral to other professionals, such as otolaryngologists or neurologists. Changes in vocal quality that accompany onset of dysphagia can point to vocal fold pathology related to reflux or perhaps to problems with vocal fold movement, including vocal fold paralysis or paresis.

## Meal Length

Another question to pose is how long it is taking the patient to consume a meal. Prolonged mealtimes are often an issue for individuals with degenerative neurological diseases such as amyotrophic lateral sclerosis or Parkinson's disease. Patients may report that they discontinue eating because they are the last to finish their meal and do not wish to eat alone or have those dining with them wait on them to finish. Food or liquid that has sat for a prolonged period of time may no longer be palatable to the patient because of changes in temperature or taste. This can result in a decreased amount of oral intake and subsequent weight loss. Additionally, prolonged mealtimes can result in fatigue, which may place patients at increased risk of swallowing difficulty.

## Patient Awareness

In some cases, patients may not be aware of their swallowing difficulty. Patient awareness may vary as a function of the underlying etiology of their dysphagia. For instance, when surveyed, only one-third of individuals with Parkinson's disease reported symptoms of dysphagia. However, up to 80% of individuals with Parkinson's disease actually present with dysphagia.[37] Additionally, individuals with dysphagia subsequent to head and neck cancer and dysphagia subsequent to stroke have also been found to have poor perceptions of dysphagia symptoms.[38,39,40] Patient awareness or lack thereof of their dysphagia symptoms can provide important information regarding the safety of recommending an oral diet. For instance, individuals who are unaware of food pocketed in the lateral sulci may choke on pocketed material if they fall asleep with it in their mouth. Others who cough frequently when taking thin liquids may continue consuming these liquids despite risks of aspiration and subsequent development of upper respiratory infection. Interviewing the patient's significant others or caregivers who are present during patient meal consumption can provide important information regarding the patient's insight and awareness of signs or symptoms of dysphagia.

## Quality of Life

Clinicians may wish to formally assess the impact of dysphagia on the patient's quality of life. Many social situations and celebrations involve consumption of food and liquid. Inability to participate fully in mealtimes because of swallowing issues, even if they are relatively mild from a physiological perspective, can result in a significant negative impact on an individual's quality of life.[41] There are several standardized assessments of swallowing-related quality of life. These include the SWAL-QOL,

a swallowing-related quality of life assessment, and the SWAL-CARE, a quality of care assessment, both developed by Colleen McHorney and colleagues.[41,42,43] Questions address issues such as social impact, symptom frequency, and swallow-related fear. The Dysphagia Handicap Index[44] is another swallow-related quality of life assessment. It consists of 25 items that are broken down into three subscales: physical, functional, and emotional.

The MD Anderson Dysphagia Inventory (MDADI) is a quality of life assessment tool that focuses specifically on individuals with dysphagia subsequent to head and neck cancer[45] The MDADI consists of 20 questions divided into three subscales: emotional, physical, and functional. Scores on the MDADI have been found to differentiate individuals who aspirate from those who do not as well as individuals who are able to tolerate an oral diet from those who cannot.[46]

## 4.11.3 Cognitive Assessment

Following the chart review and the case history, clinicians may wish to incorporate a cognitive assessment as part of their clinical swallow assessment. Cognitive assessment can be done using the clinician's own, informal assessment and should include questions regarding orientation, command following, attention, and alertness level. Clinicians wishing to use a standardized assessment may use tools such as the Mini-Mental State Exam or the Montreal Cognitive Assessment. Both of these tests are readily accessible and provide valuable information regarding patients' cognitive abilities.

The cognitive examination can provide valuable information regarding the patient's readiness for assessment. For instance, is the patient fully alert and awake? If not, a full assessment (i.e., one that includes bolus presentation) may not be possible at this time, and a nonoral means of nutrition may need to be recommended until mental status improves. Even if the patient is able to wake up sufficiently to participate in the examination, if alertness level waxes and wanes throughout the day, an oral diet may not be a safe option if the patient receives a meal when he or she is not sufficiently awake to attend to each bolus, chew thoroughly, and swallow the bolus in its entirety. When the patient is not easily awakened, clinicians should check with nursing or other staff to determine whether this is the patient's usual state or whether there are other factors involved, such as recent medication administration; other activities, such as dialysis, testing, or other therapies; or other reasons that the patient may be less awake and alert than usual. If the patient is unable to stay awake to participate in an examination, clinicians are advised to postpone the CSE until the alertness level improves.

The clinician also needs to gather information regarding the patient's executive function abilities. Many individuals with traumatic brain injury or other neurologic insult exhibit disorders of executive functioning. The clinician should consider such questions as, Is the patient easily distracted? or able to maintain attention on the task? Is the patient able to initiate actions? or is prompting required? Does the patient exhibit impulsive behavior that may affect the safety of oral intake? The answers to all these questions again point to the patient's readiness for feeding, the safety of recommending an oral diet, and the need for supervision versus independent feeding. Additionally, information gathered from the answers to these questions can assist clinicians in determining appropriate diet texture for their patients (e.g., pureed vs.

mechanical or regular) and in deciding what treatment options are appropriate. Troche and colleagues found that individuals with mild cognitive impairment experienced declines in swallow function when presented with a cognitively taxing situation, digit span testing, while individuals with more significant cognitive impairment actually had improved swallowing ability when presented with the same task.[47] They suggested the CSE be conducted in an environment that closely mimics the one in which a patient would eat (e.g., with multiple possible distractors), in order to gain a more realistic impression of swallow function.

Information regarding command following can help the clinician determine what assessment options are practical for their patients. Can the individual follow commands sufficiently to participate in therapy if therapy is indicated? Many of the compensatory strategies and rehabilitative exercises designed for the treatment of dysphagia include multiple steps to complete. Patients who cannot follow commands or retain the information necessary to follow several steps per technique may not be ideal candidates for direct treatment, and other options that require less patient effort, such as diet modification, may need to be considered. Empirical evidence suggests individuals who are unable to follow one-step commands exhibit higher odds of aspiration of thin liquids than individuals who are able to follow commands.[18]

Orientation status can also provide information regarding the patient's readiness for an oral diet. Typically, clinicians seek to determine whether the patient is alert and oriented times three (A & O × 3): to person, place, and time. Questions include "What is your full name?" "Where are you?" "What year is it?" As with command following, orientation status can provide information regarding odds of aspiration. Individuals who are oriented to person, place, and time are at lower odds of aspiration than individuals who are not oriented.[18]

## 4.11.4 Oral Mechanism Examination

The next step in the CSE should include an oral mechanism examination. During the oral mechanism examination, integrity of the following structures should be assessed: lips, tongue, facial symmetry, hard and soft palate, dentition, oral health, and jaw. Structures should be observed at rest and during functional movement. The oral mechanism examination can help the clinician form hypotheses regarding the nature of the patient's swallowing disorder. Additionally, the oral mechanism examination can indicate the presence of underlying disease. Looking in the patient's mouth may reveal underlying structural issues, such as a submucous cleft or neoplasms that are affecting swallow function. Poor dentition or oral hygiene can indicate increased risk of aspiration pneumonia.[48] Listening to the patient speak allows detection of dysarthria, the presence of which may be predictive of aspiration risk or dysphagia.[49]

The oral mechanism examination provides a means of assessing the integrity of the cranial nerves involved in swallowing and may indicate which aspects of swallow function are impaired. The cranial nerves involved in swallowing are the trigeminal (V), facial (VII), glossopharyngeal (IX), vagus (X), and hypoglossal (XII) nerves. The following is a suggested means by which clinicians can evaluate each of the cranial nerves involved in swallowing.

The trigeminal nerve (CN V) can be assessed by observing symmetry of jaw closure at rest and during jaw opening. Patients should be asked to open their mouth with and without the clinician providing resistance to movement, and move their jaw from side to side. Asymmetrical jaw opening (i.e., the jaw deviating to the right or left of midline upon opening) indicates unilateral damage to the trigeminal nerve, whereas open-mouth posture and an inability to maintain jaw closure indicate bilateral damage. Clinicians can also palpate the masseter by placing their fingers on the patient's external surface of the temporomandibular joint. Integrity of jaw movement can indicate the possibility of impaired ability to chew the bolus. This can also be assessed by having the patient attempt to masticate a solid-textured bolus at bedside. It should not be assumed individuals with poor dentition or those who are edentulous (i.e., have no teeth) are unable to chew solid textures. Many patients who are edentulous report they are able to chew solid textures, including fresh fruits and vegetables and tougher cuts of meat despite the absence of teeth. Therefore, absence of teeth should not automatically preclude the clinician from recommending a solid-texture diet, either mechanical or regular texture.

The facial nerve (CN VII) provides efferent, motor information to the facial muscles and taste sensation to the anterior two-thirds of the tongue. Observing facial symmetry at rest can assess integrity of the facial nerve. Unilateral lower facial weakness indicates unilateral damage to the ipsilateral facial nerve. Bell's palsy is a disorder in which unilateral facial nerve dysfunction can be observed. Bilateral damage to the facial nerve would be indicated by bilateral facial droop. Damage to the facial nerve can also result in perioral fasciculations. To observe facial nerve integrity during movement, clinicians can ask the patient to smile or purse his lips. Unilateral facial nerve damage resulting in reduced tone on one side of the face may indicate a risk for the bolus collecting in the lateral sulcus. Again, if the clinician is concerned that the patient is at risk for this condition, having the patient masticate a bolus and then observing whether residual material is present in the lateral sulcus after the swallow is a more functional means of assessment.

The glossopharyngeal nerve (CN IX) and the vagus nerve (CN X) are often damaged together. As such, integrity of these nerves can be assessed simultaneously. Function can be tested by observing the velum at rest and during elevation. Vocal quality can also indicate functionality of these nerves. Breathy vocal quality may indicate unilateral or bilateral vocal fold dysfunction that could place the patient at increased risk for aspiration due to decreased airway protection during the swallow. A number of studies indicate that the presence of dysphonia, including breathiness, harshness, or hoarseness, is predictive of aspiration.[49,50] Others have suggested reduced pitch elevation is predictive of dysphagia.[51] Clinicians may also want to elicit a gag response from their patients to assess integrity of CN IX and X. It is not unusual for SLPs to receive referrals to see a patient for a swallow evaluation based on absence of a gag response. The rationale for this is based on the flawed thinking that absence of a gag response indicates cranial nerve pathology and increased risk for dysphagia. However, research does not support the notion that absence of a gag response is a predictor of dysphagia or aspiration.[52] Integrity of the patient's voluntary cough can be used to assess glossopharyngeal and vagus nerve function. Objective measures of voluntary cough have been found to have high sensitivity and specificity for detecting aspiration risk.[10]

Finally, the hypoglossal nerve (CN XII) controls all tongue movements. Lower motor neuron lesions of this nerve will result in lingual atrophy, paralysis, and fasciculations on the affected side. These can be observed by viewing the tongue at rest. Clinicians should also ask the patient to protrude the tongue. Individuals with unilateral CN XII lesions will present with lingual deviation to the ipsilateral side during protrusion due to unopposed action of the intact side. Bilateral lower motor neuron lesions will result in significant inability to protrude the tongue, bilateral lingual fasciculations, and atrophy. Unilateral upper motor neuron lesions to the hypoglossal nerve may result in mild unilateral lingual weakness on the contralateral side; whereas bilateral upper motor neuron lesions of the hypoglossal nerve result in moderate-to-severe lingual dysfunction. This is often seen in individuals with pseudobulbar palsy or amyotrophic lateral sclerosis.

## 4.11.5 Bolus Administration

After the clinician has collected information from the chart review, case history, cognitive assessment, and oral mechanism examination, it is time to decide whether or not to administer a bolus. Not all patients are able to tolerate bolus administration during a clinical swallow examination. Patients who are somnolent or obtunded should not be given a bolus at bedside unless and until their alertness level improves sufficiently to allow them to participate actively in the assessment. Patients who are medically fragile to the extent that they are unable to tolerate any threat to their respiratory status, including the possibility of aspiration of a food or liquid bolus, should not be presented with boluses at the bedside. Patients who have recently had surgical procedures may not yet be ready for trials of boluses by mouth, and clinicians should check with the patient's physicians to determine the appropriateness of bolus administration. With some specific patient populations, such as those individuals who have recently been extubated or those with tracheotomy tubes, bolus administration may not be appropriate, although this is a topic of debate. This issue is addressed in more detail in Chapter 20 of this textbook.

If the clinician determines it is appropriate to give the patient a bolus, the questions of what, how much, and how many different bolus types to administer arises. There is considerable disagreement among SLPs regarding the ideal approach to bolus administration during the CSE. The decision as to what bolus types to include in the clinical assessment can be based on the patient's current oral feeding status: in other words, whether the patient is taking an oral diet already, and, if so, whether the purpose of the clinical swallow assessment is to determine appropriateness of the current diet. In this case, it would be appropriate to observe the patient taking boluses similar in texture and size to what has currently been given during meals. If the patient is currently receiving a nonoral means of nutrition and has not eaten by mouth for a prolonged period of time, it may be more appropriate to begin the evaluation with small boluses of ice chips or water. If the patient has recently had surgery, the examination may be limited to only those bolus types that have been cleared by the patient's physicians.

Assuming there are no restrictions on the type of boluses that can be administered to the patient, a standardized protocol for bolus administration is recommended. Standardization of bolus types, numbers of boluses, and bolus amounts allows for comparison of patient behavior across trials so any changes in behavior, either improvement in or worsening of function, can be systematically observed. It also ensures consistency across clinicians so patients who see one clinician for testing on one day can be assured of having the same examination done if they see a different clinician on a different day. Use of a standardized protocol does not mean clinicians cannot individualize their assessment approach. If, for instance, the patient is exhibiting overt signs or symptoms of aspiration and is clearly unable to tolerate a particular consistency, the clinician can make adjustments in the protocol to accommodate (e.g., change bolus viscosity, introduce compensatory strategies, etc.). Use of a standardized protocol simply provides a framework from which clinicians can tailor their examination.

An Internet search of the term "clinical swallow evaluation" yields hundreds of responses and various forms from a number of different clinical facilities. It seems clinicians often develop their own CSE to be used within their individual facility.[2] Although this ensures consistency across clinicians within a particular facility, it does not ensure consistency across facilities. Thus patients who receive an evaluation in one facility that yields particular results may produce different results when examined in a different facility using a different evaluation protocol. This may result in inconsistency of care, which can adversely affect patient outcomes. Additionally, there are published standardized clinical swallow assessments, including the Mann Assessment of Swallowing Ability (MASA).[53] Use of a validated clinical tool that includes items for which there is sound empirical evidence is recommended.

Typically, a CSE will include presentation of a thin liquid, often water, a pureed or pudding-type bolus, and a solid consistency. Boluses of each may be presented in varying amounts, often progressing from very small amounts—1, 3, or 5 mL—to larger amounts that are considered to be more reflective of typical patient behavior (e.g., cup sips of thin liquids or self-fed pudding or solid boluses). If patients are able to self-feed, it is recommended they be observed doing so. Allowing the patient to self-feed allows clinicians to observe the typical bolus size the patient takes and the rate of intake, and it provides a more functional indication of patient feeding/swallowing safety than clinician-provided, volume-controlled boluses do.

Some clinicians opt to provide thickened liquids, such as a nectar-thick liquid, during a CSE. However, use of thickened liquids is a compensatory treatment strategy meant to address a specific swallowing disorder, such as delayed initiation of the pharyngeal swallow. If patients do not have the specific disorder this particular treatment is meant to address, it is unclear why this treatment would be introduced as part of the standardized clinical evaluation. Additionally, there are very few naturally occurring nectar-thick liquids available to patients. Thus it is very unlikely patients would encounter this consistency in their day-to-day eating activities.

### Oral Phase of the Swallow

Once the decision is made to administer boluses, the clinician must decide what behaviors to observe and which of those behaviors is clinically meaningful. If the patient is capable of self-feeding, the clinician should note bolus amoun (in other words, bite or sip size) rate of intake, and if the patient swallows each bolus between bites or sips. These observations may indicate safety of recommending an oral diet for the patient and may point to the need for patient supervision during meals. Clinicians should observe how long it takes the patient to chew a solid bolus and the number of swallows per bolus. These observations can provide information about efficiency of swallowing. After the patient swallows, the clinician should check the patient's mouth to see whether there is residual material. If so, location of residue, tongue, and lateral sulci, and approximate amount should be noted. Patients who have a large amount of residual material in their mouth after swallowing are at risk for aspiration of residual material after the swallow. The patient's ability to seal his lips around a cup, spoon, or straw and his ability to contain the bolus in his mouth should be noted. The patient's ability to contain oral secretions can also be observed.

## Pharyngeal Phase

Very little information about the pharyngeal phase of swallowing can be gleaned from the CSE because structures in the pharynx, such as the base of the tongue, posterior pharyngeal wall, valleculae, and piriform sinuses, cannot be visualized without the aid of instrumentation, such as an endoscope or X-ray. Therefore, important physiological events, such as velar elevation, tongue base retraction, airway closure, and relaxation of the cricopharyngeus, cannot be assessed using a CSE. Additionally, bolus flow and timing of movements, including onset and duration of pharyngeal transit and duration of cricopharyngeal opening, cannot be determined with a clinical examination.

Some clinicians have suggested using a four-finger method of palpating the hyoid and larynx during the swallow to make determinations of timing of swallow initiation and adequacy of hyolaryngeal excursion.[54] This is done by placing one finger just behind the mandible, one on the hyoid bone, one at the top of the thyroid cartilage, and one at the bottom of the thyroid cartilage. Clinicians can feel for pumping of the tongue with the finger placed behind the mandible, and can thus determine the interval between tongue pumping and onset of laryngeal elevation. This is thought to give an estimate of the timing of swallow onset. Clinicians are then taught to feel for the extent of hyoid and larynx movement during the swallow in an attempt to determine adequacy of hyolaryngeal excursion. However, there is no empirical evidence to support this notion. A clinician's judgment of adequacy of hyolaryngeal excursion based on laryngeal palpation is subjective. At best, laryngeal palpation can be used to determine whether a patient has attempted to swallow. Clinicians cannot rely on laryngeal palpation to determine timing or adequacy of swallow-related events.

Signs and symptoms of aspiration can be detected during a CSE. It is important, though, to differentiate between reliable signs/symptoms of aspiration and those that are not reliable or valid. Cough is one of the most reliable signs of aspiration.[10,27,55] Wet vocal quality immediately postswallow has also been suggested to have predictive value for detecting aspiration.[26,48] However, clinicians do not reliably perceive wet vocal quality when material

is present in the larynx during phonation, and there are studies that indicate vocal quality lacks sensitivity and specificity for detection of aspiration.[56,57] Thus clinicians should be cautious in making judgments of aspiration risk based solely on changes in vocal quality. Throat clearing postswallow is another possible sign of aspiration.[27] The likelihood that a patient is going to present with overt signs/symptoms of aspiration, cough, wet vocal quality, or throat clearing appears to be dependent on bolus volume. Presentation of small bolus volumes (1–5 mL), as is often done during clinical assessment, lacks sufficient sensitivity for detection of aspiration, and patients who aspirate silently may not be identified if only small bolus volumes are presented. Larger bolus volumes (90–100 mL), have high sensitivity for detection of aspiration, and patients who aspirate silently when presented with small bolus volumes are less likely to do so when they take larger bolus volumes.[9,58]

Other behaviors that have been suggested to indicate possible aspiration include watering eyes, runny nose, hiccoughing, and sneezing. However, there is no empirical evidence that any of these behaviors reliably predict aspiration events. Rather, behaviors such as watering eyes, runny nose, or sneezing, regardless of whether or not they co-occur with eating, are reactions to a noxious stimulus in the nose or eyes, such as a chemical irritant. These behaviors should not be considered to be predictive of aspiration.

## 4.12 Instrumentation

The use of instrumentation, such as a stethoscope or pulse oximeter, has been suggested to increase accuracy of the CSE for detection of aspiration and dysphagia. Cervical auscultation involves use of a stethoscope placed at or around the level of the larynx to gather information about the pharyngeal phase of swallowing. Sounds produced during the swallow consist of two distinct components, called bursts or clunks, followed by a third, less distinct component called a puff. Clinicians are asked to make perceptual judgments of swallow function based on these sounds. A normal swallow is one that is rhythmical and has crisp clunks and dry breath sounds; an abnormal swallow is one that is nonrhythmical and has obscured clunks and noisy breath sounds. There are concerns about the use of cervical auscultation for evaluation of dysphagia. First, there are no definitive data correlating the sounds heard using cervical auscultation with specific physiological events and abnormalities.[59] Second, accuracy of this technique is affected by the perceptual skills of the listener, the quality of the stethoscope used, and patient-related factors, such as presence of noisy breath sounds associated with asthma or chronic obstructive pulmonary disease. At this time, data are insufficient to support inclusion of cervical auscultation as part of the clinical evaluation.

Pulse oximetry provides a means of measuring arterial blood oxygenation. A sensor placed on the patient's earlobe, finger, or toe monitors wavelengths emitted by a small light source as it passes through tissue and measures the amount of light absorbed by the blood in the tissue. This is then converted to a number called oxygen saturation, which indicates the percentage of oxygenized hemoglobin. The normal range is 95 to 100%; levels lower than

90% suggest significant problems. It has been suggested that declines of 2% or more from baseline levels may indicate aspiration.[60] However, more recent data indicate that changes in oxygen saturation levels detected through pulse oximetry do not correlate with aspiration events.[61] Colodny[62] found that individuals who aspirated during an instrumental swallow examination had lower resting oxygen saturation levels than nonaspirators. However, oxygen saturation levels were not affected by single aspiration events observed during swallow evaluation. Thus, oxygen saturation levels do not appear to be predictive of aspiration.

## 4.13 Next Steps

Following bolus administration and observation of patient behaviors during these trials, the clinician must decide the next steps for the patient. There are basically three choices: (1) recommend a diet without the need for further testing; (2) recommend nonoral means of nutrition pending further testing—instrumental assessment of swallowing with videofluoroscopy or endoscopy; or (3) recommend referral to another professional, such as a gastroenterologist, otolaryngologist, or neurologist. If the patient exhibits no overt signs or symptoms of aspiration or dysphagia, and if the patient is medically stable, the clinician may wish to recommend an oral diet. Choice of diet type, pureed versus mechanical or regular texture, is primarily dependent upon the patient's dentition status. As stated earlier in this chapter, lack of dentition does not necessarily preclude a patient from taking a solid-textured diet, but clinicians should be mindful of the risk of choking in patients who are weak due to their current medical status or in those who demonstrate fluctuating levels of awareness or alertness. In those instances, clinicians may wish to make the more conservative recommendation of a pureed diet. There are issues with pureed diets too. Patients often find them unpalatable, and they may be less likely to consume an adequate amount of calories. Clinicians must carefully weigh patient safety with patient wishes when making recommendations for a particular diet texture.

If patients exhibit overt signs or symptoms of aspiration or dysphagia, the clinician may wish to recommend a nonoral means of nutrition pending further assessment of swallowing. The specific indications, contraindications, advantages, and disadvantages of videofluoroscopic versus endoscopic evaluation of swallowing are discussed at length in Chapters 5 and 6 of this book. Instrumental assessment can provide information about the pathophysiology responsible for the signs and symptoms of aspiration or dysphagia that are observed at bedside. As discussed previously, neither bolus flow nor timing of swallow-related events can be observed during a CSE. In order to formulate a treatment plan that focuses on compensating for or rehabilitating disordered swallow physiology, clinicians must have the benefit of an instrumental assessment.

Finally, clinicians may opt to recommend a referral to another professional. If the patient presents with complaints of globus, difficulty swallowing solids or pills only, frequent heartburn, or other symptoms of esophageal dysphagia, referral to a gastroenterologist may be appropriate. If the patient presents with complaints of sore throat, vocal changes, or other symptoms suggesting laryngeal pathology, referral to an otolaryngologist may be indicated. Finally, if the patient presents with complaints

of soft neurological signs, such as weakness or frequent falls, or if the clinician notes behaviors suggestive of neurological pathology, such as lingual fasciculations or tremor, referral to a neurologist may be appropriate.

## 4.14 Conclusion

This chapter has provided clinicians with information regarding the purpose and method by which to conduct a CSE. Additionally, what can and cannot be determined based on findings of the CSE has been discussed. The CSE provides the clinician with valuable information regarding patient readiness and appropriateness for an oral diet. It allows clinicians to make appropriate management decisions, including the need for further assessment or referral to other professionals.

## 4.15 Questions

1. Which of the following is one advantage of screening tests when compared to full diagnostic testing?

A. Screening tests are more expensive than full diagnostic testing.

B. Screening tests are more time consuming than full diagnostic testing.

C. Screening tests offer a simple, quick, and cost-effective means of identifying individuals at risk for a particular disease or condition.

D. Screening tests require more training and expertise to administer than diagnostic tests.

E. Screening tests offer no advantage over full diagnostic testing and should not be used.

2. The current state of practice with regard to use of a dysphagia screening tool indicates which of the following?

A. Speech-language pathologists are in agreement regarding who should administer the protocol.

B. Speech-language pathologists are in agreement regarding what items should constitute a protocol.

C. Speech-language pathologists are in agreement regarding what bolus types and amounts should be administered as part of a protocol.

D. There is considerable disagreement among speech-language pathologists regarding who, how, and what should be involved in dysphagia screening.

E. Speech-language pathologists should not be using screening tools.

3. Which of the following is true regarding use of a chart review as part of a routine clinical swallow examination?

A. It can provide good information regarding aspiration risk, particularly if the patient presents with a current diagnosis of pneumonia.

B. It yields no valuable information regarding a patient's risk of aspiration.

C. It should only be done if the clinician has sufficient time in his/her schedule to complete prior to evaluating the patient.

D. It is unnecessary and should not be done.

E. It can be done in lieu of a face-to-face interview with the patient.

4. Which of the following is true regarding use of the four-finger method of hyolaryngeal palpation during the clinical swallow examination?

A. It has been found to reliably indicate the extent of hyoid anterior movement.

B. It has been found to reliably indicate the extent of laryngeal elevation.

C. It has been found to reliably indicate timing of onset of the pharyngeal phase of the swallow.

D. It has not been found to be an accurate means of assessing timing of the swallow or extent of hyolaryngeal excursion.

E. It has been found to reliably indicate the presence of aspiration.

5. Which of the following is true with regard to the clinical swallow evaluation?

A. Speech-language pathologists are in agreement regarding what items should constitute the evaluation.

B. Speech-language pathologists are in agreement regarding what bolus types should be administered as part of a clinical swallow evaluation.

C. Speech-language pathologists are in agreement regarding what specific aspects of swallowing should be observed as part of a clinical swallow evaluation.

D. Speech-language pathologists are in agreement regarding bolus sizes that should be administered.

E. There is considerable disagreement among speech-language pathologists regarding how and what should be involved in clinical swallow evaluations.

## 4.16 Answers and Explanations

1. **Correct: Screening tests offer a simple, quick, and cost-effective means of identifying individuals at risk for a particular disease or condition (C).**

   Screening tests are meant to be quick, cost-effective tools used to determine more accurately which patients do and do not need to be referred for the more time-consuming, costly diagnostic examination. Screening tests are meant to be simple to administer, and, with proper training, they can be administered by a variety of health care professionals.

2. **Correct: there is considerable disagreement among speech-language pathologists regarding who, how, and what should be involved in dysphagia screening (D).**

   There is currently considerable disagreement among speech-language pathologists regarding how and who should administer screenings. There is also disagreement regarding what boluses, if any, should be administered and what is to be screened for (i.e., dysphagia risk versus aspiration risk).

3. **Correct: can provide good information regarding aspiration risk, particularly if the patient presents with a current diagnosis of pneumonia (A).**

   Research by McCullough and colleagues indicates that information gathered during a chart review can provide information regarding the likelihood that a patient is aspirating. Specifically, current diagnosis of pneumonia, presence of a nonoral means of nutrition, and need for suctioning were all found to be predictive of aspiration.

4. **Correct: has not been found to be an accurate means of assessing timing of the swallow or extent of hyolaryngeal excursion (D).**

   Hyolaryngeal palpation during the clinical swallow examination has never been found to be a reliable indicator of integrity of swallow function, including promptness of swallow onset or adequacy of hyolaryngeal excursion. There is no empirical evidence to support its inclusion in a clinical swallow evaluation.

5. **Correct: there is considerable disagreement among speech-language pathologists regarding how and what should be involved in clinical swallow evaluations (E).**

   As with swallow screening, there is no agreement among speech-language pathologists regarding how a clinical swallow evaluation should be completed.

## References

[1] Suiter DM, Leder SB. Clinical utility of the 3-ounce water swallow test. *Dysphagia* 2008;23(3):244–250

[2] McCullough GH, Wertz RT, Rosenbek JC, Dinneen C. Clinicians' preferences and practices in conducting clinical/bedside and videofluoroscopic swallowing examinations in an adult, neurogenic population. *Am J Speech Lang Pathol* 1999;8(2):149–163

[3] American Speech-Language-Hearing Association. *Preferred Practice Patterns for the Profession of Speech-Language Pathology*. Rockville, MD; ASHA; 2004

[4] Rosenbek JC, McCullough GH, Wertz RT. Is the information about a test important? Applying the methods of evidence-based medicine to the clinical examination of swallowing. *J Commun Disord* 2004;37(5):437–450

[5] Logemann JA, Veis S, Colangelo L. A screening procedure for oropharyngeal dysphagia. *Dysphagia* 1999;14(1):44–51

[6] Leder SB, Espinosa JF. Aspiration risk after acute stroke: comparison of clinical examination and fiberoptic endoscopic evaluation of swallowing. *Dysphagia* 2002;17(3):214–218

[7] Warner HL, Suiter DM, Nystrom KV, Poskus K, Leder SB. Comparing accuracy of the Yale swallow protocol when administered by registered nurses and speech-language pathologists. *J Clin Nurs* 2014;23(13-14):1908–1915

[8] Cochrane AL, Holland WW. Validation of screening procedures. *Br Med Bull* 1971;27(1):3–8

[9] Leder SB, Suiter DM, Green BG. Silent aspiration risk is volume-dependent. *Dysphagia* 2011;26(3):304–309

[10] Smith Hammond CA, Goldstein LB, Horner RD, et al. Predicting aspiration in patients with ischemic stroke: comparison of clinical signs and aerodynamic measures of voluntary cough. *Chest* 2009;135(3):769–777

[11] DePippo KL, Holas MA, Reding MJ. Validation of the 3-oz water swallow test for aspiration following stroke. *Arch Neurol* 1992;49(12):1259–1261

[12] Daniels SK, McAdam CP, Brailey K, Foundas AL. Clinical assessment of swallowing and prediction of dysphagia severity. *Am J Speech Lang Pathol* 1997;6(4):7

[13] Martino R, Silver F, Teasell R, et al. The Toronto Bedside Swallowing Screening Test (TOR-BSST): development and validation of a dysphagia screening tool for patients with stroke. *Stroke* 2009;40(2):555–561

[14] Ramsey DJ, Smithard DG, Kalra L. Can pulse oximetry or a bedside swallowing assessment be used to detect aspiration after stroke? *Stroke* 2006;*37*(12):2984–2988

[15] Leder SB, Suiter DM, Murray J, Rademaker AW. Can an oral mechanism examination contribute to the assessment of odds of aspiration? *Dysphagia* 2013;*28*(3):370–374

[16] Leder SB, Judson BL, Sliwinski E, Madson L. Promoting safe swallowing when puree is swallowed without aspiration but thin liquid is aspirated: nectar is enough. *Dysphagia* 2013;*28*(1):58–62

[17] Suiter DM, Sloggy J, Leder SB. Validation of the Yale Swallow Protocol: a prospective double-blinded videofluoroscopic study. *Dysphagia* 2014;*29*(2):199–203

[18] Leder SB, Suiter DM, Lisitano Warner H. Answering orientation questions and following single-step verbal commands: effect on aspiration status. *Dysphagia* 2009;*24*(3):290–295

[19] Leder SB, Suiter DM, Warner HL, Kaplan LJ. Initiating safe oral feeding in critically ill intensive care and step-down unit patients based on passing a 3-ounce (90 milliliters) water swallow challenge. *J Trauma* 2011;*70*(5):1203–1207

[20] Leder SB, Suiter DM, Warner HL, Acton LM, Siegel MD. Safe initiation of oral diets in hospitalized patients based on passing a 3-ounce (90 cc) water swallow challenge protocol. *QJM* 2012;*105*(3):257–263

[21] Leder SB, Suiter DM. *The Yale Swallow Protocol: An Evidence-Based Approach to Decision Making.* Springer International Publishing. Switzerland. 2014

[22] American Speech-Language-Hearing Association. Clinical Indicators for Instrumental Assessment of Dysphagia [Guidelines]. Rockville, MD: ASHA; 2000

[23] Martino R, Foley N, Bhogal S, Diamant N, Speechley M, Teasell R. Dysphagia after stroke: incidence, diagnosis, and pulmonary complications. *Stroke* 2005;*36*(12):2756–2763

[24] Luchesi KF, Kitamura S, Mourão LF. Management of dysphagia in Parkinson's disease and amyotrophic lateral sclerosis. *CoDAS* 2013;*25*(4):358–364

[25] Cintra MT, de Rezende NA, de Moraes EN, Cunha LC, da Gama Torres HO. A comparison of survival, pneumonia, and hospitalization in patients with advanced dementia and dysphagia receiving either oral or enteral nutrition. *J Nutr Health Aging* 2014;*18*(10):894–899

[26] Hutcheson KA, Bhayani MK, Beadle BM, et al. Eat and exercise during radiotherapy or chemoradiotherapy for pharyngeal cancers: use it or lose it. *JAMA Otolaryngol Head Neck Surg* 2013;*139*(11):1127–1134

[27] McCullough GH, Rosenbek JC, Wertz RT, McCoy S, Mann G, McCullough K. Utility of clinical swallowing examination measures for detecting aspiration post-stroke. *J Speech Lang Hear Res* 2005;*48*(6):1280–1293

[28] Marik PE. Aspiration pneumonitis and aspiration pneumonia. *N Engl J Med* 2001;*344*(9):665–671

[29] Daniels SK, Foundas AL, Iglesia GC, Sullivan MA. Lesion site in unilateral stroke patients with dysphagia. *J Stroke Cerebrovasc Dis* 1996;*6*(1):30–34

[30] Robbins J, Levine RL, Maser A, Rosenbek JC, Kempster GB. Swallowing after unilateral stroke of the cerebral cortex. *Arch Phys Med Rehabil* 1993;*74*(12):1295–1300

[31] Suntrup S, Kemmling A, Warnecke T, et al. The impact of lesion location on dysphagia incidence, pattern and complications in acute stroke. Part 1: dysphagia incidence, severity and aspiration. *Eur J Neurol* 2015;*22*(5):832–838

[32] Smithard DG, O'Neill PA, Martin DF, England R. Aspiration following stroke: is it related to the side of the stroke? *Clin Rehabil* 1997;*11*(1):73–76

[33] Falsetti P, Acciai C, Palilla R, et al. Oropharyngeal dysphagia after stroke: incidence, diagnosis, and clinical predictors in patients admitted to a neurorehabilitation unit. *J Stroke Cerebrovasc Dis* 2009;*18*(5):329–335

[34] Stoschus B, Allescher HD. Drug-induced dysphagia. *Dysphagia* 1993;*8*(2):154–159

[35] Al-Shehri AM. Drug-induced dysphagia. *Ann Saudi Med* 2003;*23*(5):249–253

[36] Madhavan A, Carnaby GD, Crary MA. 'Food sticking in my throat': videofluoroscopic evaluation of a common symptom. *Dysphagia* 2015;*30*(3):343–348

[37] Kalf JG, de Swart BJ, Bloem BR, Munneke M. Prevalence of oropharyngeal dysphagia in Parkinson's disease: a meta-analysis. *Parkinsonism Relat Disord* 2012;*18*(4):311–315

[38] Rogus-Pulia NM, Pierce M, Mittal BB, Zecker SG, Logemann J. Bolus effects on patient awareness of swallowing difficulty and swallow physiology after chemoradiation for head and neck cancer. *Head Neck* 2015;*37*(8):1122–1129

[39] Parker C, Power M, Hamdy S, Bowen A, Tyrrell P, Thompson DG. Awareness of dysphagia by patients following stroke predicts swallowing performance. *Dysphagia* 2004;*19*(1):28–35

[40] Schroeder MF, Daniels SK, McClain M, Corey DM, Foundas AL. Clinical and cognitive predictors of swallowing recovery in stroke. *J Rehabil Res Dev* 2006;*43*(3):301–310

[41] McHorney CA, Martin-Harris B, Robbins J, Rosenbek J. Clinical validity of the SWAL-QOL and SWAL-CARE outcome tools with respect to bolus flow measures. *Dysphagia* 2006;*21*(3):141–148

[42] McHorney CA, Bricker DE, Kramer AE, et al. The SWAL-QOL outcomes tool for oropharyngeal dysphagia in adults: I. Conceptual foundation and item development. *Dysphagia* 2000;*15*(3):115–121

[43] McHorney CA, Robbins J, Lomax K, et al. The SWAL-QOL and SWAL-CARE outcomes tool for oropharyngeal dysphagia in adults: III. Documentation of reliability and validity. *Dysphagia* 2002;*17*(2):97–114

[44] Silbergleit AK, Schultz L, Jacobson BH, Beardsley T, Johnson AF. The Dysphagia Handicap Index: development and validation. *Dysphagia* 2012;*27*(1):46–52

[45] Chen AY, Frankowski R, Bishop-Leone J, et al. The development and validation of a dysphagia-specific quality-of-life questionnaire for patients with head and neck cancer: the M. D. Anderson dysphagia inventory. *Arch Otolaryngol Head Neck Surg* 2001;*127*(7):870–876

[46] Hutcheson KA, Barrow MP, Lisec A, Barringer DA, Gries K, Lewin JS. What is a clinically relevant difference in MDADI scores between groups of head and neck cancer patients? *Laryngoscope* 2015

[47] Troche MS, Okun MS, Rosenbek JC, Altmann LJ, Sapienza CM. Attentional resource allocation and swallowing safety in Parkinson's disease: a dual task study. *Parkinsonism Relat Disord* 2014;*20*(4):439–443

[48] Scannapieco FA, Bush RB, Paju S. Associations between periodontal disease and risk for nosocomial bacterial pneumonia and chronic obstructive pulmonary disease. A systematic review. *Ann Periodontol* 2003;*8*(1):54–69

[49] Daniels SK, Brailey K, Priestly DH, Herrington LR, Weisberg LA, Foundas AL. Aspiration in patients with acute stroke. *Arch Phys Med Rehabil* 1998;*79*(1):14–19

[50] Horner J, Massey EW, Riski JE, Lathrop DL, Chase KN. Aspiration following stroke: clinical correlates and outcome. *Neurology* 1988;*38*(9):1359–1362

[51] Malandraki GA, Hind JA, Gangnon R, Logemann JA, Robbins J. The utility of pitch elevation in the evaluation of oropharyngeal dysphagia: preliminary findings. *Am J Speech Lang Pathol* 2011;*20*(4):262–268

[52] Leder SB. Gag reflex and dysphagia. *Head Neck* 1996;*18*(2):138–141

[53] Mann G. *MASA, the Mann Assessment of Swallowing Ability.* Vol 1. Stamford, CT: Cengage Learning; 2002

[54] Logemann JA, Logemann JA. *Evaluation and Treatment of Swallowing Disorders.* Cranston, RI: College-Hill Press; 1983

[55] McCullough GH, Wertz RT, Rosenbek JC. Sensitivity and specificity of clinical/bedside examination signs for detecting aspiration in adults subsequent to stroke. *J Commun Disord* 2001;*34*(1-2):55–72

[56] Groves-Wright KJ, Boyce S, Kelchner L. Perception of wet vocal quality in identifying penetration/aspiration during swallowing. *J Speech Lang Hear Res* 2010;*53*(3):620–632

[57] Waito A, Bailey GL, Molfenter SM, Zoratto DC, Steele CM. Voice-quality abnormalities as a sign of dysphagia: validation against acoustic and videofluoroscopic data. *Dysphagia* 2011;*26*(2):125–134

[58] Brodsky MB, Suiter DM, González-Fernández M, et al. Screening accuracy for aspiration using bedside water swallow tests: A systematic review and meta-analysis. *Chest* 2016;*150*(1):148–163

[59] Leslie P, Drinnan MJ, Zammit-Maempel I, Coyle JL, Ford GA, Wilson JA. Cervical auscultation synchronized with images from endoscopy swallow evaluations. *Dysphagia* 2007;*22*(4):290–298

[60] Collins MJ, Bakheit AM. Does pulse oximetry reliably detect aspiration in dysphagic stroke patients? *Stroke* 1997;*28*(9):1773–1775

[61] Wang TG, Chang YC, Chen SY, Hsiao TY. Pulse oximetry does not reliably detect aspiration on videofluoroscopic swallowing study. *Arch Phys Med Rehabil* 2005;*86*(4):730–734

[62] Colodny N. Comparison of dysphagics and nondysphagics on pulse oximetry during oral feeding. *Dysphagia* 2000;*15*(2):68–73

# 5 Pediatric Swallow Screening and Clinical Swallow Evaluation

*Amy L. Delaney*

## Summary

A clinical swallow evaluation (CSE) has a critical role in the differential diagnosis of a pediatric feeding disorder or pediatric dysphagia. Although it is often titled differently based on the setting in which it is conducted (e.g., bedside swallow evaluation; clinical feeding evaluation), the desired outcomes of the assessment should be the same. In pediatrics, the child's oral skills and feeding expectations change rapidly throughout infancy and childhood as a result of changes in anatomy and physiology, physical growth, and development that occur. The pediatric feeding/swallowing clinician must acquire extensive knowledge in these areas in order to diagnose a feeding disorder accurately. When conducted properly and systematically, a pediatric CSE is considered a formal, diagnostic examination and not simply a screening to determine the need for an instrumental assessment. This targeted investigation can lead to identification of other red flags indicative of larger health issues warranting additional medical team investigation and intervention.

## Keywords

Clinical swallow feeding, feeding skills, feeding observation, non-nutritive sucking, nutritive sucking, sucking, infant feeding, oral feeding skills, chewing, texture transition, Cranial nerve examination, oral sensory, oral motor

## Learning Objectives

- Use typical feeding expectations and feeding principles as baseline comparisons for any child receiving a clinical swallow evaluation (CSE).
- Understand that the child's feeding progression and experiences help to determine the nature of the feeding disorder.
- Use direct assessment of the oral structure and function for speech and language to identify red flags about the function for feeding skills.
- Observe feeding to obtain key information about oral feeding abilities.
- Counsel caregivers regarding typical feeding expectations as a critical part of the CSE.

## 5.1 Introduction

Whenever possible, a formal and standardized clinical swallow evaluation (CSE) should be implemented. The CSE is a noninstrumental assessment of a child's feeding presentation. A CSE should include a chart review, interview, direct observation and assessment of oral feeding skills, screening other body systems for contributing factors, and treatment planning. The CSE can be supplemented with validated parent-report measures.[1] Unfortunately, there are only a few standardized CSEs available for use with pediatric patients that are designed and reported with sufficient psychometric rigor to ensure validity and reliability for this population. A recent systematic review of 30 noninstrumental assessments of feeding and swallowing for pediatric patients revealed significant variability in terms of target populations and assessment design and domains. This variability was most likely an indicator of the variability of the professionals who diagnose and treat pediatric feeding and swallowing difficulty as well as the complexity and diversity of the various pediatric populations that present with feeding and swallowing difficulty. None of the 30 assessments reviewed provided complete information with regard to oral motor skill, behavioral and environmental factors, feeding/swallowing activity, quality of life, and sensory integration factors.[2]

A review of 11 infant-specific noninstrumental feeding assessments revealed similar results but concluded that the Early Feeding Skills Assessment and the Bristol Breastfeeding Assessment Tool had the most psychometric development and testing of the assessment tools reviewed.[3] Similarly, in a review of noninstrumental feeding assessments for children with cerebral palsy, it was found that the Schedule for Oral Motor Assessment and the Functional Feeding Assessment, Modified had the strongest, published measures of validity and reliability; however, the Schedule for Oral Motor Assessment and the Dysphagia Disorders Survey demonstrated the strongest clinical utility.[4] It should be noted, however, that the Schedule for Oral Motor Assessment is no longer in print or available for purchase.

When faced with a lack of psychometrically validated and available instruments for CSE, clinicians must utilize knowledge of typical feeding expectations to guide their assessment of the infant or child's feeding skills.

## 5.2 Clinical Swallow Evaluation

A CSE may be requested for a variety of reasons, such as concerns about picky eating, lack of advancement in diet, and coughing with liquids. There are many possible reasons for each of those presenting concerns, including oral hypersensitivity, anxiety, inefficient chewing, introduction of inappropriately advanced textures, poor esophageal motility, poor oral control of liquids, neurologic deficits, or a laryngeal cleft. The feeding clinician's role is to determine the underlying deficits contributing to the child's presentation. Decision-making about the child's feeding difficulties is highly dependent on comparisons to *typical feeding expectations*—those age-specific goals for the successful transition through developmental progressions of textures and volumes as compared to those acquired by full-term and healthy children.[5,6,7,8,9] Feeding expectations change based on the child's age, growth, and development. Specific oral feeding skills and swallowing abilities are required to achieve these feeding transitions. Feeding clinicians must integrate these normal expectations into their skill set, just as a speech-language pathologist understands developmental expectations of typical speech and language. This is where pediatric specialty begins. Although some variability is inherent in developmental changes, some feeding expectations never change and should always be used as baseline principles during any CSE. It should be noted, however, that medical and developmental issues will impact feeding expectations. Here are five guiding principles that should always be considered during a CSE:

- Structured mealtimes: Infants and children are expected to consume all of their nutrition and calories in structured and scheduled meals and snacks. Feedings should be scheduled per the child's age. Meals should last no more than 30 minutes, with adequate time between meals to maximize hunger for the next meal. Only water should be offered between meals and snacks (except for young infants, who rely on breast milk or formula for all hydration).

- Positive mealtime experiences: Infants and children are expected to enjoy eating and have positive mealtime experiences. By nature, children are curious and interested in foods. Although first introduction to new textures or foods might result in gagging or a facial grimace, these negative reactions quickly resolve with ongoing exposure and practice. Toddlers are expected to go through a picky phase, where they prefer to eat certain foods, but this is not expected to become so limited that it impacts growth/nutrition or severely restricts the family's ability to provide food.

- Easy feeding transitions: Learning to drink and eat is a natural process that most people take for granted. Children should transition to new textures and new ways of drinking with ease. Children typically require frequent exposures to new foods before they will consume them on a regular basis. Short-term difficulties are typical in the first weeks of a new transition, but ongoing difficulties are not expected.

- Eating is a comforting/stress-free task: Infants and children are expected to be comfortable when eating and drinking. Breathing should remain stable. They should not feel pain or discomfort during or after a meal. Infants and children tend to avoid or limit intake of those food or liquids that cause distress or discomfort. These behaviors should be taken seriously.

- Achievement of feeding milestones: Children should achieve the following feeding milestones without significant difficulty, taking in appropriate volumes for age, and efficiently consuming a variety of flavors and food choices. The volume and variety of intake rapidly change from birth into school-age years; these expectations are extremely important for a clinician to know. Global milestones are expected at the following ages:
  o Drink efficiently from a bottle or the breast after the first few days of life
  o Take a measurable volume and variety of baby foods by 9 months
  o Take first finger foods by 12 months
  o Take first table foods by 15 months
  o Drink milk from a cup or straw at meals and snacks by 15 months
  o Take all food and drink during the day by 15 months

Descriptions of problems and/or variations from these feeding principles and achievement of feeding milestones will be identified through the process of the CSE, the goal of which is to identify the following:

- Possible reasons for the feeding problem
- Barriers to feeding progression
- The need for instrumental swallow assessment
- Other medical referrals that are needed
- A diet that is safe, efficient, and based on the child's skills
- The need for feeding intervention

It is of the utmost importance that the clinician provide the family with a plan for ongoing feeding that is easily implemented after they leave the assessment. To accomplish this goal, a CSE should consist of five key components: (1) preevaluation chart review, (2) caregiver/child interview, (3) direct assessment, (4) screenings (red flags), and (5) counseling, recommendations, and treatment planning.

## 5.3 CSE Procedures

A description of a CSE protocol is presented in **Table 5.1**. Each of these components should be addressed and completed regardless of the setting. When you receive a referral, your work setting, the current status of the child, and the reason for the consultation will dictate where the stronger focus will be during the evaluation. In reality, the tasks in the protocol often co-occur during the assessment period because your observations will lead to more questions, and the family's responses to questions will lead to the need for other specific observations or therapeutic trials. The evaluation will never proceed in a defined order. In an optimal situation, all the components detailed are completed. In reality, you do the best you can and gather as much information as possible. This chapter focuses on the direct assessment portion of the feeding presentation and counseling, recommendations, and treatment planning procedures of the CSE. The procedure for taking a detailed feeding history and current feeding status and the specific expectations for volume, variety, texture introduction, and mealtime process at each age are described only briefly.

### 5.3.1 Chart Review

The chart review generates possible clinical hypotheses for the child's presentation if the reason for referral has not been directly stated. The extent of this review depends on the setting where you work. The level of information available can vary from very little to extensive amounts and is intended to provide a framework for understanding contributing factors to feeding experiences and difficulties. Although all information in a review may be interesting, the focus must be on those medical and developmental issues most pertinent to the feeding and swallowing status relating to the reasons for the consult. This information enables you to begin developing hypotheses about how the child's feeding difficulties relate to underlying neurologic, respiratory, and gastrointestinal problems as well as psychosocial issues. For example, a 3-year-old child is referred

**Table 5.1** Clinical swallow evaluation procedures

| | | |
|---|---|---|
| Chart Review | | Generate possible clinical hypotheses for the child's presentation based on medical, developmental, and feeding experiences |
| Feeding Presentation | **Caregiver/child interview**<br>Feeding history<br>Current feeding status | Identify problems and barriers to typical feeding progression and expectations<br>• Provides an understanding of the timing of onset of feeding difficulties and the persistent or acute nature of problems<br>• Provides information about mealtime process related to schedule, location, specific strategies, oral and enteral intake at present time |
| | **Direct assessment**<br>Oral peripheral examination<br>Oral feeding skills<br>Therapeutic trials | Determine whether problems exist in structure and function of the swallowing mechanism; identify skill-based etiology<br>• Provides information about skill-based contributions and barriers and parent–child interactions at mealtimes |
| **Screenings/identify red flags**<br>Swallow<br>Respiratory<br>Gastrointestinal/nutrition<br>Neurologic<br>Other medical<br>Development | | Determine the need for instrumental assessment<br>Determine potential contributing factors to the feeding disorder |
| **Counseling, recommendations, and treatment planning** | | Counsel/educate caregivers on etiology, prognosis, diet, and therapy needs<br>Create a feeding plan (safe and efficient diet for child)<br>Create a treatment plan (recommended goals and strategies to advance diet and skills)<br>Make referrals (instrumental swallow assessment or other medical referrals) |

for a CSE due to concerns for picky eating. According to the chart review, the child was born at 40 weeks' gestation, with diagnoses of gastroesophageal reflux in infancy and chronic ear infections, with placement of pressure-equalization tubes at 14 months of age. Based on this history, you will want to identify further red flags regarding gastrointestinal and respiratory status.

## 5.3.2 Feeding Presentation: Caregiver Interview and Direct Assessment

Once the chart review is completed, you will begin with the interview and complete the direct assessment. The interview and direct assessment focus on understanding and describing the child's feeding presentation. The child's *feeding presentation* is a culmination of experiences starting at birth with first oral feedings (although in utero experience is relevant) and progresses to the present time (**Fig. 5.1**). Your assessment will focus on describing this child's experiences around feeding as they relate to the following:

1. Feeding history: the child's previous feeding experiences and achievement of feeding milestones
2. Current feeding status: the child's current experiences related to the mealtime process and current oral intake
3. Oral peripheral examination: the relevant structure and function of the oral mechanism
4. Feeding observation: the mealtime process and specific oral feeding skills (both oral motor skills and oral sensory processing abilities) used for eating

## 5.3.3 Caregiver Interview

First, the parents' concerns, expectations, and goals for their child's feeding difficulties should be discussed at the beginning of the evaluation. This helps you understand what the caregiver's

concerns are related to the reason for the referral. Often the caregiver's primary concern or difficulty in feeding their child is different from why a provider referred them. For example, a caregiver might struggle to get their child to drink from a cup and the provider is concerned about the child's respiratory health. The conversation with the caregivers also guides you in how you approach your counseling and recommendations later in the CSE. Next, you will conduct an interview with the caregivers and the child. As clinicians, we are anxious to observe the child eating in order to assist the child and their family. Simply observing a child eating is not adequate to determine the etiology of the feeding problem or to make a diagnosis, nor is asking questions alone adequate.

By taking a thorough *feeding history* from the parents and child, you will document the feeding experiences and progression of the child from birth until the time of the evaluation. You will start

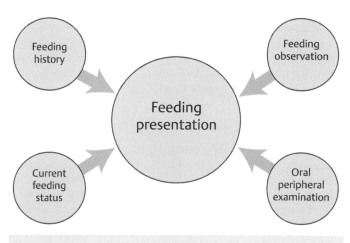

**Fig. 5.1** Schema of the feeding presentation.

from birth and inquire about each feeding transition and any problems encountered during that transition. You can determine if difficulties were present at birth, began with a particular feeding transition, or arose acutely based on a recent change in status.

The *current feeding status* of the child details exactly what the child's diet consists of at the time of CSE and includes a 24-hour diet recall and a food/liquid inventory. Through a 24-hour diet recall, you describe the feeding schedule related to onset and cessation of meals, location and seating, process for preparation and presentation of foods, diet specific to textures and methods/volume of intake, and parent–child interactions.[5,8,9,10] Throughout the interview, you will compile a list of red flags.

Your analysis of the child's feeding presentation and your list of red flags tell you whether the child is consuming an age-appropriate diet. The nature of the feeding disorder relates to the frequency and severity of problems with a particular drinking method, solid food texture, volume of intake for a particular method or texture, variety of foods accepted, mealtime schedule, or parent–child interaction.

In our case example, a 3-year-old child with a history of gastroesophageal reflux and ear infections is referred for a CSE due to concerns for picky eating. Through your discussion, the parents express that feeding their child is very stressful. They want her to eat more nutritious foods. They state that they think her feeding problems are impacting sleep; she is a restless sleeper, she snores, and she is irritable in the morning. You conduct your interview inquiring about the child's feeding history from birth and detail her current feeding status.

## 5.3.4 Feeding History

The parents report that the child drank regular formula (based on cow's milk) by bottle at birth without difficulty in sucking or swallowing. She vomited frequently from 3 to 6 months of age, at which time their pediatrician recommended changing to soy formula, which led to resolution of vomiting. She easily transitioned to smooth-puree baby foods and dissolvable solids at expected ages and to whole milk at her first birthday. She initially accepted whole cow's milk but began refusing it by 18 months. They state that she initially accepted some table foods around 10 months of age, such as pancakes and diced fruit, and appeared to attempt to tongue mash and swallow this texture. All subsequent feeding transitions to table foods were very stressful and resulted in choking and vomiting with most solid feeding attempts until 2 years of age, when she stopped accepting table foods. The parents had resorted to force feeding at times to get her to try new foods.

## 5.3.5 Current Feeding Status

The child's current feeding status consists of thin liquid by open cup, a variety of fruits and vegetables in the form of smooth baby foods and yogurt, and small volumes of dissolvable solids. She accepts these food items happily and efficiently. The parents express significant concerns about their child's nutrition because she does not drink milk or eat table foods. Instead, she drinks water and orange juice. Thus they offer three meals and two snacks each day, and food is left out all day for snacking because they are concerned about their child not eating enough. They

are frustrated that their child is acting out and being difficult by refusing table foods. They report quality of life issues because they cannot easily feed their child outside of their home without packing foods each time they leave.

You can now summarize what you know about this child's feeding presentation from the interview. She has a persistent (since infancy) feeding disorder for a specific texture (table foods). Problems are frequent (with each solid feeding) and severe (with all table foods). Her diet is consistent with that of a child less than 12 months old. She also appears to have a sensory-based issue with milk because she drinks other liquids without difficulty. It does not appear to be a problem of picky/selective eating. Now we return to the goals of the CSE:

- Possible reasons for the feeding problem: lack of chewing skill, negative feeding experiences leading to learned aversion with vomiting in infancy and choking and vomiting with solids, history of force feeding, and/or limited appetite from grazing throughout the day
- Barriers to feeding progression: long-standing problem since infancy, inappropriate mealtime schedule, negative parent–child interactions, potential underlying gastrointestinal issue, potential underlying upper airway issue
- Need for instrumental swallow assessment: unknown at this time
- Other needed medical referrals: possible gastrointestinal and ear, nose, and throat (ENT) exams pending further investigation
- Diet that is safe and efficient based on the child's skills: appears to be her current diet of thin liquids by open cup, smooth purees, and first finger foods
- Need for feeding intervention: unknown at this time but likely needed to advance diet and meet parental goals

From the interview, you have described the child's feeding presentation. You are formulating your hypothesis regarding the etiology of the problem. It appears that a variety of factors may be contributing to the feeding disorder, and you must determine whether there is a skill-based problem. You should already be anticipating what you will observe during the meal. You are expecting normal oral feeding skills for drinking, purees by spoon, and dissolvable solids. You also expect difficulties chewing table foods or simply refusal of these food items. You have already been observing the child's motor control, communication, and interaction with caregivers, and you have a good sense of normal developmental levels. You must now prove or disprove your hypothesis of chewing impairment and, if proven, determine whether the chewing impairment is due to a structural or functional problem or if there is another unknown etiology.

## 5.3.6 Feeding Presentation: Direct Assessment

The direct assessment is completed via oral peripheral examination and the feeding observation. The structure and function of the oral mechanism are critical components of the CSE because the integrity of the oral mechanism and upper airway is the foundation for oral feeding skills. The feeding observation is the second critical component to your direct assessment. It provides a window into the mealtime experience of the child and parent, and it provides you the opportunity to observe oral feeding skills directly during the meal.

## 5.3.7 Direct Assessment: Oral Peripheral Examination

The oral peripheral examination is conducted in any type of evaluation completed by a speech-language pathologist and is a procedure used to examine the cranial nerves. Although the focus is certainly on the mouth, the entire upper airway system engaged in communication typically assessed by a speech-language pathologist should also be assessed during the CSE. For example, a child with a hoarse vocal quality would lead to suspicion of vocal fold pathology and may interfere with speech intelligibility. However, in children with dysphagia, vocal fold pathology would raise a red flag for the inability to obtain complete glottic closure to protect the airway during swallowing and should lead to a referral to an otolaryngologist (ENT). As well, a child with only nonnasal speech sounds and altered resonance patterns would raise a red flag for poor velopharyngeal closure during swallowing should nasal congestion be heard during a feeding. Identifying differences in the expected structure and function of the oral mechanism may help with a differential diagnosis for other medical professionals when a clear medical or developmental etiology for the feeding disorder has not been identified. For example, an unidentified submucous cleft palate may be determined after your observation of nasal congestion and nasal leakage during feedings.

However, understanding and identifying normal structure and function will provide you the foundation for observations that vary from these expectations. Based on this, it is difficult to describe all the variations from normal that you might observe. Instead, it is more useful for you to understand normal structure and function, which allows you to note any observation that you consider different from typical expectations. It is up to you through your critical thinking to determine whether these differences contribute to the feeding presentation, if they warrant further investigation, and how they might impact the prognosis. For example, open-mouth posture, forward tongue positioning at rest, and drooling could be indicators for low tone and weakness and poor sensory awareness, or they might be indications of upper airway obstruction (such as choanal atresia or enlarged adenoids or palatine tonsils) that require medical assessment.

## 5.3.8 Structure

First you assess the external structures of the head and face. For any child, regardless of age and level of cooperation, the external structure assessment should be completed. The internal examination is often difficult to obtain, and attempts to complete this part of the assessment should be documented (see Chapter 2 on normal anatomy). This assessment focuses on the size, shape, position, condition, and tone of the structures, skin, and tissue as shown in **Table 5.2**.

For all children, structures should be proportionately sized, symmetric, appropriately positioned, and in good condition.

**Table 5.2** Examination of external facial and internal oral structures

| Structure | Size | Symmetry | Position | Condition | Tone |
|---|---|---|---|---|---|
| Head | + | + | + | + | |
| Ears | + | + | + | + | |
| Eyes | + | + | + | + | |
| Nose | + | + | + | + | |
| Mandible | + | + | - | + | |
| Lips | + | + | - | + | |
| Dentition | + | + | + | + | |
| Hard palate | + | + | + | + | |
| Tongue | + | + | + | + | |
| Soft palate | ? | ? | ? | ? | |
| Pharynx | - palatine tonsils 50% to midline | + | + | + | |
| Larynx/vocal folds | ? | ? | ? | ? | |

+ is within range of normal; − is a concern.
For the case example, the child's jaw and lips were in a slightly open position at rest.

Although these observations are not mutually exclusive, certain co-occurring observations are often indicative of a specific genetic or neurologic condition. In general, the jaw should be in a closed position, and the tongue should rest comfortably on the floor of the mouth behind the lower teeth or gums without bunching, elevation, or retraction, as often seen in children with high tone, respiratory issues, and sensory issues. The lips should be moist and should rest comfortably together, symmetrically. The nares should be symmetric with adequate opening for comfortable nasal breathing. The hard palate should be rounded but not high or arched. Dental alignment should be observed for factors related to poor chewing and general oral hygiene. Oral tissue should be pink and moist and without atypical color or condition of teeth. Neonates may have some facial asymmetry due to tightness in facial musculature or the neck and shoulder girdle from unusual positioning in utero or from the delivery process, which may impact range of motion of the jaw, lips, and tongue and should spontaneously resolve. However, these observations may also indicate an underlying neurologic or genetic etiology.

Examples of observations include the following:

- Size: microcephaly (small head), thin upper lip, macroglossia (large tongue)
- Symmetry: right labial droop
- Position: low-set ears, wide-set eyes, tongue protruding from mouth at rest
- Condition: dry or cracked lips, repaired cleft lip, atrophy of the tongue
- Tone: tight cheek tissue

## 5.3.9 Function

Next, you will assess the movements of the oral mechanism. The range of motion, coordination, and timing of oral movements

**Table 5.3** Examination of external facial and internal oral function

| Function | Symmetry | Range of motion | Coordination | Strength |
|---|---|---|---|---|
| Mandible/jaw | + | + with yawn and then on command | + repeated model but then accurate | + |
| Lips | + smile | + | + | + |
| Tongue | + | - no lateral movements | - | + |
| Soft palate/ resonance | ? | ? | hyponasal | ? |
| Vocal folds/ voice | + | + | + | + |

*+ is within range of normal; ? is unknown/unable to determine; – is a concern.*

spontaneously versus during feeding or on command provide key information of the integrity of the mechanism, as shown in **Table 5.3**. Ideally you will already have observed and noted spontaneous movements throughout the first portion of the CSE. If possible, oral movements should be observed in a structured task using verbal commands or via imitation of a model. Movements should be observed in isolation as discrete movements or in repeated or combined movements to distinguish between overall reduced function (e.g., weakness, fatigue) from impairment in the voluntary control of movements (e.g., oral apraxia). Typically developing toddlers might engage in some oral-motor imitation tasks, but preschool-aged children and beyond should attempt imitation tasks to assess for cranial nerve deficits and overall range of motion, coordination, and timing of oral movements. Some of these tasks can simply be observed in typical interaction and do not need to be elicited (e.g., vocal quality). Overall, this process can take just minutes. This has been described in detail in other sources.[11,12]

In general, spontaneous movements and movements during a structured task should be smooth and coordinated, with full range of motion and adequate strength. If the child is old enough to follow commands, prompt the following:

- Open and close your mouth; do this three times.
- Smack your lips; repeat three times.
- Smile.
- Show me a kiss; smile and kiss three times.
- Stick out your tongue.
- Open your mouth and touch your tongue to your top lip, then to your bottom lip, right lip corner, and left lip corner, and then lick your lips all around.
- Touch your tongue to the right lip corner, then the left; repeat three times.
- Push on the tongue depressor during tongue protrusion, lateral movements, etc.
- Show me your teeth; bite down.
- Click your tongue; repeat three times.
- Open your mouth and touch your tongue to the roof of your mouth, inside right cheek, inside left cheek.

- Open your mouth wide (*note the soft palate and pharynx*), say /ah/ (*note the movement of the soft palate and observe for palatine tonsils*).

It is important to document whether movements were observed spontaneously, upon command, or via modeling. If the child is unable or does not understand the task, observe for the child to perform these movements spontaneously (does the jaw open widely for a yawn or cry? do the lips fully retract for a smile or evenly purse for a kiss?). Note the accuracy in discrete (or individual) movements versus movements repeated or combined. Also note if you started with a command, visual model, and any other strategies required in order to elicit accuracy, such as repeated modeling, instruction, or tactile input.

The jaw should open evenly with full range of motion and return and maintain a closed position. The lips should retract symmetrically without tensing or curling under and should purse evenly. The tongue should smoothly protrude beyond the lower lip with tongue shape maintaining a flattened/thinned or cupped posture, elevate to upper lip and alveolar ridge independent of the jaw, and lateralize to the lip corners and to the inside of cheeks. The tongue tip should be pointed upon protrusion for licking the lips or licking foods. The soft palate should elevate evenly and the posterior pharynx should be clear. For neonates and infants, retraction of the tongue tip or the inability to protrude the tongue beyond the lower lip should be a red flag for tongue-tie (ankyloglossia) or incoordination of movements. In infants older than 6 months, spontaneous movements of the tongue to lip corners or into the cheek are positive for integrity of the mechanism but do not guarantee voluntary control of these same movements when moving a solid bolus. Saliva control expectations vary by age and eruption of dentition. A wet vocal quality might suggest pooling of secretions in the pharynx due to poor sensation, infrequent swallowing, or aspiration.

For the 3-year-old referred for picky eating, you observe overall facial symmetry and the appearance of normal facial tone. The tongue remains in the mouth at rest, but the jaw and lips are slightly open at rest. She allows a very brief look inside her mouth, and the hard palate is intact and of normal shape. Her dentition is normal. Her voice is clear, and articulation is appropriate for her age. Her nasal resonance is hyponasal, and saliva management is normal. She readily participates in oral imitation tasks. You had observed her yawning earlier in the visit and noted full range of motion of the jaw, with return to the closed position. When you tell her to open and close her mouth she opens her mouth fully but needs a verbal prompt in order to close. You repeat this twice, and by the third trial she can open and close her mouth with coordinated movements and appropriate range of motion and timing. She is able to retract and purse her lips both in isolation and in sequence. Coordination was an initial concern, with repeated modeling needed before achieving it, which is likely due to her age. She was unable to achieve lateral tongue movements even with tactile input. Completion of a form such as **Table 5.4** will assist in identification of underlying neurologic compromise.

For infants, assessment of oral reflexes and nonnutritive sucking (NNS) is appropriate during this time. Oral reflexes include rooting, transverse tongue, suck, and gag. A gloved finger or pacifier should be used to assess the response to oral stimulation

**Table 5.4** Oral peripheral/cranial nerve examination to assess integrity of the structure and function of the speech mechanism

| Task | +/− | Description of concern |
|---|---|---|
| **CN V: trigeminal** | | |
| Jaw opening/closing | | |
| Alternate open/close | | |
| Jaw resistance during closing | | |
| **CN VII: facial** | | |
| Facial symmetry | | |
| Lip closure | | |
| Lip retraction | | |
| Lip purse | | |
| Alternate retraction and purse | | |
| Intra-oral pressure | | |
| Lip smack | | |
| Show teeth | | |
| Bite | | |
| Resist eye opening | | |
| **CN X: vagus** | | |
| Palatal elevation | | |
| Gag | | |
| Vocal quality | | |
| **CN XII: hypoglossal** | | |
| Tongue protrusion | | |
| Tongue elevation to upper lip | | |
| Tongue depression | | |
| External lateralization to lip corner right/left | | |
| Alternate external lateralization | | |
| Lick lips | | |
| Tongue click | | |
| Internal lateralization right/left | | |

*+ is within range of normal; ; ? is unknown/unable to determine; − is a concern.*

throughout the oral cavity, the tone of the tongue, and strength and movement patterns of the tongue during sucking. NNS is established quickly with gagging or stress cues. In the neonatal period, the tongue first strips the nipple front to back. Changes to true up/down tongue motions for nipple compression evolve due to improved jaw stability. Lips should be flanged outward on the nipple base with little leakage of secretions from the lips (and without lip retraction or curling). Infants that have reduced range of motion of the tongue due to tongue-tie, reduced tongue-cupping ability, or increased facial tone often pull their lips inward or bite on the nipple to compensate for lack of tongue mobility. As described earlier, the tongue should easily protrude to the lower lip without retraction of the tongue tip while maintaining a thin and cupped tongue shape. NNS performance is measured as two sucks per second.[7] Sucking performance is discussed in greater detail later in the chapter.

## 5.3.10 Direct Assessment: Feeding Observation

As a feeding clinician you want to be involved from the start of the meal observation; watching the parent–child interaction during setup, initiation of the meal, and the mealtime process can be very informative. A tube feeding observation may be helpful in understanding a child's behaviors, interactions and tolerance to the feeding process. Caregivers should bring typical foods eaten, utensils and cups used, and food items that are difficult to feed. Observations of how a bottle is made, how much food is provided, how it is prepared (texture, bite size, etc.), which utensils are used, and how food is presented can lead to clues about the problem. How the child is held, seated, and positioned also provides critical information. Start with typical eating and drinking. During the feeding observation, try to observe a liquid, a puree, and a chewable solid from each texture category

**Table 5.5** Possible signs of an oral-sensory versus an oral-motor impairment for children

| Oral sensory impairment | Oral motor impairment |
|---|---|
| Refuses certain material of a spout cup | Loss of food from mouth despite attempts to contain |
| Unaware of food loss or food in mouth | Smaller than expected bolus size or bite size for age |
| Prefers certain temperature of liquid/food | Bolus scatter, oral residue unable to clear |
| Prefers bland foods or spicy foods | Slow, inaccurate chewing motions, inability to bite through foods, inadequate breakdown of foods |
| Brand-specific preferences | Gagging with foods when unable to propel or break down |
| Gags on food despite adequate skills | Lack of advancement of diet for an entire texture category |

**Table 5.6** Nutritive sucking performance measures

| Skill | Performance | Variable |
|---|---|---|
| Suck | Frequency and periodicity of sucking events | Number of sucks; bursts; pauses, sucks/burst; sucking rate; pressures |
| Swallow | Timing of swallowing events | Suck–swallow ratio; temporal physiological and bolus flow measures; pressures |
| Breathe | Respiratory patterns | Swallow apnea; oxygen saturations; rest/pause |

appropriate for age. Your goal is to determine contributions from oral sensory and oral motor impairment. Oral sensory and oral motor impairment characteristics are not mutually exclusive. This list of characteristics is meant to assist in critical thinking about the child's diet and presentation as shown in **Table 5.5**.

Note the following:

- Who feeds
- What strategies are used to initiate the meal
- Sucking organization
- How quickly bites are presented or taken
- Size of bites
- Length of time it takes to complete each bite
- Specific oral skills used
- Any difficulties in bolus manipulation or swallowing
- Parent–child interaction

Depending on your observations, you may attempt therapeutic trials (e.g., changes to positioning, types of foods, textures of foods, bolus size, utensils, presentation rate). Therapeutic trials during the feeding observation may occur, but the extent of trials is dependent on the child's age, level of cooperation, and current feeding status. For infants, only breast and/or bottle feeding will be observed, and you will rely on positioning, flow rate, and pacing techniques. For some children, the extent of the feeding observation is eliciting nonnutritive sucking on a pacifier or finger or conducting pacifier dips due to known dysphagia or identified risk factors. For preschool-aged and older children, attempts to adjust and modify those variables in the list should be completed during the therapeutic trials. Through these trials you aim to reduce identified problems and elicit increased acceptance, efficiency, and safety. The results of these trials and the critical thinking you have done throughout all components of this evaluation will help you with your differential diagnosis and help determine the next steps.

There are many different checklists and clinical tools available for tracking oral feeding skills by direct observation but limited choices that meet desired psychometric properties. Again, as with the oral peripheral examination, it is crucial that you understand and integrate normal oral feeding expectations as the baseline

for your observations. It is impossible to describe and present all possible variations from these baseline expectations, and clinicians should not rely on "recipes" for decision making. You will need to determine if variations from baseline expectations are contributing to the feeding disorder.

## Infant Feeding Observation

Unlike NNS, nutritive sucking (NS) performance is measured as one suck per second.[7] Suck–swallow–breathe coordination during NS is a highly complex skill, with increased demands on breathing when coupled with liquid swallows. Infants unable to meet expectations during NNS are at high risk for faltering with NS demands. For either NNS or NS, sucking performance is measured using three main skills as detailed in **Table 5.6**.[6,7,17,18,19,20]

Some of these variables require instrumentation and are not feasible for the average evaluation. However, direct observation is possible for several of these variables and should be considered during an infant feeding observation, primarily those variables related to sucking.[15] Sucking bursts are measured when at least two sucks occur in a row with no more than 2 or 3 seconds' pause between sucks, which marks the end of a burst. Between birth and 6 months of age, the number of sucks per burst and the duration of bursts increase, and the number of bursts per feeding and the duration between bursts decrease. That is, as infants age, they sequence a greater number of sucks together without requiring a pause, thereby decreasing the total number of bursts needed, as

**Table 5.7** Nutritive sucking performance of term, healthy infants during a 5-minute portion of a bottle feeding

| Age | Sucks/burst | Number of sucks | Number of bursts | Sucks per minute | Sucking rate |
|---|---|---|---|---|---|
| DOL 2 | 13 | 216 | 22 | 43 | 0.72 |
| 1 month | 38 | 290 | 8 | 67 | 1.1 |
| 3 months | 43 | 315 | 7 | 70 | 1.2 |
| 6 months | 82 | 372 | 5 | 81 | 1.3 |

*Summary data from [4] compiled from variety of sources. Data were calculated from available data for sucks per minute and sucking rate, and all data are rounded up/down except for sucking rate.*

**Table 5.7** summarizes. The suck–swallow ratio (SSR) is another critical measurement. The optimal SSR is 1:1, but 2 to 3:1 generally results in an efficient feeding. Increased or variable SSR is an indication of problems, such as weakness, fatigue, increased work of breathing, or incoordination. Infants not achieving this performance may have feedings that last too long, which may increase the risk for dysphagia, with or without aspiration. Referral for an instrumental assessment should occur with ongoing signs or symptoms of dysphagia, with or without aspiration, despite intervention.

It is important to initially observe the caregiver feeding the infant, if possible, to elicit the problems the infant is reported to exhibit. You may also identify compensations the caregiver has already initiated so that you can determine what intervention is needed during the therapeutic trial. Monitor the amount consumed and the duration of the feeding as an indicator of feeding efficiency. When stress cues are observed, interventions should be applied. The type of stress cues you observe will help you to decide what intervention to start with. Stress cues would include observations of gagging, eye widening, gulping, flailing, liquid loss, coughing/choking, breathing changes, pulling off the nipple, and arching. The hierarchy of interventions, listed here in order in which the interventions are generally applied, consist of the following:

- Sensory inputs (e.g., tactile, proprioceptive; to assist in oral organization, state control, latch).
- Bolus flow management (e.g., by increasing or decreasing flow with change in nipple or position)
- Pausing/stopping feeding (e.g., breathing breaks or pulling nipple from mouth)

Stress cues are not exclusively linked to a particular intervention and can suggest different problems and different needs, as shown in **Table 5.8**. The frequency and severity of these cues will dictate where you begin and how quickly you move through interventions until stress cues are minimized, organization is improved, and signs and symptoms of dysphagia, with or without aspiration, are resolved. For example, an infant might have a high SSR of 5:1 with a slow-flow nipple and three sucks per burst, but she is able to manage the flow of liquid without difficulty in a cradled, semireclined position. You change the nipple to a faster flow, with a positive outcome of a 2:1 SSR, but now the infant demonstrates stress cues (eye widening and gulping) for the increased flow rate, requiring a position change or pacing. You must then teach the caregiver how to implement the new position to ensure successful transition at home.

## Child Feeding Observation

For children transitioning to solids, oral skills are rapidly changing.[6,7,13,14,21,22,23,24,25,26,27,28,29] Between 6 and 12 months of age, oral feeding skills change from skills for liquids only to chewing and swallowing table foods. Infants first introduced to a spoon around 6 months of age will have reduced range of motion of their jaw, opening too little for the bolus and the spoon, or opening too wide. Often the spoon touches the lips before the infant opens her mouth given her lack of experience or previous sensory feedback for this new task. The spoon enters the infant's mouth without the infant closing her mouth on the spoon to clear the bolus. Thus parents often scrape the bolus off the spoon and onto the infant's upper gums. The infant may bite on the spoon as the parent tries to remove the spoon from her mouth. Lip residue is common after a spoon presentation. Infants are not aware of the residue and do not attempt to clear it, leaving parents to scrape the lips with the spoon and re-present it to the child. These infants will use strong tongue protrusion and a suckle pattern to propel the puree for

**Table 5.8** Common observations and hierarchy of interventions during infant sucking observations

| Observation/stress cues | Possible intervention | Description of intervention/therapeutic trials |
|---|---|---|
| Flailing, arm extension | Sensory input | Nonnutritive sucking, taste |
| Eyebrow furrow, arching | | Swaddle, physical pressure |
| Gagging with nipple on tongue | | Rocking, bouncing, swaying |
| Move nipple around in mouth | | Chin or cheek support |
| Slow sucking | Flow management (increase or decrease flow) | Chin or cheek support |
| Minimal sucks/burst | | Position change |
| Pauses greater than 2–3 seconds between bursts | | Tip bottle or tilt in space to slow flow |
| High suck–swallow ratio | | Tip bottle or tilt in space to stop flow for "x" number of sucks or for every "x" sucks |
| Falling asleep | | Change nipple and/or bottle |
| Liquid loss, eye widening | | Change consistency of liquid |
| Coughing, gulping | | |
| Nasal flaring | | |
| Retractions, stridor | | |
| Choking, desaturations | Pause/stop feeding | Remove nipple from mouth for "x" period of time |
| Head bobbing, breath holding | | Remove nipple from mouth and give pacifier/nonnutritive sucking |
| Frantic | | Discontinue feeding |
| Tachypnea, stridor | | |

the swallow, thereby pushing out a portion of the bolus and swallowing the rest. Some gagging and facial grimacing may occur, but generally these events are not persistent and do not result in vomiting. Within 2 to 3 weeks of spoon introduction, these events lessen, and infants begin to accommodate the amount of jaw opening for the size of the bolus and spoon, demonstrating motor learning from experience and feedback. With daily practice, by 8 months of age the oral feeding skills for spoon feeding have dramatically improved. The infant maintains mouth opening as the spoon approaches, the tongue remains in the mouth, both upper and lower lips contact the spoon, the timing and efficiency of opening for the spoon are observed, with more consistent lip contact on the spoon. The tongue protrusion has decreased or has been replaced with more intentional propulsion of the bolus with upward and backward movement of the tongue. Lip residue lessens with more accurate timing of mouth opening, but residue is still not cleared by the infant. The infant is not bothered by food on her lips or face. Although their interest in eating by spoon may vary as they are tired at the end of the day or when ill, overall infants enjoy the eating experience.

Chewing efficiency dramatically improves for solids between 6 and 18 months as the amount of time to chew a solid and the number of chewing motions both decrease. By the time children are introduced to their first chewable solid foods at 8 months of age, they demonstrate more refined skills than when first starting spoon feeding, even with little to no experience. Chewing rate is similar to nutritive sucking and is about one chewing cycle per second regardless of age.

For first finger foods, children open for a solid with more stable jaw movements and timing; they attempt biting in the front of their mouth, rather than on the side, but are often unsuccessful at biting

through the solid without multiple attempts. Multiple motions of the cheek and lips are used, with some lateral shifting of the tongue to move the solid to the molar surfaces (even though they do not have molars yet). Chewing motions are brief, with some random or unintentional movements during attempts to control and swallow the solid, resulting in some food falling out of the mouth. By 10 months of age, children learn how to vary the range of jaw opening for different-sized solids, vary the amount of force generated during the initial chewing phase based on the firmness and thickness of the solid, and build endurance for longer chewing cycles. Chewing motions are more intentional and efficient, with active lateral movement of the bolus, longer chewing motions, and less bolus loss. However, by 12 months of age, children can bite through solids in one motion, lateralize the solid to molar surfaces, and use jaw movements in varying directions to break down their first table foods.[13] If no lateral movement of the solid bolus is observed, the child is not demonstrating adequate skills to chew solid foods safely and efficiently. Children at this age may demonstrate brief chewing for first finger foods, but this skill does not automatically transfer to first table foods or regular table foods. This distinction is extremely important; children with chewing impairment often plateau at their first finger foods, but they are interpreted as being picky.

As first table foods are introduced, children may revert back to early chewing motions when attempting to manage different textures that are more difficult to control (e.g., slippery fruit). Children at this age show increased awareness of residue on their lips and face; they might begin to use their hands and lips to clear the residue, but tongue movements are not used until sometime later. The grinding and shearing motions required to break down advanced table foods do not develop until children reach or exceed 3 years of age.[29] As with the introduction to spoon feeding,

**Table 5.9** Recommended age of texture introduction, specific oral feeding skills, and possible concerning observations at each age

| Recommended age of introduction | Oral feeding skills needed | Possible concerning observations (cumulative concerns) |
|---|---|---|
| 6 and 7 months: Infant smooth puree | Inconsistently opens mouth for spoon; little attempt to close lips on spoon; bolus pushed out of mouth; may gag | Frequent gagging and vomiting or coughing and choking, increasing refusal |
| 8 and 9 months: Infant textured puree First finger foods Spout cup | More consistent mouth opening and lip closure on spoon; bolus remains in mouth Picks up solids and brings to mouth; attempts to bite pieces in front of mouth; lateral shift of solid; few chewing cycles/motions; early up-down chewing (munch) Inconsistent lip closure on cup, small individual sips, some coughing, consistent liquid loss from mouth Unable to extract from spill-proof cup or straw | No lip closure on spoon, strong tongue protrusion No attempts to bite on solid Frequent gagging and vomiting or coughing and choking, increasing refusal Chronic coughing/choking, wet vocal quality |
| 10 and 11 months: First table foods Open cup/straw | Efficient skills for spoon feeding; tongue mashing pieces; improved chewing; moves food to side with tongue Efficient drinking from spout cup, sequential swallows Inconsistent lip closure on open cup, small individual sips, some coughing, consistent liquid loss from mouth | Poor bolus maintenance for purees No lateral movement of solid bolus; only tongue mashing Only individual swallows or refusal of cup Chronic coughing/choking, wet vocal quality with any cup |
| 12 to 35 months: Regular table foods | Biting and chewing skills more efficient Bites through solids in one motion, consistently lateralizes solid to molar surfaces, and uses jaw movements in varying directions to break down Efficient drinking from cup and straw | Unable to break down solid bolus of first table foods, food loss, oral residue |
| 36+ months: Advanced table foods | Grinding and shearing motions of jaw to break down advanced table foods | Unable to break down solid bolus of regular table foods, food loss, oral residue |

Key: Infant smooth puree: cohesive smoothly blended baby or table food; First finger foods: easily dissolvable or meltable solids; First table foods: soft, cooked, table food that requires only limited chewing; Regular table foods: range of table foods and textures that require more mature chewing; Advanced table foods: fibrous meats, nuts, hard fresh vegetables, etc.

children at this age may gag as they learn to manage each new texture. Usually these gagging events are brief and do not persist. The key skills required are listed in **Table 5.9**.

## Clinical Note

Understanding a child's feeding presentation is as equally important as the direct assessment of oral feeding skills.

As you observe stress cues and skill-based problems, you may begin to modify the presentation. If concerns are for coughing with an open cup, you may reduce the sip size or alter the cup to reduce the bolus size. If the child is gagging on first finger foods with tongue mashing only, you might try lateral placement on molars for the first bite. If this is unsuccessful you might revert to nonnutritive chewing on a therapy tool.

For our 3-year-old, the parents bring a wide variety of preferred foods and refused foods. The child requests to eat during the interview. Prior to the observation, there is no coughing or throat clearing. She sounds slightly congested, but her parents report no current illness. The parents make up a plate of food consisting of two graham cracker squares, 10 pretzel sticks, two raw baby carrots, one-fourth cup cubed baked chicken, and a 6-ounce container of yogurt with an infant-sized spoon. They put two 6-ounce cups in front of her, one with water and one with milk. Both are open cups with straws. While they are preparing the plate, the child states, "No I don't want that" and refuses to sit down. The parents comment that this is typical and say that she is just being "behavioral." You have them remove the refused foods (i.e., carrot, chicken), put these on a separate plate on the table, and return the other plate to the table. The rationale is to be able to observe typical eating first in order to note skills before she completely refuses to eat. She begins by scooping half of the infant spoon, opens as the spoon approaches, closes her lips and clears the spoon, and keeps her lips closed during the swallow. When asked, the parents report that she only takes that amount on the spoon, otherwise she might gag. You ask her to take a full spoon of yogurt and she complies. She uses the same oral skills, but this time she uses a chin tuck and effortful swallow, and after the swallow you note throat clearing and a mild cough. The parent report that this is the typical gagging they observe. You ask her to repeat, and she does, with the same occurrences, but this time she takes a drink. She demonstrates good lip closure on the straw without biting, and sequential swallows without coughing or throat clearing. After the liquid swallows, she exhales loudly. She picks up the graham cracker square, places it at her front teeth, and takes a very small bite the size of a pea. She holds it for about 5 seconds on her tongue, elevates her tongue to her palate mashing the cracker on the roof of her mouth, and swallows. Some cracker crumbs remain on her tongue, which she clears with water. She repeats this until the square is completed over 10 minutes. The parents report this as being typical. She resumes eating her yogurt in her preferred way, finishing half the container, and she finishes her water without difficulty. You had established a rapport with her earlier in the interview, and partway through the feeding observation you

sit down with the family. You move the plate of table foods next to your patient. You ask her to try one of the foods. She refuses. You implement a shaping procedure to desensitize her to the food (i.e., stepwise process to engage in exploring the food); all of which she does. She complies with a request to take a small bite, which she does, surprisingly. She attempts to mash it with her tongue, fails to lateralize to her molars, gags, and vomits and refuses to complete further tasks.

You have now completed the direct assessment portion of the CSE. You must now complete subsequent screenings to identify red flags and other issues contributing to the feeding presentation.

## Clinical Note

Your counseling and recommendations should always focus on the safety and feeding efficiency of the child.

# 5.4 Consideration for Screenings

As a clinician, you determine the presence of red flags/concerns in other areas that may be contributing to the child's presentation. A failed screening warrants consideration of a referral to another provider. As speech-language pathologists do during a general language evaluation, you are screening for differences in voice, fluency, prosody, resonance, and articulation, even though you may not complete a formal assessment in those areas. During a feeding evaluation, you are responsible for screening for differences in all areas of communication. You should also identify or screen other important areas that could impact a child's feeding and swallowing abilities. Goday and colleagues (2019) have defined Pediatric Feeding Disorder as impaired oral intake that is not age appropriate and is associated with medical, nutritional, feeding skill, and/or psychological dysfunction. They define diagnostic criteria within each domain that a feeding clinician must always consider during their clinical swallow evaluation.[30] Although these screenings are not formalized surveys, they are based on pass/fail criteria for noting observations as red flags or of no concern.

## 5.4.1 Swallow Screen

Swallow screens have been proposed to identify those patients at risk for aspiration, such as the pass/fail 3-ounce water challenge.[31] Consideration for a swallowing screen in pediatrics depends on a variety of factors.[32] Every feeding evaluation should include a "screening" (either formal or informal) to determine the need for an instrumental swallowing assessment by identifying signs/symptoms of dysphagia, with or without aspiration. Possible signs/symptoms of dysphagia will be identified during your chart review, through the interview process, and through your observations. This is similar to any other medical provider screening for feeding and swallowing concerns or red flags contributing to their area of expertise.

## 5.4.2 Respiratory Screen

Respiratory screening should be performed in any evaluation. Again, the process of screening the respiratory system is to identify any factors contributing to the child's feeding difficulties. Be sure to note breathing prior to the feeding observation and specifically note changes in breathing during the meal. Changes from normal breathing expectations can lead to referrals regarding points of obstruction or restriction, which impact the child's ability to coordinate breathing and chewing and/or swallowing.[33,34] These changes would include noisy or labored breathing, retractions above or below the sternum, and stridor or high-pitched noises during inspiration and/or expiration. Increased respiratory rates negatively impact infant feeding performance by shortening sucking bursts due to the need for longer pauses for catch-up breathing, poorer swallowing coordination leading to coughing, and increased fatigue due to increased work of breathing and energy expenditure.

## 5.4.3 Gastrointestinal Screen

The gastrointestinal screening identifies underlying problems in a child's gastrointestinal tract related to motility, tolerance, and absorption.[35,36] Be sure to note difficult or effortful swallowing, discomfort, arching, and distress after swallowing or after a feeding; unusual reactions during or after feedings, such as rash, sneezing, congestion, and vomiting; and complaints of pain or discomfort.

## 5.4.4 Nutrition Screen

The nutrition screening occurs during the interview for current feeding status. You will identify variations from expected intake or differences in what the child consumes. A referral for a nutrition consult is warranted when a child has issues that include avoidance of an entire food group, refusal to drink a nutritious beverage, or growth concerns. Not only are we screening for growth but also for aspects of nutrition and hydration, which are described in greater detail elsewhere.[5,6,7,8,9,10]

## 5.4.5 Neurologic/Developmental Screen

The neurologic screening identifies any changes in muscle tone, movement coordination, and postural stability that might influence the function of the swallowing mechanism. This includes your screening of gross and fine motor skills, even in the neonatal period. As described earlier, a speech-language pathologist should always screen for aspects of communication and how those issues might impact feeding and swallowing abilities. All developmental domains should be screened because each could impact the feeding expectations.[32] These developmental levels provide the basis on which your recommendations will be based. While we know that a child's developmental level will drive the treatment recommendations and the prognosis, we do not know which developmental domain is most predictive of feeding outcomes.[32]

In our 3-year-old case example, red flags were identified for the following:

- Instrumental swallow referral
  - Possible concerns for pharyngeal dysphagia due to throat clearing and effortful swallowing, coughing, and using liquids after puree swallows
  - Concerns for negative impacts of upper airway obstruction on pharyngeal swallow
- Gastrointestinal referral
  - Concerns for milk and/or food allergy due to vomiting with formula based on cow's milk in infancy and refusal of cow's milk
  - Esophageal dysmotility due to effortful swallowing after puree swallows even though limited bolus size and throat clearing after swallow
  - Ongoing gastroesophageal reflux or other issues, such as EoE due to the foregoing concerns and restless sleeping
- ENT referral
  - Concerns for upper airway obstruction due to snoring at night and restless sleeping, loud exhale after drinking, hyponasal resonance, open jaw and lip position at rest, presence of palatine tonsil tissue during oral peripheral examination, nasal congestion in the absence of an illness
- Nutrition referral
  - Possible nutrition concerns due to lack of nutritious beverage and no table foods

## 5.5 Differential Diagnosis: Red Flags and Critical Thinking

A differential diagnosis entails a list of the possible contributing factors to the problem/s that led to the reason for referral and the child's feeding presentation. All decisions regarding your findings of the evaluation are based on typical expectations of feeding development and achievement of feeding milestones coupled with your direct assessment. Your impressions and recommendations from the CSE will be complete when you answer the following questions:

1. Is the reason for the referral the actual problem?
2. Is this a lifelong, persistent, or acute feeding disorder?
3. Is the problem based on oral-motor impairment, oral-sensory impairment, or both?
4. Is the problem related to potential swallowing impairment?
5. How do these impairments impact the child's diet?
6. Is the child capable of an age-appropriate diet?
7. What are the interfering factors to achieving diet goals and feeding milestones?
8. Would direct feeding intervention be beneficial?
9. What is a safe and efficient diet for the child?
10. What are reasonable intervention goals?

In the case of our 3-year-old "picky eater," even when inaccurate, any reason for the referral to a CSE is acceptable since it allowed the child to be seen. This child was not a picky eater but has oral skill impairment. This has been a persistent disorder since the introduction of all chewable solid foods and is based on oral-motor impairment and lack of lateral movement of a solid bolus for chewing. She also presents with reduced bolus size for preferred texture of purees that appears related to effortful swallowing and discomfort rather than an oral-sensory or oral-motor impairment. The child is not currently capable of an age-appropriate diet, which negatively impacts the quality of life for her and her family. Red flags were identified for a pharyngeal swallowing impairment that may be related to upper airway obstruction due to observation of puree swallows. There are concerns for nutrition, gastrointestinal status, and upper airway status, which could all be impacting feeding presentation. These possible medical issues may have caused discomfort and vomiting at the first texture introduction, which have led to refusals and now lack of skill development. However, lack of skill may have led to swallowing solids whole and then vomiting and subsequent refusals. Either way, medical issues must be confirmed or ruled out. From the direct assessment, oral skill impairment was confirmed and would benefit from intervention. Intervention goals should focus on development of jaw and tongue movements to support chewing skills.

## 5.5.1 Recommendations and Counseling

Finally, recommendations, counseling, and treatment planning will complete the CSE. Your therapeutic trials and integration of all the information gathered are meant to be helpful in distinguishing between a *feeding plan* and a *treatment plan*. The goal of mealtimes at home is to provide adequate nutrition and hydration for growth and development. Challenging oral skills at each meal is not advised unless there is a specific plan with a team of feeding professionals helping to monitor growth and nutrition status. Changes you make can have a negative impact that you are not capable of assessing alone.

The feeding plan consists of the recommendations you provide to the family about how to feed their child every single day. The plan should support efficiency and nutrition at each meal. The feeding plan may include specific interventions, such as the order of presentation of liquids and foods to increase volume, limiting volumes of textures that oral feeding skills do not support, or modifications to foods to increase intake.

The treatment plan is the recommendations you provide to the treating clinician for skill development and possible suggestions for the family for next steps in advancing their child's diet. The treatment plan may include specific interventions to elicit new skills, improve strength and coordination, or improve swallowing safety.

Based on our example, the ideal feeding plan would be as follows:

- Food is offered only at scheduled meals and snacks without grazing during the day.
- Offer milk-based products at each meal pending determination from a physician or dietitian on a specific product.
- Allow a small, pureed bolus with liquid after each bite to help with swallowing.
- Offer dissolvable solids only with close monitoring to avoid choking. Texture education for parents would be helpful to understand the difference between textures that melt and those that require true chewing.

- Encourage tasting of table foods without a requirement for taking bites to avoid negative feeding experiences and the risk for choking and vomiting. Education for parents on skills is needed for table foods.
- However, this is generally too much to change at once and you need to prioritize based on health and safety factors and what the caregivers feel is manageable.

## 5.5.2 Referrals

- Have a discussion with a pediatrician regarding concerns and red flags and potential referrals to nutritional, gastrointestinal, and ENT specialists and for possible completion of instrumental swallow assessment.

## 5.5.3 Counseling

The parents' goals and expectations are paramount to the next steps. As completed in the interview, the parents' concerns, expectations, and goals for their child's feeding difficulties were discussed. Sometimes parental expectations exceed those of the child's capabilities, and parents need to be counseled as to the pieces that need to be in place before their goals are reached. As well, parents often carry a great deal of guilt; feeding a child is one of the most essential and basic parental tasks. They have likely experienced criticism from others about their child's feeding differences. Recall feeding principles described at the beginning of this chapter: Children learn to eat with ease. Children with a feeding disorder do not respond to typical strategies used by parents, and parents are often confused, frustrated, and very concerned. You will use the foundation principles of typical feeding expectations to demonstrate to parents how their child's feeding abilities differ and why they were unable to resolve these differences. When parents' concerns about their child's feeding difficulties are confirmed and when they understand why their child has not met expected feeding milestones, they will partner with you to implement a feeding plan. This step in counseling a family is paramount to the child's success. Some expectations are too difficult for a family to implement; an open conversation with the parents about an ideal feeding plan will help you determine an appropriate first step. Changing the family's mealtime structure and routine is often overwhelming. Setting up a stepwise plan will be better received and more easily achieved. Strong counseling skills are essential for pediatric feeding clinicians in order to communicate essential information effectively in a caring and nonjudgmental way, to promote the child's success. You will help parents understand goals that are accurate, reasonable, achievable, and feasible. Using the framework of these expectations will provide context for the parents regarding their child's progression of eating, previous problems, next steps, and prognosis.

## 5.5.4 Evidence for Utility of Exam

There is no professional better equipped than a speech-language pathologist to conduct a feeding evaluation. Speech-language pathologists have expertise in the anatomy and physiology of feeding and swallowing mechanisms and in general development.

The differences in the anatomy and physiology that may pertain to speech and language difficulties have direct application to feeding. There is a clear progression in the developmental oral feeding skills and in achievement of feeding milestones. A comprehensive and formal CSE provides key clinical information required as the medical team makes decisions about diagnostic tests, medical procedures, and intervention recommendations.

## 5.6 Questions

1. A 2-year-old child presents to the CSE with concerns of being a picky eater. Current complaints include persistent gagging with each solid-texture transition and a diet consisting of milk by cup and pureed baby foods. What are the potential reasons for this clinical presentation?

A. Oral-motor impairment
B. Poor esophageal motility
C. Anxiety
D. All of the above
E. None of the above

2. What feeding principle/s should be used as normal expectations when evaluating a child of any age?

A. Transient gagging is expected with any transition to a new texture.
B. Children should enjoy mealtimes.
C. Free access to food during the day will encourage children to eat.
D. Both A and B
E. All of the above

3. A 3-month-old infant presents to the clinical swallow evaluation due to poor growth. The pediatrician's note indicates that the baby appears to drink the expected amount of formula each day to grow appropriately. What other variables should be considered?

A. How much formula the baby drinks at each bottle
B. How long the caregiver spends feeding the baby each bottle
C. Breathing changes that occur during the feeding
D. Both A and C
E. All of the above

4. Which of the following is the goal of the chart review as part of the clinical swallow evaluation?

A. Providing an understanding of the timing of onset of feeding difficulties and the persistent or acute nature of problems
B. Providing information about the mealtime process related to schedule, location, specific strategies, oral and enteral intake at the present time
C. Determining whether there is a problem in structure and function of the swallowing mechanism
D. Identifying skill-based etiology
E. Generating possible clinical hypotheses for the child's presentation based on medical, developmental, and feeding experiences

5. Observations of the jaw during chewing provide information about which cranial nerve?

A. IX—glossopharyngeal
B. X—vagus
C. V—trigeminal
D. VII—facial
E. XII—hypoglossal

## 5.7 Answers and Explanations

### 1. Correct: all of the above (D).
The presenting complaints may be due to oral-motor impairment, poor esophageal motility, and/or anxiety. The clinical swallow evaluation will help determine the possible cause of the child's presenting symptom of picky eating.

### 2. Correct: both A and B (D).
It is important to remember that mealtimes should be enjoyable for children and their parents and that gagging is expected as children are learning to eat new foods/textures. The gagging should be transient in nature and should not inhibit the child's exploration of the new food/texture. Free access to food during the day does not encourage the child to eat, therefore C is not correct, and E (all of the above) cannot be correct either.

### 3. Correct: all of the above (E).
The volume of formula given with each bottle may influence the time spent feeding for the infant. Excessive volume of formula may lead to reflux, which is known to affect growth. Prolonged mealtimes (feeding the infant a bottle over more than 15–20 minutes) can also impact growth over time. Breathing changes that occur during feeding may be indicative of aspiration. Chronic aspiration is also linked to poor growth. D (both A and C) excludes choice B, which is an appropriate consideration in this scenario, so D cannot be correct. Choosing either A, B, or C alone also leaves out appropriate considerations.

### 4. Correct: generating possible clinical hypotheses for the child's presentation based on medical, developmental, and feeding experiences (E).
The chart review should generate possible clinical hypotheses for the child's presentation based on medical, developmental, and feeding experiences. A and B are both goals of the caregiver interview. C and D are both expected to be gleaned during the direct assessment of the child's feeding skills.

### 5. Correct: V—trigeminal (C).
Cranial nerve V provides innervation to the muscles of mastication. Cranial nerves IX, X, VII, and XII are all important for feeding and swallowing; however, they have no direct innervation to the muscles of mastication and therefore would not be influencing jaw movement during chewing.

# References

[1] Park J, Pados B, Thoyre S, Estrem H, McComish C. (In Press). Factor structure and psychometric properties of the Child Oral and Motor Proficiency Scale (ChOMPS). *Journal of Early Intervention.* Thoyre S, Pados B, Park J, Estrem H, McComish, C, Hodges E. *Journal of Pediatric Gastroenterology & Nutrition,* 2018: 66(2), 299-305. doi: 10.1097/MPG.0000000000001765

[2] Heckathorn DE, Speyer R, Taylor J, Cordier R. Systematic review: non-instrumental swallowing and feeding assessments in pediatrics. *Dysphagia* 2016;31(1):1–23

[3] Pados BF, Park J, Estrem H, Awotwi A. Assessment tools for evaluation of oral feeding in infants younger than 6 months. *Adv Neonatal Care* 2016;16(2):143–150

[4] Benfer KA, Weir KA, Boyd RN. Clinimetrics of measures of oropharyngeal dysphagia for preschool children with cerebral palsy and neurodevelopmental disabilities: a systematic review. *Dev Med Child Neurol* 2012;54(9):784–795

[5] American Academy of Pediatrics. Accessed November 21, 2015. www.Healthy-Children.org

[6] Delaney AL, Arvedson JC. Development of swallowing and feeding: prenatal through first year of life. *Dev Disabil Res Rev* 2008;14(2):105–117

[7] Delaney AL, Rudolph CD. Nascent oral phase. In: Shaker R, Belafsky PC, Postma GN, Easterling C, eds. *Principles of Deglutition: A Multidisciplinary Text for Swallowing and Its Disorders.* New York, NY: Springer; 2012:151–162

[8] Kleinman RE, Coletta FA. Historical overview of transitional feeding recommendations and vegetable feeding practices for infants and young children. *Nutr Today* 2016;51(1):7–13

[9] Samour PQ, King K. *Handbook of Pediatric Nutrition.* Burlington, MA: Jones and Bartlett Learning; 2006

[10] USDA website. MyPlate.gov. 2016

[11] Love RJ, Webb WG. *Neurology for the Speech-Language Pathologist.* Newton, MA: Butterworth-Heinemann; 1996

[12] Robbins J, Klee T. Clinical assessment of oropharyngeal motor development in young children. *J Speech Hear Disord* 1987;52(3):271–277

[13] Delaney AL. *Oral-Motor Movement Patterns in Feeding Development.* Dissertation. University of Wisconsin. 2010

[14] Morris SE. *Pre-Speech Assessment Scale.* Clifton: J.A. Preston; 1982

[15] Thoyre SM, Shaker CS, Pridham KF. The early feeding skills assessment for preterm infants *Neonatal Netw* 2005;24(3):7–16

[16] da Costa SP, van den Engel-Hoek L, Bos AF. Sucking and swallowing in infants and diagnostic tools. *J Perinatol* 2008;28(4):247–257

[17] Lau C, Schanler RJ. Oral motor function in the neonate. *Clin Perinatol* 1996;23(2):161–178

[18] Medoff-Cooper B, Bilker W, Kaplan JM. Sucking patterns and behavioral state in 1- and 2-day-old full-term infants. *J Obstet Gynecol Neonatal Nurs* 2010;39(5):519–524

[19] Medoff-Cooper B. Nutritive sucking research: from clinical questions to research answers. *J Perinat Neonatal Nurs* 2005;19(3):265–272

[20] Arvedson JC, Delaney AL. Development of oromotor functions for feeding. In: Roig-Quilis M, Pennington L, eds. *Oromotor Disorders in Childhood.* Barcelona: Viguera Editores, SL; 2011:25–41

[21] Gisel EG. Chewing cycles in 2- to 8-year-old normal children: a developmental profile. *Am J Occup Ther* 1988;42(1):40–46

[22] Gisel EG. Effect of food texture on the development of chewing of children between six months and two years of age. *Dev Med Child Neurol* 1991;33(1):69–79

[23] Green JR, Moore CA, Ruark JL, Rodda PR, Morvée WT, VanWitzenburg MJ. Development of chewing in children from 12 to 48 months: longitudinal study of EMG patterns. *J Neurophysiol* 1997;77(5):2704–2716

[24] Le Révérend BJD, Edelson LR, Loret C. Anatomical, functional, physiological and behavioural aspects of the development of mastication in early childhood. *Br J Nutr* 2014;111(3):403–414

[25] Schwaab LM, Niman CW, Gisel EG. Comparison of chewing cycles in 2-, 3-, 4-, and 5-year-old normal children. *Am J Occup Ther* 1986;40(1):40–43

[26] Stolovitz P, Gisel EG. Circumoral movements in response to three different food textures in children 6 months to 2 years of age. *Dysphagia* 1991;6(1):17–25

[27] van den Engel-Hoek L, van Hulst KC, van Gerven MH, van Haaften L, de Groot SA. Development of oral motor behavior related to the skill assisted spoon feeding. *Infant Behav Dev* 2014;37(2):187–191

[28] Wilson EM, Green JR, Weismer G. A kinematic description of the temporal characteristics of jaw motion for early chewing: preliminary findings. *J Speech Lang Hear Res* 2012;55(2):626–638

[29] Goday PS, Huh SY, Silverman A, Lukens CT, Dodrill P, Cohen, SS, et al. Pediatric feeding disorder: consensus definition and conceptual framework. *J Pediatr Gastroenterol Nutr.* 2019 Jan;68(1): 124–129

[30] Suiter DM, Leder SB, Karas DE. The 3-ounce (90-cc) water swallow challenge: a screening test for children with suspected oropharyngeal dysphagia. *Otolaryngol Head Neck Surg* 2009;140(2):187–190

[31] Delaney AL. Special considerations for the pediatric population relating to a swallow screen versus clinical swallow or instrumental evaluation. *Perspectives on Swallowing and Swallowing Disorders (Dysphagia)* 2015;24:26–33 10.1044/sasd24.1.26

[32] Ayari S, Aubertin G, Girschig H, Van Den Abbeele T, Mondain M. Pathophysiology and diagnostic approach to laryngomalacia in infants. *Eur Ann Otorhinolaryngol Head Neck Dis* 2012;129(5):257–263

[33] Lyons M, Vlastarakos PV, Nikolopoulos TP. Congenital and acquired developmental problems of the upper airway in newborns and infants. *Early Hum Dev* 2012;88(12):951–955

[34] Kirby M, Noel RJ. Nutrition and gastrointestinal tract assessment and management of children with dysphagia. *Semin Speech Lang* 2007;28(3):180–189

[35] Rudolph CD, Link DT. Feeding disorders in infants and children. *Pediatr Clin North Am* 2002;49(1):97–112, vi

# Suggested Reading

[1] DeMatteo C, Matovich D, Hjartarson A. Comparison of clinical and videofluoroscopic evaluation of children with feeding and swallowing difficulties. *Dev Med Child Neurol* 2005;47(3):149–157

[2] Glass RP, Wolf LS. *Feeding and Swallowing Disorders in Infancy: Assessment and Management.* San Antonio, TX: Therapy Skill Builders; 1992

[3] Rommel N. Assessment techniques for babies, infants and children. In: Cichero J, Murdoch B, eds. *Dysphagia: Foundation, Theory, and Practice.* Chichester, UK: John Wiley & Sons Ltd, 2006:466–486

# 6 Adult Videofluoroscopic Swallow Evaluation

*Catriona M. Steele*

## Summary

This chapter reviews the videofluoroscopic swallowing examination in detail to equip readers with a solid understanding of the indications for and purpose of a videofluoroscopic exam. Important technical aspects of the examination are reviewed, including radiation safety, image acquisition rate, and contrast media. Various approaches to the design of videofluoroscopy testing protocols are discussed, with an emphasis on the value of standardizing the diagnostic portion of the examination. Common procedures for rating swallowing safety and postswallow residue are discussed, as well as physiologic parameters that can be measured to confirm hypotheses regarding the mechanisms behind swallowing impairment. This chapter will equip and encourage clinicians to use videofluoroscopy not only for detecting aspiration but also to reveal pathophysiology, guide treatment choices, and measure change in patients with dysphagia over time.

## Keywords

videofluoroscopy, swallowing assessment, standardization, X-ray, protocols, physiology, barium, aspiration, residue, radiation exposure.

### Learning Objectives

- Describe the indications for performing videofluoroscopy, and apply this to clinical case scenarios.
- Collaborate with radiologic personnel to determine the optimal image acquisition rates and settings used in videofluoroscopy.
- Understand the importance of preparing barium stimuli with low weight-to-volume concentration according to standard recipes.
- Design a standard testing protocol for diagnostic and therapeutic probe purposes.
- Describe the Penetration-Aspiration Scale as well as current methods for rating residue severity.
- Understand which physiologic parameters are believed to be linked to the risk of penetration and aspiration.

## 6.1 Introduction

Clinical or bedside swallowing examinations are key to evaluating swallowing function in people suspected of having dysphagia. However, the information we can collect from a clinical examination is limited, because we cannot see what happens inside the mouth, pharynx, and esophagus—the clinician forms inferences about events that are not directly observed. These inferences are often correct, but in some cases, they are only an educated guess based on the available information and may be incorrect. The presence or absence of a cough after a swallow of water is commonly weighed heavily in judging the patient's safety when swallowing, but it is widely recognized that this sign can be misleading. The absence of a cough and the observation of a clear voice quality after a swallow are used as clinical evidence that penetration and aspiration are unlikely to have occurred. Of course, if the patient has silent aspiration, in which an aspiration event elicits no observable clinical signs, then this inference would be incorrect. On the other hand, the presence of a cough after a swallow is typically interpreted as clinical evidence that aspiration may have occurred. This may also not be the case, and importantly, even if the cough does represent an aspiration event, the clinician doesn't know whether the cough was effective in expelling material from the airway. These two examples of the types of clinical inference that arise from a clinical bedside swallowing assessment may lead a clinician to follow up with an instrumental examination. The clinician may also wish to understand the physiologic mechanisms behind penetration-aspiration or residue, or to directly observe the impact of compensatory maneuvers on swallowing function, both of which require an instrumental swallowing examination.

Two types of instrumental examination are commonly performed to explore these questions:

1. The videofluoroscopic swallow study (VFSS)
2. The fiberoptic endoscopic examination of swallowing (FEES)

This chapter describes the VFSS in detail and addresses the following key topics:

- What is a videofluoroscopic exam?
- What are the indications for performing a videofluoroscopic exam?
- How does one choose between videofluoroscopy and FEES?
- Who is usually present at a videofluoroscopic exam?
- What radiation safety considerations arise with the use of videofluoroscopy?
- What are the technical aspects of a videofluoroscopic exam?
- How are contrast media used in videofluoroscopy?
- How does one design the videofluoroscopic procedure?
- How is videofluoroscopy used to evaluate swallowing safety?
- How is videofluoroscopy used to evaluate swallowing efficiency?
- How is videofluoroscopy used to determine the pathophysiology behind swallowing? impairment?
- How is videofluoroscopy used for treatment planning and outcome measurement?

## 6.2 What Is a Videofluoroscopic Exam?

Videofluoroscopy is a dynamic X-ray procedure performed using a fluoroscope and recorded to a video format. When this technique is used to study swallowing function, various procedural names may be used (**Box 6.1**). Each of these names serves to describe the focus of the examination or to distinguish this examination from other similar radiological tests (e.g., a barium swallow, which is an examination of the esophageal phase of swallowing).

---

### Box 6.1

**Various Names and Abbreviations for Videofluoroscopy**

- VFSS—videofluoroscopic swallowing study
- VFSE—videofluoroscopic swallowing examination
- MBS—modified barium swallow
- PPA—palatopharyngeal analysis
- OPMS—oropharyngeal motility study
- Cine-esophagram
- Cookie swallow (named for the Lorna Doone cookie that was used in the procedure)

---

Videofluoroscopy of oropharyngeal swallowing involves the administration of liquid and food stimuli, mixed with a radi-opaque contrast medium (e.g., barium), and the observation of swallowing with these stimuli on X-ray. Dynamic sequences of X-ray images are collected and viewed as a movie to reveal the physiology of swallowing.

In the United States, videofluoroscopy of the oropharyngeal phases of swallowing is currently reimbursed under Medicare code 92611 (Motion fluoroscopic evaluation of swallowing function by cine or video recording).[1] In addition to this code, the radiology department may request reimbursement for radiologist involvement in the procedure using Medicare code 74230 (Swallowing function, with cineradiography/videoradiography).

## 6.3 What Are the Indications for Performing a Videofluoroscopic Exam?

A videofluoroscopic examination provides an opportunity to see inside the oropharynx and to observe how structures move during the different phases of swallowing. This inside view enables the clinician to appreciate aspects of swallowing that are not externally visible in a clinical or bedside swallowing examination. This opportunity to see inside provides valuable understanding of what is wrong with a person's swallowing function, as well as a means to explore the mechanisms behind the impairment. The primary indications or purposes of the exam have been summarized in the American Speech-Language-Hearing Association (ASHA) guideline *Clinical Indications for Instrumental Assessment of Dysphagia*[2] and are listed in **Box 6.2**. In addition to these indicators, the ASHA guideline points out that there may be situations, including the following, in which videofluoroscopy is not appropriate:

- When the clinical examination suggests that the patient does not have dysphagia
- When the patient is too medically unstable to tolerate the procedure
- When the patient is unable to cooperate or participate in an instrumental examination
- When, in the speech-language pathologist's judgment, the instrumental examination would not change the clinical management of the patient

---

### Box 6.2

**Clinical Indications for an Instrumental Assessment of Swallowing[2]**

- An instrumental examination *is indicated* for making the diagnosis and/or planning effective management and treatment in patients with suspected, or who are at high risk for, oropharyngeal dysphagia based on the clinical examination when
  - The patient's signs and symptoms are inconsistent with findings on the clinical examination.
  - There is a need to confirm a suspected medical diagnosis and/or assist in the determination of a differential medical diagnosis.
  - Confirmation and/or differential diagnosis of the dysphagia is needed.
  - There is either nutritional or pulmonary compromise and a question of whether the oropharyngeal dysphagia is contributing to these conditions.
  - The safety and efficiency of the swallow remain as concerns.
  - Tthe patient is identified as a swallow rehabilitation candidate and specific information is needed to guide management and treatment.
- An instrumental examination *may be indicated* for making the diagnosis and/or planning effective treatment in patients with suspected dysphagia based on the clinical examination and the presence of one or more of the following:
  - The patient has a medical condition or diagnosis associated with a high risk for dysphagia, including but not limited to neurologic, pulmonary or cardiopulmonary, gastrointestinal problems; immune system compromise; surgery and/or radiotherapy to the head and neck; and craniofacial abnormalities.
  - The patient has a previously diagnosed dysphagia, and a change in swallow function is suspected.
  - The patient has a condition such as cognitive or communication deficits that preclude completion of a valid clinical examination.
  - The patient has a chronic degenerative disease or a disease with a known progression, or is in a stable or recovering condition for which oropharyngeal function may require further definition for management.

---

When we evaluate a person's swallowing, we need to consider two primary functional concerns in swallowing:

1. Swallowing safety
2. Swallowing efficiency

*Swallowing safety* is defined as the ability to move a bolus of liquid, food, or saliva from the mouth through the pharynx to the esophagus without any of that material entering the airway. The fact that the upper aerodigestive tract supports the multiple tasks of breathing, swallowing, and phonation means that we are susceptible to material entering the airway if the breathing passage's reconfiguration to one for swallowing takes too long or fails to happen at all. Material entering the airway is referred to as penetration-aspiration. *Swallowing efficiency* is defined as the ability to move a bolus of liquid or food from the mouth through the pharynx into the esophagus in a timely fashion, without leaving residue behind in the spaces of the oropharynx. Typically, we expect a person to completely clear a bolus through the oropharynx in one or two swallows.

Videofluoroscopy provides a means of confirming whether a person has impaired swallowing safety or impaired swallowing efficiency. The videofluoroscopic evidence is more direct than the inferences that can be made based on subjective clinical observation. For example, penetration-aspiration can be seen on videofluoroscopy, confirming or refuting suspicions that were made on the basis of clinical observation. Similarly, residue can be seen and confirmed (or ruled out) with videofluoroscopy.

In addition to confirming the presence of impairments in swallowing safety and efficiency, videofluoroscopy provides an important opportunity to probe the effectiveness of different treatment techniques designed to improve swallowing function. The selection of specific techniques will vary, depending on the mechanisms that are thought to be contributing to the impairment. Using videofluoroscopy to test interventions is a very important component of testing, which directly supports clinical decision making regarding dysphagia management.

Videofluoroscopy is usually considered to be a physiologic examination, but it will also reveal the anatomy of the oropharynx, allowing the clinician to identify structural abnormalities that may partially explain why the patient is experiencing swallowing difficulty. These can include abnormalities of the cervical spine, such as cervical osteophytes (bony spurs that can form on the corners of the cervical vertebrae, causing a protrusion into the wall of the pharynx). Other structural abnormalities that may be visible with videofluoroscopy include webs or strictures, diverticuli (pouches in the walls of the pharynx), and fistulae (abnormal connections between parts of the upper aerodigestive tract that are usually separated, such as the trachea and the esophagus).[3] Dysphagia clinicians are not typically trained to be able to detect soft tissue lesions in the oropharynx (such as tumors), but if these are present, a radiologist may recognize them. Whenever a structural abnormality is seen or suspected on a videofluoroscopic image, a radiologist should be consulted as to whether additional tests are needed to determine the nature and severity of the problem.

## 6.4 How Does One Choose between Videofluoroscopy and FEES?

Videofluoroscopy was first described as a procedure for swallowing assessment in the early 1980s through the publication of Dr. Jeri Logemann's seminal textbook on dysphagia[4] as well as articles by leading radiologists who described their approaches to the examination.[5,6,7,8,9] The fiberoptic endoscopic examination of swallowing (FEES) was introduced a few years later in 1988.[10] When the new procedure was developed, it became important to understand the strengths and limitations of each procedure so that clinicians could determine which one would be most appropriate for their patients.

Videofluoroscopy's main strength is that it allows the clinician to watch the swallow, from the moment that the bolus enters the mouth until it enters the esophagus, and to recognize features of swallowing physiology that are functioning properly or abnormally. However, this procedure must be limited to a relatively small number of boluses or tasks in order to avoid unnecessary radiation exposure. The procedure also requires the use of radio-opaque contrast media, such as barium, that differ from foods and regular liquids in taste and other important characteristics, such as viscosity. Furthermore, the procedure is conducted in a radiology suite, with equipment, noise, medical personnel, and procedures that all differ from a normal mealtime situation. Any and all of these issues might alter the patient's behavior such that the swallows seen in the examination may not represent the way the patient would swallow at a meal or outside the testing situation.

By contrast, a FEES examination does not require transportation to a radiology suite and does not involve radiation or radio-opaque contrast media. Thus the procedure may be ideal for patients who cannot easily be transported, regular foods and liquids can be used, and a longer procedure can be performed without concern for radiation exposure. However, these benefits have their own limitations. A FEES exam requires that an endoscope be passed transnasally, which may cause discomfort for some patients and potentially impact closure of the velopharyngeal port. Additionally, the view provided by a FEES exam does not allow the clinician to see biomechanical features of swallowing that may help to explain impairment, such as hyolaryngeal excursion. On the other hand, visualization of the location of preswallow pooling or postswallow residue, and its proximity to the larynx, is superb. One of the most important limitations of a FEES exam is the fact that the camera view experiences a period of "white-out" during the swallow, when constriction of the pharynx and the movement of structures causes a backward reflection of light, which blocks the camera view. There is a moment when information is not available, and one can never completely rule out the possibility that important events, including penetration-aspiration, may have occurred during that white-out period. Expert FEES clinicians are able to draw inferences about what happens during the white-out period by inspecting the laryngeal vestibule, vocal folds, and tracheal rings when the view becomes available again, but there is always some possibility that an aspiration event occurred but left no clues.

Both instrumental procedures have their strengths and their limitations. The choice of procedure will depend on a variety of considerations, including (but not limited to) the medical status of the patient; whether the patient can be easily transported to the radiology department; whether this is a first or repeat swallowing examination; how quickly and easily the facilities, equipment, and personnel for either exam can be accessed; whether there is a concern about using barium; and whether visualizing the structural integrity and appearance of the larynx is also an assessment objective.

## 6.5 Who Is Usually Present at a Videofluoroscopic Exam?

Various health care professionals may be present at a VFSS examination. They must have expertise in the following areas:

- Competency and knowledge operating a fluoroscopy machine (typically requiring either a radiologist or a suitably trained radiation technologist)
- Competency directing the videofluoroscopy protocol to reveal problems in swallowing
- Knowledge of swallowing physiology and of pathophysiological indications for specific treatment techniques

In addition to these key roles, additional personnel may be present to help with recording the exam to a video format, and to assist with feeding. For patients with complex conditions, additional personnel, such as nurses or respiratory therapists, may attend to assist with tasks like suctioning.

It is important to remember that detecting swallowing problems online in real time during the VFSS procedure is challenging. For this reason, it is strongly recommended that you do not attempt to communicate the results of the examination to the patient immediately after the procedure. Instead, the recording should be reviewed in detail so that you can be confident about the results. However, in some cases, having a second clinician present to observe the procedure (perhaps in conjunction with operating the recording equipment) provides a useful opportunity for a second set of eyes to monitor the procedure online. Dialogue between the primary clinician, radiologic personnel, and any other clinicians who may be present can serve a valuable function online for discussing the patient's swallowing and guiding choices regarding additional swallows or therapeutic maneuvers to explore.

## 6.6 What Radiation Safety Considerations Arise with the Use of Videofluoroscopy?

Radiology professionals are trained to adhere to the "ALARA" (as low as reasonably achievable) principle. According to this principle, the amount of radiation that is delivered in a medical test should be limited to the extent possible, while seeking to answer the medical questions that need to be explored. Radiation dose is measured in units called milliSieverts (mSv). Another term you may encounter is Gray or milliGray. Technically, milliSieverts are used to describe the dose received, whereas milliGrays are used to describe the amount of radiation to which the person is exposed. One milliSievert is the dose received from exposure to one milliGray. Background radiation exposure is known to occur in everyday activities, such as flying in a plane (0.005 mSv per hour) or smoking cigarettes (0.18 mSv per half-pack) as well as during medical tests, such as a chest X-ray (0.02 mSv) or a computed tomographic scan (10 mSv). In North America, the average person experiences between 2 and 4 mSv background radiation exposure each year. Most regulatory bodies recommend that occupationally exposed workers not exceed 20 mSv per year.

Several researchers have tried to quantify the levels of radiation exposure associated with a VFSS in patient populations. Of course the specific dose experienced by the patient will depend on a variety of factors, including the number of swallows collected, how long it takes the patient to complete each swallow, the size of the radiation field, the amount of radiation generated to produce a clear image, and the skill of the radiology professional in turning the fluoroscope on and off at the best times to capture relevant information. As a general rule, videofluoroscopy involves low levels of radiation exposure to the patient, and this exposure carries the risk of stochastic radiation effects (such as gene mutation and cancer). Stochastic radiation effects are effects produced at random without a threshold dose level. Their probability of occurrence increases with increased radiation dose, but their severity is independent of the dose.

Zammit-Maempel and colleagues[11] reported a median exposure time of 171 seconds and an associated dose of 0.20 mSv, while Moro and Cazzani[12] reported a median exposure time of 149 seconds and an associated dose of 0.35 mSv. Moro and Cazzani[12] showed that this dose (0.35 mSv) corresponds to a risk of 1 in 39,000 of developing a radiation-induced stochastic effect from a VFSS. In a study of healthy young adults, Molfenter and Steele[13] performed a protocol requiring participants to swallow 15 liquid boluses. The mean (± standard deviation [SD]) radiation exposure time across participants was measured to 1.75 ± 0.31 min, with a corresponding dose estimate of 0.24 ± 0.11 mSv. On average, this was estimated to translate to an extremely rare 1 in 57,000 risk of stochastic radiation effects.

In addition to considering the radiation exposure received by the patient, it is important to understand the radiation exposure risks incurred by the clinicians themselves. In reality, clinicians should be able to take measures to reduce their radiation exposure to zero. These measures include wearing protective lead aprons and thyroid collars and moving to locations inside the fluoroscopy suite where the radiation scatter has dissipated.

When protective lead aprons are not worn, the clinician runs the risk of exposure to radiation scatter. One study from Australia has estimated that a clinician who does not wear a thyroid collar will receive between 0 and 0.017 mSv of radiation dose at the thyroid in a 3- to 4-minute procedure, and that wearing a thyroid collar reduces this dose by a factor of about 40.[14] In terms of where to stand in the fluoroscopy suite, it is important to know that the radiation will scatter out from the source in radial arcs, and that the dose reduces with increasing distance from the source according to the inverse square law. For clinicians, the primary source of radiation scatter is the patient. By stepping backward and to one side, clinicians will dramatically reduce their radiation dose, compared to a position standing immediately in front of the patient. Any location that is 6 feet away from the source is considered to be a zero-exposure location (**Fig. 6.1**).

In her original *Manual for the Videofluorographic Study of Swallowing*,[15] Dr. Logemann advised that clinicians should be careful to keep their hand out of the radiation beam, and when this was not possible, that they should wear a lead-lined glove. However, in a review article in ASHA's SIG 13 Perspectives publication in October 2004,[16] radiation physicist Dr. Lisa Lemen wrote "[a] lead glove and a person's hand will attenuate part of the radiation being received by the [image intensifier] II tube, and the [fluoroscopy] system may boost the tube current to compensate for the fewer photons if a significant amount is blocked" (p. 12). This indicates that it may be in error to assume that a lead glove provides good protection to the clinician. If the attenuation of a significant portion of the image occurs due to the intrusion of a lead glove, or another attenuating object, then the fluoroscope may increase the dose of radiation to optimize the image. A greater dose to the patient will, in turn, generate a greater scatter dose to the clinician. For this reason, a lead glove should not be placed into the field.

## 6.7 What Are the Technical Aspects of a Videofluoroscopic Exam?

### Field of View

A videofluoroscopic examination of the oropharyngeal phases of swallowing typically begins in the lateral (sagittal) view, and may conclude with an anterior-posterior (coronal) view. In the lateral plane, it is important to capture the oral cavity in the field of view as well as the pharynx and the first portion of the cervical esophagus. **Fig. 6.2** illustrates the ideal boundaries of a sagittal view videofluoroscopic image. It is important to recognize that several key structures in the lateral view will move upward during the swallow. These include the hyoid, the larynx, and the upper esophageal sphincter. Consequently, the field of view should be established to capture both the lowest (starting) and the highest positions of these structures. It is ideal to set the field of view on a still frame at the beginning of the procedure, and to avoid moving the camera too much during the test. In particular, the radiological personnel should be asked to avoid chasing the bolus down through the esophagus in the lateral view, so that a clear view of the airway and pharynx is maintained after the bolus passes.

In an ideal videofluoroscopic study, the procedure will include an anterior-posterior view. This serves to illustrate the symmetry of structures and bolus movement through the pharynx, allows visualization of vocal fold movement, and enables the clinician to evaluate bolus movement through the cervical esophagus. The ideal boundaries of an anterior-posterior pharyngeal field of view are illustrated in **Fig. 6.3**. The radiologist may find that visualization in the anterior plane is improved if the table is tilted to be parallel to the cervical spine, thereby achieving a constant distance between the source of the radiation and the cervical spine along its entire length. In contrast to the lateral view, it is quite common to move the camera to follow the bolus down through the esophagus in an anterior view examination. Occasionally, the radiologist may choose additional views to further explore suspected anatomical abnormalities during videofluoroscopy. For example, an oblique view is often used to further investigate and measure diverticuli.[3]

### 6.7.1 Image Acquisition Rate

A videofluoroscopic study captures a dynamic sequence of images that can be played as a movie. This makes it important to

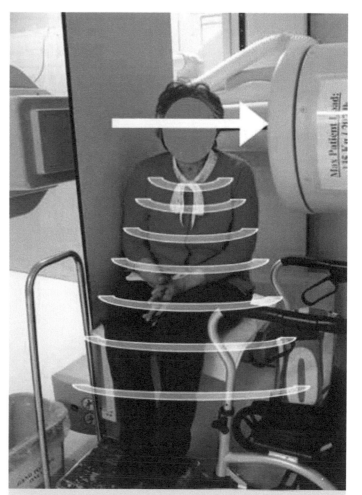

**Fig. 6.1** The typical videofluoroscopy setup, in which the patient is seated between the table and the image intensifier tube, which registers the X-ray image. The source of radiation is behind the table (to the left of the image). The white arrow shows the direction of the radiation beam, which will scatter outward from the patient in radial arcs toward the clinician. The dose will reduce asymptotic according to the inverse square law. By moving backward and to one side, clinicians will dramatically reduce their radiation dose.

think about how many images are going to be collected, and how far apart these images are spaced in time, to understand whether the procedure is accurately capturing the moving events that take place in swallowing. Several terms are used in regard to the image acquisition rate for videofluoroscopy. *Frame rate* is a term that was historically used in a generic sense to describe the number of images that were generated per second in a videofluoroscopic study. Advances in imaging technology have introduced the need to be clear about the differences between fluoroscopy rate, pulse rate, and frame rate.

*Fluoroscopy rate* refers to the number of images that are produced by the fluoroscope each second. On older, analog systems, the radiation beam that created the X-ray image was either "on" or "off," and when it was "on," the radiation was continuous. On analog systems, the number of images that are produced per second depends on the frame rate of the recording system. In North America, standard video recording systems operate at a frame rate of 30 frames per second, whereas European, Japanese,

by recording videofluoroscopy at 30 frames per second, and then manipulating the recording to delete every second image, thereby creating a version with 15 images per second.[17] There are three main findings from these studies:

1. Penetration-aspiration events are more frequently missed in recordings with only 15 images per second. This suggests that penetration-aspiration events can sometimes be extremely brief (i.e., shorter than 1/15 of a second).[17]

2. For patients who have penetration-aspiration, fewer swallows are required at 30 images per second to catch the problem than at 15 images per second. This finding has been used to suggest that radiation exposure may, in fact, *not* end up being lower at 15 pulses per second, particularly if extra swallows are needed to reveal the problem.[17]

3. Interrater agreement for Penetration-Aspiration Scale scores and overall impairment scores measured with the Modified Barium Swallow Impairment Profile (MBSImp)[18] are reported to be higher when there are only 15 images per second.[19] This last finding may actually not be an entirely unexpected result, because there is less opportunity for disagreement across raters when fewer images are being reviewed. The finding is not dissimilar to the report that interrater agreement regarding penetration-aspiration is higher when binary decisions are made compared to the full 8-point Penetration-Aspiration Scale.[20] It is important to remember that agreement and reliability across raters are not the same as rating accuracy.

Although these research findings do not provide explicit guidance for clinicians who are trying to decide on the best image acquisition rates to use in their videofluoroscopies, they do raise three important questions for you to consider:

1. How serious would it be if you missed a brief penetration-aspiration event because you were capturing only 15 (or fewer) images per second?
   - For some patients, this might not be considered to be terribly serious, because a very brief penetration-aspiration event is more likely to involve only a tiny amount of material entering the airway. If a penetration-aspiration event is not visible at 15 images per second, perhaps it is not significant enough to warrant intervention.
   - On the other hand, there may be some patients where respiratory concerns are very serious, and the clinician wants to be very confident that no penetration-aspiration events have been missed. In these cases, 15 images per second are probably inadequate to rule out penetration-aspiration as a problem. Certainly, image acquisition rates below 15 images per second should be considered inadequate in terms of sensitivity for detecting penetration-aspiration.

2. How serious is the additional radiation exposure required to generate 30 images per second?
   - This question deals directly with the ALARA radiological ideal. In some cases (e.g., working with very young children), there may be valid reasons to limit radiation exposure by using pulse rates of 15 pulses per second. However, 15 images per second should be considered the lower limit; anything lower is likely to miss important information. It

is also important to remember that you might be able to answer your clinical questions more efficiently (i.e., in fewer swallows), if you pulse and record at 30 images per second, so the argument that radiation is saved at lower pulse rates may not be valid.

3. What else can be missed when fewer than 30 images per second are captured?
   - Swallowing is a dynamic physiologic process, and one purpose of a videofluoroscopic exam is to look beyond the functional outcomes of penetration-aspiration or residue, to reveal the underlying mechanisms behind these problems. A second goal of the exam may be to explore the benefits of maneuvers for addressing pathophysiology. If fewer than 30 images per second are recorded, this will introduce constraints on the clinician's ability to discern the mechanisms behind impairment.

## 6.8 How Are Contrast Media Used in Videofluoroscopy?

A variety of contrast agents are available for medical imaging. Most commonly, these products involve either barium or iodine, and they have in common the ability to attenuate radiation, so that they appear as a contrasting black object on a videofluoroscopic image. The degree of contrast and the visibility of the radiopaque substance depend on the concentration of barium or iodine, which is typically expressed in weight per unit volume (w/v). Most contrast media used in gastrointestinal imaging have been mixed with other ingredients to aid particle suspension or reduce foaming.

In most countries, clinicians who are performing videofluoroscopic studies of oropharyngeal swallowing use contrast media that have been developed for gastrointestinal imaging procedures. If these products are barium based, they will come in either a high or low concentration, also referred to as double- or single-contrast examination products. Double-contrast barium products typically have a concentration of > 100% w/v barium, and are specifically intended to leave a coating along the lining of the gastrointestinal mucosa as they flow through tubes like the pharynx and the esophagus. Single-contrast barium products typically have a concentration of < 100% w/v barium and are supposed to flow through the gastrointestinal tract without leaving any residual coating on the walls. It is important to be aware of the concentration of the product you are using in videofluoroscopy so that you can know whether a coating that remains behind on the walls or in the spaces of the pharynx was expected or is a true clinical finding representing poor bolus clearance.[21]

The question of the ideal barium concentration for oropharyngeal swallowing studies has become a focus of research. In the late 1990s, Bracco Imaging (formerly E-Z-EM) released a new barium product in the United States known as Varibar, developed by Dr. JoAnne Robbins at the University of Wisconsin–Madison. The barium is designed to be low concentration (40% w/v), with this target providing a level of contrast that is clearly visible on videofluoroscopy but not concentrated enough to leave a coating on the walls of the pharynx. Additionally, the Varibar product line offers several consistencies of product (e.g., Thin, Nectar, and Thin-Honey products, which map to the thin, mildly thick, and moderately thick levels of the International Dysphagia Diet Standardisation Initiative Framework, www.iddsi.org) with the specific purpose of supporting dysphagia clinicians to explore the benefits of thickened liquids for people with dysphagia. Unfortunately, at the time of writing, these products are not available outside the United States.

In 2008, a paper by Fink and Ross[22] raised the possibility that slightly increased viscosity might be a side-product of a 40% w/v barium concentration, such as that used in the Varibar products. If the purpose of thin barium stimuli is to mimic the conditions that a patient would experience when drinking water, any slight thickening that occurs as a result of adding barium could alter swallowing behavior. Fink and Ross showed that some patients who were able to swallow 40% w/v barium without problems showed penetration or aspiration on a diluted 20% w/v barium liquid. They suggested, therefore, that a 20% w/v dilution was more representative of a true thin liquid. Regardless of the concentration of barium that you choose to include in your videofluoroscopies, and the different consistencies that you wish to test, it is important to develop standardized methods of preparing your test stimuli so that they are always the same. Avoid eyeballing the dilution or thickening a videofluoroscopy test material, because it leads to variable results.

In some countries, and in some research literature, there are reports of swallowing studies that have used iodine-based contrast agents. One of these products, Hypaque (also known as Gastrografin), is preferred for gastrointestinal imaging studies where the integrity of a surgical anastomosis is being evaluated. This preference arises from the fact that the product does not cause harm if it leaks through a suture line into the peritoneal cavity. However, iodinated contrast agents can cause quite serious adverse events if they are aspirated into the lungs.[23] A recent development in radiological imaging products has been the introduction of contrast agents that use iohexol or iopamidol (e.g., GE Healthcare OMNIPAQUE, Bracco Gastromiro, Bracco Isovue, Bracco Iopamiro). These products were originally developed as injectable contrast agents for angiography, but the versions intended for oral administration are in the form of a clear liquid that is water soluble and easily absorbed in the lungs without causing damage in the event of aspiration.

## 6.9 How Does One Design the Videofluoroscopic Procedure?

In her original description of the videofluoroscopic procedure,[15] Logemann recommended beginning the procedure with the administration of thin liquid barium in 1-, 3-, 5-, and 10-mL volumes. If aspiration or significant residue was not observed on the initial presentation of a bolus, that bolus would be repeated once or twice more, to confirm the result. If three presentations of a bolus were tolerated without any concern, the procedure would move to a larger volume. After demonstrated tolerance of 10-mL boluses, cup drinking would be tested. At the end of liquid testing in the lateral position, Logemann's protocol would test two boluses of pudding-thick barium and a solid stimulus (one-fourth of a cookie coated in barium paste). Once these stimuli were completed, Logemann recommended that the patient be placed in an anterior-posterior position, and that any stimuli on which concerns had been observed in the lateral plane be repeated in this position.

In the event that a significant concern was noted on a particular bolus, Logemann recommended departing from the test protocol and repeating the problematic bolus with a compensatory maneuver intended to mitigate the underlying mechanism of dysfunction. If postural maneuvers were unsuccessful, voluntary airway protection or stimulation techniques would be tried, and if none of these techniques was successful, thicker liquids would be tested. With this approach, Logemann illustrates both the diagnostic and the therapeutic purposes of videofluoroscopy. It may be of interest to note that, in Sweden, Dr. Olle Ekberg and colleagues routinely perform two videofluoroscopic examinations for each patient. The first is a diagnostic examination, which follows a standard protocol with the aim of revealing abnormal physiology. The second is a therapeutic examination, designed based on the diagnostic exam results, and intended to explore the benefits of specific intervention approaches for the patient. A seminal article by radiologists Bronwyn Jones and Martin Donner captures the dual diagnostic and therapeutic purposes of videofluoroscopy as follows: "Each patient with dysphagia is different. Although there is a routine or basic examination, as with any radiologic technique, studies of patients with swallowing problems lend themselves to tailoring. Each examination is subtly altered on the basis of a mini patient history taken by the radiologist. This history guides the entire examination, as the basic routine is modified in an attempt to reproduce symptoms by means of provocative testing."[24]

The dysphagia literature is full of articles in which authors report performing videofluoroscopy with modifications to the Logemann protocol. These modifications fall into four main categories: the order of stimulus presentation, the volumes tested, the number of tasks collected as well as the number of repetitions collected for each task, and whether swallows are cued or spontaneous. Logemann recommended beginning the videofluoroscopic exam with thin-liquid barium stimuli. The choice to begin with a thin stimulus can be rationalized based on the fact that thin liquids like water are most likely to be aspirated. If one accepts the premise that a videofluoroscopic exam would be wasted if aspiration was never observed in a person who is actually an aspirator, then Jones and Donner's principle of "provocative testing" would support a decision to begin the examination with thin liquids. Secondly, of all the stimuli included in the test, thin barium (which consists of barium and water) is least likely to cause damage to the lungs if aspirated, given that there is no acid or fat content. Many clinicians are unaware that bronchographic examinations of the lungs were historically performed by delivering barium directly into the bronchi and then taking radiographic images of the respiratory passages that were coated by the barium. If aspirated, thin stimuli are also plausibly easier to eject from the trachea and larynx by spontaneous or cued coughing, whereas thicker stimuli may be harder to expel. Nevertheless, many clinicians feel uncomfortable beginning an assessment with thin liquids with patients who are suspected to aspirate; they prefer to begin with a consistency that is expected to be safely tolerated. For example, Palmer and colleagues describe their approach to videofluoroscopy using a standardized "sequence of liquid and solid foods, starting with those that are easiest for most patients to swallow and progressing to more difficult consistencies."[25] One historic reason for this choice to begin a videofluoroscopic exam with thicker consistencies relates to the number of aspiration events that should be allowed before the procedure is terminated in the interest of patient safety. Many clinicians report that their colleagues in radiology are reluctant to continue the test once the first episode of aspiration has occurred. Although this decision is clearly motivated by concerns for patient safety, it does not show an appreciation for the goal of the examination to determine both the underlying reasons for aspiration and the effectiveness of therapeutic interventions intended to limit aspiration. Clearly, an exam should be terminated if a significant aspiration event occurs. An alarming 2012 report in the *New England Journal of Medicine*[26] illustrates one such case where a procedure was not terminated quickly enough, and the patient aspirated a very large volume of barium, leading to hypoxemia, respiratory failure, and ultimately death. However, if videofluoroscopy is being performed in a controlled manner according to a standard protocol, the volume of each stimulus tested should progress cautiously from a small amount to larger amounts, such that an unexpected large aspiration event should be unlikely.

Logemann recommended beginning videofluoroscopy with 1-mL volumes of thin-liquid barium. She argued that this volume was similar to the volume of saliva swallows. However, subsequent research has shown that this volume falls far below the volume of a typical swallow, and questions have been raised about whether such a small volume will be enough to elicit a representative swallow. Recent studies suggest that adults will take sips averaging approximately 16 mL when instructed to take a single sip out of a cup of water.[27,28] If the same instruction is used with thin-liquid barium, most adults take slightly smaller sips, averaging about 12 mL. These findings suggest that it is important to include sips of at least 10 mL in the videofluoroscopy protocol. Given the need to conduct an efficient examination without unnecessary radiation exposure, it may be most appropriate to start with "small sips" of 5 mL and then move to natural or large sips in order to test swallowing under conditions that mimic real mealtime swallowing behaviors as closely as possible. A further question is whether to tightly control the volumes administered or allow the patient to take a more natural sip. Although research studies have traditionally controlled volume, it must be recognized that a 5 mL bolus may be relatively large for a small person but small for a larger person. Allowing each person to take a natural sip, perhaps with an upper limit, may be the most ecologically valid approach.

Logemann's original protocol description encouraged clinicians to repeat each thin-liquid bolus for a total of two to three examples of each task. This is an important recommendation, designed to ensure that the results of the examination capture problems (if they occur) as well as representative behavior. Several studies confirm that people who aspirate will not necessarily aspirate on every swallow. Although we do not know exactly how many repetitions of a task are required in order to completely rule out aspiration, the literature points to a minimum of three repetitions being required as a general rule. In recent work from my own lab, we asked patients to take six sips of thin-liquid barium. We discovered that 8% of patients in our study did not show problems until sips 4, 5, or 6.[29]

Logemann's *Manual for the Videofluorographic Study of Swallowing* describes the process of administering boluses in videofluoroscopy as follows: "With each swallow, the patient is told to hold the material in his or her mouth until given the command to swallow."[15] This type of instruction has become known as the command swallow or cued swallow. Cued swallows serve the practical purpose of providing time for clinicians to remove their hand from the radiation field and to step backward out of the direct scatter field. However, some patients may be unable to contain the bolus in their mouth, either due to cognitive factors or to oral motor control difficulties. In these cases, the fluoroscope may be turned on too late to capture relevant events. Two research studies have explored differences between cued and noncued swallows.[30,31] In both of these studies, it was shown that the cued swallowed condition led to the bolus being located higher up in the oropharynx at the time of pharyngeal swallow initiation, with corresponding impact on timing measures of swallow response. Additionally, Martin-Harris and colleagues[32] observed that healthy adults quite frequently initiate the pharyngeal swallow with the bolus located further into the pharynx on spontaneous, noncued swallows. These findings point to an important conclusion, that the use of a deliberate oral bolus hold or a command swallow may be an effective intervention technique for limiting premature spillage and preswallow aspiration. On the other hand, the findings also point to the fact that use of a command swallow paradigm during videofluoroscopy changes the location of the bolus at swallow initiation compared to a spontaneous swallow. It is currently recommended that clinicians make sure to include some spontaneous, noncued swallows in their videofluoroscopy protocol in order to properly capture the risk of aspiration associated with spontaneous swallowing outside the examination context.

In 2008, an important paper was published by Martin-Harris and colleagues, introducing the MBSImp (Modified Barium Swallow Impairment Profile).[18] This tool defines a new standard approach to performing and scoring a videofluoroscopic exam. The standardized protocol comprises only the diagnostic portion of an examination and involves 11 tasks, as summarized in **Box 6.3**. An important aspect of the work behind the MBSImp is the fact that all videofluoroscopies used for determining reference standards were performed using the same barium product line, Varibar with a 40% w/v concentration. The MBSImp protocol does not require three repetitions of each task–volume combination, but rather embeds the repetition of tasks within the process of administering increasing volumes of each stimulus consistency. Martin-Harris and colleagues used this protocol with a large prospective sample of patients referred for swallowing evaluation, as well as in a sample of asymptomatic healthy adult control participants. Their results show that swallows of thin and nectar-thick stimuli were sensitive for eliciting and revealing abnormal function on the majority of parameters scored using the MBSImp protocol.

Regardless of the choices you make with respect to designing your videofluoroscopy protocol, it is important to take the time to develop a standard approach in your facility. Using the same approach across examinations enables you to identify impairment efficiently and also creates a context in which you can objectively measure change in a patient over time, either due to disease progression or as a function of successful treatment.

## Box 6.3

**Protocol for the MBSImp Videofluoroscopic Evaluation of Swallowing[18]**
- Thin liquid barium
  - 5 mL by teaspoon
  - 5 mL by teaspoon
  - Cup sip
  - Sequential drinking
- Nectar-thick barium
  - 5 mL by teaspoon
  - 5 mL by teaspoon
  - Cup sip
  - Sequential drinking
- Honey-thick barium
  - 5 mL by teaspoon
- Pudding-thick barium
  - 5 mL by teaspoon
- Solid
  - Cookie smeared with pudding-thick barium
- Explorations of compensatory maneuvers
- Additional tasks as determined by the clinician

In my own practice, we adopt a hybrid approach involving a standard core of nine swallowing tasks and a variable set of up to nine therapeutic tasks as described in **Box 6.4**. We adopted the limit of 18 tasks based on a 6-month quality improvement audit project, which showed us that most videofluoroscopies in our facility used 18 or fewer tasks. Rather than strictly controlling the radiation exposure, we aim to perform efficient quality examinations by answering our questions within 18 tasks. If we find ourselves considering 19 or more tasks, we feel it is appropriate to require a clear justification for the additional radiation exposure. Our studies begin with a saliva swallow, without any barium administered. Although we cannot expect to see penetration-aspiration on this task, this gives us a baseline reference of structural movement to which later swallows can be compared. We then perform a bolus-hold challenge, in which we ask patients to take a sip of thin liquid barium and hold it in their mouth for 5 seconds before swallowing. The clinician counts out loud from 1 to 5 and then cues the patient to swallow. This test is intended to challenge the patient's cognitive and motor ability to control the bolus in the oral cavity without premature spillage into the pharynx. We use a 10 mL volume of thin barium for this task, which may not be enough to truly challenge the patient's capacity for oral bolus control but gives us important preliminary information. If the patient is unable to demonstrate oral containment of this bolus for 5 seconds, this provides a warning that bolus control for either cognitive or motor reasons may be a concern. The core of our standardized examination then continues with up to four naturally sized sips of thin-liquid barium using spontaneous, noncued swallows. These tasks provide our context for identifying impairment on thin stimuli, with a particular interest in confirming or ruling out penetration and aspiration. Later in the examination, we collect three 5 ml boluses of extremely thick barium administered by teaspoon, again with the goal of defining

impairment on this consistency, and with a particular purpose of confirming or ruling out postswallow residue. The remaining tasks in our protocol may fall in between the thin and extremely thick barium stimuli and are tailored to the particular patient. These tasks may involve larger volumes of thin liquid, for the purpose of stress-testing the system to rule out penetration and aspiration, or they may involve the exploration of compensatory maneuvers and/or thickened liquids to reduce aspiration or residue. If time permits, and if it is appropriate given the goals of the patient, solid stimuli, pills, or mixed consistencies may be included in these additional tasks. Anterior-posterior views may also be included in these additional tasks to address questions about symmetry of bolus flow, pharyngeal constriction, or residue.

## Box 6.4

**Steele Swallowing Lab Protocol for the Videofluoroscopic Evaluation of Swallowing**
- Diagnostic exam
  - Saliva swallow
  - Bolus "hold" challenge with 10 mL thin-liquid barium
- Up to seven core swallows (no maneuvers)
  - Natural sip of thin-liquid barium
  - Natural sip of thin-liquid barium
  - Natural sip of thin-liquid barium[a]
  - Natural sip of thin-liquid barium[a]
  - 5 mL of extremely thick barium
  - 5 mL of extremely thick barium
  - 5 mL of extremely thick barium[a]
- Therapeutic exam
  - Up to nine other tasks (other consistencies, maneuvers), which may be inserted between the thin liquid and spoon-thick sets of the diagnostic exam
- The third or fourth task in each set may be omitted or modified in case of serious safety or efficiency concerns on previous tasks.

## 6.10 How Is Videofluoroscopy Used to Evaluate Swallowing Safety?

A primary purpose of videofluoroscopy is to rule out penetration-aspiration or to confirm its presence and severity. Penetration is defined as entry of material into the supraglottic space (extending down as far as the true vocal folds), whereas aspiration is defined as entry of material into the airway, below the true vocal folds. In 1996, Rosenbek and colleagues[33] introduced the 8-point Penetration-Aspiration Scale (PAS) as a standard method for scoring the severity of airway invasion. The scale describes penetration and aspiration with respect to the deepest point reached by the aspirated material, and whether or not this material is subsequently ejected from that location to a higher position. The first two levels on the scale are considered normal and are seen in healthy people[34]: level 1 (no entry of material into the airway) and level 2 (brief and transient entry of material into the supraglottic space with subsequent ejection

and McCullough[44] reported average distances of superior hyoid excursion in healthy liquid swallows in the range of 14 to 16 mm with mean measures of anterior hyoid excursion ranging from 10 to 18 mm. However, a subsequent review of measurements of healthy hyoid excursion in the swallowing literature[45] revealed huge variation in reported measures, with the 95% confidence interval limits for superior excursion ranging from 2 to 28 mm and corresponding measures for anterior excursion ranging from 5 to 20 mm. Against this backdrop of highly variable normative references, it becomes practically impossible to determine whether hyoid excursion is abnormal in a patient. In their discussion of this dilemma, Molfenter and Steele[46] identified several methodological choices that could contribute to variations in measures of hyolaryngeal excursion. Among these, measurement of the distance moved between minimum and maximum hyoid (or laryngeal) position was identified as a parameter susceptible to methodological artifacts. In particular, the identification of minimum hyoid position may differ depending on whether a pre- or postswallow frame is used. Many people show an early, anticipatory partial elevation of the hyolaryngeal complex, even before the bolus is delivered to the pharynx, and this position is considerably higher than the position achieved at rest after the swallow. A second factor contributing to variation in normative reference measures of hyolaryngeal excursion was identified to be the size of the oropharynx, which appears to be correlated with a person's height. Molfenter was able to show that the amount of

hyolaryngeal excursion, measured in millimeters, was correlated with the length of the cervical spine; that is, tall people show larger hyoid movements than short people.[45] Taking these two factors into consideration, Molfenter proposed that hyolaryngeal excursion should be measured on a single frame (the frame of maximum excursion or peak position), as a distance relative to the anterior inferior corner of the C4 vertebra, in units normalized to an anatomic scalar (the length of the C2–C4 cervical spine), which also defines the y-axis of the coordinate system for measurement. Using this approach, subsequent measures in healthy adults have suggested a normative reference of not less than 150% of the C2–C4 cervical spine reference distance on thin and nectar-thick liquid swallows of 5 to 20 mL.[45,47] Precise measurements of peak hyoid position can be made using image analysis software, such as ImageJ,[48] and are illustrated in **Fig. 6.5**.

In terms of timing measures that clearly delineate the probability of aspiration, several studies point to an increased risk whenever the bolus reaches the pharynx (below the ramus of the mandible) before the patient achieves airway protection in the form of laryngeal vestibule closure (LVC). Nativ-Zeltzer and colleagues[49] have measured this parameter, defining the onset of the interval as opening of the glossopalatal junction (GPJO). This parameter (GPJO-LVC) was identified to be significantly shorter (< 350 milliseconds) in people with no penetration-aspiration compared to mean interval measures of 600 to 800 milliseconds in individuals with penetration or aspiration in a retrospective

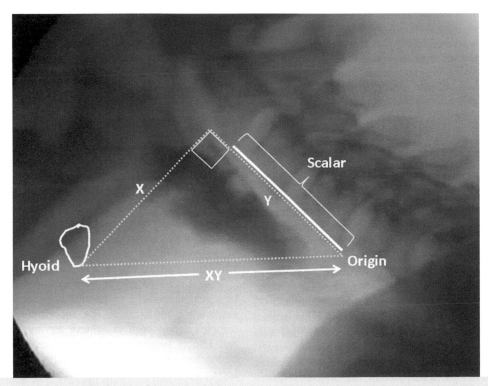

**Fig. 6.5** The recommended method for measuring the location of the hyoid at peak excursion. In this case, the patient is leaning forward, so the vertical (y) axis of the measurement is defined by the cervical spine. The horizontal (x) axis is defined at 90 degrees to the y-axis. The location of the hyoid is measured in pixels in ImageJ[48] software, relative to a measurement origin at the anterior inferior corner of the C4 vertebra. The pixel distance from origin to hyoid position (either x, y, or xy planes of measurement) is then divided by the pixel length of a cervical spine scalar, measured as the distance between the anterior inferior corners of the C2 and C4 vertebrae.

cohort study of male patients and controls undergoing videofluoroscopy. Humbert and colleagues have studied a similar measure, labeled Laryngeal Vestibule Closure Reaction Time, in which the onset event is the beginning of the hyoid burst movement.[50] Interestingly, once laryngeal vestibule closure has been achieved, research suggests that the duration of laryngeal vestibule closure does not differentiate between individuals with and without penetration-aspiration.[51]

To date, we do not have much evidence pointing to pathophysiologic explanations for the accumulation of residue in the valleculae and piriform sinuses after the swallow. Dejaeger and colleagues[52] pointed to three potential factors: ineffective bolus propulsion by the tongue, reduced pharyngeal constriction, and reduced pharyngeal shortening. Further research is needed to better understand these possible predictors. As mentioned earlier, a recent study by Stokely and colleagues[39] has identified an inverse correlation between the degree of pharyngeal constriction and the subsequent severity of postswallow residue measured using the Normalized Residue Ratio Scale.

## 6.13 How Is Videofluoroscopy Used for Treatment Planning and Outcome Measurement?

The clinician's understanding of the pathophysiologic mechanisms behind impairments in swallowing safety and efficiency becomes the basis for selecting intervention techniques that may be effective in improving swallowing function for people with dysphagia. For example, in cases where a person experiences penetration or aspiration due to late laryngeal vestibule closure relative to the timing of bolus arrival in the pharynx, several potential interventions might be tried. A command swallow, intentional oral hold, or chin-down posture may help to keep the bolus in the oral cavity for longer and delay the delivery of the bolus to the pharynx. A chin-down posture may also alter the dimensions of the oropharynx sufficiently to compress the area of the laryngeal vestibule and make laryngeal vestibule closure easier to achieve in a timely fashion.[53] If these mechanisms fail, thickening the bolus so that it travels more slowly may be an effective method of preventing aspiration. The indications for specific intervention techniques will be discussed in the treatment section of this textbook.

Regardless of the interventions chosen, videofluoroscopy provides an objective method for measuring the immediate impact of compensatory maneuvers, progression of a patient either toward recovery or with advancing disease, as well as the posttreatment impact of rehabilitative techniques. In order to draw valid conclusions regarding changes in a patient's swallowing across repeated videofluoroscopies, it is crucial that the testing conditions be standardized and held constant. Paying attention to the careful mixing of barium stimuli is particularly important in this regard, as well as following the same standardized protocol in both examinations. However, even when strict standardization is used, it can be challenging to decide how to capture a patient's

overall impairment status for each examination. The conservative approach, recommended within the MBSImp protocol, is to define the level of impairment based on the worst performance seen in an examination. Here, it is particularly important to set a level playing field for comparison in terms of the number of boluses tested. If a patient aspirates once on a set of three thin boluses at the initial examination, but does not aspirate until presented with a sixth or seventh bolus during an outcome examination, it is challenging to determine whether or not this reflects a clinically relevant improvement. These challenges are commonly encountered in dysphagia research, and the delineation of a set number of standard tasks that will serve as the unit of measurement, together with rating of both pre- and posttreatment recordings by raters who are blinded to the time point of each recording, is a method for reducing potential bias in outcome measurement.

## 6.14 Questions

1. Which of the following scenarios suggests that videofluoroscopy is not appropriate?

A. The clinician wishes to confirm the severity of aspiration.
B. The clinician wishes to rule out silent aspiration.
C. The patient is too medically unstable to tolerate the procedure.
D. The clinician wishes to confirm whether texture modification reduces aspiration.
E. The clinician wishes to determine whether a chin-down posture prevents aspiration.

2. Which levels on the 8-point Penetration-Aspiration Scale[33] are considered normal, and may be seen in healthy people without dysphagia?

A. Levels 1 and 2
B. Only level 1
C. Levels 1, 2, and 3
D. Levels 6, 7, and 8
E. Levels 3, 4, and 5

3. Which of the following statements is true regarding radiation exposure in videofluoroscopy?

A. The radiation exposure received annually by a clinician should not exceed 5 mSv.
B. The radiation dose received by the clinician will increase as the clinician moves away from the patient.
C. The radiation dose received by the patient during videofluoroscopy is usually more than the 10 mSv radiation dose typically received in a computed tomographic scan.
D. Wearing a thyroid collar reduces the radiation dose received by the clinician's neck.
E. The radiation dose received by the patient during videofluoroscopy is about the same as the dose received during a chest X-ray.

**4.** Which of the following contrast media is most likely to leave a coating on the walls of the pharynx?

A. 40% w/v nectar-thick Varibar

B. 40% w/v thin Varibar

C. Thin Varibar diluted to a 20% w/v ratio using water

D. 105% w/v Liquid Polibar diluted to a 40% w/v ratio using water

E. 105% w/v Liquid Polibar.

**5.** Which of the following statements is true regarding swallowing physiology seen on videofluoroscopy?

A. Hyoid excursion, measured in millimeters, will tend to be larger in tall people than in short people.

B. A command swallow is likely to lead to the bolus accumulating in the vallecular space before pharyngeal swallow initiation.

C. Aspiration risk is higher in individuals with a short laryngeal vestibule closure reaction time.

D. Piriform sinus residue is likely to be higher in individuals with good pharyngeal constriction.

E. Patients who aspirate on their first bolus of thin liquid are also likely to aspirate on all subsequent boluses of thin liquid.

# 6.15 Answers and Explanations

## 1. Correct: the patient is too medically unstable to tolerate the procedure (C).

ASHA's guideline "Clinical Indications for Instrumental Assessment of Dysphagia"[2] identifies four situations in which videofluoroscopy may be inappropriate:

1. When the clinical examination suggests that the patients does not have dysphagia

2. When the patient is too medically unstable to tolerate the procedure

3. When the patient is unable to cooperate or participate in an instrumental examination

4. When, in the speech-language pathologist's judgment, the instrumental examination would not change the clinical management of the patient

Answers **A**, **B**, **D**, and **E** each provide a valid rationale for performing videofluoroscopy. A full list of reasons for performing videofluoroscopy, as outlined in ASHA's guideline "Clinical Indications for Instrumental Assessment of Dysphagia,"[2] can be found in **Table 5.2**.

## 2. Correct: levels 1 and 2 (A).

Levels 1 and 2 on the 8-point Penetration-Aspiration Scale[33] indicate that material does not enter the airway (level 1) or enters briefly into the supraglottic space and is then ejected (level 2). These levels are considered normal and are seen in healthy people.[34]

Answers **B**, **C**, **D**, and **E** are incorrect. Level 1 on the 8-point Penetration-Aspiration Scale[33] indicates that no material enters the airway. This level is considered normal and is seen in healthy people, but level 2 is also considered normal. Level 2 indicates that material enters briefly into the supraglottic space and is then ejected. Levels 3, 4, and 5 represent penetration of material into the supraglottic space and are considered abnormal. Levels 6, 7, and 8 represent aspiration of material below the true vocal folds and are considered abnormal.

## 3. Correct: wearing a thyroid collar reduces the radiation dose received by the clinician's neck (D).

An Australian study[14] has estimated that a clinician who does not wear a thyroid collar will receive between 0 and 0.017 milliSieverts of radiation dose at the thyroid in a 3- to 4-minute procedure, and that wearing a thyroid collar reduces this dose by a factor of about 40.

Answers **A**, **B**, **C**, and **E** are incorrect. Annual limits for radiation exposure of occupationally exposed health workers are set at 20 mSv. Clinicians can dramatically reduce their exposure during videofluoroscopy by moving further away from the source of radiation, and by wearing appropriate protective garments such as lead aprons. The dose received by the patient during a 2- to 3-minute examination has been shown in different studies to be approximately 0.2 to 0.4 mSv. This compares to a typical dose of 0.02 mSv for a chest X-ray.

## 4. Correct: 105% w/v Liquid Polibar (E).

Higher-concentration barium products (i.e., > 100% w/v) are designed to leave a coating along the walls of the gastrointestinal tract. This should not be confused with residue.

Answers **A**, **B**, **C**, and **D** are incorrect. These products are considered to have a low concentration of barium (< 100% w/v) and are less likely than the 105% w/v concentration Liquid Polibar suspension to leave a coating on the walls of the gastrointestinal tract.

## 5. Correct: hyoid excursion, measured in millimeters, will tend to be larger in tall people than in short people (A).

Molfenter has shown that the amount of hyolaryngeal excursion (in millimeters) is correlated with the length of the cervical spine; that is, tall people tend to show larger hyoid movements than short people.[45]

Answers **B**, **C**, **D**, and **E** are incorrect. A command swallow is likely to keep the bolus in the mouth for longer and will reduce the chance of preswallow accumulation of material in the vallecular space. Laryngeal vestibule closure reaction time (i.e., the time that the bolus is in the pharynx prior to laryngeal vestibule closure) has been shown to be a factor predictive of aspiration. When this timing measure is longer, there is a greater risk of aspiration. Postswallow residue has been shown to be more likely when pharyngeal constriction is poor. Aspiration is not a constant phenomenon: individuals who aspirate may not do so on every swallow.

# References

[1] American Speech-Language Hearing Association. Medicare-Physician-Fee-Schedule-SLP. 2013; https://www.asha.org/uploadedFiles/2018-Medicare-Physician-Fee-Schedule-SLP.pdf Accessed December 6, 2018

[2] American Speech-Language Hearing Association. Clinical Indications for Instrumental Assessment of Dysphagia. 2000; https://www.asha.org/Practice-Portal/.

[3] Jaffer NM, Ng E, Au FW, Steele CM. Fluoroscopic evaluation of oropharyngeal dysphagia: anatomic, technical, and common etiologic factors. *AJR Am J Roentgenol* 2015;*204*(1):49–58

[4] Logemann JA. *Evaluation and Treatment of Swallowing Disorders.* 2nd ed. San Diego, CA: College Hill Press; 1997

[5] Donner MW. Radiologic evaluation of swallowing. *Am Rev Respir Dis* 1985;*131*(5):S20–S23

[6] Jones B, Kramer SS, Donner MW. Dynamic imaging of the pharynx. *Gastrointest Radiol* 1985;*10*(3):213–224

[7] Ekberg O, Hillarp B. Radiologic evaluation of the oral stage of swallowing. *Acta Radiol Diagn (Stockh)* 1986;*27*(5):533–537

[8] Ekberg O, Nylander G. Cineradiography of the pharyngeal stage of deglutition in 250 patients with dysphagia. *Br J Radiol* 1982;*55*(652):258–262

[9] Ekberg O, Nylander G. Cineradiography of the pharyngeal stage of deglutition in 150 individuals without dysphagia. *Br J Radiol* 1982;*55*(652):253–257

[10] Langmore SE, Schatz K, Olsen N. Fiberoptic endoscopic examination of swallowing safety: a new procedure. *Dysphagia* 1988;*2*(4):216–219

[11] Zammit-Maempel I, Chapple CL, Leslie P. Radiation dose in videofluoroscopic swallow studies. *Dysphagia* 2007;*22*(1):13–15

[12] Moro L, Cazzani C. Dynamic swallowing study and radiation dose to patients. *Radiol Med (Torino)* 2006;*111*(1):123–129

[13] Molfenter SM, Steele CM. Variation in temporal measures of swallowing: sex and volume effects. *Dysphagia* 2013;*28*(2):226–233

[14] McLean D, Smart R, Collins L, Varas J. Thyroid dose measurements for staff involved in modified barium swallow exams. *Health Phys* 2006;*90*(1):38–41

[15] Logemann JA. *Manual for the Videofluorographic Study of Swallowing.* Austin, TX: Pro-Ed; 1986

[16] Lemen LC. A discussion of radiation in videofluoroscopic swallow studies. *Radiation Safety for Speech-Language Pathologists* 2004:7

[17] Bonilha HS, Blair J, Carnes B, et al. Preliminary investigation of the effect of pulse rate on judgments of swallowing impairment and treatment recommendations. *Dysphagia* 2013;*28*(4):528–538

[18] Martin Harris B, Brodsky MB, Michel Y, et al. MBS measurement tool for swallow impairment—MBSImp: establishing a standard. *Dysphagia* 2008;*23*(4):392–405

[19] Martino R, Shaw S, Greco E, et al. Comparing physiological swallow measures captured on videofluoroscopy at different frame rates: A reliability analysis. *Dysphagia* 2015

[20] Hind JA, Gensler G, Brandt DK, et al. Comparison of trained clinician ratings with expert ratings of aspiration on videofluoroscopic images from a randomized clinical trial. *Dysphagia* 2009;*24*(2):211–217

[21] Steele CM, Molfenter SM, Péladeau-Pigeon M, Stokely S. Challenges in preparing contrast media for videofluoroscopy. *Dysphagia* 2013;*28*(3):464–467

[22] Fink TA, Ross JB. Are we testing a true thin liquid? *Dysphagia* 2009;*24*(3):285–289

[23] Harris JA, Bartelt D, Campion M, et al. The use of low-osmolar water-soluble contrast in videofluoroscopic swallowing exams. *Dysphagia* 2013;*28*(4):520–527

[24] Jones B, Donner MW. How I do it: examination of the patient with dysphagia. *Dysphagia* 1989;*4*(3):162–172

[25] Palmer JB, Kuhlemeier KV, Tippett DC, Lynch C. A protocol for the videofluorographic swallowing study. *Dysphagia* 1993;*8*(3):209–214

[26] Albeldawi M, Makkar R. Images in clinical medicine. Barium aspiration. *N Engl J Med* 2012;*366*(11):1038

[27] Bennett JW, Van Lieshout PH, Pelletier CA, Steele CM. Sip-sizing behaviors in natural drinking conditions compared to instructed experimental conditions. *Dysphagia* 2009;*24*(2):152–158

[28] Steele CM, Peladeau-Pigeon M, Tam K, Zohouri-Haghian N, Mukhurjee R. Variations in sip volume as a function of pre-sip cup volume. *Dysphagia* 2015

[29] Steele CM, Nagy A, Tapson M, et al. Prevalence of impaired swallowing with thin and gum-thickened barium stimuli. *Dysphagia* 2015

[30] Daniels SK, Schroeder MF, DeGeorge PC, Corey DM, Rosenbek JC. Effects of verbal cue on bolus flow during swallowing. *Am J Speech Lang Pathol* 2007;*16*(2):140–147

[31] Nagy A, Leigh C, Hori SF, Molfenter SM, Shariff T, Steele CM. Timing differences between cued and noncued swallows in healthy young adults. *Dysphagia* 2013;*28*(3):428–434

[32] Martin-Harris B, Brodsky MB, Michel Y, Lee FS, Walters B. Delayed initiation of the pharyngeal swallow: normal variability in adult swallows. *J Speech Lang Hear Res* 2007;*50*(3):585–594

[33] Rosenbek JC, Robbins JA, Roecker EB, Coyle JL, Wood JL. A penetration-aspiration scale. *Dysphagia* 1996;*11*(2):93–98

[34] Daggett A, Logemann J, Rademaker A, Pauloski B. Laryngeal penetration during deglutition in normal subjects of various ages. *Dysphagia* 2006;*21*(4):270–274

[35] Langmore SE, Terpenning MS, Schork A, et al. Predictors of aspiration pneumonia: how important is dysphagia? *Dysphagia* 1998;*13*(2):69–81

[36] Pikus L, Levine MS, Yang YX, et al. Videofluoroscopic studies of swallowing dysfunction and the relative risk of pneumonia. *AJR Am J Roentgenol* 2003;*180*(6):1613–1616

[37] Pearson WG Jr, Molfenter SM, Smith ZM, Steele CM. Image-based measurement of post-swallow residue: the normalized residue ratio scale. *Dysphagia* 2013;*28*(2):167–177

[38] Molfenter SM, Steele CM. The relationship between residue and aspiration on the subsequent swallow: an application of the normalized residue ratio scale. *Dysphagia* 2013;*28*(4):494–500

[39] Stokely SL, Peladeau-Pigeon M, Leigh C, Molfenter SM, Steele CM. The relationship between pharyngeal constriction and post-swallow residue. Dysphagia 2015; DOI 10.1007/s00455-015-9606-5. http://link.springer.com/artcle/10.1007/s00455-015-9606-5

[40] Kendall KA, McKenzie S, Leonard RJ, Gonçalves MI, Walker A. Timing of events in normal swallowing: a videofluoroscopic study. *Dysphagia* 2000;*15*(2):74–83

[41] Leonard R, McKenzie S. Hyoid-bolus transit latencies in normal swallow. *Dysphagia* 2006;*21*(3):183–190

[42] Leonard RJ, Kendall KA, McKenzie S, Gonçalves MI, Walker A. Structural displacements in normal swallowing: a videofluoroscopic study. *Dysphagia* 2000;*15*(3):146–152

[43] Steele CM, Cichero JA. Physiological factors related to aspiration risk: a systematic review. *Dysphagia* 2014;*29*(3):295–304

[44] Kim Y, McCullough GH. Maximum hyoid displacement in normal swallowing. *Dysphagia* 2008;*23*(3):274–279

[45] Molfenter SM, Steele CM. Use of an anatomical scalar to control for sex-based size differences in measures of hyoid excursion during swallowing. *J Speech Lang Hear Res* 2014;*57*(3):768–778

[46] Molfenter SM, Steele CM. Physiological variability in the deglutition literature: hyoid and laryngeal kinematics. *Dysphagia* 2011;*26*(1):67–74

[47] Nagy A, Molfenter SM, Péladeau-Pigeon M, Stokely S, Steele CM. The effect of bolus volume on hyoid kinematics in healthy swallowing. *BioMed Res Int* 2014;*2014*:738971 10.1155/2014/813084

[48] National Institutes of Health. ImageJ Release 1.48. 2013; http://rsb.info.nih.gov/. Accessed June 11, 2015

[49] Nativ-Zeltzer N, Kahrilas PJ, Logemann JA. Manofluorography in the evaluation of oropharyngeal dysphagia. *Dysphagia* 2012;*27*(2):151–161

[50] Humbert IA, Christopherson H, Lokhande A, German R, Gonzalez-Fernandez M, Celnik P. Human hyolaryngeal movements show adaptive motor learning during swallowing. *Dysphagia* 2013;*28*(2):139–145

[51] Park T, Kim Y, Ko DH, McCullough G. Initiation and duration of laryngeal closure during the pharyngeal swallow in post-stroke patients. *Dysphagia* 2010;*25*(3):177–182

[52] Dejaeger E, Pelemans W, Ponette E, Joosten E. Mechanisms involved in postdeglutition retention in the elderly. *Dysphagia* 1997;*12*(2):63–67

[53] Macrae P, Anderson C, Humbert I. Mechanisms of airway protection during chin-down swallowing. *J Speech Lang Hear Res* 2014;*57*(4):1251–1258

# 7 Pediatric Videofluoroscopic Swallow Evaluation

*Melanie P. Hiorns and Martina Ryan*

## Summary

Videofluoroscopic swallow studies (VFSSs) in children differ from those in adults. The practitioner is reminded that "Children are not mini adults requiring smaller beds and smaller portions of food."[1] Although assessing the anatomy of the oropharynx and the swallow function has the same objective in adults and children, the route to the end point is very different. This chapter explains the key differences in the VFSS assessment in children, and how to complete a meaningful examination in children from newborns to teenagers, with guidance on preassessing and preparing the child, preparing and offering the foodstuffs, interpreting the images, and using the lowest radiation dose possible. Some of the congenital conditions that affect swallowing that are unique to the pediatric population are discussed, in addition to assessment in acquired conditions that may be the result of surgery or neurologic impairment. Attention to radiation dose is critical, and radiographic techniques must be adapted to the size of the patients; these issues are discussed in detail.

### Keywords

videofluoroscopy swallow study, tracheal aspiration, pediatric dysphagia, radiographic technique, swallow fatigue, radiation dose

### Learning Objectives

- Understand why videofluoroscopic swallowing studies are different in children
- Understand the different range of conditions for which a videofluoroscopic swallow study (VFSS) may be helpful in either diagnosis or management of feeding
- Understand how to assess a child's suitability for VFSS
- Understand how to perform VFSS in children
- Understand how to evaluate the images
- Understand the radiation dose considerations in performing VFSS in children of all ages

## 7.1 Introduction

The videofluoroscopic swallow study (VFSS) in children is different from that in adults, both in the way it is performed and in the way it is interpreted. It is important to recognize this from the outset because this affects the approach to the assessment and improves the chance of obtaining a meaningful and contributory examination that may have long-lasting implications for the child. The conditions and pathology in children differ from those in adults; thus searching specifically for pediatric swallowing issues will yield far more useful information than a "one size fits all" approach.

Pediatric VFSS should include collaboration between the speech-language pathologist (SLP) and the radiologist. The SLP brings knowledge of specific swallowing problems, as well as the confidence of the parents and their child. The radiologist brings expertise in other conditions that may manifest during the study (e.g., a previously unidentified tracheoesophageal fistula) and knowledge of the equipment and radiation issues.

The VFSS assessment in children is undertaken with the same objective as in adults: to define the anatomy of the oropharynx, which in children varies with age, and physiology, which in children varies with maturation; and to assess and identify aspiration risk. It is recognized as an essential adjunct to the clinical feeding assessment, demonstrating tracheal aspiration, which can be silent on clinical assessment. The outcomes aims are, where possible, to identify clinical adaptions to facilitate safe feeding and allow a management protocol to be agreed to.[2] The dynamic procedure, however, differs at several levels from the adult assessment and is not simply a scaled-down version for "mini adults."

## 7.2 Preinvestigation Evaluation

The challenges of undertaking pediatric VFSS start with consideration as to whether this is the best test for that child. VFSS is not always the assessment of choice, and the decision-making process will take into account not only the concerns around the nature of the feeding difficulties and indicators of unsafe swallow but whether the child will be able to comply adequately with the procedure in order for the clinician to answer the clinical question. The literature unanimously recommends that all children undergo a clinical feeding assessment by an appropriately qualified SLP before being referred for VFSS. This allows the clinician to determine the nature of the difficulty, the optimal timing of the study, and whether there are indications of pharyngeal-stage dysphagia. It also allows the child's optimum positioning for feeding, likely cooperation, and the foods/liquids to be assessed. Skilled pediatric clinical assessment can often identify problems without the automatic need for a VFSS.

## 7.3 Preinvestigation Preparation

An important part of preparing the child for this examination will be the information and guidance given to parents/caregivers. The best results are achieved with maximal cooperation. For many children and their families, coming to hospital for a procedure can be stressful and cause high levels of anxiety,[3] potentially resulting in a nonrepresentative profile of the child's swallow function. There can be concern that the outcome of the test will bring bad news and that the procedure could be uncomfortable or distressing for the child. Providing sufficient verbal and written information prior to the study will help to allay some fears around the procedure itself and allow parents/

caregivers to consider how best to prepare the child to achieve optimal cooperation.[4,5]

## 7.4   Pediatric Elements to Identify

A key difference between the assessment protocols for adults and children will be the consideration of rapid changes in feeding and swallowing skills, anatomical growth, and neuromotor maturation in the first 3 years of life. The examination should be appropriate for the child's size and developmental level, and SLPs performing VFSS in children should consider where those children are in the process of anatomical change as well as their developmental abilities.[6] Additionally the diseases and disorders seen in children differ from those commonly seen in adults with dysphagia. Structural abnormalities of the oropharynx, larynx, or esophagus are more likely to be primary and congenital. Examples of such anomalies are cleft palate, macroglossia, laryngeal cleft, and tracheoesophageal fistula. A VFSS can be diagnostic for some structural pathologies. Aspiration can be common in congenital anatomical variants, such as craniofacial syndromes, Pierre Robin sequence, and laryngeal clefts or vocal fold palsy.[7,8] Young infants may present with cardiorespiratory compromise; VFSS can identify the dynamic impact on the infant's ability to successfully coordinate the suck-swallow-breathe sequence for nipple feeding with subsequent aspiration demonstrated on VFSS.[9]

Feeding problems are common in children with static and progressive neuromotor impairments. In a community-based survey, oromotor dysfunction was demonstrated in more than 90% of a sample of 49 children with cerebral palsy[10] and evidence of chronic aspiration in 41% in a separate community study.[11] Estimates of silent aspiration in children with severe cerebral palsy and dysphagia undergoing VFSS range from 31% to 97%.[12,13] Children with neuromuscular conditions such as spinal muscular atrophy may eventually develop dysphagia with aspiration.[14]

In contrast to the adult population, there is no agreed protocol for carrying out pediatric VFSS. The procedure may therefore be technically challenging, and pragmatic adaptations are often necessary. These may include extending the time of the procedure to give the child and family more time in the fluoroscopy suite to familiarize themselves with the environment and feel comfortable. The importance of a child-friendly room cannot be overstated. The availability of toys and distracters, including touch-screen devices (smartphones or tablets), which are both popular and effective, will help to create an environment in which the child can feel at ease. Parents/caregivers are requested to be present because they will be most familiar with how the child feeds at home. Children are generally more compliant with a familiar adult, and a more representative study is likely to be obtained.

## 7.5   The Clinical Procedure

### 7.5.1   Presentation of Foods

As a general rule children should be moderately hungry when attending for the study so they will be willing to try the foods offered, albeit with altered taste being unavoidable with the addition of a contrast material. The effect of this can be lessened by the use of predefined acceptable/favorite foods. There

is variability in the literature regarding the correct order of presentation of the different food and liquid consistencies to be assessed. For adult studies a uniform protocol of liquid followed by paste then cookie was described early by Logemann,[15] with the procedure starting with very small volumes of the thinnest liquid and moving systematically to larger bolus sizes and thicker consistencies. The principle behind this approach is that if a thin liquid is aspirated it will be less damaging to the lungs and will also not block the airway as could happen if a more solid consistency is aspirated. Due to the cooperation issues that can frequently sabotage the pediatric study, a more pragmatic approach is sometimes adopted whereby offering a favorite food at the beginning of the study can be reassuring to gain the child's confidence and make it more likely that a less preferred food or liquid will subsequently be acceptable. However, where it is strongly suspected that cooperation is likely to be poor throughout, the clinician may feel that it is more important to start with the consistency about which there is most concern so as not to miss evaluating this if compliance ceases after the first two or three swallows as the child senses the altered taste of the barium-impregnated food or liquid. Whenever possible, a standard protocol should be used to allow for between patient and within patient comparisons when there are repeat studies. The suggested order for introduction of consistencies during the VFSS mirrors that of the original Logemann protocol offered from developmentally appropriate bottles/nipples, cups, and utensils to ensure that test consistencies are representative of the patient's diet (thin fluid, pureed, and solids as appropriate). If there is evidence of dysphagia, then the clinician should introduce evidence-based strategies to improve swallowing function and document the patient's response in swallowing function. Strategies may include change in speed of liquid flow, change in position, verbal cueing, and increasing the viscosity of the offered liquid. The appropriate strategy depends on the swallowing function observed.

It is not possible to force this dynamic investigation, because the child must be ready to accept food by mouth and make some voluntary attempts to swallow. Attempts to force the investigation are highly likely to result in nonrepresentative findings. Specifically, there should be no attempt to push food or drink into the child's mouth, which will only increase the risk of aspiration, give an inaccurate impression of the swallow, and make the child adverse to any further studies. Children who have preexisting aversive feeding difficulties and who are refusing food and liquid will not be able to comply; these children should not even be taken to the fluoroscopy room. Those who are primarily fed by a nonoral route (e.g., gastrostomy tube) should have had some recent experience with swallowing food or liquid.

Children with severe behavioral problems or who may be hospital-phobic may need preparation to reduce anxiety and become acclimatized to the fluoroscopy room (e.g., with a play specialist), in order to accept food and drink in this unfamiliar environment. Some groups of children, such as those with a diagnosis of autism spectrum disorder, have a high prevalence of specific fears, including fear of medical procedures.[16,17] Additionally, children with autism spectrum disorder may only accept a narrow range of foods[16] in specific mealtime environments. Therefore, this procedure may provoke extreme anxiety and a refusal to participate.

## 7.5.2 The Effect of Fatigue on Swallow Function

One of the features that may become evident during VFSS is fatigue. In a study of 43 infants under 12 months of age[9] undergoing VFSS, no abnormalities were seen in the first few swallows, but gradual deterioration was evident as they continued to feed. In order to assess for fatigue, the use of interval X-ray screening is recommended (i.e., allowing the child to continue to feed for a period during the study without X-ray screening and after an interval returning to X-ray screening) to judge any changes in swallow function as the child tires. This technique is recommended for infants whose medical diagnosis may make them susceptible to fatigue when bottle feeding (e.g., cardiorespiratory conditions). It can also be used for older children with conditions such as neuromuscular disease who may decompensate with prolonged effort.

## 7.5.3 Positioning

Achieving a successful position for a child undergoing VFSS will depend on the age and size of the child, the neurodevelopmental level of the child's postural control, and whether the child requires a supportive seating system to manage altered muscle tone or movement disorders. It is generally agreed that, ideally, children should be assessed in the position in which they would usually eat,[18] but that part of the scope of the study may be to find the optimal position for that child to feed safely.[19] In general, the child should be upright or slightly reclined with the head in a stable, midline position. For infants < 3 months of age, an elevated side-lying position on the X-ray table may need to be considered if neck and trunk support is not adequate for the infant to sit in a small preformed seat. For children up to around 4 to 5 years of age who have good trunk stability, a preformed foam or polystyrene seat, such as a Tumbleform chair (Sammons Preston Rolyan) can be mounted on the plinth of the X-ray table. These seats must be virtually radiolucent, must allow the child to sit securely without being completely restrained, and must be both removable from the X-ray equipment and completely cleanable (**Fig. 7.1**). Children who come in wheelchairs or supportive seating can remain in these provided the radiopaque parts of the chair, such as the headrest or handles, can be removed from view. However, even with a seating system, some children will be difficult to position due to spinal deformities, excessive involuntary movement patterns, or fixed contractures. These issues should be evident at the clinical feeding assessment and identified by the SLP as likely to contraindicate a successful VFSS.

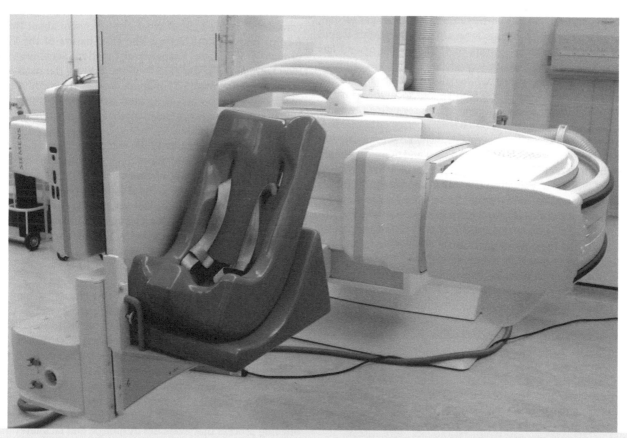

**Fig. 7.1** A Tumbleform seat positioned on the plinth of the fluoroscopy table. The X-ray source is as far away from the child as possible (seen on the righthand side of the image), and the seat is as close to the image intensifier as possible (seen behind the upright fluoroscopy table). This allows plenty of space around the patient, which is less stressful for the child and the caregiver, while reducing the radiation dose. Most small children accept the straps without difficulty because they are used to car seats.

anomalies. Hospitals typically employ billing and coding specialists to ensure seamless and accurate billing of all services, including pediatric VFSS.

### 5. Correct: All of the above (D).

A key difference between the assessment protocols for adults and children is the consideration of rapid changes in feeding and swallowing skills, anatomical growth, and neuromotor maturation in the first 3 years of life. The items in **A**, **B**, and **C** in isolation are not complete.

## References

[1] Kennedy PI. The Report into the Public Enquiry into Children's Heart Surgery at the Bristol Royal Infirmary. London, UK: The Stationery Office; 2001:48

[2] Benson J, Lefton-Greif MA. Videofluoroscopy of swallowing in pediatric patients: A component of the total feeding evaluation. In: Tuchman D, Walter R, eds. Disorders of Feeding and Swallowing in Infants and Children. San Diego, CA: Singular Publishing Group; 1994:187–200

[3] Coyne I. Children's experiences of hospitalization. *J Child Health Care* 2006;*10*(4):326–336

[4] Hiorns MP, Ryan MM. Current practice in paediatric videofluoroscopy. *Pediatr Radiol* 2006;*36*(9):911–919

[5] Ardveson JC, Brodsky L. Instrumental evaluation of swallowing. In: Ardveson JC, Brodsky L, eds. Pediatric Swallowing and Feeding: Assessment and Management. Dysphagia Series. San Diego, CA: Singular Publishing Group; 2002:341–388

[6] Practice Portal: Pediatric Dysphagia Assessment. American Speech-Language-Hearing Association website. http://www.asha.org/PRPSpecificTopic.aspx?folderid=8589934965&section=Assessment. Accessed September 18, 2015

[7] Evans JN. Management of the cleft larynx and tracheoesophageal clefts. *Ann Otol Rhinol Laryngol* 1985;*94*(6 Pt 1):627–630

[8] Monasterio FO, Molina F, Berlanga F, et al. Swallowing disorders in Pierre Robin sequence: its correction by distraction. *J Craniofac Surg* 2004;*15*(6):934–941

[9] Newman LA, Keckley C, Petersen MC, Hamner A. Swallowing function and medical diagnoses in infants suspected of dysphagia. *Pediatrics* 2001;*108*(6):E106

[10] Reilly S, Skuse D, Poblete X. Prevalence of feeding problems and oral motor dysfunction in children with cerebral palsy: a community survey. *J Pediatr* 1996;*129*(6):877–882

[11] Del Giudice E, Staiano A, Capano G, et al. Gastrointestinal manifestations in children with cerebral palsy. *Brain Dev* 1999;*21*(5):307–311

[12] Rogers B, Arvedson J, Buck G, Smart P, Msall M. Characteristics of dysphagia in children with cerebral palsy. *Dysphagia* 1994;*9*(1):69–73

[13] Arvedson J, Rogers B, Buck G, Smart P, Msall M. Silent aspiration prominent in children with dysphagia. *Int J Pediatr Otorhinolaryngol* 1994;*28*(2-3):173–181

[14] Allen J. Pulmonary complications of neuromuscular disease: a respiratory mechanics perspective. *Paediatr Respir Rev* 2010;*11*(1):18–23

[15] Logemann J. Evaluation and Treatment of Swallowing Disorders. 2nd ed. Austin, TX: PRO-ED; 1998

[16] Gillis JM, Natof TH, Lockshin SB, Romanczyk RG. Fear of routine physical exams in children with autism spectrum disorders: prevalence and intervention effectiveness. *Focus Autism Other Dev Disabl* 2009;*24*(3):156–168

[17] Mayes SD, Calhoun SL. Symptoms of autism in young children and correspondence with the DSM. *Infants Young Child* 1999;*12*(2):90–97

[18] Mirrett PL, Riski JE, Glascott J, Johnson V. Videofluoroscopic assessment of dysphagia in children with severe spastic cerebral palsy. *Dysphagia* 1994;*9*(3):174–179

[19] Arvedson J, Lefton-Grief M. Pediatric Videofluoroscopic Swallow Studies: A Professional Manual with Caregiver Guidelines. San Antonio, TX: Communication Skill Builders/Psychological Corporation; 1998

[20] Mercado-Deane MG, Burton EM, Harlow SA, et al. Swallowing dysfunction in infants less than 1 year of age. *Pediatr Radiol* 2001;*31*(6):423–428

[21] Chan CB, Chan LK, Lam HS. Scattered radiation level during videofluoroscopy for swallowing study. *Clin Radiol* 2002;*57*(7):614–616

[22] Cohen MD. Can we use pulsed fluoroscopy to decrease the radiation dose during video fluoroscopic feeding studies in children? *Clin Radiol* 2009;*64*(1):70–73

[23] Zammit-Maempel I, Chapple CL, Leslie P. Radiation dose in videofluoroscopic swallow studies. *Dysphagia* 2007;*22*(1):13–15

[24] Weckmueller J, Easterling C, Arvedson J. Preliminary temporal measurement analysis of normal oropharyngeal swallowing in infants and young children. *Dysphagia* 2011;*26*(2):135–143

[25] Gosa MM, Suiter DM, Kahane JC. Reliability for identification of a select set of temporal and physiologic features of infant swallows. *Dysphagia* 2015;*30*(3):365–372

[26] Wallis C, Ryan MM. Assessing the role of aspiration in pediatric lung disease. *Pediatr Allergy Immunol Pulmonol* 2012;*25*(3):132

# 8 Adult Fiberoptic Endoscopic Evaluation of Swallowing

*Susan Brady and Steven B. Leder*

## Summary

Fiberoptic endoscopic evaluation of swallowing (FEES) is a reliable and validated evaluation technique that is used to diagnose pharyngeal dysphagia, rate pharyngeal residue severity, and implement appropriate rehabilitation interventions to promote safe and efficient swallowing. Patients of all ages, in different environmental settings, and with diverse diagnoses can benefit from FEES. The skilled swallowing specialist knows when to recommend additional testing methods for appropriately managing an individual who presents with suspected dysphagia. Future research will include the precise reliability of FEES both in comparison to other currently used objective testing procedures (e.g., videofluoroscopic swallow study [VFSS]), as well as with tests not currently used in the diagnostic armamentarium (e.g., functional magnetic resonance imaging and real-time computed axial tomography).

## Keywords

deglutition, dysphagia, endoscopy, evaluation, fiberoptic, laryngoscope, secretions, swallow

> ### Learning Objectives
> - Gain an understanding of the standard protocol for fiberoptic endoscopic evaluation of swallowing (FEES)
> - List FEES training requirements
> - Describe indications for use, advantages, and disadvantages of endoscopic evaluation of swallowing
> - Discuss why FEES should be considered a criterion standard for evaluating the pharyngeal phase of the swallow

## 8.1 Introduction: History of the Transnasal Laryngoscopic Swallowing Evaluation

The development of improved camera technology capable of interfacing with arrayed bundles of ever smaller flexible optical fibers has permitted visualization of anatomical areas that were previously too remote to be inspected routinely for the determination of potential medical conditions. The first of these instruments was a flexible transoral gastroscope, patented in 1956, and in less than 10 years Sawashima and Hirose[91] reported the development of a smaller flexible array of optical fibers designed specifically to view the pharynx and larynx.[2] Continued improvements in both camera and fiberoptic technologies have resulted in improved laryngoscopic imaging. More recent evolution from analog to digital technology and the even newer development of the digital "distal-chip" camera rivals the images achieved with rigid telescopes. During the past 25 years there has been an ever increasing body of research describing the use of flexible fiberoptic transnasal laryngoscopy (hereafter fiberoptic endoscopic evaluation of swallowing [FEES]) for patients presenting with dysphagia. This chapter describes the unique educational training needed to perform and interpret the FEES, explains the use of FEES in the assessment of swallowing, reviews relevant findings, and stimulates further research.

## 8.2 Clinical Utility of Endoscopic Evaluation of Swallowing

The use of FEES to diagnose and treat pharyngeal dysphagia has become a criterion standard in both inpatient and outpatient settings. The first reports of the use of FEES to assess the pharyngeal swallow were reported by Langmore et al[3] and Bastian.[4] In the 25 years since these initial reports, FEES has become a reliable and validated technique to evaluate the pharyngeal phase of swallowing.[5,6,7,8,9,10] These studies demonstrated that FEES has equivalent, and at times better, sensitivity and specificity, compared with the videofluoroscopic swallowing study (VFSS), for the detection of critical variables of delay in initiation of the pharyngeal swallow, preswallow pooling in the valleculae and piriform sinuses, pharyngeal residue after the swallow, as well as laryngeal penetration and tracheal aspiration of various consistencies of foods and liquids.

An instrumental swallow evaluation has two purposes: to diagnose dysphagia and to make recommendations and implement strategies to enable safe eating. A complete FEES examination includes evaluating pharyngeal and laryngeal anatomy and physiology, identifying the presence of preswallow pooled secretions in the valleculae, piriform sinuses, laryngeal vestibule, and trachea; determining bolus flow characteristics before, during, and after the swallow; and silent aspiration status. Various food consistencies, ranging from thin liquids to nectar-like thickened liquids, purees, and solids, and different volumes (e.g., single 5 mL and 10 mL boluses and sequential bolus drinking) are tried. To ensure consistency across examiners and across clinical facilities, a standardized protocol is recommended, although such a protocol can be adjusted based on clinical findings and patient needs. A suggested protocol is provided in **Table 8.1**. If dysphagia is identified, various therapeutic interventions are implemented (with the endoscope in place) to determine whether postural adjustments (e.g., head position), dietary changes (e.g., bolus volume and consistency), and behavioral modifications (e.g., effortful swallow or two swallows per bolus) are successful in promoting safer and more efficient oral alimentation.

**Table 8.1** Suggested fiberoptic endoscopic evaluation of swallowing protocol

| Step | Rationale/additional considerations |
|---|---|
| 1. Equipment setup | 1. Clinicians need to ensure proper decontamination and testing of endoscope and other FEES equipment per facility and manufacturer's guidelines prior to the exam. Universal precautions should always be followed during the FEES procedure. |
| 2. Preparation of food/liquid for exam | 2. Use of blue food coloring is optional to enhance the visualization of the bolus. Clinicians need to be mindful of local rules and regulations for using blue food coloring; potential for cross contamination; and sepsis and other adverse/allergic reactions following use of blue food coloring. |
| 3. Explain procedure and obtain patient consent per facility standards | 3. Clinicians need to understand local rules and regulations surrounding the consent process. Although some facilities may not require a separate/specific written informed consent document for the FEES procedure, the clinician still has an obligation to explain the procedure to the patient and if possible obtain verbal consent. |
| 4. Application of a topical nasal anesthetic and/or use of a decongestant (optional) | 4. Verification of any allergies to medications is required. Clinicians should be cognizant of local rules and regulations regarding the administration of these medications. |
| 5. Passage of the nasal endoscope | 5. Clinicians should assess both nasal passages to determine the most patent route. |
| 6. Anatomical and physiological observations prior to the presentation of any bolus | 6. The purpose is to identify any potential abnormalities that may interfere with swallow function. If a clinician identifies any suspected abnormality, a referral to the appropriate medical specialist is warranted. |
| 7. Assessment of accumulated oropharyngeal secretions prior to the presentation of any bolus | 7. Clinicians should use a standardized, validated accumulated oropharyngeal secretion scale to assess the relative risks of various bolus presentations. |
| 8. Presentation of a small ice chip (recommend this step be repeated up to three times) | 8. To "prime" the swallow (especially important for patients who are given nothing by mouth); thin, copious, thick secretions; evaluate bolus flow (optional to dye ice chip blue); and further assess the relative risks of further bolus presentations |
| 9. Bolus presentation of liquids<br><br>a. ½ teaspoon of thin liquid via spoon<br><br>b. Full teaspoon of thin liquid via spoon<br><br>c. Small sip of thin liquid via cup<br><br>d. Large, uncontrolled sip of thin liquids<br><br>e. Multiple, consecutive swallows of thin liquid | 9. Consistency, volume, and presentation mode should be based upon the performance and risk to the patient. If a consistency, volume, or presentation method is deemed unsafe based on the patient's clinical presentation, it should be deferred. If the patient demonstrates no airway invasion with the ice chip trials, it is generally recommended to start with thin-liquid trials. If the patient demonstrates airway invasion with the ice chip trials or with the thin-liquid trials, then the examiner may wish to attempt thickened liquids with the patient. For the teaspoon and small-sip bolus presentations, it is generally recommended to use at least three administrations (depending on safety). Swallowing safety strategies should be incorporated into the exam as needed based on the clinical presentation of the patient. |
| 10. Bolus presentation of solids<br><br>a. ½ teaspoon of puree<br><br>b. Full teaspoon of puree<br><br>c. ½ teaspoon of semisolid/chopped food item<br><br>d. Full teaspoon of semisolid chopped food item<br><br>e. Self-administered bite of a bread item and/or cookie<br><br>f. Self-administered bite of a hard, raw vegetable<br><br>g. Self-administered bolus of a mixed consistency (e.g., sandwiches, soup, and whole pill with liquid) | 10. Again, presentations of the solid items should be based on the clinical presentation of the patient and relative risks. Each solid bolus presentation is normally repeated two to three times. As with the liquid presentations, swallowing safety strategies should be incorporated into the exam as needed based on the clinical presentation of the patient (e.g., liquid wash and/or chin tuck to clear pharyngeal residue) and thus may require additional bolus presentations of a consistency. One of the main advantages of the FEES procedure is it allows for the use of "real" food during the procedure. Therefore, if a patient is reporting difficulty with a specific food item, the clinician should attempt to evaluate it during the exam. A second advantage of the FEES procedure is that it allows the clinician to evaluate for fatigue. If appropriate, the clinician may want to readminister some of the thin-liquid bolus presentations a second time following the solid trial items to further assess for swallow fatigue. |
| 11. Observations of bolus flow in the preswallow segment | 11. Bolus flow before the initiation of the swallow response may be analyzed. |
| 12. White-out segment observations | 12. Events that occur during the white-out segment are inferred. |
| 13. Postswallow segment observations | 13. The Yale Pharyngeal Residue scale is one example of a tool available to assess postswallow airway invasion risk. |
| 14. Introduction of therapeutic swallowing safety and rehabilitative strategies during FEES | 14. Postures, swallowing maneuvers, sensory enhancements, and bolus modifications should be introduced into the exam as appropriate to identify the optimal swallow function and appropriate diet level. Additionally, the use of various treatment techniques can be assessed during FEES by capitalizing on the biofeedback component of the procedure to facilitate rehabilitation efforts (e.g., voluntary breath-hold to increase airway closure). |
| 15. Debrief with patient results and recommendations based on the findings of the FEES exam | 15. Clinicians should record the FEES procedure and review the video recording with the patient. Results and recommendations should be discussed with the patient. The clinician should ensure the patient and/or family has a clear understanding of the findings of the exam and has had an opportunity to ask questions, discuss concerns, and have input into the treatment options available. |
| 16. Documentation of findings | 16. The FEES report should include a complete description of the exam findings and recommendations. |

*Abbreviation:* FEES, fiberoptic endoscopic evaluation of swallowing.

*Sources:* Adapted from Langmore et al., [3] & ASHA [17].

## 8.3  Educational Training Needs for FEES

To acquire the necessary skills to perform and interpret the FEES procedure, the swallowing specialist must develop two distinct skills for the effective and competent performance of the procedure. The first skill is primarily technical in nature and requires hands-on management of the equipment and successful transnasal passage of the flexible endoscope, then advancing the endoscope into the high position of the hypopharynx and properly handling the endoscope during and after the swallow (i.e., advancing the endoscope into the low position). This skill is also known as the psychomotor component of the procedure.[11]

The second skill is cognitive in nature and requires the correct interpretation of findings observed during the procedure in order to accurately diagnose the swallowing disorder as viewed by endoscopy, implement appropriate swallowing interventions, and recommend further medical referrals as needed.[12] The cognitive skills component includes both rule-based and knowledge-based behavior. The rule-based components involve following complex sets of specific procedural steps, which are performed according to preexisting rules. An examiner must learn to identify specific signs to activate the next procedural step from the preexisting rule. In clinical situations, such as a medical complication or an unexpected anatomical variation, knowledge-based behavior is engaged when no rules are available for the given situation in order for the examiner to address the issue effectively.[13] The knowledge-based component requires both the correct sequence of steps to perform the procedure and the critical thinking skills necessary to make the appropriate decisions related to intervention, treatment, and management of the swallowing disorder.[11]

Given the advanced skills and knowledge required to perform and interpret the FEES procedure, the novice provider may face many challenges during FEES training.[14] Guidelines available from the American Speech-Language-Hearing Association (ASHA)[12] suggest a three-step process involving observations, practice under direct supervision, and independent practice with indirect supervision. The training approach recommended by ASHA is consistent with the surgical training approach of the master–apprentice model, where a trainee learns how to perform the procedure under the supervision of a qualified surgeon. However, with advances in surgical training techniques, the master–apprentice model, is no longer appropriate for the novice learner because the risk to the patient may be too high to accommodate a trainee's learning curve.[13] Novice learners need to acquire knowledge of the procedure itself, knowledge of the potential pitfalls of the procedure, and appropriate intervention strategies when an unforeseen problem arises.[13] Teaching, learning, and mastering these behaviors is a complex and interactive process. A training program for the novice examiner should provide both the foundational cognitive knowledge necessary to interpret the procedure effectively and the motor skills, with practice on human patient simulator manikins leading to supervision with actual patients.

## 8.4  Purposes of Dysphagia Testing

The response to a consultation for the evaluation of a patient with suspected dysphagia should always include a complete medical review and use of a valid and reliable swallow screen.[15] If the patient fails the swallow screen, an instrumental assessment should be performed.[15,16] The goals of the two most widely used instrumental assessments (i.e., FEES and VFSS) are similar in construct. In the course of these examinations the clinician attempts to identify normal and abnormal anatomy relative to the swallow function, discern discrete physiological structural movements associated with the swallow, determine temporal coordination of structural movements relative to pharyngeal bolus flow, assess the trajectory of the bolus through the pharynx, ascertain the severity of pharyngeal bolus residue patterns, and implement appropriate therapeutic interventions and diet recommendations when indicated. **Fig. 8.1** shows simultaneous image comparisons of VFSS (on the left) and FEES (on the right) showing spillage of material into the valleculae and piriform sinuses bilaterally. Additional differences between FEES and VFSS are discussed later in this chapter.

During FEES the swallowing specialist is alert to the major findings of retention of food and liquid in the valleculae and piriform sinuses and penetration of food and liquid into the laryngeal vestibule and trachea, either before or after the initial or subsequent clearing swallows have been completed. During the examination, the clinician will make adjustments to bolus volume, viscosity, and rate of delivery, as well as adjustments in patient positioning and implementation of maneuvers to determine whether these changes have a positive effect on the safety or efficiency of the pharyngeal swallow. The ultimate goals are safe oral alimentation for maintenance and enhancement of quality of life.

ASHA has developed a comprehensive triad of documents related to the performance of FEES. Specifically, *Knowledge and Skills for Speech-Language Pathologists Performing Endoscopic Assessment of Swallowing,*[17] *Role of the Speech-Language Pathologist in the Performance and Interpretation of Endoscopic Evaluation of Swallowing* Guidelines[12] and *The Use of Endoscopy by Speech-Language Pathologists* Position Statement.[18] Readers are encouraged to familiarize themselves with the information provided in these reports.

## 8.5  Endoscopic Equipment

The flexible laryngoscope is constructed to cast a "cold" light delivered from a halogen or xenon light source. The light travels along fiberoptic bundles that traverse the length of the scope. Depending on the configuration, the light is diffused through one or two lenses at the tip of the scope to illuminate the area of interest. An analog laryngoscope has a separate lens on the distal end of the scope that collects the reflected image and projects it along another bundle of light fibers to the eyepiece. The swallowing specialist can visualize the image by looking directly through the eyepiece or by using a distal-chip camera, which converts the image to a video signal, allowing the now much larger image to be viewed on a monitor and recorded.

A digital distal-chip scope also requires a bundled array of light fibers to illuminate the anatomy of interest, but it does not have an eyepiece for viewing. Instead, the image is captured on an optical chip and then projected to a video display/recorder. Ideally, when performing a transnasal laryngoscopic swallowing examination, the swallowing specialist should be freed from viewing the image

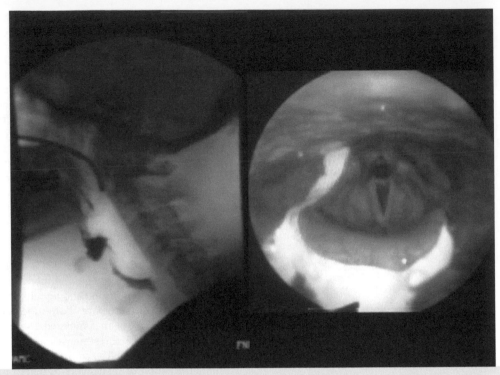

**Fig. 8.1** Simultaneous comparison of videofluoroscopic swallowing study (left) and fiberoptic endoscopic evaluation of swallowing (right) showing spillage into the valleculae and piriform sinuses bilaterally. (Reprinted from Leder SB, Murray JT. Fiberoptic endoscopic evaluation of swallowing. Phys Med Rehabil Clin N Am 2008;19(4):787–801 with permission from Elsevier, Philadelphia, PA.)

through the eyepiece. With the distal-chip camera in place, patient positioning becomes less restrictive because close proximity of the patient and swallowing specialist is no longer necessary. In addition, the image is much larger on the video monitor, allowing for better identification of potential abnormalities. It is advantageous to record the study digitally for archiving and later review for both clinical and research purposes.[19]

There are many fine flexible laryngoscopes on the market that are suitable for the performance of FEES. The typical laryngoscope has a flexible insertion shaft that is approximately 40 cm long, with the diameter ranging from 3.2 to 4 mm. Smaller pediatric laryngoscopes, with diameters ranging from 1.6 to 2.2 mm, provide diminished, but adequate, illumination capabilities for good visualization of the anatomical structures, swallow physiology, and bolus flow patterns of interest. The operation of the angulation lever on the control portion of the scope adjusts the degree of deflection. The distal tip of the scope deflects > 90 degrees to allow dynamic control of the image being viewed. Generally, the FEES examination rarely requires deflection beyond 90 degrees. For the management of the endoscope, clinicians should be aware of the manufacturer's decontamination guidelines and their institutional policies.

New technology has enabled clinical use of smartphone applications to provide a larger image and recording capabilities for later examination and visual biofeedback. Emerging technologies and interfaces will result in less expensive equipment, thereby enabling more clinicians to perform FEES in varied environments (e.g., extended-care facilities and outpatient medical offices).

## 8.6 Endoscopic Visualization of the Pharyngeal Swallow

Both nares should be examined first, and the scope is gently inserted transnasally along the path of least resistance in the most patent naris. This path is generally along the nasal floor below the inferior turbinate or, less frequently, between the inferior and middle turbinates. Blood flow to each naris and its respective inferior, middle, and superior turbinates alternates every 4 hours, resulting in a change in patency during the day. It is therefore not unusual for the most patent naris to alternate if repeat FEES evaluations are performed on the same patient over time. Once the most patent naris has been determined, the scope is gently but continuously inserted until the nasopharyngeal vault is visualized. The clinician should first position the scope just superior to the velopharyngeal port in order to determine velar function. The patient is instructed to say "money" (velopharyngeal port open) and "cookie" (velopharyngeal port closed) at this time. The patient is then instructed to breathe through the nose or hum, causing the velum to drop, thereby opening the velopharyngeal port. At this point the angulation control lever is manipulated to angle the scope downward and allow for easy insertion into the nasopharynx in order to view the base of the tongue and the laryngeal inlet. After insertion, rotation of the endoscope clockwise or counterclockwise (not movement of the swallowing specialist's arm to the left or right) combined with deflection of the endoscope tip permits the swallowing specialist to view the entire pharynx and larynx.

For the observation of pharyngeal swallowing function, the distal end of the scope is placed superior to the epiglottis at the level of the uvula. This is customarily called the high position. This position provides a view of the base of the tongue, posterior pharyngeal wall, lateral pharyngeal walls, epiglottis, valleculae, larynx, and piriform sinuses.

It is important to remember that, because the swallowing specialist and patient are facing one another, the endoscopic image is reversed (i.e., the right side in the image is actually the left side anatomically and the left side in the image is actually the right side anatomically). As the scope is advanced more distally into the pharynx, fewer structures peripheral to the larynx are included in the field of view. The scope may be advanced to the tip of the epiglottis for optimal viewing of the piriform sinuses, laryngeal vestibule, and subglottis/trachea. This is the ideal position for observing airway closure patterns during the swallow. The laryngoscope is typically placed at a depth no greater than 15 cm from the tip of the nares, which allows an adequate view of the swallow function and aspiration. Care must be taken to avoid touching any of the pharyngeal structures with the tip of the endoscope, which will cause coughing.

Flexible laryngoscopy allows visualization of the anatomy and biomechanical movements that are immediately in front of the objective lens. The oral, upper esophageal, and esophageal stages of the swallow will not be visualized during this procedure. During the height of the pharyngeal swallow there is a very brief period when the image is obliterated due to the apposition of tissue, usually the base of the tongue or the velum to the posterior pharyngeal wall, around the objective lens. This is commonly termed the white-out period. In exchange for these disadvantages, the skilled swallowing specialist will be rewarded with an unequaled view of airway protective patterns with a very sensitive tool for detecting laryngeal penetration and aspiration as well as an invaluable mechanism for biofeedback and patient education. **Fig. 8.2** shows a FEES image of diffuse spillage of liquid (milk) into the valleculae and piriform sinuses bilaterally.

It is essential to sustain discipline in positioning the endoscope before and after the swallow to augment the visualization of findings. Because the field of view is limited, findings must be pursued actively through the dynamic placement of the scope. Prior to each presentation of food or liquid the swallowing specialist must endeavor to achieve a field of view that includes the areas of interest. Following the swallow the scope should quickly be placed deeper into the pharynx to allow for visualization of the laryngeal vestibule, piriform sinuses, and subglottic region in order to determine evidence of penetration or aspiration that may have occurred during the white-out period.

Often, the tip of the endoscope will be covered by mucus or food debris, resulting in a blurry image quality. The swallowing specialist has two options when this occurs. First, wiping the tip against the posterior nasopharyngeal wall is usually successful for clearing the image. If not, the second option is to simply remove the endoscope, clean the tip with a damp paper towel, and reinsert.

Conventional wisdom has held that a bolus should not enter the pharynx prior to the onset of hyolaryngeal elevation, and in some cases the swallowing specialist may not see the bolus enter the pharynx in a nondysphagic subject who is holding a bolus intraorally while preparing to swallow spontaneously or waiting for a command to swallow. However, recent research has suggested

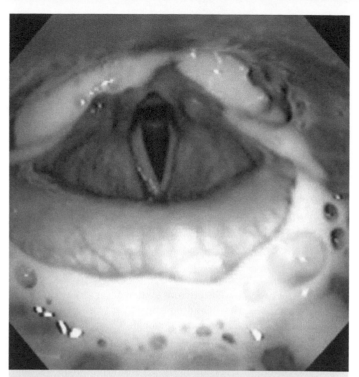

**Fig. 8.2** Fiberoptic endoscopic evaluation of swallowing image of diffuse spillage of a liquid (milk) into the valleculae and piriform sinuses bilaterally. (Reprinted from Leder SB, Murray JT. Fiberoptic endoscopic evaluation of swallowing. Phys Med Rehabil Clin N Am 2008;19(4):787–801 with permission from Elsevier, Philadelphia, PA.)

that natural feeding and swallowing (i.e., without commands to swallow), yield a different bolus flow pattern.[20] In a study of 15 healthy, young, normal subjects, 60% of liquids and 76% of solid food boluses entered the pharynx, sometimes as deep as the piriform sinus, prior to initiating a successful pharyngeal phase of the swallow.[21]

### 8.6.1 Presence/Absence of a Foreign Body in the Pharynx: Does It Matter?

There has been concern that the presence of the flexible portion of the laryngoscope in the pharynx may have a deleterious effect on pharyngeal swallow physiology. However, this has been shown not to be the case. Suiter and Moorhead[22] reported that the presence of a flexible fiberoptic endoscope in the pharynx during swallowing in 14 normal adults did not significantly affect pharyngeal swallow physiology of three swallow duration measures, number of swallows necessary to clear the bolus, or penetration-aspiration scale scores.

### 8.6.2 Assessment of Pharyngeal and Laryngeal Anatomy and Physiology

FEES not only identifies the signs and symptoms of dysphagia; it is also capable of providing a view of the anatomy and physiology of the swallow. Prior to the presentation of any food or liquid, the examiner must first conduct an assessment of the anatomical and physiological observations in order to identify any potential bolus obstruction or bolus flow interference. For example, the observation of a reduced vocal fold movement that is resulting in a large glottal gap may place the patient at increased risk for aspiration with thin liquids. This type of reduction in vocal fold mobility (i.e., unilateral vocal fold movement in the lateral position) has been associated with increased incidence of aspiration.[29] It is important to note that, depending on the clinical background of the examiner, it may not be within the scope of the FEES exam to diagnose the specific anatomical abnormality or physiological disorders. For nonphysician examiners, any suspected abnormality should prompt a referral to the appropriate medical professional.

## 8.7 Use of Topical Anesthesia

The use of a topical nasal anesthesia during FEES may be included as part of the protocol. The current evidence regarding the use of a topical nasal anesthetic and its impact on comfort during the procedure remains somewhat equivocal. A systematic review of the literature[31] found no evidence to support reduced pain or discomfort when using a topical treatment before nasal endoscopy. Leder and colleagues[32] conducted a prospective, double-blinded, randomized study on the use of a topical nasal anesthetic with 152 subjects and found no difference in patient comfort level between the various conditions.

The effects of a topical nasal anesthetic and its impact on swallowing ability also remain equivocal. A study in 2015 by Fife and colleagues[33] revealed that the use of a topical nasal anesthetic did not result in statistically significant higher penetration and aspiration scores. However, Lester and colleagues[34] found that the use of a topical nasal anesthetic resulted in significantly worse swallow function, as evidenced by higher airway invasion on the penetration-aspiration scale.

If an examiner chooses to use a topical nasal anesthetic during FEES, a comprehensive review of the patient's medical history and allergies is required in order to avoid any potential allergic reactions or adverse events related to the administration of the topical nasal anesthetic. Further, for the nonphysicians performing FEES, the administration of a topical anesthetic varies by state laws, and clinicians need to be aware of local rules and regulations.[12]

## 8.8 Pharyngeal Secretion Level

A clinical benefit of performing FEES is the suspected or observed difficulty in swallowing saliva or secretions. Most FEES clinical protocols include an observation of secretions, including the amount and location, before any bolus presentation.[12] The rationale for evaluating secretion levels with a reliable measure is to provide the examiner with a mechanism to differentiate safe or acceptable levels from accumulated secretions that are dangerously large. Further, by having a method for the examiner to discern the secretion levels, the examiner is potentially able to provide more appropriate treatment, thus reducing the incidence or complication of aspiration pneumonia and its associated health care costs.[35,36,37] Various secretion scales are available in the literature,[35,36,37] and **Table 8.2** summarizes the three-point

**Table 8.2** Three-point secretion scale

| Level | Estimated amount of secretions |
|---|---|
| 1 | Functional: ≤ 25% pooling in piriform sinuses and/or vallecular space |
| 2 | Severe: Penetration of secretions above the true vocal folds; intermittent penetration of secretions during inhalation; no aspiration of secretions; endolaryngeal secretions |
| 3 | Profound: Secretions on vocal folds and/or aspiration of secretions |

*Reproduced with permission of SAGE Publications.*

secretion scale developed by Donzelli and colleagues,[37] which measures the presence, amount, and location of oropharyngeal secretions. With this three-point secretion scale, the higher score, 3, represents more secretions. Further, the score that the patient receives is the point of maximum secretions present (no transition score is available). This three-point secretion scale also distinguishes between laryngeal penetration and tracheal aspiration of secretions. The predictive validity of the three-point secretion scale in relation to aspiration was moderately correlated ($r_s = 0.516$, $P < 0.0001$) and highly correlated to diet outcome recommendations ($r_s = 0.72$, $P < 0.0001$) because patients receiving a higher secretion level were more likely to aspirate and also to receive a lower diet level or be recommended to be given nothing by mouth.[37]

## 8.9 Indications for FEES Testing

Following a failed swallow screening, the clinician should determine the field of view necessary to reveal the pathophysiology of the suspected dysphagia most completely. A VFSS evaluation should be performed if questions regarding oral stage impairments cannot be answered following the swallow screening or if there is a suspicion of an esophageal component to the dysphagia.

There are a number of clinical signs and symptoms of dysphagia that can be confidently assessed with FEES. For example, ideal candidates are patients with hypernasality and suspected nasal regurgitation, laryngeal penetration or aspiration before the swallow is initiated, abnormal vocal quality, and increased swallowing difficulty over the duration of a meal secondary to fatigue. The practical reasons for employing FEES are more numerous given that a swallowing specialist can perform the examination at bedside and on short notice. Some practical reasons for choosing FEES include testing individuals who may have safety issues associated with radiation exposure (e.g., women with confirmed or possible pregnancy) or patients with radiation limitations, and retesting individuals with documented dysphagia on the endoscopic or fluoroscopic evaluation.[38,39] Because transportation to the radiology suite is often difficult for many patients (e.g., if mechanical ventilation or orthopedic traction is required), FEES may be the test of choice for bedridden or weak patients; patients with open wounds, contractures, fractures, or pain; and patients with quadriplegia or ventilator dependency. Additionally, patients who are morbidly obese, require special positioning, or are wheelchair dependent are challenging to assess with VFSS. In the authors' experience, patients who are in the intensive care unit, are heavily monitored, or require mechanical ventilation via a tracheotomy tube present the greatest opportunities for choosing FEES.

Contraindications for FEES include cases of facial trauma, recent refractory epistaxis, bilateral obstruction of the nasal passages due to packing or choanal atresia, severe agitation, and inability to cooperate with the examination.

## 8.10 Risk Assessment: FEES *Before* Administration of Liquid and Food

Following proper positioning of the fiberoptic endoscope in the pharynx but prior to the administration of any food and liquid, the clinician has the opportunity to survey the anatomy, elicit physiological movements, observe the management of secretions, and monitor spontaneous swallows. Edema, postsurgical anatomical changes, and tissue changes secondary to radiation treatment can affect the configuration of the protective mechanisms of the pharynx and larynx and influence the size and shape of the valleculae and piriform sinuses. These changes can potentially have an impact on the success of the pharyngeal swallow and the ability to contain spilled material before the swallow and retained bolus after the swallow.

The collection of persistent pharyngeal secretions located within the laryngeal vestibule prior to the presentation of food and liquid is an important sign of potential poor swallowing performance (i.e., increased aspiration risk) later on in the examination. Murray et al,[35] in a study comparing elders with neurogenic disease with age-matched controls, reported that the combination of secretions in the laryngeal vestibule with reduced frequency of swallowing were highly predictive of aspiration of food and liquid. Link et al,[36] in a study of pediatric patients with dysphagia, found that pooled secretions in the laryngeal vestibule correlated with later development of aspiration pneumonia. Therefore, it is recommended that the swallowing specialist have the patient phonate and cough at the onset of the examination to provide an impression of airway protection abilities before giving any food or liquid. **Fig. 8.3** documents copious secretions, indicating an increased risk of aspiration later on during FEES.

The objective of diagnostic testing for dysphagia is to show ability as well as disability. The initial careful presentation of measured stimulus volumes limits the amount of penetration and aspiration early in the examination so as to reduce patient distress and thus the likelihood of an aborted examination. Small bolus volumes ranging from 5 to 10 mL are given first. FEES should not be stopped when a small amount of aspiration occurs. Discontinuing the examination prevents the implementation of adjustments to swallowing behavior that may alleviate future aspiration events. When the findings of copious secretions in the vestibule and reduced frequency of swallowing occur at the onset of the examination, there are a number of options available. Murray[16] recommends that food and liquid boluses be momentarily deferred and that the examination proceed with the more cautious offering of ice chips to further determine aspiration status. This reduces the chance of severe aspiration that may truncate the examination and reduce the degree and quality of any findings. Also, limiting swallowing to single, small (5 mL) bolus volumes of puree gives the patient the

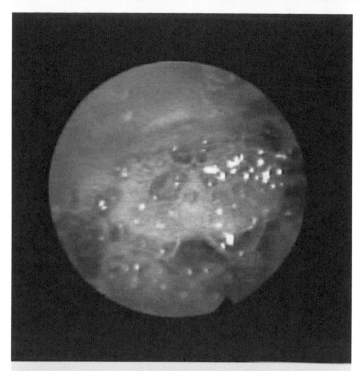

**Fig. 8.3** Fiberoptic endoscopic evaluation of swallowing image of documentation of copious secretions, indicating increased risk of aspiration later on in the examination. (Reprinted from Leder SB, Murray JT. Fiberoptic endoscopic evaluation of swallowing. Phys Med Rehabil Clin N Am 2008;19(4):787–801 with permission from Elsevier, Philadelphia, PA.)

best opportunity to swallow successfully. Alternatively, the experienced swallowing specialist should abort a FEES exam for safety issues if prandial aspiration is deemed inevitable.

## 8.11 Conducting FEES

The patient can be positioned sitting in a procedure chair or wheelchair or can be positioned sitting upright (or as upright as possible) in bed. The swallowing specialist usually stands during the procedure. It is recommended that the swallowing specialist master the performance of transnasal endoscopy while standing on either side of the patient, to allow for greater flexibility when the examination is performed at the bedside.

Following transnasal passage of the endoscope and performing the initial risk assessment, food and liquid are presented. Ideally, the potentially dysphagic patient can self-feed during the examination, allowing for a natural delivery of food and liquid, in a volume and at a rate that typify the patient's self-feeding behaviors. However, self-feeding is not the norm. Should the patient be unable to self-feed due to cognitive disability or physical limitations, an assistant can deliver the boluses to the patient's mouth via a spoon, straw, or cup. In either case, the swallow is elicited by providing food and liquid of varying volumes and consistencies to the patient. When possible, no command to swallow is given, which provides a more natural representation of the eating process.[20] However, neurologically impaired patients may benefit from a verbal cue to swallow.

The food and liquid should be light in color to enhance visibility.[40] Foods that are translucent (water and most juices), dark, or colored red or brown (many meats) may be more difficult to visualize because they will blend in when viewed against the pharyngeal mucosa. Milk, puddings, yogurt, breads, and cheeses as well as many of the commercially available liquid nutrition formulas are light in color and reflect light well. Given that the direct entry of food and liquid can occur during the period when the view of the larynx and pharynx is obliterated (i.e., at the height of the swallow due to tissue apposition to the objective lens), the reflective properties of the bolus are especially important. Highly reflective food and liquid are easily observed in the pharynx and laryngeal vestibule as well as subglottically along the anterior tracheal wall after the brief period of visual obliteration has resolved.

## 8.11.1 Use of Blue Dye and Other Food Colorings

The rationale for dyeing food blue (or green or red or yellow), usually with the use of FD & C Blue No. 1, to help identify aspiration appears to be based on tradition, intuition, acceptance, and assumptions rather than on objective analyses of available evidence.[3] Because blue is not a color found in oropharyngeal secretions, blue dye has been used to detect aspiration without feeding trials,[4] as well as being added to enteral feedings of critically ill patients[5,6] and to oral feedings of patients with suspected dysphagia,[7,8] for over 25 years. New concerns, however, have developed over the safety of using blue (or any) dye, especially for patients at risk for increased gastrointestinal permeability (e.g., sepsis, burns, trauma, shock, renal failure, celiac sprue, and inflammatory bowel disease).[42,43] However, the small volumes of blue dye used during FEES have not given rise to reports of adverse events.[42,43]

The reliability of FEES to detect the critical features of pharyngeal dysphagia and aspiration is consistently high using either blue-dyed or non-blue-dyed foods. A study by Leder and colleagues[40] found that FEES maintained high intrarater and interrater reliability in detecting the critical features of pharyngeal dysphagia and aspiration with or without the use of blue dye. As a result, the swallowing specialist can reliably identify depth of bolus flow, bolus retention, laryngeal penetration, and tracheal aspiration using regular, non-blue-dyed foods (e.g., yellow custard and white skim milk). It was thus recommended that the use of blue dye during FEES be abandoned as a marker of pharyngeal dysphagia and aspiration.[41,40] Even though the swallowing specialist can be assured of reliable FEES results using regular, non-dyed food trials, it is still recommended to use foods that are highly reflective and contrast well against the pharyngeal mucosa during the FEES procedure.[42,40]

## 8.11.2 Swallow Function and Bolus Flow during FEES

When presenting a bolus, the FEES procedure is described as having three distinct components: the preswallow segment, the white-out segment, and the postswallow segment. During the preswallow segment, the swallowing specialist examines the anatomy and physiology of the hypopharynx and larynx, assesses accumulated oropharyngeal secretion levels, and analyzes bolus flow before the initiation of the swallow response. Bolus flow events that may be observed in the preswallow segment include premature spillage to the valleculae, piriform sinuses, and laryngeal vestibule; a delayed triggering of the reflexive pharyngeal swallow; and tracheal aspiration. The white-out period occurs at the height of the pharyngeal phase due to tissue apposition to the objective lens at the distal tip of the endoscope. During the white-out period, a view of the hypopharynx is not possible; therefore, events that occur during this period are inferred. In the postswallow segment, the endoscope is then advanced to the low position to evaluate for airway invasion, which may have occurred during the white-out segment. Additionally, in the postswallow segment, an assessment of pharyngeal residue in the valleculae and piriform sinuses, as well as the presence of any airway invasion from the residue, is noted.

## 8.11.3 Detection of Laryngeal Penetration and Aspiration

Interestingly, FEES has proven to be more precise in identifying laryngeal penetration and aspiration compared to VFSS. Kelly et al[9] investigated 15 simultaneous VFSS and FEES tests with 15 independent raters. They reported significant differences between FEES and VFSS regarding pharyngeal residue severity scores. In a follow-up study, Kelly et al,[10] using the Penetration-Aspiration Scale (PAS),[45] found that the judges ranked the PAS score significantly higher when the swallow was viewed with FEES than with VFSS. This may be due to the fact that the swallowing specialist can visualize very small amounts of food particulate and mucosal coating with the laryngoscope that may not carry enough barium sulfate to cause an impression on the fluoroscopic image and are thus not perceived by the examiner during VFSS. It was suggested that, because both residue and PAS scores were consistently higher with FEES than with VFSS, clinicians using both instruments in their practice should make every effort to calibrate their ratings for the two examinations and not treat results as interchangeable.[9,10] **Fig. 8.4** is a FEES image of tracheal aspiration.

## 8.11.4 The Importance of Pharyngeal Residue

Pharyngeal residue, defined as preswallow secretions and postswallow food residue in the pharynx not entirely cleared by a swallow, is a clinical predictor of prandial aspiration.[3] An accurate description of pharyngeal residue severity is an important but difficult clinical challenge.[4] Pharyngeal residue occurs in either the valleculae (spaces between the base of the tongue and the epiglottis) or the piriform sinuses (spaces formed on both sides of the pharynx between the fibers of the inferior pharyngeal constrictor muscle and the sides of the thyroid cartilage and lined by orthogonally directed fibers of the palatopharyngeus muscle and pharyngobasilar fascia).[5]

The Yale Pharyngeal Residue Severity Rating Scale[46] provides reliable and valid information regarding the location and severity (i.e., none, trace, mild, moderate, and severe) of vallecular and piriform sinus residue observed during FEES. Because the Yale Pharyngeal Residue Scale is anatomically defined and image

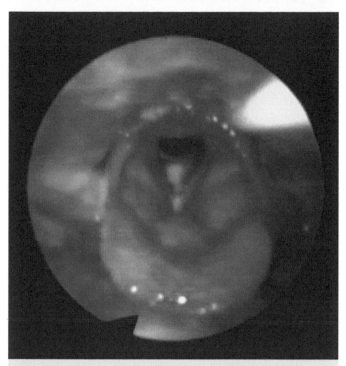

**Fig. 8.4** Fiberoptic endoscopic evaluation of swallowing image of tracheal aspiration. (Reprinted from Leder SB, Murray JT. Fiberoptic endoscopic evaluation of swallowing. Phys Med Rehabil Clin N Am 2008;19(4):787–801 with permission from Elsevier, Philadelphia, PA.)

based, the severity rating is not affected by either the shape or the size of the valleculae and piriform sinus. Variations across body size, age, and gender are irrelevant because individuals serve as their own controls. This generalizability makes it possible to determine pharyngeal residue severity for any given person.

The Yale Pharyngeal Residue Rating Scale[46] works well for any swallow, whether it is the first swallow, subsequent clearing swallow, or last swallow. The clinician simply has to match the chosen swallow with its scale mate. In this way, it is possible to determine whether spontaneous or volitional clearing swallows or a throat-clearing maneuver are actually helpful in reducing the amount of residue in the valleculae and piriform sinuses. Because an important therapeutic goal is to aid pharyngeal clearing, this information can guide intervention strategies and promote safer swallowing. For example, it is now possible to determine objectively whether drinking a small liquid bolus after a puree/solid bolus, an effortful swallow, a double-swallow/bolus, a head turn to the left or right, and a chin tuck are successful in reducing residue in the valleculae and piriform sinus.

In summary, the Yale Pharyngeal Residue Severity Rating Scale[46] is a reliable, validated, anatomically defined, image-based tool to determine residue location and severity based on FEES. Proficiency can be readily achieved with minimal training and at high levels of intra- and interrater reliability and validity. Clinical uses include, but are not limited to, accurate classification of valleculae and piriform sinus residue severity patterns as none, trace, mild, moderate, or severe for diagnostic purposes, determination of functional therapeutic change, and precise dissemination of shared information. Research uses include, but are not limited to,

tracking outcome measures, demonstrating efficacy of interventions to reduce pharyngeal residue, investigating morbidity and mortality in relation to pharyngeal residue severity, and improving training and accuracy of FEES interpretation by students and clinicians.

## 8.12 Therapeutic Interventions with FEES

FEES is ideally suited for implementation of various therapeutic interventions prior to recommending oral feedings. The endoscope can be safely and atraumatically inserted via the most patent naris[47] and, if necessary, reinserted during an evaluation for optimal visualization. Scope placement can also be tolerated for relatively long periods of time (e.g., 15 minutes or longer), while different food consistencies, bolus sizes, and therapeutic interventions are tried. Thickening agents can be added to thin liquids to assess success with nectar-, honey-, or custard-like consistencies using real food during the initial as well as the follow-up FEES.[38] Gum-based, rather than starch-based, thickeners are recommended because they maintain the desired consistency for longer periods of time. Volume adjustments can also be tried to determine optimal bolus volumes to promote safe swallowing.

Additionally, various postural changes can be assessed (e.g., chin tuck or head turn to left or right), in combination with different bolus consistencies and volumes and with different swallow strategies, such as an effortful swallow, two swallows/bolus, or swallow—clear throat—swallow again, in an attempt to determine optimal safe and successful feeding strategies. Lastly, in patients who can benefit from visual biofeedback, placing the monitor in their visual field and instructing them to swallow twice, swallow hard, or swallow—throat clear—swallow again, or perform a super-supraglottic swallow[48] may provide enough reinforcement for successful swallowing of at least one consistency or adequate success on which to base ongoing rehabilitation. **Fig. 8.5** demonstrates the change in anatomy with a head turn to the left (i.e., close off the left piriform sinus and lateral pharyngeal area) with the goal of promoting more efficient pharyngeal clearing and a safer and more successful swallow.

## 8.13 Cost Comparisons between FEES and VFSS

Even though the primary rationale as to which instrumental swallow exam to use with the patient should be based on clinical needs, health care costs may be a concern for the provider and/or patient. Aviv and colleagues[49] reported that FEES is more cost-effective than VFSS for the management of dysphagia with inpatients following therapy for head and neck cancer. In the United States, performing VFSS results in three separate charge codes (i.e., one each for the radiation room, the physician/professional interpretation, and the speech-language pathologist). FEES has only one charge code (i.e., for either the speech-language pathologist or the physician performing the examination). Because reimbursements for health care services are constantly changing, this information may be different in the future.

## 8.14 Visual Biofeedback with FEES

The swallowing specialist can initially be a passive observer to determine whether patients will swallow on their own dependent upon bolus location in the pharynx (e.g., triggering of the pharyngeal swallow reflex when the bolus contacts the rim of the aryepiglottic folds). Once a pattern of swallowing is observed, the swallowing specialist can be directive and inform the patient of the most successful swallow steps or strategies. For example, to aid in pharyngeal clearing the patient may be instructed to swallow hard two times in rapid succession, swallow—clear throat—swallow again, or alternate a small liquid bolus after every puree bolus. These therapeutic interventions may be helpful in transitioning the patient from a status of nothing by mouth to a safe and more efficient oral diet, or in changing from a puree to a more palatable solid consistency diet.

Real-time visual feedback is a powerful intervention strategy uniquely provided by FEES. It is very helpful in providing the patient with objective input regarding targeted laryngeal adduction maneuvers and confirmation of attainment of successful physiology and bolus status in the pharynx.[50] The patient and relevant caregivers are positioned in front of the video monitor in order to be able to view their own oropharyngeal swallow. This enables the patient to understand the exact nature of the swallowing impairment rather than relying only on the swallowing specialist's descriptions. Then different bolus consistencies and

bolus volumes as well as targeted therapeutic interventions (e.g., head turn), can be explored. The patient and caregivers become direct participants in swallow rehabilitation and are able to immediately see successful as well as unsuccessful outcomes.

### 8.14.1 Compensatory Strategies/ Swallowing Interventions

The FEES examiner must possess the experience and critical thinking skills necessary to make the appropriate decisions related to specific interventions for compensatory swallowing safety strategies and swallowing intervention. The various compensatory strategies and swallowing interventions (e.g., postures, maneuvers, bolus modifications, and sensory enhancements) are summarized in **Table 8.3**. It is vital for the FEES examiner to understand the swallowing physiology of the patient in order to select the most appropriate intervention. Further, the FEES examiner should evaluate whether the desired effect of the intervention was achieved and, if not, identify other potential strategies. Although various compensatory strategies may be used during FEES or VFSS, some strategies are procedure specific. For example, although a breath-hold maneuver with a goal of increased airway protection can be used during both FEES and VFSS, only during FEES is it possible to see whether the patient is accurately performing the voluntary airway closure during the breath-hold maneuver.[51] Conversely, use of the Mendelsohn maneuver may be better visualized during VFSS because of the tissue apposition with the objective lens at the height of the swallow resulting in the white-out. The FEES examiner should also recognize the potential advantage of using multiple strategies simultaneously (e.g., chin tuck with head turn).

## 8.15 Use of FEES in Specific Patient Populations

The applicability of FEES to both diagnose and treat pharyngeal swallowing disorders has grown as clinicians have investigated its efficacy in different patient populations. The categories are varied and include broad patient descriptors as well as specific patient diagnoses. Broad patient descriptors include trauma,[52,53,54] pediatrics,[8,55] nursing home residents,[56] patients in intensive care units,[57] and long-term care settings.[58] More specific patient diagnoses include head and neck cancer,[59,60] inhalation injuries,[61] developmental disabilities,[62] acute stroke,[63] respiratory failure,[64] amyotrophic lateral sclerosis,[65] vocal fold immobility,[29,30] and posttranshiatal esophagectomy.[66] This literature attests to the generalizability of FEES. It has gained widespread acceptability and utility for the diagnosis and treatment of pharyngeal stage swallowing disorders.

## 8.16 Future Research

Regardless of the testing method used to assess the pharyngeal swallow, precision in establishing the exact pathophysiology of the dysphagia in a patient is poor.[16,67,68] Recent research investigating pharyngeal residue[9] and laryngeal penetration and

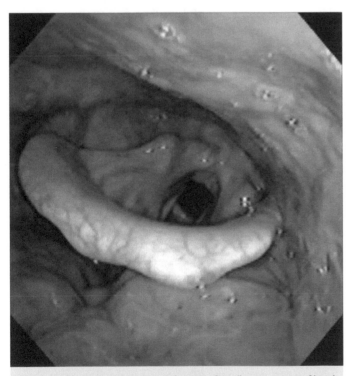

**Fig. 8.5** Fiberoptic endoscopic evaluation of swallowing image of head turn to left compensatory maneuver to close off the left piriform sinus and lateral pharyngeal area to aid in pharyngeal clearing and promote safe swallowing. (Reprinted from Leder SB, Murray JT. Fiberoptic endoscopic evaluation of swallowing. Phys Med Rehabil Clin N Am 2008;19(4):787–801 with permission from Elsevier, Philadelphia, PA.)

**Table 8.3** Compensatory strategies used during the fiberoptic endoscopic evaluation of swallowing and videofluoroscopic swallowing study

| Compensatory strategy | Rationale/indication | VFSS | FEES |
|---|---|---|---|
| Chin tuck posture | Premature spillage, laryngeal penetration, aspiration, pharyngeal residue | X | |
| Head rotation posture | Unilateral pharyngeal weakness to close off weaker side (turn head to weaker side); enhance opening of upper esophageal sphincter (UES) | X | X |
| Head tilt posture | Unilateral pharyngeal weakness. Tilt head to stronger side (ear to shoulder) to use gravity to divert bolus down the stronger side. | X | X |
| Throat clear | Clearing penetrated or aspirated material | X | X* |
| Mendelsohn maneuver | Used to increase vertical and anterior laryngeal motion and increase UES opening | X* | X |
| Effortful swallow | Improve tongue base motion, reduce pharyngeal residue | X | X |
| Ice chips | Dried secretions | | X |
| Breath-holding (supraglottic and super-supraglottic swallow) | Increase airway protection/glottal closure | X | X* |
| Multiple swallows | Used to eliminate or reduce oral and pharyngeal residue by completing a second "dry" swallow | X | X |
| Liquid wash or alternating liquids | Used to eliminate or reduce oral and pharyngeal solid bolus residue | X | X |
| Oral hold | Used with liquid boluses to reduce premature spillage and reduce swallow response delay | | |

*Abbreviations:* FEES, fiberoptic endoscopic evaluation of swallowing; VFSS, videofluoroscopic swallowing study.
*Source:* Reprinted from Brady S, Donzelli D. The modified barium swallow and the functional endoscopic evaluation of swallow. Otolaryngol Clin N Am 2013;46(6):1009–1022. doi: 10.1016/j.otc.2013.08.001 with permission from Elsevier, Philadelphia, PA.
*Indicates the preferred exam to use/view the effectiveness of the compensatory strategy.

aspiration[10] using simultaneous FEES and VFSS concluded that the examinations are not interchangeable because of the unequal judgments made by clinicians when judging pharyngeal residue, laryngeal penetration, and tracheal aspiration. On the contrary, some clinicians would argue that FEES and VFSS, although not interchangeable, are quite complementary,[69,70] because visualization of the pharyngeal swallow is achieved from different perspectives. The mucosal surface of the pharynx is very well visualized endoscopically, whereas the submucosal elements are better visualized fluoroscopically. Future research pairing the two instruments should focus on reliable and accurate identification of focal disorders of the propulsive components of the oropharyngeal swallow. Every effort should be made to link signs and symptoms from each examination so that firm inferences can be made regarding the presence of a focal swallow disorder.

## 8.17 Questions

1. A complete FEES examination includes all of the following except:

A. Evaluating pharyngeal and laryngeal anatomy and physiology
B. Identifying the presence and location of preswallow pooled secretions in the valleculae, piriform sinuses, laryngeal vestibule, and trachea
C. Determining bolus flow characteristics before, during, and after the swallow
D. Use of fluoroscopy to evaluate for silent aspiration
E. Use of endoscopy to evaluate for pharyngeal residue

2. Which of the following statements regarding the use of a topical nasal anesthetic during the FEES procedure is true?

A. Nonphysicians administering a topical anesthetic need to be aware of local rules and regulations regarding administration policies.
B. The use of a topical nasal anesthetic will improve comfort during the procedure.
C. The use of a topical nasal anesthetic will usually improve swallowing function.
D. The use of a topical nasal anesthetic will usually reduce swallow function.
E. The use of a topical nasal anesthetic requires a physician order and does not require a review of the patient's medical history and allergies by the person administering the anesthetic.

3. Potential clinical indications for FEES generally include all of the following except:

A. Hypernasality
B. Abnormal vocal quality
C. Lateral buccal stasis
D. Difficulty managing secretions
E. Issues with transportation to radiology

4. Potential contraindications for FEES generally include all of the following except:

A. Facial trauma
B. Pregnancy
C. Recent refractory epistaxis
D. Bilateral obstruction of the nasal passages
E. Severe agitation

5. Which of the following statements is true regarding the FEES procedure?

A. The FEES procedure requires the use of food that is dyed blue to assist with the visualization of the bolus.

B. The FEES procedure should not be used with infants and young children.

C. The FEES procedure is not as sensitive for detecting aspiration as other instrumental swallow exams.

D. The FEES procedure requires only advanced motor skill training in order to appropriately perform and interpret the results.

E. The FEES procedure may include the use of compensatory swallow safety strategies and other swallowing trial interventions.

# 8.18   Answers and Explanations

## 1. Correct: use of fluoroscopy to evaluate for silent aspiration (D).

A FEES examination does not include the use of fluoroscopy. This does not mean, however, that FEES cannot be used to determine the presence of silent aspiration. Research comparing the accuracy of FEES for determining aspiration to that of videofluoroscopic evaluation of swallowing has found that FEES is as sensitive as videofluoroscopy.[10]

## 2. Correct: nonphysicians administering a topical anesthetic need to be aware of local rules and regulations regarding administration policies (A).

Clinicians should be aware of potentially negative side effects of topic anesthesia and contraindications for its use. Before administering topical anesthesia, it is essential that clinicians be aware of their facilities' policy on the use of anesthesia by nonphysician health care professionals and what the policy is for handling adverse events.

## 3. Correct: lateral buccal stasis (C).

This is generally *not* a potential clinical indication for FEES. Because the oral cavity is bypassed by the endoscope, lateral buccal stasis would not be observed on the endoscopic imaging. Additionally, oral phase problems alone often do not warrant the use of instrumental assessment (e.g., difficulty chewing or lateral buccal stasis can be observed during clinical swallow assessment).

## 4. Correct: pregnancy (B).

Pregnancy is generally not a potential contraindication for the FEES procedure, and FEES is often used instead of a modified barium swallow for individuals who are pregnant.

## 5. Correct: the FEES procedure may include the use of compensatory swallow safety strategies and other swallowing trial interventions (E).

FEES is useful for teaching patients the use of many compensatory swallow strategies, including the super-supraglottic swallow. The ability to view immediately what effects a strategy has enabled the swallowing specialist to provide feedback to that patient and facilitate improved execution of that strategy.

# References

[1] Sawashima M, Hirose H. New laryngoscopic technique by use of fiber optics. *J Acoust Soc Am* 1968;43(1):168–169

[2] Hecht J. *City of Light*. New York, NY: Oxford University Press; 1999:67

[3] Langmore SE, Schatz K, Olsen N. Fiberoptic endoscopic examination of swallowing safety: a new procedure. *Dysphagia* 1988;2(4):216–219

[4] Bastian RW. Videoendoscopic evaluation of patients with dysphagia: an adjunct to the modified barium swallow. *Otolaryngol Head Neck Surg* 1991;104(3):339–350

[5] Langmore SE, Schatz K, Olson N. Endoscopic and videofluoroscopic evaluations of swallowing and aspiration. *Ann Otol Rhinol Laryngol* 1991;100(8):678–681

[6] Wu CH, Hsiao TY, Chen JC, Chang YC, Lee SY. Evaluation of swallowing safety with fiberoptic endoscope: comparison with videofluoroscopic technique. *Laryngoscope* 1997;107(3):396–401

[7] Leder SB, Sasaki CT, Burrell MI. Fiberoptic endoscopic evaluation of dysphagia to identify silent aspiration. *Dysphagia* 1998;13(1):19–21

[8] Leder SB, Karas DE. Fiberoptic endoscopic evaluation of swallowing in the pediatric population. *Laryngoscope* 2000;110(7):1132–1136

[9] Kelly AM, Leslie P, Beale T, Payten C, Drinnan MJ. Fibreoptic endoscopic evaluation of swallowing and videofluoroscopy: does examination type influence perception of pharyngeal residue severity? *Clin Otolaryngol* 2006;31(5):425–432

[10] Kelly AM, Drinnan MJ, Leslie P. Assessing penetration and aspiration: how do videofluoroscopy and fiberoptic endoscopic evaluation of swallowing compare? *Laryngoscope* 2007;117(10):1723–1727

[11] Tjiam IM, Schout BM, Hendrikx AJ, Scherpbier AJ, Witjes JA, van Merriënboer JJ. Designing simulator-based training: an approach integrating cognitive task analysis and four-component instructional design. *Med Teach* 2012;34(10):e698–707. doi: 10.3109/0142159X.2012.687480

[12] American Speech-Language-Hearing Association. The role of the speech-language pathologist in the performance and interpretation of endoscopic evaluation of swallowing: guidelines, 2004

[13] van Det MJ, Meijerink WJ, Hoff C, Middel LJ, Koopal SA, Pierie JP. The learning effect of intraoperative video-enhanced surgical procedure training. *Surg Endosc* 2011;25(7):2261–2267. doi: 10.1007/s00464-010-1545-5

[14] Benadom EM, Potter NL. The use of simulation in training graduate students to perform transnasal endoscopy. *Dysphagia* 2011;26(4):352–360 http://dx.doi 10.1007/s00455-010-9316-y

[15] Leder SB, Suiter DM. Five days of successful oral alimentation for hospitalized patients based upon passing the Yale Swallow Protocol. *Ann Otol Rhinol Laryngol* 2014;123(9):609–613 10.1177/0003489414525589

[16] Murray J. Manual of Dysphagia Assessment in Adults. San Diego, CA: Singular Publishing Group; 1999

[17] American Speech-Language-Hearing Association. Knowledge and skills for speech-language pathologists performing endoscopic assessment of swallowing. *ASHA Suppl* 2002;22:107–112

[18] American Speech-Language Hearing Association. (2008). Use of endoscopy by Speech-Language Pathologist: Position Statement. Available from www.asha.org/policy

[19] Gallivan G. FEES/FEEST and videotape recording. *Chest* 2002;122:1513–1515

[20] Daniels SK, Schroeder MF, DeGeorge PC, Corey DM, Rosenbek JC. Effects of verbal cue on bolus flow during swallowing. *Am J Speech Lang Pathol* 2007;16(2):140–147

[21] Dua KS, Ren J, Bardan E, Xie P, Shaker R. Coordination of deglutitive glottal function and pharyngeal bolus transit during normal eating. *Gastroenterology* 1997;112(1):73–83

[22] Suiter DM, Moorhead MK. Effects of flexible fiberoptic endoscopy on pharyngeal swallow physiology. *Otolaryngol Head Neck Surg* 2007;137(6):956–958

[23] Gomes GF, Pisani JC, Macedo ED, Campos AC. The nasogastric feeding tube as a risk factor for aspiration and aspiration pneumonia. *Curr Opin Clin Nutr Metab Care* 2003;6(3):327–333

[24] Huggins PS, Tuomi SK, Young C. Effects of nasogastric tubes on the young, normal swallowing mechanism. *Dysphagia* 1999;14(3):157–161

[25] Wang TG, Wu M-C, Chang Y-C, Hsiao T-Y, Lien I-N. The effect of nasogastric tubes on swallowing function in persons with dysphagia following stroke. *Arch Phys Med Rehabil* 2006;87(9):1270–1273

[26] Leder SB, Suiter DM. Effect of nasogastric tubes on incidence of aspiration. *Arch Phys Med Rehabil* 2008;89(4):648–651

[27] Fattal M, Suiter DM, Warner HL, Leder SB. Effect of presence/absence of a nasogastric tube in the same person on incidence of aspiration. *Otolaryngol Head Neck Surg* 2011;145(5):796–800

[28] Leder SB, Ross DA. Incidence of vocal fold immobility in patients with dysphagia. *Dysphagia* 2005;20(2):163 167, discussion 168 169

[29] Leder SB, Suiter DM, Duffey D, Judson BL. Vocal fold immobility and aspiration status: a direct replication study. *Dysphagia* 2012;*27*(2):265–270 doi: 10.1007/s00455-011-9362-0

[30] Burton MJ, Altman KW, Rosenfeld RM. Extracts from The Cochrane Library: Topical anaesthetic or vasoconstrictor preparations for flexible fibre-optic nasal pharyngoscopy and laryngoscopy. *Otolaryngol Head Neck Surg* 2012;*146*(5):694–697

[31] Leder SB, Ross DA, Briskin KB, Sasaki CT. A prospective, double-blind, randomized study on the use of a topical anesthetic, vasoconstrictor, and placebo during transnasal flexible fiberoptic endoscopy. *J Speech Lang Hear Res* 1997;*40*(6):1352–1357

[32] Fife TA, Butler SG, Langmore SE, et al. Use of topical nasal anesthesia during flexible endoscopic evaluation of swallowing in dysphagic patients. *Ann Otol Rhinol Laryngol* 2015;*124*(3):206–211 doi: 10.1177/0003489414550153

[33] Lester S, Langmore SE, Lintzenich CR, et al. The effects of topical anesthetic on swallowing during nasoendoscopy. *Laryngoscope* 2013;*123*(7):1704–1708 doi: 10.1002/lary.23899

[34] Murray J, Langmore SE, Ginsberg S, Dostie A. The significance of accumulated oropharyngeal secretions and swallowing frequency in predicting aspiration. *Dysphagia* 1996;*11*(2):99–103

[35] Link DT, Willging JP, Miller CK, Cotton RT, Rudolph CD. Pediatric laryngopharyngeal sensory testing during flexible endoscopic evaluation of swallowing: feasible and correlative. *Ann Otol Rhinol Laryngol* 2000;*109*(10 Pt 1):899–905

[36] Donzelli J, Brady S, Wesling M, Craney M. Predictive value of accumulated oropharyngeal secretions for aspiration during video nasal endoscopic evaluation of the swallow. *Ann Otol Rhinol Laryngol* 2003;*112*(5):469–475

[37] Leder SB. Serial fiberoptic endoscopic swallowing evaluations in the management of patients with dysphagia. *Arch Phys Med Rehabil* 1998;*79*(10):1264–1269

[38] Brady S, Donzelli J. The modified barium swallow and the functional endoscopic evaluation of swallowing. *Otolaryngol Clin North Am* 2013;*46*(6):1009–1022 doi: 10.1016/j.otc.2013.08.001

[39] Leder SB, Acton LM, Lisitano HL, Murray JT. Fiberoptic endoscopic evaluation of swallowing (FEES) with and without blue-dyed food. *Dysphagia* 2005;*20*(2):157–162

[40] Leder SB, Murray JT. Fiberoptic endoscopic evaluation of swallowing. *Phys Med Rehabil Clin N Am* 2008;*19*(4):787–801, viii–ix

[41] Brady S. The use of blue dye and glucose oxidase reagent strips for detection of pulmonary aspiration: efficacy and safety update. *Perspectives (Dysphagia)* 2005;*14*(4):8–13

[42] Acheson DWK. FDA Public Health Advisory: Subject: reports of blue discoloration and death in patients receiving enteral feedings tinted with the dye, FD&C Blue no. 1. September 29, 2003. https://www.fda.gov/ForIndustry/ColorAdditives/ColorAdditivesinSpecificProducts/InMedicalDevices/ucm142395.htm

[43] Rosenbek JC, Robbins JA, Roecker EB, Coyle JL, Wood JL. A penetration-aspiration scale. *Dysphagia* 1996;*11*(2):93–98

[44] Neubauer PD, Rademaker AW, Leder SB. The Yale pharyngeal residue severity rating scale: an anatomically defined and image-based tool. *Dysphagia* 2015;*30*(5):521–528 10.1007/s00455-015-9631-4

[45] Aviv JE, Kaplan ST, Thomson JE, Spitzer J, Diamond B, Close LG. The safety of flexible endoscopic evaluation of swallowing with sensory testing (FEESST): an analysis of 500 consecutive evaluations. *Dysphagia* 2000;*15*(1):39–44

[46] Logemann JA, Gibbons P, Rademaker AW, et al. Mechanisms of recovery of swallow after supraglottic laryngectomy. *J Speech Hear Res* 1994;*37*(5):965–974

[47] Aviv JE, Sataloff RT, Cohen M, et al. Cost-effectiveness of two types of dysphagia care in head and neck cancer: a preliminary report. *Ear Nose Throat J* 2001;*80*(8):553–556, 558

[48] Denk DM, Kaider A. Videoendoscopic biofeedback: a simple method to improve the efficacy of swallowing rehabilitation of patients after head and neck surgery. *ORL J Otorhinolaryngol Relat Spec* 1997;*59*(2):100–105

[49] Donzelli J, Brady S. The effects of breath-holding on vocal fold adduction: implications for safe swallowing. *Arch Otolaryngol Head Neck Surg* 2004;*130*(2):208–210

[50] Leder SB, Cohn SM, Moller BA. Fiberoptic endoscopic documentation of the high incidence of aspiration following extubation in critically ill trauma patients. *Dysphagia* 1998;*13*(4):208–212

[51] Leder SB. Fiberoptic endoscopic evaluation of swallowing in patients with acute traumatic brain injury. *J Head Trauma Rehabil* 1999;*14*(5):448–453

[52] Ajemian MS, Nirmul GB, Anderson MT, Zirlen DM, Kwasnik EM. Routine fiberoptic endoscopic evaluation of swallowing following prolonged intubation: implications for management. *Arch Surg* 2001;*136*(4):434–437

[53] Hartnick CJ, Hartley BE, Miller C, Willging JP. Pediatric fiberoptic endoscopic evaluation of swallowing. *Ann Otol Rhinol Laryngol* 2000;*109*(11):996–999

[54] Pelletier CA. Use of FEES to assess and manage nursing home residents. In: Langmore SE, ed., Endoscopic Evaluation and Treatment of Swallowing Disorders. New York, NY: Thieme; 2001:201–212

[55] Langmore SE. Dysphagia in neurologic patients in the intensive care unit. *Semin Neurol* 1996;*16*(4):329–340

[56] Spiegel JR, Selber JC, Creed J. A functional diagnosis of dysphagia using videoendoscopy. *Ear Nose Throat J* 1998;*77*(8):628–632

[57] Denk DM, Swoboda H, Schima W, Eibenberger K. Prognostic factors for swallowing rehabilitation following head and neck cancer surgery. *Acta Otolaryngol* 1997;*117*(5):769–774

[58] Leder SB, Sasaki CT. Use of FEES to assess and manage patients with head and cancer. In: Langmore SE, ed., Endoscopic Evaluation and Treatment of Swallowing Disorders. New York, NY: Thieme; 2001:178–187

[59] Muehlberger T, Kunar D, Munster A, Couch M. Efficacy of fiberoptic laryngoscopy in the diagnosis of inhalation injuries. *Arch Otolaryngol Head Neck Surg* 1998;*124*(9):1003–1007

[60] Migliore LE, Scoopo FJ, Robey KL. Fiberoptic examination of swallowing in and young adults with severe developmental disability. *Am J Speech Lang Pathol* 1999;*8*:303–308

[61] Leder SB, Espinosa JF. Aspiration risk after acute stroke: comparison of clinical examination and fiberoptic endoscopic evaluation of swallowing. *Dysphagia* 2002;*17*(3):214–218

[62] Leder SB. Incidence and type of aspiration in acute care patients requiring mechanical ventilation via a new tracheotomy. *Chest* 2002;*122*(5):1721–1726

[63] Leder SB, Novella S, Patwa H. Use of fiberoptic endoscopic evaluation of swallowing (FEES) in patients with amyotrophic lateral sclerosis. *Dysphagia* 2004;*19*(3):177–181

[64] Leder SB, Sasaki CT, Bayar S, et al. Fiberoptic endoscopic evaluation of swallowing in the evaluation of aspiration following transhiatal esophagectomy. *J Am Coll Surg* 2007;*205*:581–585

[65] Ekberg O, Nylander G, Fork FT, Sjöberg S, Birch-Iensen M, Hillarp B. Interobserver variability in cineradiographic assessment of pharyngeal function during swallow. *Dysphagia* 1988;*3*(1):46–48

[66] Kuhlemeier KV, Yates P, Palmer JB. Intra- and interrater variation in the evaluation of videofluorographic swallowing studies. *Dysphagia* 1998;*13*(3):142–147

[67] Schroter-Morasch H, Bartolome G, Troppmann N, et al. Values and limitations of pharyngolaryngoscopy in patients with dysphagia. *Folia Phoniatr Logop* 1999;*51*:172–178

[68] Kidder TM, Langmore SE, Martin BJW. Indications and techniques of endoscopy in evaluation of cervical dysphagia: comparison with radiographic techniques. *Dysphagia* 1994;*9*(4):256–261

# 9 Pediatric Fiberoptic Endoscopic Evaluation of Swallowing

*Claire Kane Miller and Jay Paul Willging*

## Summary

The anatomical relationships of the oral cavity, pharynx, and larynx undergo a continuous transition during the first several years of life. Likewise, the neurologic control mechanisms that coordinate swallowing with respiratory activity are modified as infants develop. Thus, application of fiberoptic endoscopic evaluation of swallowing (FEES) in infants and children requires in-depth knowledge of the trajectory of oral/motor feeding skill development and recognition of the changes that simultaneously occur in feeding and swallowing dynamics. Endoscopic evaluation of the pediatric upper aerodigestive tract requires proficiency in the identification of normal and abnormal pediatric velopharyngeal and laryngopharyngeal anatomy and function. Both congenital and acquired nasopharyngeal, oropharyngeal, and laryngeal anomalies may have an impact on the efficiency of feeding, airway protection, and swallowing function; the conditions vary widely. In addition, comorbidities, if present, may require careful consideration of multiple and interacting neurologic, inflammatory, structural, and cardiorespiratory variables that affect the ability to achieve and maintain airway protection during feeding and swallowing.

## Keywords

dysphagia, pediatric dysphagia, fiberoptic endoscopic evaluation of swallowing, FEES, instrumental assessment of swallowing

## Learning Objectives

- Describe clinical signs, symptoms, and conditions that indicate the use of fiberoptic endoscopic evaluation of swallowing (FEES) in the pediatric population to assess airway protection and swallowing function
- Identify anatomical landmarks and key structures in the upper aerodigestive tract in infants and children as viewed during the endoscopic examination
- Define the examination protocol used in pediatric FEES
- Increase knowledge of age-related differences in feeding and swallowing parameters as viewed endoscopically
- Recognize the indications and utility of pediatric FEES in special populations, including medically fragile patients, infants in the neonatal intensive care unit (NICU), and patients undergoing surgical procedures (e.g., cardiac procedures, airway reconstruction)

## 9.1 Introduction

The use of fiberoptic endoscopic evaluation of swallowing (FEES) in the pediatric population requires comprehensive knowledge of the structural and functional changes that occur in the pediatric aerodigestive tract with maturation. The process of feeding and swallowing evolves as the central nervous system develops, and anatomical changes in oral and pharyngeal structural relationships occur simultaneously. Therefore, recognition of age-related neurological and structural differences in the feeding and swallowing process is key to accurate interpretation during the pediatric FEES examination.

FEES enables the examiner to directly visualize anatomical and physiological abnormalities that have an impact on airway protection integrity during swallowing in pediatric patients. Diseases and conditions include, but are not limited to, congenital structural anomalies of the head and neck, congenital or acquired neurologic issues, and cardiorespiratory compromise associated with feeding. The integrity of the laryngeal adductor reflex (LAR), central to airway protection, can be judged in the context of a pediatric FEES procedure. The portability of the examination makes it possible to complete examinations in the neonatal intensive care unit (NICU) or at the bedside of patients who are too medically fragile to be transported to the clinic setting.

This chapter defines the indications and contraindications for the use of FEES in the pediatric population, describes the pediatric FEES examination protocol, delineates how examination results are interpreted, and identifies how subsequent treatment recommendations are determined.

## 9.2 Application of FEES in the Pediatric Population

The use of FEES in the pediatric population was first explored at Cincinnati Children's Hospital in 1993. Twenty children between 3 and 7 years of age were undergoing nasopharyngoscopy for evaluation of resonance issues, with no history of feeding or swallowing concerns.[1] The institutional review board (IRB) granted permission to extend the typical nasopharyngoscopy exam to include advancement of the scope into the hypopharynx during the presentation of food and liquid so that swallowing parameters could be viewed. The patients were evaluated in terms of their ability to tolerate passage of the scope into the hypopharynx and to comply with eating and drinking during the examination. The patients tolerated the exam well, adapting easily to advancement of the scope to allow visualization of swallowing, and readily ate and drank during the exam.

A pilot study was then developed to compare findings and recommendations between FEES and videofluoroscopy to ensure there was good validity and reliability for judgments of swallowing parameters that are common to each exam (oral control/bolus transfer, swallowing onset time, laryngeal penetration, aspiration, residue). The pilot study design included simultaneous FEES and videofluoroscopic swallowing studies on six children between the ages of 4 months and 6 years.[2] Comparison of findings and recommendations in the studies revealed a high level of agreement for findings of penetration and aspiration. Small differences were found in the judgments of swallowing onset time and degree of pharyngeal residue following swallows. Overall, FEES results were correlative to findings of the video-fluoroscopic swallowing examination; moreover, FEES could be performed easily and safely in children. Subsequent investigations of the utility of FEES in a variety of contexts confirmed the procedure's usefulness in a wide range of pediatric patients and settings.[3,4,5,6,7,8] FEES is now established as feasible and useful for pediatric swallowing assessment, particularly to obtain information regarding sensory threshold, glottic competence, and repeated interval examinations of swallowing function while avoiding additional radiation.

## 9.3 Indications and Contraindications for Pediatric FEES

FEES offers a means to visualize swallowing function and airway protection ability directly in infants and children who present with clinical signs and symptoms of swallowing dysfunction, including coughing, choking, color changes, and gagging during secretion management or during nutritive intake. In-depth assessment of the structural and functional integrity of the nasal, pharyngeal, and laryngeal regions is possible. Direct visualization of swallowing during the exam gives clear information about the efficiency and safety of swallowing and defines the ability to achieve and maintain airway protection during swallowing. Additionally, interpretation of the swallowing parameters during the exam guides the use of direct and indirect compensatory strategies (to be discussed). The efficacy of the compensatory interventions is assessed, and treatment recommendations can be formulated.

The pathophysiology of feeding and swallowing issues differs in pediatric patients as compared with adults. Conditions with concomitant dysphagia may be congenital or acquired and include a wide array of structural, neurologic, metabolic, and cardiorespiratory factors.[9,10,11] With maturation, major changes occur in the oral, pharyngeal, and laryngeal anatomy in terms of size and anatomical relationships and in the integration of sucking, swallowing, and respiratory sequencing. Evaluation of swallowing function via FEES offers an opportunity to visualize structures and function and to determine the impact of the aforementioned conditions on swallowing function. Anatomical contrasts between the infant and the toddler, older child, and adult, as well as differences in swallowing dynamics, are described later in this chapter.

### 9.3.1 Overview: Etiologies of Swallowing Dysfunction in Infants and Children

Although the etiologies of dysphagia in infants and children generally fall into neurologic, structural, cardiorespiratory, metabolic, and inflammatory categories, categories do overlap, and comorbidities are often present.[12] As in adults, neurologic issues are a common cause of pediatric dysphagia. Congenital and acquired neurologic lesions (e.g., cerebral palsy, intraventricular

hemorrhage, anoxic brain injury, traumatic brain injury, Chiari malformation) and progressive neurologic conditions (e.g., muscular dystrophy, spinal muscular atrophy, and congenital myopathies) affect the efficiency and safety of feeding and swallowing. Congenital syndromes often have accompanying cranial nerve abnormalities that adversely affect the sensory and motor aspects of feeding and swallowing function. Cardiorespiratory compromise as a consequence of prematurity, cystic fibrosis, or upper airway obstruction is characterized by the inability to achieve and sustain a coordinated respiratory and swallowing pattern during feeding, thus affecting airway protection integrity. Metabolic abnormalities (e.g., glycogen storage disease) or disorders of fatty acid, nitrogen, or carbohydrate metabolism may limit the type of feeding regimen allowed, preventing exposure to nutritive input at critical times for acquiring feeding skills. Lastly, inflammatory conditions, such as eosinophilic esophagitis, candida pharyngitis, or esophagitis, may create discomfort with feeding and have an impact on the coordination and efficiency of swallowing. Early and accurate identification and management of pediatric dysphagia is essential for adequate nutrition, growth, and respiratory health.

## 9.4 Indications for Pediatric FEES

Indications for the use of FEES in the diagnostic protocol include clinical signs and symptoms of swallowing dysfunction, abnormal videofluoroscopic evaluation findings that warrant further analysis, suspected secretion management issues, and the need to confirm the adequacy of swallowing function and safety of swallowing in patients who have never eaten orally or who ingest insufficient volumes for an adequate video swallowing study.[13] Indications for a pediatric FEES examination are summarized in **Box 9.1**.

### Box 9.1

**Indications for Pediatric FEES Examinations**
- Patient has never eaten orally or has not eaten orally for an extended period; medically fragile, need to assess readiness for transition to oral feeding
- Suspected difficulty with secretion management, questionable swallowing function
- Patient has known or suspected structural abnormality in the pharynx or larynx that may impact ability to achieve or maintain airway protection during swallowing
- Need to evaluate patient's swallowing function for determination of surgical candidacy for airway reconstruction
- Abnormal videofluoroscopic swallowing study results; need to further investigate swallowing function and the efficacy of compensatory strategies to improve airway protection/swallowing
- Patient who cannot be transported to radiology for videofluoroscopic swallowing study
- Patient who cannot be positioned adequately for a videofluoroscopic study
- Patient who requires repeated interval swallowing examinations; want to avoid radiation exposure

In conditions whereby upper airway obstruction is present due to structural or physiological anomalies, problems with the coordination of respiration and swallowing may arise. Inadequate airflow and the increased respiratory demand of feeding may compromise the infant or child's ability to maintain airway protection during feeding and increase the risk of aspiration. The increased respiratory demands of feeding may also result in episodes of **apnea** and/or **bradycardia** in some cases. The etiologies of upper airway obstruction are varied and include congenital or acquired nasopharyngeal, oropharyngeal, and laryngeal anomalies, as outlined in **Table 9.1**.

Craniofacial malformations in infants and children that are frequently associated with feeding and swallowing difficulty include **choanal atresia**, nasal cavity deformities, **micrognathia** (small mandible), **retrognathia**, **glossoptosis** (posterior displacement of the tongue), macroglossia, and decreased oropharyngeal space. **Pierre Robin sequence** (PRS) is a well-recognized craniofacial condition and is characterized by micrognathia, glossoptosis, and airway obstruction. A **U**-shaped posterior cleft palate may also occur as part of the sequence. Feeding difficulties are common in PRS due to the degree of upper airway obstruction present, though there is a subset of patients who do not experience significant respiratory issues with the respiratory effort of feeding or difficulty with coordination of feeding and swallowing.[14]

**Laryngomalacia** (**Fig. 9.1**) is the most common congenital laryngeal anomaly and etiology of inspiratory stridor in infants, and may occur in isolation or as part of a neurologic condition or genetic syndrome, such as Down syndrome.[15,16] Laryngomalacia is characterized by floppy arytenoid cartilages, relatively short aryepiglottic folds, and an infantile, omega-shaped epiglottis. Infolding of the aryepiglottic folds with collapse of structures into the airway occurs during inspiration and is identified during flexible endoscopy. Infants may demonstrate difficulty in coordinating respiration, swallowing, and airway protection as a result, which can be visualized during a FEES examination. Severe cases of laryngomalacia may require surgical intervention to relieve upper airway obstruction; improvement of feeding often follows. Prolapse of the arytenoid mucosa may be treated by surgical excision of the redundant mucosa; excision of short aryepiglottic folds alleviates tethering of the supraglottic structures. Division of the **glossoepiglottic ligament** with suture suspension of the epiglottis to the base of the tongue is used to treat prolapse of the epiglottis.

Oher laryngeal conditions associated with concurrent feeding and swallowing problems include **vocal fold paralysis**, **vallecular cyst**, and **laryngeal webs**. Vocal fold paralysis (VFP) is the second most frequent cause of airway obstruction in pediatric patients and may be congenital or acquired.[17] Congenital VFP may occur in conjunction with developmental anomalies of the central nervous system, including Chiari malformation, **cerebral agenesis**, and **hydrocephaly**. VFP is clearly visualized during the FEES exam; the effects of VFP on airway protection and the efficacy of compensatory strategies, such as postural maneuvers or viscosity changes, can be identified. Acquired VFP is most commonly the result of a traumatic or infectious process. Inflammation from infections or compression from tumor growth may injure the vagus nerve and thus interfere with innervation of the laryngeal muscles. Endotracheal intubation or injury to the recurrent laryngeal nerve following surgical repair of thoracic or cardiovascular anomalies may also result in VFP. Vallecular cysts (cyst formation in the

**Table 9.1** Etiologies of upper airway obstruction: nasopharyngeal, oropharyngeal, laryngeal

| Nasopharyngeal | Oropharyngeal | Laryngeal |
|---|---|---|
| Choanal atresia | Retrognathia and posterior displacement of the tongue (glossoptosis) | Laryngomalacia |
| Nasal cavity deformities | Macroglossia | Vocal fold paralysis |
| | Vallecular cyst | Laryngeal web |
| | Pharyngeal stenosis (congenital or acquired as in caustic ingestion) | |

vallecular space) are rare but may be associated with feeding and swallowing difficulty as well as inspiratory stridor and failure to thrive.[18] The respiratory and feeding difficulties are typically immediately resolved once the vallecular cyst is identified and surgically removed. A laryngeal web occurs when there is a lack of complete separation of the connective tissue of the vocal folds during embryonic development of the larynx and may occur in conjunction with genetic syndromes, such as **velocardiofacial syndrome**.[16] Large webs obstruct the glottis and are life threatening, requiring surgical intervention. Smaller webs may result in inspiratory stridor that increases with the respiratory effort of feeding. Once the obstruction is relieved, feeding improves rapidly in the absence of other conditions.

**Laryngotracheoesophageal** (LTE) **clefts** develop when the fusion of the posterior trachea fails to develop normally in the fetus.[19,20,21] Depending on when the process of separating the trachea from the esophagus stops, a small (type I or II) or large (types III and IV) defect develops.[22] As described by Myer and Shott, a

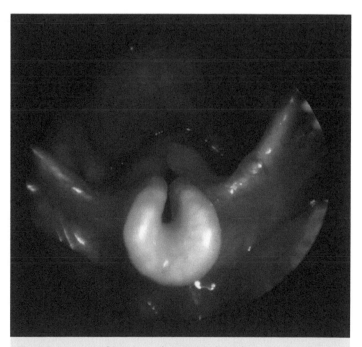

**Fig. 9.1** Laryngomalacia. Note the omega-shaped appearance of the epiglottis and shortening of the aryepiglottic folds

type I cleft is defined as a supraglottic interarytenoid defect above the level of the posterior cricoid cartilage; type II clefts involve the **cricoid lamina** and extend below the level of the vocal folds; type III clefts involve the entire cricoid with extension into the cervical trachea; and type IV clefts extend through the posterior wall of the thoracic trachea and may continue to the **carina**, as seen in **Fig. 9.2**. LTE clefts are associated with aspiration and the development of chronic lung disease if they are not surgically corrected.

FEES offers a way to assess both the sensory and the motor aspects of the swallowing process that may be compromised in the aforementioned conditions. In addition, readiness to transition to oral feeding can be assessed in medically fragile populations, such as premature infants, or in infants who have undergone cardiac procedures. The adequacy of airway protection and swallowing function can be confirmed preoperatively in patients seeking surgical intervention for airway reconstruction that may involve altering laryngeal anatomy. Information from the examination is used to inform the patient's surgical and treatment plan.[23]

In summary, indications for the use of FEES in the diagnostic protocol include clinical signs and symptoms of swallowing dysfunction, abnormal videofluoroscopic evaluation findings that warrant further analysis, suspected secretion management issues, and the need to confirm the adequacy of swallowing function and safety of swallowing in patients who have never eaten orally or who ingest insufficient volume for an adequate video swallowing study.[13]

## 9.5   Contraindications

There are few contraindications to the use of FEES in infants and children; the majority relate to the ability to mechanically perform the test, not to the medical condition of the patient. Anatomical conditions that limit visualization include nasal obstruction, choanal atresia (blockage by bone or tissue of the nasal passages

(choana) leading from the back of the nose to the throat), retrognathia, and **pharyngeal stenosis**; conditions that preclude adequate visualization of the hypopharyngeal and laryngeal areas. Medical conditions that contraindicate the use of FEES include extreme medical fragility; in that circumstance, the rationale for a FEES examination request would need to be carefully evaluated by the medical team. Patients with underlying sensory integration and processing issues may have some difficulty with the tactile stimulation during the transnasal passage of the scope and may display strong behavioral resistance initially during the examination. On most occasions, once the scope is advanced from the nasopharynx, the stimulation of the nasal mucosa subsides and the patient becomes more comfortable. **Subacute bacterial endocarditis**, an infection of the inner lining of the heart and the heart valves, is a concern for children with cardiac abnormalities who are undergoing dental treatment or surgical intervention of the upper respiratory tract, where breaks in the lining of the tract are likely to allow bacteria to enter the blood stream and attach to various structures within the heart. In such circumstances, **prophylactic antibiotic treatment** is indicated. Subacute bacterial endocarditis is *not* considered a concern for patients undergoing FEES because there is little risk of causing a break in the mucosa of the nose or pharynx. Contraindications to pediatric FEES are summarized in **Box 9.2**.

### Box 9.2

**Contraindications to Pediatric FEES**
- Extreme medical fragility
- Choanal atresia
- Nasal obstruction
- Oropharyngeal stenosis
- Hypopharyngeal stenosis/collapse

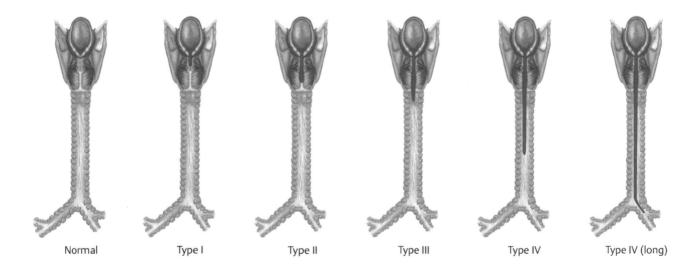

| Normal | Type I | Type II | Type III | Type IV | Type IV (long) |

**Fig. 9.2** Types of laryngeal clefts. Type I is a supraglottic interarytenoid defect above the level of the posterior cricoid cartilage; type II involves the cricoid lamina and extends below the level of the vocal folds; type III involves the entire cricoid with extension into the cervical trachea; type IV extends through the posterior wall and may continue to the carina.

## 9.6 Pediatric FEES Examination Protocol

The protocol for a pediatric FEES procedure includes review of the medical and feeding history, oral motor assessment, anesthetic preparation, execution of the FEES exam, interpretation of the examination findings, determination of recommendations, and a plan for treatment during collaborative discussion with the caregiver. The components are described in the following section. The overall advantages and disadvantages of pediatric FEES are summarized in **Table 9.2.**

### 9.6.1 Preassessment Interview and Preparation for FEES

Previsit planning involves offering education and instruction to the caregiver and sometimes the patient (depending on cognitive status) about the FEES procedure, prior to the actual appointment. Providing verbal and written instructions and information about what to expect increases the chance for a successful procedure. In our experience, it has been beneficial to use a simple patient education booklet that explains the pediatric FEES procedure in simple terms and includes instructions for what to bring to the examination (usual nipple, bottle, formula, typical foods). The patient's medical history and diagnoses are carefully reviewed prior to the FEES visit and confirmed during a preexamination interview by a nurse and the speech pathologist.

### 9.6.2 Medical play therapy

Prior to medical procedures to help decrease anxiety and increase cooperation is helpful in some circumstances.[24] Allowing the child to see and gently touch the endoscope, and to watch how it moves, is effective in allaying concerns and increasing cooperation during the exam. The use of a child life specialist to help with preparation prior to the examination and to provide visual and auditory distraction techniques during the examination is an option.

The speech pathologist reviews the results of prior clinical oral motor and instrumental assessments and past and current feeding history and completes an examination of oral structures and function prior to the FEES examination. Overall level of alertness, basic posture and position, and control of secretions are assessed. Food allergies are reviewed and documented in the medical record. Preparation of equipment, foods, and liquids to be used during the examination is completed as the patient undergoes anesthetic preparation prior to the examination, as described in the following section. The physician reviews the patient's medical history and current status to confirm the medical appropriateness of the FEES exam and also confirms the type of anesthesia to be used.

### 9.6.3 Anesthetic Preparation

The use of topical anesthesia helps to maximize cooperation in children; the options include a nasal spray of 1:1 mixture oxymetazoline and 2% tetracaine and/or the use of topical 2% viscous lidocaine on the distal end of the endoscope. Only viscous lidocaine is used in infants less than 1 year of age and in children with severe neurologic impairment, seizures, and questionable ability to manage secretions. Otherwise, nasal spray in conjunction with viscous lidocaine is used per dosing guidelines. The combination of oxymetazoline and 2% tetracaine is administered via a hand-activated atomizing dispenser to the right and left nares by the nurse, who directs the spray upward to avoid anesthetizing the hypopharynx. The use of oxymetazoline promotes nasal decongestion and eases scope passage; this is an advantage to using it in combination with topical lidocaine during the examination.[23]

**Table 9.2** Advantages and disadvantages of pediatric fiberoptic endoscopic evaluation of swallowing

| Nasopharyngeal | Oropharyngeal |
|---|---|
| Clear view of structures and functional ability to protect the airway | Some discomfort may be associated with passage of the scope; usually subsides once the scope moves from the nasopharynx and the stimulation of the nasal mucosa ceases |
| Allows assessment of a child's ability to manage secretions | Presence of the scope may trigger gagging and or vomiting during the exam |
| No time limits | View disappears briefly during the moment of the swallow as structures contract during swallowing and deflect the light |
| Effect of compensatory strategies to improve airway protection/swallowing function can be identified | Focus is limited to the pharyngeal phase of the swallow |
| Portability | Requires special training |
| Can identify indirect signs of reflux irritation | Pediatric exams require two professionals: one to pass the scope, and one to feed the patient and initiate compensatory strategies |
| Provides mechanism to assess sensory response | |
| Can help determine readiness and safety of advancing oral feeding | |
| Does not require alteration of foods and liquids with barium | |
| Allows assessment of swallowing function without intake of significant volume | |
| No radiation exposure | |

## 9.6.4 Endoscopic Equipment

There are a variety of scope options available for use in pediatric FEES. Differences in anatomy from infants and children to adolescents and young adults require the use of varied endoscope sizes. Standard size endoscopes (3.5–4 mm) work well in the majority of infants and children, though the use of a smaller endoscope (approx. 2 mm) may be indicated if structural abnormalities of the nasal passageway or midface are present. Passage of the endoscope may be done by either the otolaryngologist or the speech pathologist, depending on the laws governing the scope of practice for speech-language practitioners in a particular state.

## 9.7 Performing the FEES Examination

### 9.7.1 Positioning

To assist with maintaining optimal and static positioning during the examination, the parent or caretaker is seated in a standard clinical examination chair with the infant or child positioned upright in his or her lap as the scope is passed transnasally. The parent or caretaker is coached on how to help maintain positioning of the infant or child during the exam and how to assist with helping to keep arms and hands away from the scope. Positioning is then adjusted to reflect the typical feeding position if needed. For infants, this may include repositioning in a side-lying, semireclined, or cradle position; for older children, adjustment to semireclined positioning may be necessary. The nurse present during the exam helps to position and support the child's head in order to keep the scope positioned for optimal viewing. Older children may be independent in sitting in the examination chair with the parent or caretaker in close proximity as needed to assist with maintaining positioning during the evaluation.

## 9.7.2 Anatomical Landmarks and Assessment—Infants and Children

Evaluation of the pediatric upper aerodigestive tract requires medical expertise and experience in recognition of normal and abnormal velopharyngeal and laryngopharyngeal anatomy. Additionally, a thorough understanding of the changes in structure and function that occur with maturation is required for accurate interpretation of events during the examination. The anatomical contrasts between the infant and the older child are summarized in **Table 9.3**.

### Nasopharynx

The evaluation is done under direct visualization and begins with assessment of the nasal cavity and nasopharynx. In pediatric FEES, the endoscope is guided either above the inferior turbinate into the middle meatus or along the floor of the nose, depending on which area will most easily accommodate the scope. The maxillary crest is prominent in children and often

**Table 9.3** Summary of anatomical contrasts among infant, child, and adult

| Infant | Toddler/child | Adult |
|---|---|---|
| • Small oral cavity, forward resting posture of the tongue<br>• Prominent buccal pads facilitate sucking | • Buccal pads decrease in size, downward, forward growth of mandible<br>• Position of tongue descends within oral cavity | • Growth of mandible is complete |
| • Tongue maintains approximation with the lips, gums, hard/soft palate | • Increased space of the oral cavity allows differentiated movements of the tongue within oral cavity | • Oral cavity accommodates range of tongue motion during biting and mastication |
| • Uvula may rest against the tip of the epiglottis | • Palatal contact with the epiglottis begins to decrease around 18 months of age | • Separation between structures is complete |
| • Tongue base, soft palate, and pharyngeal walls are in close approximation, the pharynx has a curve<br>• Accelerated growth of structures from birth to 18 months | • Space between tongue base, soft palate and pharyngeal walls increases as structures elongate and separate<br>• Pharynx elongates | • Elongation of structures to vertical orientation |
| • Epiglottis is proportionally more narrow, vertical, tubular, omega shaped compared to adult | • Separation of the epiglottis and soft palate facilitates oral breathing | • Epiglottis loses bulk, becomes broad and flatter in appearance |
| • Larynx is in a high position, adjacent to C1–C3<br>• Hyoid is not ossified | • Larynx begins to descend<br>• Hyoid at the level of C2–C3<br>• Hyoid ossifies | • Larynx descends to the level of C6–C7<br>• Complete ossification of the hyoid |
| • Larynx at birth is one-third of the adult size<br>• Vocal folds: membranous folds = 1.3–2 mm; cartilaginous folds = 1.4 mm | • Growth of the larynx continues<br>• Cricoid loses bulk, arytenoids decrease in relative size, vocal folds elongate to span the distance between the arytenoids and growing thyroid cartilage<br>• Gradual descent of the larynx | • Larynx descends to the level of the cervical vertebrae<br>• Ossification is complete by ~ 20 years of age<br>• One-third or less of vocal fold is cartilaginous<br>• Vocal folds reach maximal length |
| • Trachea is short and narrow compared to adult, 5.7 cm long in first 3 months of life | • Trachea grows from 5.7 to 8.1 cm between 12 and 18 months of age | • Trachea reaches adult size (~ 8.5–15 cm) |

narrows the floor of the nose in the pediatric patient. Passage into the middle meatus provides an optimal angle for assessment of the **velopharyngeal sphincter** function.

Nasal patency, **posterior choanal aperture** size, mucosal hypertrophy, and adenoid size are assessed by the physician during transnasal passage of the endoscope. Because infants (for the first several months of life) are obligate nasal breathers, any degree of nasal obstruction has implications for coordination of respiration and swallowing. The function of the velopharyngeal sphincter is assessed as the scope is passed through the choanae, during speech in children with language, or during vocalization or crying for those who do not have language skills. Though velopharyngeal closure may not be complete during speech, closure may be complete during swallowing. It is important to note that, if inadequate velopharyngeal closure does occur during swallowing, some degree of **pharyngonasal backflow** or reflux is likely to occur during feeding. Though episodes of pharyngonasal reflux may be developmental and transient in nature, frequent episodes of large amounts may signal the presence of a structural problem, such as a **submucous cleft**, an overt cleft of the secondary palate, or a neuromuscular issue. Depending on the degree of frequency and amount, pharyngonasal retrograde flow has the potential to be disruptive to the rhythm and overall coordination of feeding.[25,26]

## Oropharynx

The endoscope is advanced through the nasopharynx into the oropharynx. **Palatine and lingual tonsil** size, the uvula, and the position of the tongue base relative to the posterior pharyngeal wall are assessed at this point in the examination. Patients with craniofacial anomalies may have **glossoptosis** (posterior displacement of the tongue) or relative glossoptosis secondary to micrognathia. **Macroglossia** (enlarged tongue) or relative macroglossia is assessed in the context of feeding in terms of the impact on the feeding coordination and airway protection maintenance.

## Hypopharynx

The scope is advanced beyond the free margin of the soft palate for viewing the hypopharyngeal and laryngeal region. The lateral and posterior pharyngeal walls, pharyngoepiglottic band, epiglottis, glossoepiglottic fold, valleculae (right and left), piriform sinuses, aryepiglottic folds, arytenoids, interarytenoid space, false vocal folds, true vocal folds, anterior and posterior commissure, and postcricoid area are identified.

The location of the larynx varies with the age of the patient (**Fig. 9.3**). In newborns, the larynx projects upward into the oropharynx, with the tip of the epiglottis often extending into the nasopharynx, above the level of the free margin of the soft palate. There is a gradual descent of the larynx with maturity, and the final resting position of the larynx at the level of the sixth cervical vertebra occurs after puberty. The shape and position of the epiglottis are observed. The piriform sinuses are evaluated for masses and asymmetry that may affect swallowing dynamics. Signs of possible reflux irritation are noted, including **erythema** (redness), **edema** (swelling), or interarytenoid pachydermia (thickening or tissue redundancy). At this point during the anatomical examination, careful attention is given to laryngeal anomalies, such as laryngomalacia, deepening between the arytenoids suggestive of possible laryngeal cleft, presence of a ventricular/ saccular cyst, and vocal fold paralysis; each of these conditions can have a negative impact on the child's ability to maintain airway protection during swallowing, and all require evaluation and possible intervention by the pediatric otolaryngologist.

## 9.7.3 Assessment of Secretion Management

As the scope is advanced into the hypopharynx during the anatomical assessment, consideration is given to any standing secretions that may be present and whether there are spontaneous swallowing efforts to clear secretions. Secretions that are present at the onset of the exam and that accumulate during

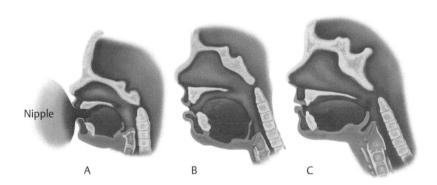

**Fig. 9.3** Relationship of the larynx to the cervical vertebrae: infancy to adult. **(a)** Note the small size and shape of the oral cavity relative to the tongue, high position of the larynx, and close proximity of the epiglottis to the uvula. **(b)** Increased size of the oral cavity and elongation of the pharynx, gradual descent of the larynx in a child. **(c)** Note the relative size of the tongue in relation to the oral cavity, the position of the epiglottis, and the descent of the larynx to the adult level (C6).

(From Myer CM, Cotton RT, Schott SR. The Pediatric Airway: An Interdisciplinary Approach. Philadelphia, PA: JB Lippincott; 1995. Reprinted by permission.)

the examination without spontaneous swallow efforts to clear are of concern, because this finding has been associated with significant swallowing abnormality.[27] Reaction to penetrated and aspirated secretions is noted; the absence of a protective response indicates swallowing deficits. As described earlier in the chapter, there is a white-out period that occurs during swallowing that is reflective of contractile function of the hypopharyngeal musculature and light deflection from the scope. The patient's reaction to accumulated secretions and the degree of white-out and subsequent clearance ability with swallowing efforts furnish some initial information regarding the patient's sensory responsiveness to secretions and to the adequacy of the contractile force of the swallow. Symmetry of pharyngeal contraction during the swallow should be noted. If structural or functional abnormalities are found in the supraglottic or glottic larynx, the implications for airway protection should be described.

At this point during the exam, taste (citrus or carbonation) or thermal stimulation (ice chips, cold liquid) may be introduced to increase sensory input for activation of swallowing.[13,28,29] The effect of sensory input on secretion management and spontaneous swallow initiation is noted; if the patient demonstrates improved secretion management and increased frequency of swallowing, small amounts of nutritive stimulus may be introduced later in the examination.

### 9.7.4 Evaluation of Airway Protection Integrity and Sensory Assessment

Assessment of vocal fold mechanics and analysis of laryngopharyngeal sensation gives important, predictive information about the patient's ability to achieve and maintain airway protection during swallowing. Protection from aspiration is mediated through the LAR, characterized by immediate glottic closure in response to mechanical or chemical stimulation of the laryngeal mucosa. Elevated sensory thresholds and impairment of the LAR have been found to be associated with numerous conditions with concomitant dysphagia.[4,30] The integrity of the LAR in the pediatric patient can be assessed by delivering a puff of air, of calibrated duration and controlled intensity, from an endoscope positioned 1 to 2 mm above the arytenoid mucosa during the FEES examination. Responses that occur at > 4 mm Hg are considered to be abnormal.[4,31] Alternatively, functional assessment of the LAR can be achieved by gentle tapping in the region of the aryepiglottic fold and lateral aspect of the epiglottis with the tip of the endoscope to observe for reflexive glottic closure.

### 9.7.5 Assessment of Swallowing Parameters in the FEES Protocol

The feeding portion of the pediatric FEES protocol is conducted by the speech-language pathologist, using liquids, foods, and utensils that are typical and consistent with the patient's level of oral motor skills. A minimal amount of food coloring (green) (< 1 mL in total) is mixed with food and liquid during the exam to enhance visualization of swallowing dynamics. Blue dye no. 1 has been associated with **methemoglobinemia** (decreased availability of oxygen to tissues); therefore, patients with

increased gut permeability (premature infants, celiac disease, inflammatory bowel conditions) should avoid this compound. A bright orange multivitamin suspension, AquADEKS (Allergan), may be used to color secretions, breastmilk, or formula in place of food colorant during FEES studies in the NICU, considering the medical fragility of the neonate and the potential implications with the use of food color.[32]

Assessment of airway protection and swallowing function during breastfeeding as part of the pediatric FEES protocol is a special advantage of FEES because videofluoroscopic analysis is not possible during breastfeeding. During the FEES examination of breastfeeding, the scope is passed transnasally with the infant initially in the upright position. The infant is then repositioned in their typical position for breastfeeding. No food color or use of AquADEKS is necessary during the assessment of breastfeeding via FEES. The translucent nature of the breastmilk can be adequately visualized.

## 9.8 Interpretation of Swallowing Parameters during Pediatric FEES

Specific swallowing parameters are assessed during the pediatric FEES examination, some of which are similar to the adult parameters described previously in this chapter.

### 9.8.1 Oral Control and Transfer

The pre-FEES oral motor assessment with the patient provides information in regard to the patient's overall oral motor control during the oral phase of swallowing. Though FEES does not provide a view of the oral stage of the swallow per se, the consequences of poor oral control are visualized during the exam. For example, inadvertent transfer of the bolus into the hypopharynx over the base of the tongue or transfer of unmasticated or poorly masticated solids prior to airway closure and swallowing onset can be identified.

### 9.8.2 Swallowing Onset Time

Judging the timeliness of swallowing onset differs between infants, toddlers, and older children. During typical infant bottle or breastfeeding, sequential filling and contraction of the hypopharynx occur in the context of a rhythmic suck–swallow–breathe pattern. The small size of the infant oral cavity relative to the tongue facilitates rhythmic alternation of compression, suction, expression, and swallow-breathe. Nasal airflow during breathing is maintained during sucking and feeding, but at the moment of swallow, there is a distinct apneic interval.[33,34] The relative frequency of swallowing during sequential swallowing sequences causes frequent white-out or loss of view during the FEES assessment. Therefore, judgments of airway protection must be made during pause intervals between chain-swallowing sequences. If the swallowing response is latent during bottle feeds, episodes of penetration or aspiration may be detected prior to swallowing onset; however, because the view is obscured at the moment of the swallow, it is possible that penetration and even aspiration may occur during the periods that the view is obliterated. In older infants, toddlers, and children, onset of swallowing can be judged in the context of single-bolus presentations by spoon, or by single sips by cup. Sequential swallowing may also be assessed if the infant or toddler is still using a nipple/bottle or toddler sipper cup.

Delay in the onset of the swallowing response may not always signify swallowing abnormality.[13] The overall pattern of the swallow, degree of latency, and adequacy of the vallecular space and piriform sinus region to accommodate the bolus prior to swallowing onset before overflow into the endolarynx can be judged in the context of each individual patient scenario, as in the adult.

### 9.8.3 Laryngeal Penetration

Laryngeal penetration identified during pediatric FEES is defined as passage of secretions, liquid, or food within the confines of the endolarynx. In pediatric patients, the larynx is in a relatively higher position than the adult and is essentially an "island" within the hypopharynx, surrounded by the piriform sinuses, valleculae, and postcricoid area.[23] The endolarynx is protected by the epiglottis anteriorly, the aryepiglottic folds laterally, and the arytenoids posteriorly. Penetration is generally described in terms of depth and frequency of occurrence and in the context of patient response. If secretions or nutritive materials travel into the endolaryngeal area and continue to accumulate in these regions, there is risk of overflow into the larynx with subsequent aspiration.

In infants and children, the most common area for liquids to gain entrance to the endolaryngeal area is through the interarytenoid notch because this is the lowest point in the protective system. However, it is possible for penetration into the endolarynx at any anatomical point (e.g., over the aryepiglottic fold, over or beneath the epiglottis) prior to activation of the swallowing response and the subsequent closure of the airway.

### 9.8.4 Aspiration

As in adults, aspiration during a FEES examination can only be visualized prior to the swallow, or detected after the swallow. Food or liquid that travels into the laryngeal area and below the level of the vocal folds prior to onset of the swallowing response can clearly be visualized. However, aspiration cannot be identified during the actual swallow because of the upward excursion of the larynx, deflection of the epiglottis, contraction of the pharynx, and the subsequent deflection of light or white-out. Evidence of aspiration may be detected after the swallow either by visualization of aspirated material in the subglottic area or when the patient expels material from the airway, through spontaneous or volitional coughing or protective reaction.

### 9.8.5 Residue

The degree of residue in the hypopharynx following the swallow is easily discerned during the FEES exam. The amount of residue and the initiation and effectiveness of secondary clearing swallows, throat clearing, or coughing are noted. The effectiveness of compensatory strategies to assist with clearance of pharyngeal residue is judged; strategies to improve pharyngeal clearance

and other aspects of the swallow are described in the following section.

## 9.9 Compensatory Strategies During the Pediatric FEES Examination

The introduction of compensatory strategies to modify the swallowing process during pediatric FEES is an integral part of the procedure. The types of techniques that are used in the pediatric population differ in some respects from the strategies used with adults, though there are some commonalities, depending on age and cognitive ability. For example, the postural changes used in adults (e.g., the chin tuck maneuver, or head turns to the right or left to narrow the piriform sinus and lateral pharyngeal area) may be of benefit in older children and adolescents as well. However, there are certain compensatory strategies that are specific to infants and younger children, including, but not limited to, adaptations in positioning, methods to assess readiness to transition to oral feeding, implementation of **pacing** (feeder-imposed pause intervals) during breast or bottle feeding, modification of liquid flow rate, and use of a modified supraglottic swallowing sequence.

### 9.9.1 Positioning and Postural Alterations

Positional adaptations can be implemented at any point in the examination to assess the effect on swallowing function. For infants, a position can be quickly modified during the examination; for example, from semireclined to side-lying, or from semireclined to upright. Positioning modifications may be appropriate to address issues with head hyperextension that result in loss of oral control and subsequent problems with airway protection during swallowing. Side-lying positioning may facilitate more anterior positioning of the tongue in infants with retrognathia and posterior tongue displacement that interferes with coordination of respiration and swallowing.

### 9.9.2 Strategies for Determining Readiness for Oral Feeding

FEES offers a mechanism to assess swallowing function without requiring intake of barium contrast. This is particularly useful when the patient has never taken any oral volume or the oral intake has been minimal. In the pediatric population, this scenario occurs in a variety of medical conditions that preclude oral feeding. For example, oral feeding may be delayed for weeks or months until surgery can be performed or until recovery is complete in patients with esophageal conditions (**long gap esophageal atresia**, severe caustic ingestion injury, or tumor). Patients who are status posttraumatic brain injury with subsequent swallowing deficits are candidates for FEES to assess readiness to begin with oral trials, as discussed in the adult section of the chapter. Infants undergoing cardiac procedures to repair congenital anomalies, such as **hypoplastic left heart syndrome**, or other cardiac anomalies may experience a period of nonoral feeding status preoperatively as well as postoperatively during the recovery period. Postoperative instrumental assessment with FEES when physiological status is stable is useful in this particular group of patients because the cardiac surgical interventions may affect recurrent laryngeal nerve innervation to the vocal folds.[35,36] FEES affords an opportunity to assess vocal fold mobility/airway protection ability during swallowing and the efficacy of compensatory feeding strategies.

Premature infants or extremely medically fragile infants represent an additional group of patients who do not have exposure to oral feeding or oral feeding trials until an appropriate level of physiological readiness is reached. In such cases, readiness for oral feeding trials can be assessed safely via FEES. Key factors that indicate an infant's readiness to advance with nutritive trials include the presence of oral reflexes (root, suck, swallow), the ability to maintain state regulation (reach and maintain a quiet alert state), and capability to maintain an appropriate respiratory rate (~ 20–50 breaths per minute).[37,38,39] The level of sensory awareness in the hypopharynx and the infant's ability to achieve and maintain airway protection during nonnutritive swallowing can be ascertained prior to presentation of any nutritive stimulus. Appropriate management of secretions and the ability to generate spontaneous, clearing swallows can be clearly visualized. Introduction of very small volumes (minuscule) of either formula or breastmilk alongside the pacifier by use of a flexible dropper or 1 mL syringe controls the amount of nutritive stimulus during the exam. A small syringe (1–3 mL) may also be placed inside a nipple, which allows the clinician to carefully control the amount of formula contained within the nipple. The infant's ability to manage the nutritive input within the context of the suck–swallow–breathe triad can be determined; physiological responses can be monitored to assess for any stress reaction, such as increased heart or respiratory rate. As suck/swallow competence with small amounts of nutritive intake is established, volume can be gradually increased.

## Implementation of Pacing Intervals

In infants, coordination of respiration and swallowing can be problematic because feeding places additional demands on the coordinative relationships between breathing and swallowing. Though the exact neural controls that determine the onset and duration of the respiratory pause are unknown, patterns of respiratory activity surrounding swallowing can be an indicator of maturity and stabilization.[34] There are five respiratory phase categories in which swallowing may occur in healthy infants: during inspiration, in between inspiration and expiration, in the middle of expiration, between expiration and inspiration, and during prolonged respiratory pauses. Investigations of the developmental time course of respiratory phase and swallowing coordination suggest that respiratory rhythm becomes more stable with maturity.[40,41,42,43] The frequency of respiratory pauses during sequential swallowing characteristic of infant bottle or breastfeeding can be documented during FEES. Infants that engage in repeated suck–swallow cycles without respiratory pauses may be susceptible to aspiration when ventilatory needs override and interrupt the suck–swallow cycle.[34,44] The lack of appropriate respiratory pauses during sequential swallowing

and the effect on airway protection during swallowing can be detected. It is possible to gauge the effect of introducing feeder-imposed respiratory pauses, or pacing, during feeding to help facilitate appropriate respiratory pauses and adequate ventilation during sequential chain swallowing sequences. Close inspection of the endolaryngeal area during respiratory pauses facilitates detect evidence of aspiration; however, there is frequent loss of view during sequential swallowing chains secondary to white-out. Therefore, both videofluoroscopy and FEES may be needed to confirm swallowing safety and the effect of compensatory strategies, such as pacing.

## Modification of Liquid Flow

In infants, the use of a slower-flow nipple may help to decrease the volume of the bolus and the overall rate of swallowing, thereby facilitating appropriate respiratory pauses during feeding.[44] Likewise, in older infants, toddlers, and older children, a slower flow rate and a decreased overall rate of swallowing may help facilitate airway protection during the swallowing. The flow rate may slowed by modifying the intake mode (type of nipple, type of cup) or by increasing the viscosity of the liquid. However, the efficacy of these strategies has not been systematically studied across various conditions and disorders.[45] In particular, the implications for infants in terms of the possible nutritional compromise that occurs when changing the viscosity and composition of infant formula must be considered. There may be other factors to consider as well, such as the effects on hydration and digestion and in regard to the increased sucking effort required to extract a thickened liquid from a nipple or sipper cup spout. Changes in the viscosity of liquid must be considered in the context of each individual patient, and carefully considered by the members of the medical team including a registered dietitian. Thus recommendations about changing the viscosity of formula should not be made unilaterally by the speech-language pathologist.

## 9.9.3 Strategies to Improve Hypopharyngeal Clearance

Patients with weak tongue base retraction and/or reduced strength of pharyngeal contraction secondary to structural or neurologic etiologies present with varying locations and degrees of residue postswallow. The relative amount of residue and location (vallecular space, piriform sinus region, diffusely through the hypopharynx, interarytenoid region, surface of vocal fold, etc.) can be easily discerned during FEES. Some of the strategies to enhance hypopharyngeal clearance as previously described for adults may also be applicable for children. For instance, children who are able to follow directions may respond to verbal cues to generate additional swallows to clear residue, or to "squeeze" and "swallow hard" for production of an effortful swallow. The patient's ability to view the FEES examination enables immediate feedback regarding the effectiveness of the compensatory swallowing strategies. Combining verbal cues to use an effortful swallow in combination with chin flexion may be useful in some circumstances. Alternating sips of liquid with each presentation of solid food may also help the pediatric patient to achieve some improvement in hypopharyngeal clearance.

### 9.9.4 Modified Supraglottic Swallowing Sequence

In pediatric patients, there are both congenital conditions (laryngeal atresia, subglottic stenosis, bilateral vocal fold paralysis, laryngeal webs) and acquired conditions (subglottic and/or tracheal stenosis, hypopharyngeal stenosis, vocal fold paralysis) that require tracheotomy for airway patency.[46,47] Laryngotracheal reconstruction procedures are often necessary for expansion of the airway before **decannulation** (removal of the tracheostomy tube). The necessary surgical procedures involve alteration of the laryngeal anatomy, and compensatory swallowing actions are often developed as children adjust to the changes in anatomy.[48,49] The airway reconstruction may be done in a series of staged procedures with grafts and stents to maintain expansion of the airway, and continual adaptations in swallowing must occur. Preoperative FEES assessment delineates the patient's baseline swallowing function and permits some preliminary judgment regarding risk of swallowing dysfunction following surgical intervention. Significant premorbid swallowing dysfunction, such as delayed swallowing onset, poor pharyngeal clearance ability, and poor airway protection ability, is factored into the decision regarding the patient's surgical candidacy.[23]

Patients who demonstrate adequate swallowing function preoperatively undergo varied surgical reconstructive procedures depending on the underlying condition. As previously noted, airway stenting may be necessary, forcing the vocal folds to assume a lateral position in the postoperative period. Therefore, sufficient contraction of supraglottic structures and shielding by epiglottic inversion are critical during swallowing to maintain airway protection. Postoperatively, patients who have undergone airway reconstruction have been found to respond favorably to a variety of compensatory swallowing strategies, including the use of a modified supraglottic swallowing sequence.[49] The modified supraglottic sequence is composed of five steps: gentle cough/throat clear prior to intake of bolus, oral "holding" of the bolus prior to swallow initiation, effort to hold the breath prior to bolus transfer and swallowing, and swallow followed by gentle cough/throat clear. Use of a simple sequential series of pictures facilitates teaching the modified supraglottic swallowing sequence. In addition, slightly thickened fluid boluses can help the patient to maintain bolus control while learning the steps to the supraglottic sequence.[48,49] The use of FEES at intervals in the peri- and postoperative period contributes objective information regarding the effectiveness of the modified supraglottic sequence as a compensatory strategy.

### 9.10 Interpretation of Pediatric FEES

When the pediatric FEES assessment of anatomy and swallowing function is complete, the scope is withdrawn and the caregiver and patient are escorted from the FEES examination room to an adjacent examination room in the clinic. The speech-language pathologist and otolaryngologist review the results of the examination and record the findings in a pediatric FEES template report. Consensus is reached regarding overall impressions and recommendations. The otolaryngologist and the speech-language pathologist then meet with the caregiver and patient to discuss the examination findings and recommendations. The safety of feeding, the appropriate types of foods and liquids, and the options for compensatory strategies to improve swallowing function are discussed. Recommendations for further testing or consultations are made. Once consensus is reached with the caregiver regarding the recommendations, the plan is documented in the pediatric FEES report template, and a report is generated. It is helpful to allow the caregiver to view the FEES images during the discussion and explanation of swallowing dynamics and the rationale for the types of recommendations that are made. A sample pediatric FEES report template is located in **Appendix 9.1**.

### 9.11 Treatment Planning

Subsequent treatment recommendations are dependent on each patient's constellation of issues. The patient's response to compensatory strategies is often the basis for recommending additional dysphagia treatment, as well as referral for additional consultative services or tests. For example, patients who present with interarytenoid pachydermia, erythema, and nodularity throughout the hypopharynx may be referred to gastroenterology for consideration of possible reflux-related issues. If the safety of feeding appears to be severely compromised, consultation with the managing physician is indicated to determine the appropriate course of action. The need for an interval FEES examination to assess a patient's response to treatment recommendations is determined and is included in the overall recommendations.

### 9.12 Safety of FEES in the Pediatric Population

Flexible endoscopic examinations are performed in pediatric otolaryngology practices for a variety of reasons (assessment of anatomy, analysis of velopharyngeal function, voice analysis). We have not experienced any serious complications or adverse events in our experience of performing thousands of FEES examinations in patients ranging from neonates to young adults since the development of the procedure and examination protocol in 1993.

Careful review of the patient's medical history prior to the examination is essential. Patients who have significant pulmonary disease or respiratory distress known to be associated with oral feeding attempts should ideally be monitored with pulse oximetry during pediatric FEES. Patients with a history of cardiac arrhythmia or cardiac anomalies in which stress is contraindicated need to be medically cleared for FEES. Children with seizure disorders, known or suspected secretion management issues, need for frequent tracheal suctioning, or overall medical fragility need to be closely monitored during the FEES examination. Suction equipment should be readily accessible during the examination, as should pediatric resuscitation equipment and personnel. In particular, suctioning equipment must be accessible for children with tracheostomy tubes or neurologic conditions with accompanying secretion management issues who require frequent suctioning under normal circumstances.

Care should be taken when using nasal spray (oxymetazoline and 2% tetracaine) prior to the exam; the spray should be directed upward toward the middle meatus with the patient positioned in an upright position. Otherwise, inadvertent anesthesia of the hypopharynx may occur, which interferes with the validity of the examination. The effect of the nasal spray lasts 90 minutes or less; this should be explained to the caregiver and, if appropriate, to the patient.

During the examination, care should be taken to keep the infant or child's head in a static position. Passage of the endoscope under constant visualization precludes trauma to the nose; however, septal deflections, narrow middle meatus dimensions, or frequent motion of the child's head during insertion can lead to localized trauma and bleeding. Epistaxis (nose bleed) is an infrequent occurrence that can occur during any instrumentation of the nose, and it does not interfere with conducting the FEES procedure.

The threat of **laryngospasm** is a problem associated with flexible laryngoscopy. Laryngospasm (involuntary vocal fold adduction in response to laryngeal stimulation associated with intense vagal discharge leading to bradycardia and bronchospasm) is a well-known complication associated with induction or emergence from general anesthesia. It does not occur in the awake state. As mentioned, no adverse events, including laryngospasm, have occurred over thousands of pediatric FEES examinations in our office setting. Resuscitation equipment and personnel trained in establishing an emergency airway are essential for centers where pediatric FEES is performed because of the compromised medical status of patients requiring a FEES exam, not because of the FEES procedure.

## 9.13 Pediatric FEES Training

Knowledge, skills, and training guidelines for the use of FEES in clinical practice with both adult and pediatric patients are outlined by the American Speech-Hearing-Language Association (www.asha.org). When FEES is used in the pediatric population, collaboration with a pediatric otolaryngologist is essential in the consideration of anatomical, functional, and medical aspects that are outside the scope of the speech pathology practice. Pediatric speech pathologists who are considering integrating FEES into their clinical dysphagia practice may benefit from collaboration with a pediatric ear, nose, and throat specialist affiliated with their institution. Attending a dedicated pediatric FEES training course or workshop, observation of a pediatric FEES clinic, and ongoing collaboration with a mentor who has experience with FEES will be of benefit in establishing a dedicated pediatric FEES service.

## 9.14 Questions

1. A method to deliver oral taste stimulation during FEES to infants who have little or no experience with oral feeding is to

A. Intermittently replace the pacifier with a full bottle once nonnutritive sucking activity has been established

B. Present small drops of formula alongside the pacifier or within a nipple during nonnutritive stimulation with close monitoring of the infant's reaction

C. Present tastes prior to nonnutritive stimulation whenever possible

D. Use a syringe to present formula intraorally and then follow up with a full bottle

2. The feeder can use pacing intervals during FEES to

A. Increase the overall rate of feeding in order to increase volume of intake

B. Facilitate maintenance of sequential swallowing without respiratory pauses

C. Determine how much actual volume has been ingested

D. Impose respiratory pause intervals during sequential swallowing to facilitate maintenance of airway protection

3. Infants who present with increased inspiratory stridor with the respiratory effort of feeding may have laryngomalacia, which can be identified during FEES and is characterized by which of the following?

A. Bulky or "floppy" arytenoid cartilages, relatively short aryepiglottic folds, infantile omega-shaped epiglottis

B. Either right or left true vocal fold paralysis

C. Prolapse of the tongue base

D. Widely spaced arytenoid cartilages

4. Laryngotracheoesophageal clefts occur when the process of separation of the trachea from the esophagus stops in utero and are classified by type A type I laryngeal cleft is described as

A. A cleft that extends through the cricoid lamina that extends to the vocal folds

B. A cleft that begins in the interarytenoid area and extends to the carina

C. A cleft that involves the entire cricoid with extension into the cervical trachea

D. A cleft that presents as a defect in the interarytenoid area above the level of the posterior cricoid cartilage

5. Infants and children with craniofacial anomalies who are undergoing FEES may present with glossoptosis, which refers to

A. Posterior displacement of the tongue secondary to micrognathia

B. Habitual forward-resting tongue posture

C. Habitual elevation of the tongue tip, precluding visualization during fees

D. Enlargement of the entire tongue body

## 9.15 Answers and Explanations

1. **Correct: present small drops of formula alongside the pacifier or within a nipple during nonnutritive stimulation with close monitoring of the infant's reaction (B).**

2. **Correct: impose respiratory pause intervals during sequential swallowing to facilitate maintenance of airway protection (D).**

3. **Correct: bulky or "floppy" arytenoid cartilages, relatively short aryepiglottic folds, infantile omega-shaped epiglottis (A).**

4. **Correct: a cleft that the presents as a defect in the interarytenoid area above the level of the posterior cricoid cartilage (D).**

5. **Correct: posterior displacement of the tongue secondary to micrognathia (A).**

# Appendix 9.1: Pediatric FEES Examination

**Pertinent History:** [name, age, sex] [weeks gestation if pertinent] presents with [primary diagnosis, secondary diagnosis] and a medical history [pertinent medical history]. Prior surgical history includes: [ ]. (Patient) is currently receiving [oral feedings, diet level, viscosity level of fluid, enteral feedings, a combination of oral and enteral feeding, other]. Respiratory history was reported to be [unremarkable, significant for frequent respiratory infections, significant for pneumonia, tracheostomy, other]. (Patient) is currently receiving [early intervention therapies, speech therapy services, occupational therapy services, no therapy services, other]. Current concerns regarding feeding and swallowing [ ]. Clinical signs and symptoms of swallowing dysfunction: [ ]. Results of prior instrumental examinations [prior videofluoroscopic studies, prior FEES].

The following FEES study was requested to assess [airway protection/swallowing function, the ability to manage secretion]. The topical anesthesia of [Afrin/tetracaine, viscous lidocaine] was administered. The position during the examination was [upright, in a semireclined position, other]. The scope was passed transnasally by [ ].

## Summary of Examination (*** represents other, free field)

### Oral Motor Assessment

- **Orofacial symmetry and tone at rest:** [normal, abnormal, ***]
- **Range of oral motor movements:** [no restrictions in range of cheek, jaw, lip, tongue motion, limited active movements, significant limitation in active movements, ***]
- **Strength of oral motor movements:** [within normal limits, reduced, ***]
- **Current oral intake:** [tastes of no appreciable volume, liquids, pureeds, solids, ***]
- **Vocal quality:** [normal, intermittent wet vocal quality, consistent wet vocal quality, ***]

### Physical Examination

- **Appearance of hypopharynx and larynx at rest:** [symmetrical, asymmetrical, erythema, edema, prominent postcricoid venous plexus, pachydermia, ***]
- **Vocal fold mobility:** [normal mobility bilaterally, immobility, limited abduction, unable to visualize vocal folds, vocal folds fixed in midline, ***]
  - **Left vocal fold:** [normal, immobile, in paramedian position, in lateral position, arytenoid prolapse, ***]
  - **Right vocal fold:** [normal, immobile, in paramedian position, in lateral position, arytenoid prolapse, ***]

### Secretion Management and Swallow Frequency

- **Frequency of spontaneous swallowing:** [within normal limits, reduced, ***]
- **Location of secretions in the hypopharynx:** [vallecula, piriform sinus (R, L, Both), diffusely throughout hypopharynx***]
- **Response to aspiration of secretions:** [clearing response, inconsistent clearing, no protective response, ***]

### Sensation

- **Sensory response:** [normal threshold, decreased threshold, response to light touch of pharyngeal walls, response to light touch of epiglottis, ***]
- **Sensory response to formal sensory testing**: ___ response at ___.

### Bolus Presentations
The following consistencies were presented during the examination:

- **Liquids:** [thin, nectar consistency, honey consistency, pudding consistency, ***] via [flexible dropper, bottle, sipper cup with valve, sipper cup without valve, straw, cut-out cup, spoon]. Overall volume presented: [no appreciable volume, 5 mL, 10 mL, 15 mL, 20 mL, ***].
- **Pureed:** [pudding, applesauce, stage 1 puree, stage 2 puree, stage 3 puree, ***]. Overall volume of intake was [< 1 ounce, 2 ounces, 3 ounces, ***].
- **Solids:** [graham cracker, vanilla wafer, toddler puff snack, cookie, ***]. Overall volume of intake was [***].

## Swallowing parameters:

- **Oral manipulation and transfer skills:** [within normal limits, impaired, ***]
- **Onset of swallow:** The bolus was noted to collect in the [valleculae, piriform sinus region, overflow to laryngeal vestibule, ***] prior to initiation of the swallow response to [solids, liquids, pureed].
- **Laryngeal penetration (passage of material into the larynx that does not pass below the vocal folds):** [not identified; identified with bolus type: liquid, pureed, solid]
  - o **Depth of laryngeal penetration (degree of proximity to the true vocal folds):** [bolus type: liquid, pureed, solid; at depth of: laryngeal surface of epiglottis, aryepiglottic fold, interarytenoid notch, level of the true vocal folds; consistent, inconsistent, ***]
  - o **Sensory response to penetration:** [no response; swallow response with clearance, cough, cough with swallow, throat clear, progression to aspiration; consistent, inconsistent, ***]
- **Aspiration (defined as passage of material below the vocal folds):** [not identified; identified with: liquid, pureed, solid, ***]
  - o **Amount of aspiration:** [minimal, inconsistent, moderate, significant, consistent, ***]
  - o **Sensory responses to aspiration:** [no response, delayed response, effective cough; consistent, inconsistent, ***]
- **Pharyngeal residue following swallows:** [not noted; clearance was: complete through the hypopharynx following swallows, minimal following swallows of [liquid, pureed, solid] of a [mild, moderate, significant, ***] degree of residue following the initial swallow]

## Response to Compensatory Strategies to Improve Airway Protection/Swallowing Function

The patient was noted to be responsive/not responsive to the following compensatory strategies:

- **Clearance of pharyngeal residue:** [responsive, not responsive] to verbal cues to use [additional swallows, effortful swallow] to clear; improved clearance noted with: [alternation of solids and liquid boluses, ***]
- **Modification of liquid:** [improved, did not improve] airway protection was noted with presentation of [thickened liquid, ***]
- **Modification of positioning:** [effective, not effective] in facilitation of airway protection in [upright, semireclined, side-lying, ***]
- **Postural maneuvers:** [effective, not effective] in improving swallowing function/airway protection in [chin tuck, head turn, head tilt, effortful swallow, ***]
- **Use of pacing to impose pauses during intake:** [facilitated, did not facilitate] airway protection
- **Supraglottic swallow sequence:** [improved, did not improve] airway protection during swallowing
- **Other**

## Impressions

(Patient) demonstrated: [normal vocal fold mobility, vocal fold immobility, ***]. Secretion management was [within normal limits, impaired]. (NAME) demonstrated [normal swallowing parameters, abnormal swallowing parameters as characterized by ***]. Child [would, would not, ***] be at risk for aspiration following airway reconstruction surgery.

## Recommendations

The findings of the FEES examination were discussed, and the following recommendations were made:

- **Feeding position:** [continue to position upright, semireclined, side-lying, ***]
- **Diet recommendations:** [consider an alternative source of nutrition; continue with therapeutic/recreational tastes only; implement compensatory feeding strategies, including ***; continue ad lib intake of liquid, pureed foods, mechanical soft foods, easy-to-manage toddler food items, regular table foods, ***]
- **Compensatory strategies:** [use of effortful swallow, supraglottic swallowing sequence, implementation of pacing strategies, alternation of solids and liquids, limited bolus sizes, head turn, chin tuck, limited volume (***) of intake, neutral head position, chin tuck, other positioning, ***]
- **Further referrals:** [video swallow study, gastroenterology, psychology, occupational therapy, speech pathology, nutrition, interdisciplinary feeding team (IFT), ***]
- **Additional**

## References

[1] Willging JP. Endoscopic evaluation of swallowing in children. *Int J Pediatr Otorhinolaryngol* 1995;32(Suppl):S107–S108

[2] Miller CKWJ, Strife JL, Rudolph CD. Fiberoptic endoscopic examination of swallowing in infants and children with feeding disorders. *Dysphagia* 1994;9(4):266

[3] Leder SB, Karas DE. Fiberoptic endoscopic evaluation of swallowing in the pediatric population. *Laryngoscope* 2000;110(7):1132–1136

[4] Link DT, Willging JP, Miller CK, Cotton RT, Rudolph CD. Pediatric laryngopharyngeal sensory testing during flexible endoscopic evaluation of swallowing: feasible and correlative. *Ann Otol Rhinol Laryngol* 2000;109(10 Pt 1):899–905

[5] Willging JPMC, Hogan MJ, Rudolph CD. Fiberoptic endoscopic evaluation of swallowing in children: A preliminary report of 100 procedures. *Dysphagia* 1996;11:2

[6] Hartnick CJ, Hartley BE, Miller C, Willging JP. Pediatric fiberoptic endoscopic evaluation of swallowing. *Ann Otol Rhinol Laryngol* 2000;109(11):996–999

[7] Manrique D, Melo EC, Bühler RB. Fiberoptic endoscopic swallowing disorders in chronic encephalopathy [in Portuguese]. *J Pediatr (Rio J)* 2002;78(1):67–70

[8] Thottam PJ, Silva RC, McLevy JD, Simons JP, Mehta DK. Use of fiberoptic endoscopic evaluation of swallowing (FEES) in the management of psychogenic dysphagia in children. *Int J Pediatr Otorhinolaryngol* 2015;79(2):108–110

[9] Arvedson AB. L. Pediatric Feeding and Swallowing. New York, NY: Singular Publishing; 2001

[10] Rommel N, De Meyer AM, Feenstra L, Veereman-Wauters G. The complexity of feeding problems in 700 infants and young children presenting to a tertiary care institution. *J Pediatr Gastroenterol Nutr* 2003;37(1):75–84

[11] Newman LA, Keckley C, Petersen MC, Hamner A. Swallowing function and medical diagnoses in infants suspected of dysphagia. *Pediatrics* 2001;108(6):E106

[12] Burklow KA, Phelps AN, Schultz JR, McConnell K, Rudolph C. Classifying complex pediatric feeding disorders. *J Pediatr Gastroenterol Nutr* 1998;27(2):143–147

[13] Willging JP, Miller CK, Link DT, Rudolph CD. Use of FEES to assess and manage pediatric patients. In: Langmore SE, ed. Endoscopic Evaluation and Treatment of Swallowing Disorders. New York, NY: Thieme Medical; 2001:102–127

[14] Saal H. The genetics evaluation and common craniofacial syndromes. In: Kummer AW, ed. Cleft Palate and Craniofacial Anomalies: Effects on Speech and Resonance. 2nd ed. San Diego, CA: Singular; 2008:73–100

[15] Landry AM, Thompson DM. Laryngomalacia: disease presentation, spectrum, and management. Int J Pediatr 2012;2012:753526

[16] Rutter MJ. Congenital laryngeal anomalies. Rev Bras Otorrinolaringol (Engl Ed) 2014;80(6):533–539

[17] Rutter MJ. Evaluation and management of upper airway disorders in children. Semin Pediatr Surg 2006;15(2):116–123

[18] Miller CK, Willging JP. The implications of upper-airway obstruction on success-ful infant feeding. Semin Speech Lang 2007;28(3):190–203

[19] Lim TA, Spanier SS, Kohut RI. Laryngeal clefts: a histopathologic study and review. Ann Otol Rhinol Laryngol 1979;88(Pt 1):837–845

[20] Moungthong G, Holinger LD. Laryngotracheoesophageal clefts. Ann Otol Rhinol Laryngol 1997;106(12):1002–1011

[21] Myer CM III, Cotton RT, Holmes DK, Jackson RK. Laryngeal and laryngotra-cheoesophageal clefts: role of early surgical repair. Ann Otol Rhinol Laryngol 1990;99(2 Pt 1):98–104

[22] Myer CM III, Cotton RT, Shott SR, eds. The Pediatric Airway: An Interdisciplinary Approach. Philadelphia, PA: JB Lippincott; 1995

[23] Willging JP. Benefit of feeding assessment before pediatric airway reconstruction. Laryngoscope 2000;110(5 Pt 1):825–834

[24] Kool R, Lawver T. Play therapy: considerations and applications for the practi-tioner. Psychiatry (Edgmont) 2010;7(10):19–24

[25] Oestreich AE, Dunbar JS. Pharyngonasal reflux: spectrum and significance in early childhood. AJR Am J Roentgenol 1984;142(5):923–925

[26] Park JW, Kwon BS, Chang JH, Sim KB. Nasal backflow and the difficulty of relax-ation in the upper esophageal sphincter. Laryngoscope 2013;123(4):966–968

[27] Murray J, Langmore SE, Ginsberg S, Dostie A. The significance of accumulated oropharyngeal secretions and swallowing frequency in predicting aspiration. Dysphagia 1996;11(2):99–103

[28] Steele CM, Miller AJ. Sensory input pathways and mechanisms in swallowing: a review. Dysphagia 2010;25(4):323–333

[29] Humbert IA, Joel S. Tactile, gustatory, and visual biofeedback stimuli modulate neural substrates of deglutition. Neuroimage 2012;59(2):1485–1490

[30] Aviv JE, Martin JH, Kim T, et al. Laryngopharyngeal sensory discrimina-tion testing and the laryngeal adductor reflex. Ann Otol Rhinol Laryngol 1999;108(8):725–730

[31] Willging JP, Thompson DM. Pediatric FEESST: fiberoptic endoscopic evaluation of swallowing with sensory testing. Curr Gastroenterol Rep 2005;7(3):240–243

[32] Adler A, Groh-Wargo S. Transitioning the preterm neonate from hospital to home: nutritional discharge criteria. NICUCurrents 2012;3(2):1–11

[33] Kelly BN, Huckabee ML, Jones RD, Frampton CM. Nutritive and non-nutritive swallowing apnea duration in term infants: implications for neural control mechanisms. Respir Physiol Neurobiol 2006;154(3):372–378

[34] Kelly BN, Huckabee ML, Jones RD, Frampton CM. The early impact of feed-ing on infant breathing-swallowing coordination. Respir Physiol Neurobiol 2007;156(2):147–153

[35] Skinner ML, Halstead LA, Rubinstein CS, Atz AM, Andrews D, Bradley SM. Laryn-gopharyngeal dysfunction after the Norwood procedure. J Thorac Cardiovasc Surg 2005;130(5):1293–1301

[36] Pereira KdaR, Firpo C, Gasparin M, et al. Evaluation of swallowing in infants with congenital heart defect. Int Arch Otorhinolaryngol 2015;19(1):55–60

[37] Lau C, Hurst N. Oral feeding in infants. Curr Probl Pediatr 1999;29(4):105–124

[38] Thoyre SM, Shaker CS, Pridham KF. The early feeding skills assessment for preterm infants. Neonatal Netw 2005;24(3):7–16

[39] Pickler RH. A model of feeding readiness for preterm infants. Neonatal Intensive Care 2004;17(4):31–36

[40] Kelly BN, Huckabee ML, Jones RD, Frampton CM. The first year of human life: coordinating respiration and nutritive swallowing. Dysphagia 2007;22(1):37–43

[41] Gewolb IH, Bosma JF, Reynolds EW, Vice FL. Integration of suck and swallow rhythms during feeding in preterm infants with and without bronchopulmonary dysplasia. Dev Med Child Neurol 2003;45(5):344–348

[42] Goldfield EC, Richardson MJ, Lee KG, Margetts S. Coordination of sucking, swal-lowing, and breathing and oxygen saturation during early infant breast-feeding and bottle-feeding. Pediatr Res 2006;60(4):450–455

[43] Gewolb IH, Vice FL. Maturational changes in the rhythms, patterning, and coor-dination of respiration and swallow during feeding in preterm and term infants. Dev Med Child Neurol 2006;48(7):589–594

[44] Mathew OP. Breathing patterns of preterm infants during bottle feeding: role of milk flow. J Pediatr 1991;119(6):960–965

[45] Gosa M, Schooling T, Coleman J. Thickened liquids as a treatment for children with dysphagia and associated adverse effects: a systematic review. Infant Child Adolesc Nutr 2011;3(6):344–350

[46] Carron JD, Derkay CS, Strope GL, Nosonchuk JE, Darrow DH. Pediatric tracheoto-mies: changing indications and outcomes. Laryngoscope 2000;110(7):1099–1104

[47] Lewis CW, Carron JD, Perkins JA, Sie KC, Feudtner C. Tracheotomy in pe-diatric patients: a national perspective. Arch Otolaryngol Head Neck Surg 2003;129(5):523–529

[48] Miller CK, Linck J, Willging JP. Duration and extent of dysphagia following pediat-ric airway reconstruction. Int J Pediatr Otorhinolaryngol 2009;73(4):573–579

[49] Miller CK, Kelchner LN, de Alarcon A, Willging JP. Compensatory laryngeal func-tion and airway protection in children following airway reconstruction. Ann Otol Rhinol Laryngol 2014;123(5):305–313

# 10 High-Resolution Manometry in the Evaluation and Treatment of Oropharyngeal Dysphagia

*Molly A. Knigge, Sudarshan R. Jadcherla, and Susan L. Thibeault*

## Summary

Manometry has long been applied as a research tool in systematic investigation of swallowing pressures, and it remains a cornerstone in the gastroenterologist's armamentarium for assessment of esophageal pressures. Technologic advances leading to the development of high-resolution manometry (HRM) have introduced opportunities for application in the clinic setting for the evaluation and treatment of oropharyngeal dysphagia. Models are emerging for use of HRM by speech-language pathologists (SLPs) to provide a detailed analysis of a patient's ability to generate swallowing pressures from the nasopharynx through the upper esophageal sphincter (UES). Manometry measures may augment analysis of imaging studies, providing an additional dimension of assessment to assist in treatment planning. This chapter outlines developing models for HRM use by the SLP. The pressure topography plots that display swallowing data will be defined for the reader to become more familiar with the unique depiction of pressure events. Future directions for development of HRM in standard dysphagia practice are also discussed.

## Keywords

deglutition disorders, deglutition, pharynx, upper esophageal sphincter

## Learning Objectives

- List swallowing pressures that can be measured using high-resolution manometry (HRM) in the pharynx and upper esophageal sphincter (UES).
- Become familiar with eligibility criteria for application of HRM in oropharyngeal dysphagia.
- Recognize pharyngeal and UES swallowing pressure events on a topographic plot of the pharyngeal phase of swallowing.
- Identify clinical models for use of HRM by the speech pathologist in evaluation and treatment of complex pharyngeal and UES dysphagia.

## 10.1 Introduction

Imaging studies (the videofluoroscopic swallow study [VFSS] and fiberoptic endoscopic evaluation of swallowing [FEES]) are the gold standards for evaluation of pediatric and adult oropharyngeal dysphagia. Such studies are unparalleled in assessment of aspiration and bolus residuals, though they sometimes fall short in achieving objective measurement of certain aspects of swallowing, including pressures generated during swallowing, to guide treatment planning in complex dysphagia. High-resolution manometry (HRM) has emerged as a diagnostic tool that may be used clinically to augment imaging assessment of pharyngeal and upper esophageal sphincter (UES) function. This chapter outlines the evolution of manometry application from dysphagia research to clinical practice.

## 10.2 High-Resolution Manometry in the Evaluation and Treatment of Oropharyngeal Dysphagia

Oropharyngeal swallowing is a neurophysiologic response comprising exquisitely timed pressures to drive a food or liquid bolus through the upper aerodigestive tract. The structures of the upper aerodigestive tract are designed to serve multiple functions, including breathing, swallowing, and speech. In this multitasking environment, there are openings that must be regulated during swallowing to prevent losses of pressure as the bolus is passed to the esophagus. Swallowing pressures are propagated in the oral cavity and pharynx. Muscles that generate and contribute to swallowing pressures include the tongue, velum, pharyngeal musculature, and UES. Although some muscular efforts in the pharynx and UES press directly against the bolus tail, other muscular contractions serve to preserve swallowing pressures as the head of the bolus passes. For example, the pharynx serves swallowing efficiency by contracting both lengthwise and circumferentially, creating a shortened, rigid structure through which the bolus can pass easily to the UES.

Swallowing pressures may be positive or negative. Positive pressure results when musculature in the oral cavity and pharynx contracts against adjacent structures, such as the tongue base or pharyngeal walls contracting against each other. When this occurs in a precisely timed manner, a wave of muscular contraction presses against the tail of the bolus to achieve clearance of material to the esophagus. Lower or negative pressures are needed to provide an open pathway for the head of the bolus to advance. Lowered pressures occur when structures move away from adjacent structures, such as anterior movement of the cricoid cartilage away from the cervical spine during UES opening.

To date, imaging studies have represented the standard assessment for oropharyngeal swallowing evaluation across the age spectrum. VFSS and FEES offer visualization of swallowing physiology for analysis of anatomic spatial relationships, timing of physiologic events, and presence of residual contrast in the upper aerodigestive tract signaling inefficiency. VFSS promises reliable assessment of contrast entry into the airway using the Penetration-Aspiration Scale (PAS).[1] FEES offers higher sensitivity for identifying bolus material in the larynx and trachea compared to VFSS.[2,3] However, imaging studies cannot provide objective measurement of the pressures that serve swallowing. Imaging studies can yield only subjective judgments, such as residual contrast in the valleculae or piriform sinuses representing inefficiency of bolus clearance.

A manometer is a tool that can be used to measure pressures. Manometers are used throughout medicine to measure esophageal, gastric, and anorectal functions. Medical manometers consist of a catheter containing a number of sensors that interface with a computer application to collect pressure data. Manometers used for measuring esophageal pressures have historically come in several forms, including solid-state and water-perfused types. Prior to the last decade, manometry catheters contained a limited number of sensors, and they measured pressures exerted from only one direction. Advances in technology allowed sensors to be spaced 1 cm apart along the catheter for up to 36 sensors, averaging pressures circumferentially from 8 different directions, and manometers became capable of high resolution (**Fig. 10.1**).

In oropharyngeal swallowing research, manometers have long been used to measure pressures in the pharynx and UES in normal and disordered adults. Early research featured combined manometry with VFSS, referred to as manofluorography. Normative data were collected to characterize swallowing in healthy adult subjects[4,5,6,7,8,9,10,11] and facilitate modeling of swallowing physiology.[12] Radiation exposure associated with VFSS precluded systematic normative data collection during manofluorography in normal infants and children. Abnormal pressures resulting from various dysphagia etiologies in adults were investigated with this novel combination of technology, including pressure differences following surgical remodeling of the upper aerodigestive tract[4,13,14,15]; nonsurgical head/neck treatment modalities, such as chemoradiation[16]; and in neurologic and neurodegenerative disease.[17,18] Manofluorography also presented opportunities for study of analysis strategies that may improve VFSS interpretation to include inferences about swallowing strength.[19,20] Visions for clinical applications of manofluorography in complex oropharyngeal dysphagia were proposed but never achieved in standard practice during the era of lower-resolution manometers.[21,22]

Challenges in achieving accurate placement of a limited number of sensors to measure pharyngeal swallowing events were acknowledged by researchers pioneering use of pharyngeal manometry, including vertical movement of the catheter during palatal elevation, vertical movement of the UES and pharynx along the catheter during swallows, and asymmetry in the pharynx and UES requiring multidirectional sensors.[23,24] HRM permits researchers to measure swallowing pressure events simultaneously within the pharynx and UES with a contiguous representation of pressure propagation along the catheter. It has largely replaced traditional manometry in the research of pharyngeal and UES pressures, with normative data collected on young adults[25,26,27] and premature infants,[28] setting the stage for clinical application of HRM.

HRM has become a standard in the evaluation of esophageal motility disorders in pediatrics and adults.[29,30,31] Application of HRM in standard clinical care for oropharyngeal dysphagia is now emerging. Speech-language pathologists (SLPs) specializing in swallowing disorders have trained in performing HRM and analyzing the collected pressure data to serve diagnosis as well as treatment planning.[32] Use of HRM in standard pediatric dysphagia care remains a comprehensive assessment focused primarily on esophageal function. It has also been identified as a developing diagnostic tool in the evaluation of pediatric dysphagia.[33]

## 10.3 High-Resolution Manometry Eligibility and Patient Selection

HRM is an invasive diagnostic procedure and requires selective application. Passage of the manometer catheter through the nasal cavity warrants taking precautions similar to those for transnasal endoscopic evaluation for voice or swallowing (FEES).

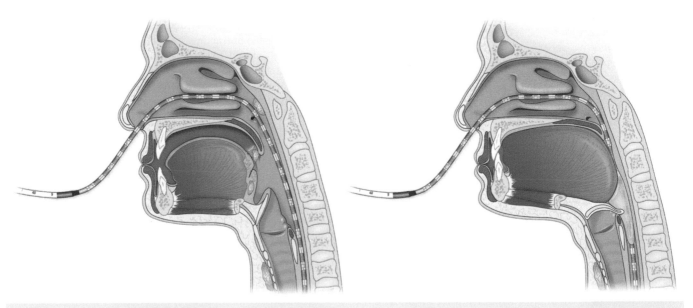

**Fig. 10.1** High-resolution manometer.

Indications and contraindications for HRM are listed in **Table 10.1**. Eligibility assessment for HRM should include medical history review to assure the patient has not had recent facial or nasal fractures or procedures. Due to the catheter advancement through the UES and into the proximal esophagus, patients considered for HRM must not have undergone recent surgical procedures in the pharynx, UES, or esophagus. HRM following surgical procedures to measure postoperative outcome should be pursued only with the surgeon's approval. Patients undergoing HRM should be cognitively capable of following directions and reconciling the sensations of catheter passage. Patients with painful conditions of the pharynx or esophagus, such as acute chemoradiation-induced mucositis, are unlikely to tolerate HRM catheter placement.

It is standard practice in esophageal manometry to perform a "blind" placement of the catheter by coaching the patient to swallow the catheter and assessing placement based on the resultant pressure topography plots. This technique of catheter placement can also be used in pharyngeal manometry. The clinician can identify the resting pressure of the UES against the catheter, the stereotypical pressure propagation of the pharyngeal swallow, and the quiescence of pressures against the catheter during UES opening to verify correct placement. However, inherent to pharyngeal and UES dysphagia is the possibility for impaired laryngeal closure or UES opening when swallowing. Either can inhibit successful placement of the manometry catheter to the esophagus. Imaging studies allow the clinician to judge carefully whether a patient may undergo blind catheter placement or requires visualization of catheter placement to ensure avoidance of laryngeal entry. HRM should be performed in conjunction with either fluoroscopic or endoscopic guidance if visualization is needed for catheter passage. Several clinical models for application of HRM in standard adult dysphagia care have been developed as a guide for the SLP.[32]

## 10.4 Guiding Treatment in Complex Pharyngeal/UES Dysphagia

Patients with complex pharyngeal or UES dysphagia will often demonstrate stasis of residual bolus material within the pharynx after swallowing. This sign on imaging studies may be related to impaired swallowing pressures, but there may be other factors that account for residual contrast that preclude making such assumptions.[34] Only HRM can measure swallowing pressures to verify whether reduced pressures may be contributing to swallowing inefficiency. Performing the VFSS or FEES first allows the clinician to assess for pharyngeal stasis and identify those individuals who may benefit from further evaluation of swallowing pressures.

Measurements of pharyngeal and UES pressures may guide the clinician in designing treatment, which may include compensatory feeding or postural strategies, exercise regimens, and surgical interventions. The set of manometric measurements serves not only as a treatment planning tool but also as an objective baseline against which future measures may be compared over time.

Table 10.1  High-resolution manometry eligibility criteria and contraindications

| Indications for high-resolution manometry | Contraindications |
| --- | --- |
| Complex pharyngeal dysphagia Pharyngeal stasis on videofluoroscopic swallow study or fiberoptic endoscopic evaluation of swallowing | Recent aerodigestive tract surgery Nasal fracture or trauma |
| Pre- and posttherapy measurement of upper esophageal sphincter dysfunction | Pharyngeal/esophageal perforation Known obstruction to catheter passage Cognitive impairment Unstable medical status |

## 10.5 Postintervention Outcome Measurement

Following completion of an exercise regimen or surgical intervention, manometric measurements may be repeated and compared to preintervention HRM to verify whether physiologic change in swallowing function was achieved. This becomes especially important when sensory impairment is part of the patient's dysphagia profile. Patient-reported quality of life outcome scales play a critical role in capturing patient perceptions of changes in swallowing function that have an impact on daily oral intake. However, it may be difficult for patients to report changes in swallowing function due to silent aspiration or inability to sense pharyngeal stasis. Pairing patient-reported outcomes with imaging and HRM can establish a postintervention measurement for both patient and payer justification of rendered dysphagia care.

### 10.5.1 Biofeedback

Sensorimotor awareness of pharyngeal swallowing events may be difficult for patients during a pharyngeal exercise. Biofeedback strategies used in training complex maneuvers, such as the Mendelsohn maneuver,[35] have drawn criticism for false-positive feedback provided to clinicians and patients during treatment sessions.[36] HRM can provide biofeedback for patients in treatment where complex manipulation of swallowing, including timing and amplitude of movement, needs to be visually represented. Preliminary research has suggested that normal participants show potential for modifying swallowing timing and peak pressures with HRM biofeedback training.[37] Systematic study of the effectiveness of HRM as a biofeedback tool is needed, though the modality shows promise for providing patients with an interactive training platform for motor learning.

### 10.5.2 Pressure Topography Plots

HRM can provide the clinician with a profound amount of data for each recorded swallow. The computer interface archives data and allows detailed review of pressure measurements. A feature of HRM systems is the representation of pressure data in a pressure topography plot, also referred to as a Clouse plot,[38] shown in **Fig. 10.2**. Along the horizontal axis, the plot features

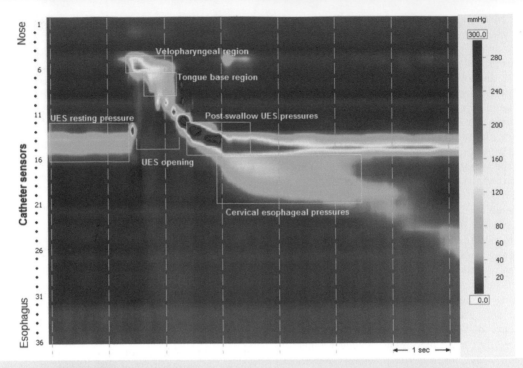

**Fig. 10.2** Pressure topography plot of a normal swallow.

time measured in seconds. The sensors along the catheter are represented along the vertical axis. The sensors at the top of the plot will be in the nasal cavity, whereas the sensors at the bottom of the plot are in the esophagus. The pharyngeal and UES swallow will require approximately 12 to 14 sensors along the HRM catheter to measure pressures from the nasopharynx to the resting level of the UES (**Fig 10.3**). A third dimension of pressure is then represented in a color-coded index, where "cool" colors of blue and green are used to show lower pressures and "hot" colors of yellow, red, and fuchsia show high pressures. Clinicians can also measure selected areas of the plot with analysis tools provided by the software applications. Classic line plots used to depict pressures along individual sensors can also be displayed. Tabulated data over selected time intervals can also be obtained with system software.

The pressure topography plot for a pharyngeal swallow will display a stereotypical pattern of pressures that comprise events from the nasopharynx through the UES. UES resting pressure is easily recognized as a running band of recorded pressure. Pharyngeal swallow initiation will interrupt this displayed pressure against the catheter, representing relaxation of the cricopharyngeus, lateral distension of the UES during bolus passage, and mechanical forces assisting anteroposterior opening of the UES. At the initiation of the swallow, pressures against the catheter in the nasopharyngeal region should display approximately 10 to 12 sensors above the level of the UES resting pressure. Pressure propagation, or fine coordination of pressure over time, between the nasopharynx and UES will create a diagonal line of displayed pressures, with resumption of resting UES pressure occurring after the pharyngeal swallow. Pressure events of interest have

been defined as nasopharyngeal region pressures, tongue base region pressures, postswallow pressures (as the UES contracts and descends upon the bolus tail), and UES opening minimum pressures. Duration of events, such as total swallow duration or UES opening duration, can also be measured. Functional comparisons can be made by having patients perform compensatory positioning or swallowing maneuvers to determine the physiologic impact on peak pressures or UES function. Examples of such comparisons are depicted in **Fig 10.4**.

## 10.6 Application of High-Resolution Manometry in Infants

Manometry applications, either alone or in concurrence with impedance and respiratory and cardiac rhythms, are being used to study pharyngoesophageal pressure topography and bolus transits.[39,40] Integrating cardiorespiratory rhythms permits the study of changes and adaptations in the regulation of breathing and cardiac rhythms, a function regulated by the vagus nerve, which also regulates foregut function and peristalsis. Prolonged studies are possible in infants at the point of care to recognize the pathophysiology of dysphagia-related symptoms under various states of oropharyngeal provocations, such as may happen under clinical settings of sucking and swallowing, feeding, choking and coughing, gastroesophageal reflux, or cardiorespiratory events should they happen during a study. The quality of data generated during such combined modalities depends largely on the skills

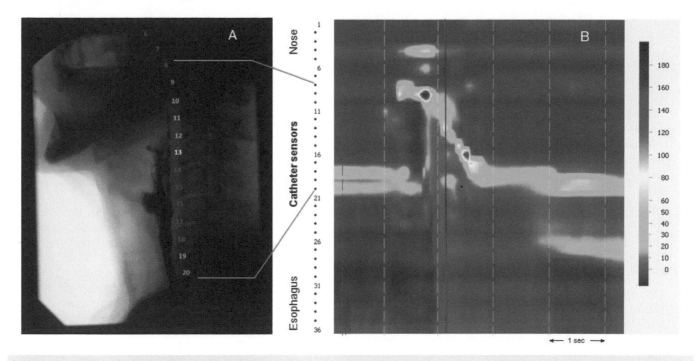

**Fig. 10.3** **(a)** Lateral fluoroscopy image of manometry catheter placement with sensors labeled and color-coded to reflect the pressure index plotted in **(b)**. The highest pressures, in yellow and green, are measured at the catheter sensors where the tongue base region, epiglottis, and upper esophageal sphincter are in contact with the catheter. **(b)** Pressure topography plot depicting pharyngeal swallow propagation. The red line represents the time point of the radiographic still shown in **(a)**.

and experience of the individual performing the procedure. Proper applications have the potential to document oropharyngeal function objectively, as well as assess the responses to therapies.

Objective assessment should be the key point for investigation into the sucking–swallowing rhythms, feeding, and swallowing abilities of infants. HRM is an innovative technique that provides the ability to characterize the pathophysiologic basis of dysphagia when attention is paid to the pressure-flow biomechanical events. Pertinent to oropharyngeal and upper esophageal sphincter functions in infants, the following definitions can be useful: (1) pharyngeal contractility and posterior tongue thrust; (2) upper esophageal sphincter basal tone (mm Hg), which is an average resting pressure; (3) onset of upper esophageal sphincter relaxation (in seconds); (4) duration of upper esophageal sphincter relaxation (in seconds).

## 10.7 Future Directions

HRM is just emerging as a tool in advanced dysphagia practice. Clinical research will need to demonstrate effective application in the use of HRM by speech pathologists in pharyngeal and UES dysphagia. Standardized competency training is needed to support skill development as HRM practice expands among clinical centers. Use of HRM by speech pathologists in pediatric and infant dysphagia practice should be explored as a distinct competency apart from adult HRM practice, because the

indications and protocol will be unique to this vulnerable population. Further development and clinical investigation of HRM assessment models in pediatric care may define a standard best practice, especially in the realm of complex dysphagia.

Gastroenterology practices have developed sophisticated computer analysis platforms (the Chicago Classification) to support the diagnosis of esophageal motility disorders.[29] The classification has been validated in adult populations, with limited application in pediatrics at this time.[41] It seems possible that as HRM in the assessment of pharyngeal and UES dysphagia develops, such a classification may evolve for the upper aerodigestive tract. The integration of impedance data has shown promise in evaluation of esophageal dysphagia in adults and pediatrics,[42,43,44,45] and it may hold potential for analysis of bolus flow as it relates to pressure measurements above the esophagus.[39,46,47] Automated HRM analysis designed specifically for pharyngeal and UES data will reduce the burden of manual analysis and allow for sophisticated calculations that integrate peak pressures and duration to better capture swallowing function. As normative data across the age spectrum emerge, clinical HRM practice can be uniquely tailored to serve individuals at any point in life. It is inevitable that technology will continue to evolve, with three-dimensional HRM already being applied in research examining asymmetric phenomena in pharyngeal dysphagia. With technological advances leading to higher resolution of pressure data, smaller catheter diameters, and automated pharyngeal and UES analysis, HRM can become a highly specialized diagnostic tool for the speech pathologist.

## 10.8 Questions

**1.** Limitations of early manometers included which of the following?

A. Too few sensors to adequately capture the range of pressure events in the pharynx and upper esophageal sphincter
B. Sensors that only measured pressure from one direction around the catheter
C. Inadequate pressure measurement to serve esophageal dysphagia
D. A and B
E. A and C

**2.** A pressure topography plot, or Clouse plot, is characterized by which three dimensions making up the display of swallowing events?

A. Bolus volume, time, and color-coded pressure index
B. Distance along the catheter, time, and gray-scale pressure index
C. Distance along the catheter, time, and color-coded pressure index
D. Bolus volume, bolus type, and age of the patient
E. Catheter diameter, catheter length, and duration of exam

**3.** Pressure events measured during high-resolution manometry include which of the following?

A. Upper esophageal sphincter (UES) postswallow pressures
B. Nasopharyngeal region pressures
C. Tongue base region pressures
D. UES minimum pressures
E. All of the above

**4.** Which of the following is a role served by high-resolution manometry in clinical application for pharyngeal dysphagia?

A. Measurement of oral pressures in planning swallowing therapy
B. Outcome measurement of pharyngeal pressures before and after swallowing therapy
C. Assessment of esophageal pressures to compare to pharyngeal pressures
D. All of the above
E. None of the above

**5.** Which of the following is not a contraindication to doing manometry?

A. Recent nasal fracture
B. Recent surgery in the upper aerodigestive tract
C. Cognitive impairment without ability to follow directions
D. Pharyngeal weakness
E. Acute mucositis of the pharynx following radiation treatment for head and neck cancer

## 10.9 Answers and Explanations

**1. Correct: A and B (D).**
Prior to the last decade, manometry catheters contained a limited number of sensors and measured pressures exerted from only one direction. As technology advanced, the high-resolution manometer was developed to allow sensors spaced 1 cm apart along the catheter for up to 36 sensors averaging pressures circumferentially from eight different directions.

**2. Correct: Distance along the catheter, time, and color-coded pressure index (C).**
Along the horizontal axis, the plot features time measured in seconds. The sensors along the catheter are represented along the vertical axis. The sensors at the top of the plot will be in the nasal cavity, whereas the sensors at the bottom of the plot are in the esophagus. A third dimension of pressure is then represented in a color-coded index, where "cool" colors of blue and green are used to show lower pressures and "hot" colors of yellow, red, and fuchsia show high pressures.

**3. Correct: All of the above (E).**
Pressure events of interest have been defined as nasopharyngeal region pressures, tongue base region pressures, postswallow pressures (as the UES contracts and descends on the bolus tail), and UES opening minimum pressures. Duration of events, such as total swallow duration or UES opening duration, can also be measured.

**4. Correct: Outcome measurement of pharyngeal pressures before and after swallowing therapy (B).**
Measurements of pharyngeal and UES pressures may guide the clinician in designing treatment, which may include compensatory feeding or postural strategies, exercise regimens, and surgical interventions. The set of manometric measurements serves not only as a treatment planning tool but also as an objective baseline against which future measures may be compared over time.

**5. Correct: Pharyngeal weakness (D).**
Pharyngeal weakness is not a contraindication for manometry. In fact, manometry can provide useful information regarding extent of pharyngeal weakness based on the measures of pressure it provides.

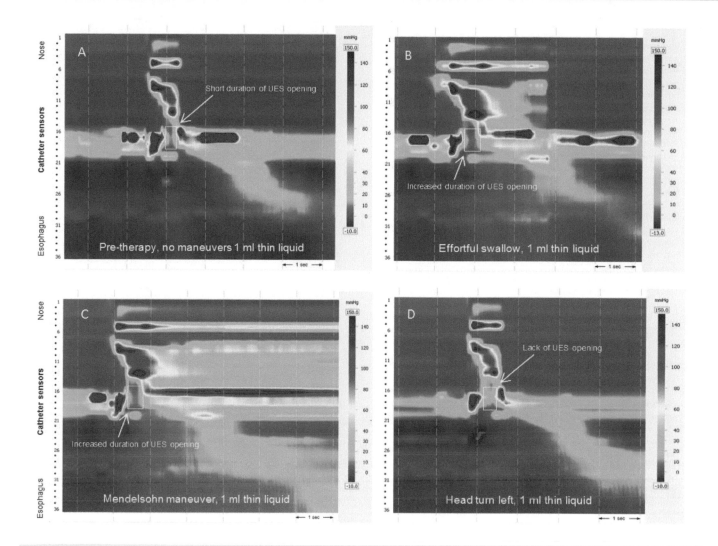

**Fig. 10.4** **(a)** Pre-therapy pressure topography plot showing impaired upper esophageal sphincter (UES) opening of shortened duration (0.1 s) and UES minimum pressures of 4.1 mm Hg during 1 mL thin-liquid bolus flow. **(b)** Effortful swallow during biofeedback therapy demonstrating a small increase in duration of UES opening (0.2 s) with lowered minimum UES pressures of − 0.8 mm Hg for a 1 mL bolus. **(c)** Mendelsohn maneuver during biofeedback therapy showing prolonged pharyngeal pressures, further increase in duration of UES opening (0.3 s), and reduced minimum UES pressures at 1.6 mm Hg during 1 mL bolus flow. **(d)** Head turn left with 1 mL bolus volume demonstrating no discernible opening with heightened minimum UES pressures at 21.5 mm Hg. These measures reveal the poor compensatory effect of the head turn strategy for this patient.

# References

[1] Rosenbek JC, Robbins JA, Roecker EB, Coyle JL, Wood JL. A penetration-aspiration scale. *Dysphagia* 1996;*11*(2):93–98

[2] Wu CH, Hsiao TY, Chen JC, Chang YC, Lee SY. Evaluation of swallowing safety with fiberoptic endoscope: comparison with videofluoroscopic technique. *Laryngoscope* 1997;*107*(3):396–401

[3] Langmore SE. Role of flexible laryngoscopy for evaluating aspiration. *Ann Otol Rhinol Laryngol* 1998;*107*(5 Pt 1):446–446

[4] McConnel FMS, Cerenko D, Mendelsohn MS. Manofluorographic analysis of swallowing. *Otolaryngol Clin North Am* 1988;*21*(4):625–635

[5] McConnel FMS, Cerenko D, Jackson RT, Guffin TN Jr. Timing of major events of pharyngeal swallowing. *Arch Otolaryngol Head Neck Surg* 1988;*114*(12):1413–1418

[6] Cerenko D, McConnel FMS, Jackson RT. Quantitative assessment of pharyngeal bolus driving forces. *Otolaryngol Head Neck Surg* 1989;*100*(1):57–63

[7] Olsson R, Nilsson H, Ekberg O. Simultaneous videoradiography and computerized pharyngeal manometry--videomanometry. *Acta Radiol* 1994;*35*(1):30–34

[8] Dejaeger E, Pelemans W, Bibau G, Ponette E. Manofluorographic analysis of swallowing in the elderly. *Dysphagia* 1994;*9*(3):156–161

[9] Zamir Z, Ren J, Hogan WJ, Shaker R. Coordination of deglutitive vocal cord closure and swallow in elderly. *Eur J Gastroenterol Hepatol* 1996;*8*:425–429

[10] Dejaeger E, Pelemans W, Ponette E, Joosten E. Mechanisms involved in postdeglutition retention in the elderly. *Dysphagia* 1997;*12*(2):63–67

[11] Steele CM, Huckabee ML. The influence of orolingual pressure on the timing of pharyngeal pressure events. *Dysphagia* 2007;*22*(1):30–36

[12] Ku DN, Ma PP, McConnel FMS, Cerenko D. A kinematic study of the oropharyngeal swallowing of a liquid. *Ann Biomed Eng* 1990;*18*(6):655–669

[13] McConnel FMS, Mendelsohn MS, Logemann JA. Examination of swallowing after total laryngectomy using manofluorography. *Head Neck Surg* 1986;*9*(1):3–12 doi: 10.1002/hed.2890090103

[14] Mendelsohn MS, McConnel FMS. Function in the pharyngoesophageal segment. *Laryngoscope* 1987;*97*(4):483–489 doi: 10.1288/00005537-198704000-00014

[15] McConnel FMS, Hester TR, Mendelsohn MS, Logemann JA. Manofluorography of deglutition after total laryngopharyngectomy. *Plast Reconstr Surg* 1988;*81*(3):346–351

[16] Pauloski BR, Rademaker AW, Lazarus C, Boeckxstaens G, Kahrilas PJ, Logemann JA. Relationship between manometric and videofluoroscopic measures of swallow function in healthy adults and patients treated for head and neck cancer with various modalities. *Dysphagia* 2009;*24*(2):196–203

[17] McConnel FMS, Cerenko D, Hersh T, Weil LJ. Evaluation of pharyngeal dysphagia with manofluorography. *Dysphagia* 1988;*2*(4):187–195

[18] Ali GN, Wallace KL, Schwartz R, DeCarle DJ, Zagami AS, Cook IJ. Mechanisms of oral-pharyngeal dysphagia in patients with Parkinson's disease. *Gastroenterology* 1996;*110*(2):383–392

[19] Leonard R, Belafsky PC, Rees CJ. Relationship between fluoroscopic and manometric measures of pharyngeal constriction: the pharyngeal constriction ratio. *Ann Otol Rhinol Laryngol* 2006;*115*(12):897–901

[20] Leonard R, Rees CJ, Belafsky P, Allen J. Fluoroscopic surrogate for pharyngeal strength: the pharyngeal constriction ratio (PCR). *Dysphagia* 2011;*26*(1):13–17

[21] Ravich WJ. The unrealized potential of pharyngeal manometry. *Dysphagia* 1995;*10*(1):42–43

[22] Cook IJ. Investigative techniques in the assessment of oral-pharyngeal dysphagia. *Dig Dis* 1998;*16*(3):125–133

[23] McConnel FMS, Guffin TN Jr, Cerenko D. The effect of asymmetric pharyngoesophageal pressures on manofluorographic measurements. *Laryngoscope* 1991;*101*(5):510–515 doi: 10.1288/00005537-199105000-00012

[24] Salassa JR, DeVault KR, McConnel FMS. Proposed catheter standards for pharyngeal manofluorography (videomanometry). *Dysphagia* 1998;*13*(2):105–110

[25] Hoffman MR, Ciucci MR, Mielens JD, Jiang JJ, McCulloch TM. Pharyngeal swallow adaptations to bolus volume measured with high-resolution manometry. *Laryngoscope* 2010;*120*(12):2367–2373 doi: 10.1002/lary.21150

[26] Yoon KJ, Park JH, Park JH, Jung IS. Videofluoroscopic and manometric evaluation of pharyngeal and upper esophageal sphincter function during swallowing. *J Neurogastroenterol Motil* 2014;*20*(3):352–361 doi: 10.5056/jnm14021

[27] Omari TI, Kritas S, Cock C, et al. Swallowing dysfunction in healthy older people using pharyngeal pressure-flow analysis. *Neurogastroenterol Motil* 2014;*26*(1):59–68 doi: 10.1111/nmo.12224

[28] Rommel N, van Wijk M, Boets B, et al. Development of pharyngo-esophageal physiology during swallowing in the preterm infant. *Neurogastroenterol Motil* 2011;*23*(10):e401–e408 doi: 10.1111/j.1365-2982.2011.01763.x

[29] Kahrilas PJ, Sifrim D. High-resolution manometry and impedance-pH/manometry: valuable tools in clinical and investigational esophagology. *Gastroenterology* 2008;*135*(3):756–769 doi: 10.1053/j.gastro.2008.05.048

[30] Fox MR, Bredenoord AJ. Oesophageal high-resolution manometry: moving from research into clinical practice. *Gut* 2008;*57*(3):405–423 doi: 10.1136/gut.2007.127993

[31] Pandolfino JE, Fox MR, Bredenoord AJ, Kahrilas PJ. High-resolution manometry in clinical practice: utilizing pressure topography to classify oesophageal motility abnormalities. *Neurogastroenterol Motil* 2009;*21*(8):796–806 doi: 10.1111/j.1365-2982.2009.01311.x

[32] Knigge MA, Thibeault S, McCulloch TM. Implementation of high-resolution manometry in the clinical practice of speech language pathology. *Dysphagia* 2014;*29*(1):2–16 doi: 10.1007/s00455-013-9494-5

[33] Rommel N, Omari T. Abnormal pharyngoesophageal function in infants and young children: diagnosis with high-resolution manometry. *J Pediatr Gastroenterol Nutr* 2011;*52*(Suppl 1):S29–S30 doi: 10.1097/MPG.0b013e318213a4b8

[34] Knigge MA, Thibeault S. Relationship between tongue base region pressures and vallecular clearance. *Dysphagia* 2016;*31*(3):391–397 doi: 10.1007/s00455-015-9688-0

[35] Kahrilas PJ, Logemann JA, Krugler C, Flanagan E. Volitional augmentation of upper esophageal sphincter opening during swallowing. *Am J Physiol* 1991;*260*(3 Pt 1):G450–G456

[36] Azola AM, Greene LR, Taylor-Kamara I, Macrae P, Anderson C, Humbert IA. The relationship between submental surface electromyography and hyo-laryngeal kinematic measures of Mendelsohn maneuver duration. *J Speech Lang Hear Res* 2015;*58*(6):1627–1636 doi: 10.1044/2015_JSLHR-S-14-0203

[37] Lamvik K, Jones R, Sauer S, Erfmann K, Huckabee ML. The capacity for volitional control of pharyngeal swallowing in healthy adults. *Physiol Behav* 2015;*152*(Pt A):257–263

[38] Clouse RE, Staiano A, Alrakawi A, Haroian L. Application of topographical methods to clinical esophageal manometry. *Am J Gastroenterol* 2000;*95*(10):2720–2730

[39] Omari T, Tack J, Rommel N. Impedance as an adjunct to manometric testing to investigate symptoms of dysphagia: What it has failed to do and what it may tell us in the future. *United European Gastroenterol J* 2014;*2*(5):355–366 doi: 10.1177/2050640614549096

[40] Shubert TR, Sitaram S, Jadcherla SR. Effects of pacifier and taste on swallowing, esophageal motility, transit, and respiratory rhythm in human neonates. *Neurogastroenterol Motil* 2016;*28*(4):532–542 doi: 10.1111/nmo.12748

[41] Singendonk MMJ, Smits MJ, Heijting IE, et al. Inter- and intrarater reliability of the Chicago Classification in pediatric high-resolution esophageal manometry recordings. *Neurogastroenterol Motil* 2015;*27*(2):269–276 doi: 10.1111/nmo.12488

[42] Chen CL, Yi CH, Liu TT, Hsu CS, Omari TI. Characterization of esophageal pressure-flow abnormalities in patients with non-obstructive dysphagia and normal manometry findings. *J Gastroenterol Hepatol* 2013;*28*(6):946–953 doi: 10.1111/jgh.12176

[43] Nguyen NQ, Holloway RH, Smout AJ, Omari TI. Automated impedance-manometry analysis detects esophageal motor dysfunction in patients who have non-obstructive dysphagia with normal manometry. *Neurogastroenterol Motil* 2013;*25*(3):238–245, e164 doi: 10.1111/nmo.12040

[44] Omari TI, Wauters L, Rommel N, Kritas S, Myers JC. Oesophageal pressure-flow metrics in relation to bolus volume, bolus consistency, and bolus perception. *United European Gastroenterol J* 2013;*1*(4):249–258 doi: 10.1177/2050640613492157

[45] Rommel N, Omari TI, Selleslagh M, et al. High-resolution manometry combined with impedance measurements discriminates the cause of dysphagia in children. *Eur J Pediatr* 2015;*174*(12):1629–1637 doi: 10.1007/s00431-015-2582-9

[46] Omari TI, Dejaeger E, Van Beckevoort D, et al. A novel method for the nonradiological assessment of ineffective swallowing. *Am J Gastroenterol* 2011;*106*(10):1796–1802

[47] Rommel N, Selleslagh M, Hoffman I, et al. Objective assessment of swallow function in children with suspected aspiration using pharyngeal automated impedance manometry. *J Pediatr Gastroenterol Nutr* 2014;*58*(6):789–794 doi: 10.1097/MPG.0000000000000337

# 11 Treatment: Compensatory, Postural, and Rehabilitation Strategies

*Nancy B. Swigert*

## Summary

Planning and implementing successful treatment for a person with dysphagia or a feeding/swallowing disorder, based on a careful analysis of the evaluation findings, requires the clinician to select and utilize appropriate compensatory, postural, and rehabilitation strategies. Compensatory and postural strategies are not expected to improve issues related to the underlying physiology, whereas rehabilitation strategies are designed to achieve a specific change in a physiological function. For some persons with dysphagia (PWD) only one type of strategy will be indicated, whereas others will need a combination of two or three types. The treatments' effectiveness should be measured. Selection of appropriate treatment strategies requires an understanding of the physiology of swallowing, the principles of motor learning, typical development in infants and children, and the role of neural plasticity. This chapter discusses the use of these strategies across the life span, although treatment for certain specific populations (e.g., neonates, patients with progressive disorders) will be discussed in greater detail in each of the disorder-specific chapters. This chapter addresses treatment of oral and pharyngeal dysphagia and some differences in treating children versus adults with dysphagia. Determining the frequency, intensity, and timing of treatment is as important as selecting appropriate treatment strategies. Clinicians should consider specific compensatory, postural, and rehabilitation strategies and the examples of available evidence for the strategy, when such evidence exists. When evidence does not exist, the clinician should consider whether a technique should work given an understanding of physiology and related principles.

## Keywords

compensation, postural, rehabilitation, motor learning, physiology, neuromuscular, sensorimotor, neural plasticity, evidence

### Learning Objectives

- Differentiate compensatory, postural, and rehabilitation strategies
- State strategies for different phases of swallow
- Describe relationship between impaired physiology and specific strategies
- Discuss principles of neural plasticity, motor learning, and neuromuscular treatments related to dysphagia
- State examples of available evidence for strategies

## 11.1 Introduction

Treatment of dysphagia in all ages and treatment of feeding/swallowing disorders in children require the clinician to possess extensive knowledge and skills. First and foremost, to develop an effective treatment plan for impaired swallowing, one must fully grasp the normal anatomy and physiology of the upper **aerodigestive** tract and swallowing mechanism. Failure to understand how the mechanism functions when it is working well will inevitably lead to an inability to plan treatment for a mechanism that is impaired or not developing normally. Treating dysphagia across the life span also requires understanding of typical development in infants and children; effects of specific diseases and disorders in children and adults; differences in acute, chronic, and neurodegenerative diseases; and changes that are seen in normal aging. Other chapters in this book provide detailed information about dysphagia in specific populations and address considerations when treating those populations. The effectiveness of the strategies described in this chapter might be affected by the nature of the disorder. For example, the treatment for a person with dysphagia (PWD) who has had an acute event (e.g., cerebrovascular accident), from which some spontaneous recovery is expected, will differ from treatment for someone with a neurodegenerative disease. The treatment for a child with developmental delay is not the same as the treatment for a child with cerebral palsy. In addition, the age and cognitive skills of the PWD and information about the person's support system must be considered when treatment strategies are being planned and implemented. Postural and compensatory strategies might be applied successfully despite the PWD's inability to use the strategy independently, whereas some rehabilitation strategies require the individual to follow a complex, multistep command.

Thus planning treatment for dysphagia and feeding/swallowing disorders is a multifaceted endeavor. All of these factors must be considered as the clinician selects strategies and collaborates with the PWD and caregivers to establish goals. With that in mind, we begin with a discussion of the three main types of treatment strategies: compensatory, postural, and rehabilitative, as described in **Box 11.1**.

## 11.2 Compensatory, Postural, and Rehabilitative Strategies

### Box 11.1

**Types of Strategies**

- Compensatory—compensate for impaired function
- Postural—compensate for impaired function
- Rehabilitative—some can compensate for impaired function but they are intended to make lasting improvements in physiology

When one is developing a treatment plan for a PWD, it is helpful to think of four main types of strategies that can be used: compensatory, postural, rehabilitative, and diet/texture modifications. In most cases, the treatment plan will use a combination of these strategies.

## 11.2.1 Compensatory Strategies

Compensatory strategies are those designed to compensate for lost or impaired function. They are not designed to improve the impaired anatomy or physiology but to help the PWD have a more functional, effective, safe, and efficient swallow. Bolus modifications and some postural changes can be considered as subtypes of compensatory strategies, though this text describes these as distinct strategies. Compensatory strategies are effective only when in use, and immediate response to the compensation can be observed.

An example of a compensatory strategy might be applying external pressure to the impaired side of the lips if the PWD is losing liquids from the front of the mouth. Placing your fingers under the lower lip to help the individual close the lips on the rim of the cup may help the PWD take a sip without anterior loss. Another example might be to have the PWD who has a unilateral lingual weakness place the bolus of food into the oral cavity on the stronger side. This will help keep the bolus on the chewing surface where the PWD has more control. How a bolus is presented can also be considered compensatory. For example, some PWDs may handle a bolus of thin liquid more efficiently or safely when it is delivered from a cup instead of a straw. None of these compensatory strategies will have any impact on the actual function of the lips and tongue. They might, however, help the PWD eat and drink more efficiently and thus compensate for the impairment.

A physical therapy example might help solidify the concept of compensation. A person who has had a stroke might have permanently impaired neural pathways, resulting in the inability to lift the toes up when walking. To maintain safe and efficient ambulation, the physical therapist may have the patient wear a brace that holds the foot up to compensate for the patient's inability to control the foot. The brace serves as a compensatory strategy to enable the patient to return to day-to-day activities despite the long-term neural impairment.

Swallowing is a sensorimotor act. The sensory strategies that have been studied (e.g., taste changes, temperature changes) are compensatory in nature. These are used with the expectation that they will lead to changes in motor output, but if the changes in motor output are only temporary (e.g., improvement on that one swallow), then the strategy would appropriately be considered compensatory. The motor output may or may not involve a swallow. Data on sensory stimulation are insufficient to indicate that there is anything but a transient effect. Most sensory strategies involve changes in the bolus that is being presented (e.g., taste, temperature) and will be discussed in Chapter 12.

For individuals with apraxia of the swallow, a compensatory strategy is to allow the PWD to self-feed. It may be that the hand to mouth movement provides increased sensory input (and if long-term gains are achieved, it could be considered a rehabilitative strategy) or it may be that self-feeding is a more natural, automatic task and thus helps the PWD motor-plan for eating.

Some individuals, for example those with advanced dementia, can present with **agnosia**. It appears they do not recognize the bolus placed in their mouth as food; thus they simply hold the bolus in the oral cavity and do not begin to manipulate it. Sometimes increasing sensory input through downward pressure from the spoon, or bringing another spoonful of food to touch the lips, cues the individual to begin the manipulation or propulsion of the bolus.

## 11.2.2 Postural Changes

Postural changes generally have no effect that changes anatomy or physiological function of the swallow. In most cases, these postural changes are used to redirect bolus flow in the oral and/or pharyngeal phases. For example, the PWD with unilateral facial weakness or who has had surgical removal of one side of the tongue might tilt (not turn) the head toward the strong side, to keep the bolus on the side where it can be manipulated. Chin tuck is an example of a postural strategy applied for the pharyngeal phase. In some instances, chin tuck provides added airway protection as the bolus travels through the pharynx. As with compensatory strategies, no matter how often the postural change is applied, no change in function, and of course no change in anatomy, would be expected.

The use of postural changes in pediatrics, particularly those with overall impaired sensorimotor function, such as in cerebral palsy, are thought to achieve a somewhat different outcome than that described in the previous paragraph. For example, a child with cerebral palsy who has increased tone may exhibit jaw thrust or jaw retraction when trying to take a bite from a spoon. Placing the child in a prone position may result in better jaw control as compensation. However, if used consistently, it may help reduce tone so that a change in function is sustained even when the posture is not used.

Some postural changes used with infants and children, however, have only the same compensatory effect as that described in use with adults. An example of such a postural change might be placing an infant in a side-lying position to provide more stability. The infant's suck–swallow–breathe sequence might be more coordinated with longer sucking bursts because the infant feels more stable in this position. There is no evidence that use of this posture is actually facilitating physiological change. The posture can be used until the infant's physiological system matures enough to enable a safe suck–swallow–breathe pattern in an upright position.

An example of a postural change for physical therapy might be one applied to a person who experienced a back injury after a fall and who complains of pain when soft tissues of the spine are under stress from a prolonged slouched sitting position. The physical therapist might alleviate the pain by correcting the sitting posture with a roll placed behind the lower back and the person's feet planted on the floor. This postural correction will provide relief from the pain, but does it actually help with healing the injury? Likely it does not, but one might argue that sitting with a better posture might facilitate a better balance between the flexors and extensors in the back and aids in reducing the low back pain.

## 11.2.3 Rehabilitative Strategies

Rehabilitative strategies are techniques that are designed to, and in some cases have been demonstrated to, effectively change the physiology of the swallow, not just when the strategy is in use, but so that the swallow is more efficient and safe after a period of therapy. The effortful swallow, for example, has been shown to result in long-term clinical improvement in the swallow.[1,2] The effortful swallow is also a good example of a rehabilitative strategy that addresses more than one aspect of physiology. It has been shown to improve linguapalatal pressure, tongue base to pharyngeal wall pressure, **hyolaryngeal** excursion, and **submental** muscle activity.[3,4,5]

The strategies should target underlying physiological impairment identified during assessment. Strategies thought to be rehabilitative in nature should have evidence to support the claims of a change in physiology. However, there are many strategies that have some evidence of change with healthy individuals, but not with PWDs. Other strategies have evidence related to one population of PWDs but not another. Still others do not have empirical evidence to support their use, but they are used by clinicians because they are based on principles of **neural plasticity** or motor learning, theoretically make sense, and address physiological impairment. When this chapter describes the strategies, examples of available empirical evidence will be cited.

These strategies are typically used during a treatment session and not during meals, although some rehabilitation strategies can also be used as compensations. For example, the Mendelsohn maneuver can be used by a PWD on each swallow in order to sustain hyolaryngeal elevation, reducing piriform sinus residue and thus perhaps enabling a safe swallow. In this way, it is being used as compensation. However, studies have also shown that, in some populations, use of the Mendelsohn maneuver as a rehabilitative strategy results in an actual long-term improvement in hyolaryngeal excursion and an improved, functional swallow.[1,6]

Unlike postural and compensatory strategies, which can often be applied or used without the active participation of the PWD, rehabilitation strategies require that the PWD be able to understand, follow directions, and perform sometimes very complex actions. For example, the super-supraglottic swallow requires that the individual take a breath, let a little out, hold the breath tightly in the throat, swallow hard, breathe out, cough, and swallow again. There are certainly many children and adults for whom following such a multistep command might be far too challenging.

When selecting strategies that the PWD will be expected to use during meals, consider the impact that the use of the strategies will have on the PWD. Is it a strategy that requires careful attention to remember? Will the PWD remember to use it with every swallow? Does the strategy require physical effort (e.g., effortful swallow, super-supraglottic swallow) that might cause the PWD to fatigue? And if it requires too much effort, will the PWD not be able to finish the meal, thus compromising nutritional status because of the extra work required? Will the PWD be able to use the strategy consistently throughout the meal, or will cues be needed? If cues are needed, who will be able to provide these cues consistently?

## 11.2.4 Combining Strategies

The skilled clinician most often uses a combination of the different types of strategies when developing a treatment plan. Using the physical therapy model as an example, immediately after surgery (e.g., knee replacement), compensations such as the use of crutches along with postural changes (e.g., starting up the steps on the leg that did not have surgery, while starting down the steps on the leg that did) might be used. However, during the therapy sessions, the therapist might be conducting rehabilitative strengthening exercises. As the client improves, crutches may no longer be needed, and the types of exercises used in therapy might change in complexity and intensity.

Consider these three swallowing examples demonstrating the combination and timing of applying different strategy types.

### Example 1

An adult in the acute phase after a cerebrovascular accident has impaired oral and pharyngeal swallow and is having some difficulty following commands. The instrumental assessment of swallowing revealed that use of the postural strategy of head turn to the left improves the safety of the pharyngeal swallow. The compensatory strategy of the clinician placing fingers on the cheek on one side helps keep the bolus on the chewing surface of the stronger side. These strategies combine to enable the PWD to consume an altered diet safely. The PWD also needs to improve laryngeal elevation but, at this time, cannot follow directions to complete rehabilitation strategies such as the Mendelsohn maneuver, so initially the treatment plan is focused on the use of the postural and compensatory strategies to enable the PWD to eat safely until the PWD can more actively participate in treatment, or until spontaneous recovery results in improved pharyngeal function.

### Example 2

A 13-year-old with traumatic brain injury was unable to eat safely during the initial phases of recovery and was fed via **percutaneous endoscopic gastrostomy tube**. Then, at the rehabilitation hospital, instrumental assessment revealed impaired hyolaryngeal excursion, impaired tongue base, pharyngeal wall movement, and impaired timing of the pharyngeal response. However, the postural change of chin tuck and bolus modifications enabled safe consumption of a modified diet without any further compensation. At that point the adolescent was able to actively participate in treatment; a variety of specific rehabilitation strategies were used in treatment sessions and by the adolescent when practicing between sessions. After a period of time, a repeat instrumental assessment revealed significantly improved pharyngeal skills, and at that point the chin tuck was no longer needed, though some bolus modifications were still required. The diet was upgraded to a normal diet, and only a few remaining rehabilitation strategies were continued in treatment.

### Example 3

An 82-year-old woman with midstage dementia was having trouble chewing solids and clearing the oral cavity. She had no pharyngeal deficits. The initial treatment plan included bolus modifications and a compensatory strategy of using a second dry swallow as well as a sip of liquid after every few bites. A small sign with these cues was placed at the resident's table in the dining room. No rehabilitation strategies were recommended due to the progressive nature of the disease and the resident's inability to follow directions in treatment. As the disease progressed, she was no longer able to understand the written or picture cues; therefore the treatment plan was changed to manage the dysphagia solely with bolus modifications.

The percentage of each type of strategy to be used, the order in which to apply the strategies, and the determination of when to discontinue a strategy are related to factors such as age and development (in a child), the etiology of the impairment, the nature (e.g. acute, chronic, progressive) of the disorder, the cognitive abilities of the PWD, the setting in which the services are provided, and the support systems available to the PWD within the setting. Although matching strategies to the impaired anatomy and physiology is crucial, these other factors will also determine in large part how successful the treatment will be.

Specific compensatory, postural, and rehabilitation strategies are described in detail later in the chapter, and organized to help the reader relate a specific strategy to impaired physiology.

## 11.3 Principles to Consider When Planning Treatment

Swallowing involves a series of highly coordinated, volitional, and reflexive skilled sensorimotor movements in the mouth, larynx, and pharynx, as well as coordination between the respiratory and swallowing functions of the upper aerodigestive tract. The clinician must have an understanding of muscle function and should grasp many related principles in order to understand how **neuromuscular** treatment for swallowing might or might not work. When treatment techniques are supported by evidence, the evidence should help the clinician determine whether the technique will be beneficial. However, the clinician should also use the knowledge of these principles to understand why a particular exercise was attempted for that impaired physiology. When there is a lack of evidence, the clinician uses information about these related principles to determine whether a treatment strategy should work, or, put more simply, given what is known about swallow physiology, does the technique make sense? These related principles include such factors as motor control, motor learning, and neural plasticity, as described in **Box 11.2**. Regarding treatment of children, the relationship between neuromuscular rehabilitation and normal development must also be considered. Information from these areas of study can help inform the decisions the clinician makes when establishing a treatment plan. Consider these important questions, which will require such information to answer:

- Can the impaired physiology in a particular PWD actually be changed?
- Is there a possibility that an exercise could cause more harm than good?
- How frequently should the exercise be practiced?

- How many repetitions of the exercise are needed in order to obtain a benefit?
- Should the practice be spaced out or massed together?
- Are typically developing peers performing the skill you are trying to teach?
- At what point in recovery will dysphagia intervention be most beneficial?

### 11.3.1 Principles of Neural Plasticity

> **Box 11.2**
>
> **Principles of Neural Plasticity**
> - Use it or lose it.
> - Use it and improve it.
> - Specificity.
> - Repetition matters.
> - Intensity matters.
> - Time matters.
> - Salience matters.
> - Age matters.
> - Transference
> - Interference

Neural plasticity describes the brain's ability to change, to alter neuronal systems in response to changes in input.[7,8] When utilizing specific rehabilitation strategies for improved swallowing, the clinician intends to achieve not only a change in strength, speed, and coordination of specific muscle movements or sensorimotor responses, resulting in a behavioral change, but also a change in the underlying neural pathways that guide the movement. Martin (p. 219) points out the mounting evidence that "(1) swallowing neural substrates can undergo plastic changes as a function of experience, and (2) these swallowing neuroplastic changes may be associated with modulated swallowing behavior."[9]

Changes in behavior and neural pathways are not necessarily reciprocal. That is, although changes in neural pathways may result in a behavioral change, only sometimes does the behavioral change indicate that neural plasticity occurred.[10] For example, compensatory strategies do not intend to change the neural pathways but perhaps to use a different neural pathway to compensate for loss.

Robbins et al[10] describe 10 principles of neural plasticity and the relationship to rehabilitation strategies used in swallowing.[10,11] These principles, as related to swallowing, are being studied in some **translational research**, but definitive information is not known. However, the clinician would benefit from being mindful of these principles and concepts when developing a plan to manage the PWD's dysphagia.

- Use it or lose it—If a certain brain function is not used, then the behavioral response can degrade. If a PWD is fed nothing by mouth, using the swallowing mechanism only for swallowing saliva, does this disuse of the mechanism result in reduced cortical representation?[10]

- Use it and improve it—Function can be improved through use, especially if the activity involves not just practicing, but practicing designed to improve the performance of the activity. This would imply that repetitive swallowing alone might not result in a change, but that the practice should involve having the PWD work to change some aspect of the swallow, such as increased strength or coordination.

- Specificity—Plasticity is related to the specific skill being practiced. Practicing one skill will not necessarily result in a change to a different area of the brain.

Specificity indicates that the movement being trained should be close to the movement needed during the functional target task. For example, practicing bringing an empty spoon to the lips would not likely result in a more efficient liquid swallow from a cup. Clark demonstrated evidence of specificity for lingual strength training because training on an **isotonic exercise** endurance task did not increase endurance on an isometric exercise endurance task.[12]

- Repetition matters—In order to change neural substrates, practice must be extensive and continue for a period of time. What is not known is how many repetitions of an exercise should be performed or how long an **isometric exercise** position (e.g., the Mendelsohn maneuver) should be sustained.

- Intensity matters—In order to achieve neural change, practice must occur frequently enough and the activity must force the body beyond the typical level of activity in order to achieve neuromuscular adaptation.[13] Related to specific swallowing rehabilitation strategies, although we do not know how much is enough, Burkhead et al suggest we should focus on working to the point of fatigue rather than having the PWD perform a specific number of repetitions or sets.[14] When the term *intensity* is used related to sensory treatment, the meaning differs, and refers to the intensity of the sensory stimulus being applied.

- Time matters—Long periods of training and continuous training (rather than intermittent training) may result in maximal neural change.[15] The clinician must apply this concept at the right time during the PWD's treatment, perhaps using compensatory strategies in the earlier phases of recovery and waiting until the PWD can fully participate in therapy and benefit most from the use of rehabilitative strategies.

- Salience matters—The movement being practiced has to be important, functional, and related to the behavior being trained.[16,17] A single repetitive movement (e.g., tongue tip elevation) does not likely enhance skilled movement such as collecting a bolus on the tongue and moving it posteriorly in the oral cavity. If the clinician intends to change swallowing, then the exercises taught must be related to swallowing. Motor output that involves a swallow (e.g., effortful swallow) is more salient than motor output without a swallow (e.g., tongue press).

- Age matters—The younger brain is more adaptive and plastic, so that training in children, for example, is more likely to result in neural plasticity than training in an individual who is elderly. And younger children may be more likely to display neural changes than older children. Neural plasticity does occur across the life span, though the response decreases with age.[18,19]

- Transference—Plasticity in response to training one behavior can enhance acquisition of similar behaviors. Training tongue lateralization to clear the sulci might enhance acquisition of tongue lateralization to place food on the chewing surface.

- Interference—Plasticity within a given neural structure can impede that structure from other, more beneficial, plasticity. A PWD might learn a maladaptive compensation, which then might impede the use of the same neural circuitry to learn an appropriate behavior.

For more detailed information, readers are directed elsewhere.[20]

## 11.3.2 Principles of Motor Learning and Neuromuscular Treatments

Humbert and German provide insights into the importance of the relationship of motor control and motor learning to swallowing, while indicating that research in the field of dysphagia lags behind research in areas such as limb movement.[21] Several principles of motor learning are listed in **Box 11.3**.

### Box 11.3

**Principles of Motor Learning**
- Sensory feedback is necessary for learning and making corrections to movements.
- Swallowing uses top-down and bottom-up processing.
- Swallowing is reflexive and volitional.
- Feedback and feedforward loops are used for adapting movements.

Although we need a better understanding of the neurological control of swallowing and how it relates to specific movements and ways to improve those movements, cursory mention of several principles is included here to challenge the reader to consider this information as specific rehabilitation strategies are later described.

- Sensory feedback is important for learning a motor movement, predicting the accuracy of the movement, and making corrections to the movement.
- Swallowing involves both top-down (cortical control) and bottom-up (peripheral input to the cortex) processing.[22,23,24,25,26]
- Swallowing movements occur on a continuum of reflexive to volitional.[27]
- Motor learning involves both feedback and feedforward control loops as the individual adapts motor movements.[28,29]

In 2003, Clark[30] published a tutorial on neuromuscular treatments for speech and swallowing in which she described types of neuromuscular impairments and neuromuscular treatment, and then discussed why some neuromuscular treatments do or do not make sense when applied to the oral musculature. Much of the work on neuromuscular treatments is derived from the work of physical therapists, who work on large muscles in the limbs. Muscle fiber types in these large muscles often differ from the muscle fiber types found in the small muscles of the lips, tongue, cheek, and soft palate; therefore, the same types of treatments cannot be applied to the oral musculature to achieve the same results. For example, it is known that muscle weakness is seen in dysphagia,[31,32,33] but the impact of that weakness on a functional swallow has not been determined.[30]

Another difference in limb muscles and muscles of the oral mechanism is that, in the limb system, it is fairly easy to identify a single muscle group (e.g., biceps) and work just on that muscle. In the oral mechanism and pharynx, many muscle groups overlap in structure and function. In addition, there is less lateralization in function of the brain for oropharyngeal function compared to limb function.[34,35]

The possible consequences in failing to understand and apply knowledge of motor control and neuromuscular treatment appropriately could mean that the PWD does not benefit from the treatment. An even more serious consequence is that the PWD's swallowing might worsen as a result of the treatment applied. For example, strength training is a form of active exercise. Strength training can produce fatigue, and in a PWD who has a disease like amyotrophic lateral sclerosis, working to the point of fatigue might actually reduce strength reserves.[36] Strength training can also increase muscle tone, so if a strengthening exercise is used in someone with spasticity, tone might be further increased. Conversely, there are instances in which it is appropriate to use strengthening techniques. Oral phase dysphagia is more often seen in PWDs who have lingual weakness.[31,32,33]

When one is treating children with dysphagia, a more in-depth understanding of principles of neuromuscular treatment is indicated in order to make informed choices about appropriate treatment strategies for oral phase problems. Sheppard[37] provides an excellent summary of five basic treatment principles, described in **Box 11.4**, that are essential for successful habilitation or rehabilitation of functional motor tasks and the role of sensorimotor therapy in the treatment of dysphagia in children: (1) select therapy strategies to address specific neuromuscular impairments that were identified during assessment; (2) maintain optimum postural alignment and postural control to achieve the best results; (3) apply the therapy strategies prior to or during the functional task of eating, making the task more specific; (4) train developmental skills in the sequence in which they are acquired by typically developing children; and (5) increase task demands while reducing facilitation strategies to help the child generalize the skill.

---

## Box 11.4

**Treatment Principles for Teaching Motor Tasks to Children with Dysphagia**

1. Select therapy strategies to address the specific neuromuscular impairment.
2. Maintain optimal postural alignment and control.
3. The best practice for the task is natural eating practice (specificity).
4. Train developmental skills in the sequence in which they were typically acquired.
5. Increase demands as you reduce facilitations/cues.

---

## 11.4 Evidence Base for Treatment of Dysphagia

Research in dysphagia, particularly translational research, continues to provide more evidence for the use of specific treatment strategies, but the field has far to go to reach the point at which the clinician can confidently select well-supported strategies to treat dysphagia in all ages and populations. The American Speech-Language-Hearing Association's (ASHA's) National Center for Evidence-Based Practice in Communication Disorders produced a three-part, evidence-based systematic review of oropharyngeal dysphagia behavioral treatments.[38,39,40] Part I provides the background and methodology, Part II describes the impact of dysphagia treatment on normal swallow function, and Part III discusses the impact of dysphagia treatment on populations with neurologic disorders. A later publication discusses outcomes for PWDs post–cancer treatment.[41] This series of articles makes clear some of the challenges clinicians face when trying to determine whether a particular treatment strategy is appropriate for a particular client:

- Many studies are completed on individuals with a normal swallow. This makes it difficult, if not impossible, to translate the findings to individuals with swallowing deficits.
- Some techniques (e.g., effortful swallow) have been studied more than others.
- Many studies are in the exploratory stages of research and are not efficacy studies.
- When a study is completed on one population (e.g., stroke), the results cannot necessarily be generalized to another population (e.g., neurodegenerative disorder).
- The studies vary in subjects and methods of analyses and "have been conducted more for pre-experimental exploration rather than for substance, direction, and advancement of science" (p. 201).[41]

The results of these systematic reviews described the research supporting behavioral interventions of postures or maneuvers as "young and sparse and use of these interventions should be considered and weighed with other important aspects of clinical decisions, which include the expertise of the treating clinician and patient preferences" (p. 203).[40] Though this series of articles was published in 2009, the statement remains accurate. A 2010 review by Speyer et al[42] came to essentially the same conclusions.

Lack of evidence does not necessarily mean that a compensation, posture, or rehabilitation technique does not work. Rosenbek pointed out that dysphagia is not the only area where clinical practice moves more quickly than the science that supports practice.[43] However, when specific evidence is lacking, the clinician must use knowledge of anatomy and physiology, normal development, neuromuscular dysfunction, and the principles discussed earlier to decide whether a technique makes sense for a particular PWD at a specific point in the person's care.

### 11.4.1 Outcomes Data

Outcomes data can be used to inform answers to questions about the structure and timing of treatment. Outcomes data answers questions about the results of typical treatment rendered in typical situations. That is, there are no control groups or prescribed methodologies. Because of this lack of controls, one cannot conclude that the changes were the result of the treatment, but simply that the outcomes occurred during the time the treatment was given. Outcomes data can be a helpful adjunct to the efficacy data as the clinician develops a treatment plan.

Questions such as these can be answered using outcomes data:

- How often should treatment be given to achieve maximum gain?
- How long should the treatment sessions be?
- Is treatment more effective when provided one on one or in a group?

For each of those questions, more specific questions might be posed as to how the outcome would differ

- For PWDs with different diagnoses
- At different points in the continuum of care
- For PWDs of different age
- For PWDs whose dysphagia is more severe

ASHA has a National Outcomes Measurement System that collects data on adults and on children 3 to 5 years of age.[44]

## 11.5 Treatment for Different Phases of Swallowing

Treatment for problems in the phases of swallowing must be based on information obtained during the assessments performed, both clinical and instrumental. Treatment for the oral preparatory phases can be determined largely from the clinical assessment, whereas treatment for the oral, and certainly for the pharyngeal, phases are based almost solely on information obtained during instrumental assessment. The speech-language pathologist (SLP) has only a tangential role in the treatment of disorders of the esophageal phase. Although the SLP must understand the relationship between symptoms presented in the pharyngeal and esophageal phases, most intervention for esophageal disorders is medical or surgical in nature. The SLP is, however, often involved in counseling and educating PWDs in both the adult and pediatric populations regarding management of gastroesophageal and laryngopharyngeal reflux and their impact on swallowing and making appropriate referrals to medical specialists for management of the disorder.

In the pediatric population, children are often treated for disorders in the oral phases. These might be due to sensorimotor deficits or related to behaviorally based feeding problems, more accurately called Avoidant-Restrictive Feeding Disorder (ARFID). Infants and children can present with deficits in the pharyngeal phase, particularly children with cerebral palsy or significant delays in development of motor skills. A major challenge to treating pharyngeal disorders in pediatrics is that the age and cognitive level of the child often precludes the use of complex rehabilitation strategies and instead requires the use of postures, compensations, and bolus modifications. In addition to basing

treatment for oral and pharyngeal dysphagia in pediatrics on the evaluation results, the clinician must also compare the results to the typical sequence of development needed for a variety of skills, such as suckle; suck—swallow—breathe; lip closure for spoon and cup drinking; and jaw, lip, and tongue movements involved in biting and chewing.

In the adult population, the clinician presumes that the PWD had normal oral and pharyngeal skills before the onset of the dysphagia. Therefore, the clinician compares the PWD's current skills with those of an adult with normal swallowing when determining targets for treatment.

## 11.6 Categorizing the Different Treatment Strategies for the Oral Phases

This chapter describes each strategy as it relates to the physiological impairment it is designed to address. In the oral phases, the information is grouped by the part of the oral mechanism that is impaired (e.g., lips, jaw). In addition, each strategy is also described as compensatory, postural, or rehabilitative (note the C, P, and/or R after each strategy). There is no definitive evidence that any of these oral strategies are rehabilitative (resulting in long-term changes in physiology), but they are characterized as such if that is the intent. To highlight the sensorimotor nature of swallowing, compensatory strategies are then further described to indicate whether the strategy employs sensory input (S) and what kind of motor response is expected (M or MS). For example, lip strength training would be indicated with R/M, meaning it is intended to be rehabilitative and includes a motor response (but not a motor response with swallow). Head tilt is postural and thus marked with P. Placing the bolus on the stronger side would be compensatory but would also employ sensory input (C/S). **Box 11.5** lists the categories of treatment strategies. For the oral phases, the information is indicated in parentheses after each strategy.

### Box 11.5

**Categorizing the Treatment Strategies**

- P = postural
- C = compensatory
- R = rehabilitative
  - S = sensory
  - M = motor response expected
  - MS = motor response with swallow expected

### 11.6.1 Oral Phases—Treatment

Treatment for problems in the oral preparatory phase is designed to help the PWD get the bolus into the oral cavity, prepare it for transit to the back of the oral cavity, and place it on the midtongue, while preventing spillage over the back of the tongue or from the front of the mouth. In the oral (transit) phase, the PWD must propel a cohesive bolus from the midtongue to the back of the oral cavity and over the back of the tongue. This requires intact structures and coordinated movements of the lips, jaw, tongue, and soft palate. All three types of strategies (postural, compensatory, and rehabilitative) can be used to treat problems in the oral preparatory and oral (transit) phases. However, evidence is lacking as to the effectiveness of many rehabilitation exercises for oral motor movements, and many times the clinician relies on postural and compensatory strategies, as well as utilizing bolus modifications to address deficits in these phases.

An evidence-based systematic review of the effects of oral-motor exercises (OMEs) on swallowing in children examined four clinical questions about the effect of OMEs used with children on swallowing physiology, pulmonary health, functional swallowing outcomes, and drooling management. Mixed results were found, mostly due to the diversity of the populations studied and methodological weaknesses in the studies. There was insufficient evidence to determine the effects of OMEs on swallowing physiology. Results were also equivocal on the impact of OMEs on functional swallowing outcomes and on drooling management. There were no studies on the impact of OMEs on pulmonary health of children.[45]

Keeping in mind Rosenbek's[44] admonition that lack of evidence does not necessarily mean a treatment technique does not work, information is provided on commonly used postural, compensatory, and rehabilitative strategies used to address functional deficits in the oral phases of swallowing.

## Lips

The lips must close on a spoon, straw, or cup for efficient intake of the bolus and must remain closed to keep the bolus in the oral cavity during preparation and transport. Strengthening exercises used for reduced lip closure are generally not supported by any studies demonstrating a change in function as a result of exercise. Hägg and Anniko[46] found improved lip strength and swallowing capacity in patients with stroke after training with a device called a lip screen, whereas Shelton[47] saw no change in lip or cheek strength following 4 weeks of training with high-resistance straws. To measure the effectiveness of any of the following strategies by objectively measuring change in lip strength, the Iowa Oral Performance Instrument (IOPI)[48] could be used. If the bulb is placed between the lips, it can measure lip compression strength. What is not known is how an increase in lip strength impacts the functional movement of the lips for eating, drinking, and swallowing. Strategies for improved lip function include the following:

- Closing the lips around a Life Saver on a string while the clinician provides resistance by pulling on the string (R/M)
- Lip strength training using a device called an oral screen[46] (R/M)
- Puckering the lips and then retracting them in a smile (R/M)
- Puffing the cheeks and keeping the lips tightly closed, with the clinician providing resistance by lightly squeezing on the cheeks (R/M)
- Sucking from straws of increasingly smaller diameters, designed to increase resistance[49] (R/MS)

- Using form and texture on a series of spoonlike shapes to place in the oral cavity to improve accuracy and strength of lip movements[50] (R/M)
- Providing external support to the weak side of the lips by placing fingers on the lower and/or upper lip while taking a bite from a spoon or drinking from a cup or through a straw (C/S)

## Jaw

Horizontal, vertical, and rotary jaw movements are necessary for effective biting and chewing solid boluses. The jaw interacts with tongue movements with solids and when liquids are swallowed.[51] Therefore, the clinician should consider this interaction when identifying deficits in bolus manipulation and selecting treatment strategies. Exercises for the jaw tend to be used in the pediatric population much more than with adults. Although there are numerous devices on the market that purport to increase jaw strength, and subsequently improve chewing, there is no reported evidence on outcomes with use of these devices. Several studies have been done on the use of chewing gum to strengthen the jaw. Tzakis et al[52] had healthy adults chew high-resistance chewing gum and found no long-term benefit; in fact they found an immediate decrease in chewing efficiency. However, Kiliaridis et al[53] found an increase in the functional capacity of the masticatory muscles and their strength in healthy adults after chewing the extra-hard chewing gum.

The following are some strategies for jaw weakness:

- Opening the jaw against resistance provided by the clinician placing a hand under the jaw (R/M)
- Closing the jaw against resistance provided by the clinician holding the jaw open with a hand on the chin (R/M)
- Providing support under the jaw to reduce the range of jaw opening and provide stability (C/S)

## Cheeks

If the cheeks have normal tone, they remain tight against the gums, keeping the bolus from falling into the lateral sulci. Some of the exercises used for the lips (e.g., puffing the cheeks, puckering and retracting) use muscles in the cheeks as well as in the lips. These exercises are also not generally supported in the literature. For example, Clark et al[54] found no change in cheek strength in healthy adults following 9 weeks of training with the IOPI. However, most strategies to address reduced tone in the cheeks are compensatory or postural in nature:

- Pucker and retract the lips (as in an exaggerated "oo" "ee") (R/M)
- Provide external pressure to the cheek to reduce pocketing (C/S)
- Place the bolus of food on the stronger side (C/S)
- Clean the buccal cavity periodically during a meal with the tongue (or finger) (C)
- Rinse and clear the oral cavity after eating (C)
- Tilt the head toward the stronger cheek to keep the bolus on that side for manipulation (P)

## Soft Palate

The soft palate is generally against the back of the tongue during the oral phases to help maintain the bolus in the oral cavity, though there is some cyclic motion of the soft palate during chewing.[55] During the pharyngeal phase, the soft palate elevates to seal the nasopharynx off tightly and prevent nasal backflow during the swallow. Tight closure of the nasopharynx presumably helps create pharyngeal pressure to aid bolus flow. Although movement of the soft palate is more integral in the pharyngeal phase, the soft palate is discussed here because it is typically considered as part of the oral musculature. There are no studies of exercises for improved velopharyngeal closure for swallowing, nor are there any postures or compensations that might reduce nasal backflow.

## Tongue

The tongue is very active in the oral preparatory and oral (transit) phases. The tongue lateralizes to place a bolus on the lateral chewing surfaces and then returns the bolus to midline. The tongue tip elevates to the alveolar ridge and the lateral borders of the tongue seal with the teeth or gums to maintain the bolus on the tongue. The back of the tongue remains elevated to keep the bolus from falling prematurely into the hypopharynx. The entire tongue, in a coordinated anterior-posterior movement, propels the bolus into the hypopharynx to begin the pharyngeal phase. (The base of the tongue plays an important role in the pharyngeal phase, helping to propel the bolus through the hypopharynx. This will be discussed in the pharyngeal phase section.)

Rehabilitative strategies for the tongue have been more extensively studied than those for the other parts of the oral musculature, and evidence continues to emerge demonstrating positive effects from strengthening exercises for the tongue. Unfortunately, with few exceptions, most of these studies were performed with adults. More recent studies have demonstrated that some exercises of the tongue have also resulted in improvements in certain aspects of the pharyngeal phase of the swallow, and those results will be mentioned in that section. Lingual strengthening is the subject of much recent research. Many of these strength studies have demonstrated increased tongue strength, whereas others have demonstrated increased lingual volume, improved swallowing pressures in healthy aging,[56] increased swallowing pressures, and reduced airway invasion,[57] as well as improved bolus control and functional dietary intake.[58]

When using tongue strength as a measure of improvement from a lingual strengthening exercise program, subjective measures may not be adequate. Clark et al[31] found that inexperienced and experienced raters judged tongue strength differently, and that correlations to specific functional aspects of the oral swallow differed between these rater groups. Several devices allow for objective measures of tongue strength. IOPI[48] measures the strength of the tongue by measuring the maximum pressure that an individual can produce on a disposable standard-sized tongue bulb by pressing the bulb against the roof of the mouth with the tongue. The peak pressure achieved is displayed on a screen. The SwallowSTRONG Device (Swallow Solutions)[59] also measures maximum tongue pressures, but instead of a bulb it uses a custom-molded mouthpiece with four separate sensors at the front and back of the hard palate and either side of the hard palate. It is a newer model of a device called the Madison Oral Strengthening Therapeutic (MOST) device (Swallow Solutions).[60] These devices can also be used as a biofeedback device during therapy.

Other "devices" have been suggested for improving lingual function, though the evidence is either nonexistent or not compelling. For examples, Ora-Light (Kapitex Healthcare) is a series of spoonlike shapes designed to provide tactile proprioceptive feedback to achieve accurate tongue placement and increase strength.[50] No research is available on the outcomes with use of the device. High-resistance straws by TheraSip[49] are suggested for improving tongue strength and increasing effort of the swallow. Shelton[48] demonstrated that with healthy adults training with the high-resistance straws improved only effortful sips and did not improve sipping strength. In a small series of case studies, Yeates et al[58] demonstrated that, in addition to training tongue strength, training accuracy may be important as well. They measured accuracy as the subject's ability to get close to the amplitude target using the IOPI.

Robbins et al studied a small group of subjects with stroke, acute and chronic. All subjects significantly increased isometric and swallowing pressures after an 8-week training program using the IOPI. Airway invasion was reduced for liquids. Two subjects increased lingual volume.[57] These studies demonstrate the principles of intensity and specificity.

Sensory strategies have not typically been employed to elicit changes in the tongue, but Pelletier and Dhanaraj[61] found that moderately sweet and high-intensity sour and salty concentrations yielded higher lingual swallowing pressures. However, Miyaoka et al found no changes in swallowing by healthy volunteers as a result of altering taste.[62]

It is difficult to draw specific training protocols from these studies because many used healthy subjects, almost all were performed with adults, and the training regimens differed (e.g., number of days/week; lingual targets). However, it generally appears that the tongue responds to strength training and that functional improvements in the oral and pharyngeal phases of the swallow can result.

Rehabilitative, compensatory, and postural strategies for reduced/impaired tongue movement include the following:

- Press the tongue tip out or up against a tongue depressor for increased strength for protrusion or elevation (R/M)
- Sweep the tip of the tongue from front to back along the hard palate (R/M)
- Push the blade of the tongue up against a tongue depressor for increased strength for bolus propulsion (R/M)
- Lateralize the tip of the tongue to the corner of the lips or either buccal cavity or cheek; for the latter, provide resistance by placing fingers on the cheek and pushing against the tongue (R/M)
- Push the lateral border of the tongue against a tongue depressor for increased strength for lateralization (R/M)
- Push the back of the tongue up against a tongue depressor (R/M)
- Forcefully produce words ending in /k/ (R/M)
- Use graduated straws for increased tongue strength (R/MS)

- Use the form and texture of a series of spoonlike shapes placed in the oral cavity to improve accuracy and strength of tongue movements with the Ora-Light[50] (R/M)
- Place a bolus of food on the stronger side (C/S)
- Tilt the head toward the stronger side if the tongue cannot lateralize food to the chewing surface (P)
- Use multiple swallows to clear the oral cavity (C)
- Provide sensory input to the tongue with downward pressure of the spoon when placing a bolus on the tongue (C/S)
- If the PWD won't open the mouth, touch a spoon of food to the lips to help initiate tongue movement of the bolus already in the oral cavity (C/S)
- Use the chin down/chin tuck position to keep the bolus from spilling prematurely over the back of the tongue (P)
- Tip the chin up to facilitate movement of the bolus to the back of the oral cavity (use this technique only if an instrumental examination has determined this posture will not compromise the airway; this head-extended position could send the bolus on a direct route to the airway. In addition, this position alters the coordination of pressures in the pharynx and pharyngoesophageal segment, perhaps exacerbating pharyngeal problems)[63] (P)
- Take a sip of liquid periodically to clear any residue (sometimes called a liquid wash) (C)

## 11.7 Categorizing the Different Treatment Strategies for the Pharyngeal Phase

Swallowing in the pharyngeal phase must be both safe and efficient. A safe swallow is one in which the bolus does not enter the airway. An efficient swallow is one in which the bolus is effectively cleared from the pharynx. Treatment of deficits in the pharyngeal phase comprises techniques to address timing of movements as well as effectiveness of these movements for airway protection and bolus clearance.

**Table 11.1** provides information on the pharyngeal strategies discussed and categorizes each as compensatory, postural, and/or rehabilitative. The rehabilitative strategies are further delineated as motor without swallow or motor with swallow. Motor output with a swallow is more salient. The table also indicates whether a device is used. If the rehabilitative strategy (e.g., supersupraglottic swallow) can also be used during intake of food, with the intent to improve each swallow, then the compensatory column is checked in addition to the rehabilitative column. Keep in mind that many of the strategies checked as rehabilitative may have minimal or no significant evidence to support that they are actually rehabilitative. If a compensatory strategy relies heavily on sensory input, an S is placed in the column along with the X. Furthermore, the strategies are marked to indicate the impaired physiology they are intended to address. For example, the Mendelsohn maneuver is marked as addressing timing, anterior and superior movement of the hyolaryngeal complex, and pharyngeal wall movement.

In the early years of dysphagia management, the phases of the swallow were viewed as distinct, with no overlap; when one phase ended, the next began. More recent investigations of the swallow have demonstrated that the phases do overlap and are well integrated.[64] There is increasing understanding of the relationship between the oral (transit) phase and the pharyngeal phase, with a recognition that the movement of the tongue initiates the pharyngeal phase. Some studies summarized earlier regarding effects of lingual exercise demonstrated how improved tongue strength resulted in a change in pharyngeal swallowing physiology.[57]

The pharyngeal phase is composed of intricately coordinated movements of the tongue, soft palate, pharyngeal walls, laryngeal muscles and cartilages, and muscles of the upper esophageal sphincter. These movements might be grouped into two main safety and efficiency functions that must occur in the pharyngeal phase: (1) airway closure for protection of the airway before and during the swallow and (2) efficient movement of structures for clearance of the bolus, which allows protection of the airway after the swallow (**Box 11.6**).

Airway closure can be affected by problems in timing and coordination of movements or by impairments in the actual movements. And of course, either can be affected by surgical changes in the structures of the mouth, pharynx, or larynx. Timing and coordination impairments affecting airway closure in the pharyngeal phase include the following:

- Delayed initiation of the pharyngeal response (with the bolus too low in the hypopharynx before closure occurs, also described as increased stage transition duration
- Mistiming of the pharyngeal response (such that closure does not occur at the correct time during bolus movement, but the bolus does not dwell long enough in the pharynx to be considered a delay)

Movement impairments that impact airway closure can include the following:

- Poor back-of-tongue control (which can allow the bolus to enter the airway prematurely)
- Reduced closure at the level of the arytenoids and vocal folds (which may result in aspiration during the swallow)
- Reduced closure at the entrance to the airway (reduced tipping of the arytenoids and the epiglottis, leaving the laryngeal vestibule exposed)
- Reduced hyolaryngeal excursion
  - Reduced hyolaryngeal elevation/superior movement (which results in lower position of the larynx before and during the swallow, allowing penetration and/or aspiration)
  - Reduced hyolaryngeal anterior movement (which also leaves the airway exposed)

Efficient movements of structures for bolus clearance, some of which are important for efficiently moving the bolus through the pharynx so there is no postswallow residue to compromise the airway, include the following:

- Reduced hyolaryngeal excursion
  - Reduced hyolaryngeal elevation/superior movement (which can contribute to residue in the piriform sinuses and somewhat to residue in the vallecula)
  - Reduced hyolaryngeal anterior movement (which can contribute to residue in piriform sinuses)

**Table 11.1** Compensatory, postural and rehabilitative strategies for pharyngeal phase

| Strategy | Compensatory (S = added sensory) | Postural | Rehabilitative | | | Can be used to address this impaired physiology | | | | | | | |
|---|---|---|---|---|---|---|---|---|---|---|---|---|---|
| | | | Motor without a swallow | Motor with a swallow | Device | Timing | Back of tongue | Closure airway vocal folds/arytenoids | Closure airway entrance | Anterior hyolaryngeal complex | Superior hyolaryngeal complex | Tongue base pressure | Pharyngeal wall pressure |
| Thermal-tactile application | X/S | | | | | X | | | | | | | |
| Taste changes | X/S | | | | | X | | | | | | | |
| Carbonated beverages | X/S | | | | | X | | | | | | | |
| Temperature changes | X/S | | | | | X | | | | | | | |
| Smaller bolus/other bolus modifications | X | | | | | X | X | X | X | X | X | X | X |
| Liquid wash | X | | | | | | | | | X | X | X | X |
| Utensil change | X | | | | | X | X | | | | | | |
| Chin tuck | | X | | | | X | X | X | X | | | | |
| Supraglottic | X | | | X | | X | | X | | | | | |
| Supraglottic with sEMG | X | | | X | X | X | | X | | | | | |
| Super-supraglottic | X | | | X | | X | | X | X | | X | | |
| Mendelsohn maneuver | X | | | X | | X | | | | X | X | | X |
| Mendelsohn maneuver with sEMG | X | | | X | X | X | | | | X | X | | X |
| Effortful swallow | X | | | X | | X | | | | X | X | X | X |
| Effortful swallow with sEMG | X | | | X | X | X | | | | X | X | X | X |
| Preparatory tasks | X/S | | | X | | X | X | | | | | | |
| Head rotation | | X | | | | | | X | | X | X | | |
| Valsalva maneuver/breath hold | | | X | | | | | X | X | | | | |
| Multiple swallows | X | | | | | | | | | X | X | X | X |
| Effortful pitch glide | | | X | | | | | | | X | X | | X |
| Head lift | | | X | | | | | | | X | X | | |
| Tongue press | | | X | | | | | | | X | X | | |
| Tongue retraction against resistance | | | X | | | | | | | | | X | |
| Pretend to gargle | | | X | | | | | | | | | X | X |
| Pretend to yawn | | | X | | | | | | | | | X | X |
| Tongue hold (Masako) | | | | X | | | | | | | | | X |
| EMST | | | X | | X | | | | | X | X | | |
| Chin tuck/jaw opening against resistance | | | X | | X | | | | | X | X | | |
| NMES | | | | X | X | | | | | X | X | | |

*Abbreviations:* EMST, Expiratory Muscle Strength Trainer; NMES, neuromuscular electrical stimulation; sEMG, surface electromyography.

- Reduced tongue base pressure against the pharyngeal walls (which can result in residue in the vallecula and/or on the pharyngeal walls)
- Reduced pressure of the pharyngeal walls (which can result in residue in the vallecula and on the pharyngeal walls)

---

## Box 11.6

**Safety and Efficiency Functions in the Pharyngeal Phase**

- Airway closure (Safety)
  - Timing and coordination (See **11.7.1**)
    - Delay (increased stage transition duration)
    - Mistiming
  - Movement for closure at all levels (See **11.7.2**)
    - Back-of-tongue control
    - Closure at the level of the vocal folds
    - Closure at the entrance to the airway
    - Reduced hyolaryngeal excursion
      - Superior
      - Anterior
- Movement of structures for bolus clearance (Efficiency) (See **11.7.3**)
  - Reduced hyolaryngeal excursion
    - Superior
    - Anterior
  - Reduced tongue base pressure
  - Reduced pharyngeal wall pressure

---

Rehabilitative strategies in the pharyngeal phase often address more than one physiological problem. For example, the super-supraglottic swallow addresses airway closure, timing of closure, and movement.[65,66] The effortful swallow has been found to affect movement, timing, duration, bolus flow, and pressures.[4,5,67,68,69] Postural and compensatory strategies can also have an impact on more than one physiological and functional problem. For example, the chin tuck posture can compensate for reduced excursion of the **hyolaryngeal complex** as well as for impaired timing of closure. Multiple swallows can compensate for reduced movement of a variety of structures. Sometimes two postural strategies are used, such as head rotation (also called head turn) with chin tuck. The clinician should be selecting techniques to treat impaired physiology, not based on a sign or symptom. For example, the clinician may observe residue in the piriform sinuses and wonder what strategies are designed to prevent or eliminate the residue. Instead, the clinician should understand what impaired physiology has resulted in residue in the piriform sinuses and treat that physiology. In order to keep the focus on the impaired physiology and not on a sign or symptom, the description of strategies (compensatory, postural, and rehabilitative) to use in the pharyngeal phase will be categorized under the impaired physiology they are intended to address.

When a strategy addresses more than one aspect of physiology, it will be mentioned briefly again in subsequent sections. As a strategy is described, some examples of the evidence to support its use are included. It is beyond the scope of this chapter to list all related evidence for a particular strategy. Many of the studies cited here were completed with healthy adults. When they were done with a particular group of PWDs, one cannot necessarily generalize the findings to other groups. At times, underlying principles (e.g., neural plasticity, motor learning) will be mentioned to encourage the reader to continue to think about the rehabilitation strategies in that way. Because different PWDs respond in different ways to a particular strategy, clinicians are encouraged to try different strategies for the pharyngeal phase during the instrumental exam to determine their effectiveness, how easily the PWD can perform the strategy, and what effect use of the strategy might have on the functional swallow during meals.

For more detailed information on how to perform the strategies, other clinician resources contain directions for the PWD with pictures of some of the strategies.[70,71] The National Foundation on Swallowing Disorders, a consumer advocacy group, has video of how some of the exercises are performed on their website.[72]

## 11.7.1 Airway Closure—Timing and Coordination Impairments

Airway closure occurs not just at the level of the true vocal folds. Complete airway closure is achieved through coordinated movements that must be precisely timed.

### Delayed Pharyngeal Response or Mistiming of Movements for Closure

Several sensory strategies, which are paired with a motor response with a swallow, have been investigated to see whether the initiation of the swallow response will become more timely. *Thermal tactile application* (originally called thermal tactile stimulation) was first described by Logemann[73] to reduce the delay in the initiation of the pharyngeal response. Subsequent studies have only inconsistently found that the use of thermal application reduces swallow delay, and then only temporarily.[74,75,76,77] That is, the gains do not hold after the therapy session is over. Several studies have looked at the combination of cold and taste or of cold, taste, and touch but also found that the results were only temporary, reducing delay on only the stimulated swallows.[78,79] Therefore, the strategy is probably best considered compensatory.

Altering *taste* alone (not with temperature) has been explored by several investigators. Logemann et al found that a bolus that was 50% barium and 50% lemon juice used in PWDs of neurogenic nature resulted in changes in the swallow.[80] For all patients, faster oral onset was observed, whereas in patients with stroke, decreased pharyngeal delay was seen, and in patients with other neurogenic disorders there was reduced aspiration frequency.

Another aspect of sensory stimulation that has been explored is the use of *carbonated beverages*. Sdravou et al[81] found that carbonated thickened liquids decreased penetration and aspiration on 5 mL boluses during instrumental exams. Presenting a smaller bolus can sometimes compensate for an issue with timing of the pharyngeal response, not because it changes the timing but because the bolus is then small enough to rest in the vallecula (or sometimes even in the piriform sinuses) during the delay and not spill into the airway. Results vary among individuals depending on the size of these pharyngeal spaces.

The *chin tuck* posture (previously mentioned in the section on the tongue) is also used to compensate for impairments in timing. This posture helps maintain the bolus in the oral cavity until the PWD is ready to attempt the swallow. In some PWDs, this posture also widens the vallecula and provides a space for the bolus to pause during the delay in the initiation of the pharyngeal response.[73] The position also serves to position the epiglottis over the entrance to the airway in some PWDs, providing added protection. Several studies found that chin tuck eliminated aspiration.[82,83] Chin tuck was also one of the strategies studied in Protocol 201, a large, randomized trial,[84] and was found to be less effective in eliminating aspiration than thickened liquids in the patients with dementia with or without Parkinson's disease. These are temporary anatomical changes, which, in some studies, resulted in a safer swallow by reducing or eliminating aspiration, but there is no evidence that any permanent physiological changes occur.

Other compensatory strategies can be tried to help the PWD protect the airway during the mistiming or delay. Controlling the size of the bolus and presenting the bolus with a different utensil (e.g., a spoon instead of a cup) can compensate for impaired timing.

The *supraglottic* and *super-supraglottic* swallow strategies are completed by having the PWD take a breath, let a little out, hold the breath, swallow, and then cough/swallow again. The cough is designed to clear any residue from the airway. The difference in the super-supraglottic swallow is to ask the PWD to do this with as much force as possible. Although originally intended to improve closure, these strategies were also found to have some impact on timing, with earlier and longer laryngeal closure, higher position of the hyoid bone at swallow onset,[66] longer pharyngoesophageal segment (PES) opening and a longer duration of hyolaryngeal complex movement in healthy volunteers.[65] Also, in healthy volunteers, Miller and Watkin[85] also reported longer duration of pharyngeal wall movement. There are no studies documenting long-term improvement with these techniques.

The *Mendelsohn maneuver* occurs at the height of the swallow. That is, the PWD is told to swallow and, when the larynx is at its highest point in the throat, to push the tongue forcefully against the roof of the mouth to keep the hyolaryngeal complex in that elevated position. The maneuver was also originally targeted for another change in physiology (prolong and hold the hyolaryngeal excursion),[86] but Lazarus et al[87] also found an impact on timing in a single subject. In healthy volunteers, the *effortful swallow* showed preswallow elevation of the hyoid, which would affect the timing.[68]

Several other techniques, *preparatory tasks*, have been used to alert the system to be ready to swallow. These are based on the understanding of how the nervous system works. When a person anticipates a physical action, such as preparing to hit a golf ball, the neurons that control the task adopt a state of readiness. *Three-second prep* is completed by telling the PWD that the clinician will count to three and then say "swallow." The PWD is asked to think about getting ready to swallow during the count. The *suck–swallow gesture* accomplishes the same thing, but asks the PWD to pretend to suck as if on a straw for a few seconds and then swallow. Still another strategy uses the *suck–swallow with added sensory input*. The finger of a glove is filled with crushed ice (and the glove tied off so no liquid escapes), and the PWD is asked to suck on the finger of the glove for a few seconds before swallowing.[70] Langmore[88] uses a *three-step swallow* in which the PWD is told to (1) hold the bolus in the mouth and not let any spill into the throat, (2) hold the breath, and (3) swallow it all at once. She trains PWDs to perform this maneuver using endoscopy.

It seems logical that strategies such as supraglottic, Mendelsohn, and these preparatory tasks could help improve overall coordination and timing of the events of the swallow. The PWD is being asked to exert some cortical control of these movements by thinking about the steps of the movement, thus using more of the top-down principle of motor learning. In addition, the principle of using sensory feedback to improve performance of an action is at play in these step-by-step swallowing techniques.

## 11.7.2 Airway Closure—Movement Impairments That Impact Airway Protection Before and During the Swallow

Even if the movements are timed in a coordinated fashion, they may not be adequate to provide airway protection. That is, the movements of different structures may be reduced or inaccurate.

### Poor Back-of-Tongue Control

If the PWD has poor back-of-tongue control, the bolus may fall over the back of the tongue prematurely and enter the airway. The *chin tuck* maneuver changes the position of the larynx and thereby improves closure of the laryngeal vestibule,[89] narrows the oropharynx,[90] and reduces the distance between the hyoid bone and larynx.[68] In some patients it widens the vallecular space. The strategy is used for PWDs who have poor back-of-tongue control for two reasons. It may help patients maintain control of the bolus in the oral cavity until they are ready to begin the pharyngeal phase, in which case it is actually a strategy for the oral phase but has a direct impact on the safety of the pharyngeal phase. In those patients for whom the vallecular space is widened, if the bolus is lost over the back of the tongue, it can pause in the vallecula while the pharyngeal response is initiated rather than falling directly into the airway. Several studies have revealed a difference in how the posture is actually performed (e.g., chin tight against chest vs. leaning head forward) and of the terms *tuck* and *down* used interchangeably.[91,92] The instructions used in most studies are for the PWD to tuck the chin tightly against the chest.

As a compensatory strategy, presenting a *smaller bolus* is sometimes helpful. The PWD may be able to keep the smaller bolus from falling over the back of the tongue. Sometimes a change in the *utensil* used to present the bolus can help the PWD maintain control of the bolus in the oral cavity. For example, some patients do better with sips from a cup rather than a straw or with small amounts of liquid from a spoon rather than a cup. Oral exercises for the back of the tongue were described in the oral phase.

### Reduced Closure at the Level of the Vocal Folds

The supraglottic swallow appears to close the larynx at the level of the vocal folds.[23,93,94] Thus the supraglottic swallow might be useful in addressing aspiration during the swallow, if closing the vocal folds would prevent the aspiration. The super-supraglottic swallow would accomplish not only closure of the vocal folds but also tight closure above the level of the folds. Some clinicians have taken one of the steps, *breath hold* (sometimes called Valsalva) of the supraglottic and used it in isolation as a rehabilitative strategy. That is, they have the PWD practice a tight breath hold without an accompanying swallow.[94] The breath hold is part of the swallowing movement and thus could be considered specific. This might be a helpful first step if the PWD is having trouble learning how to perform the full maneuver. However, to increase salience of the action, include all the steps with the swallow.

*Head rotation* (also called *head turn*) is typically used with PWDs who have a unilateral pharyngeal weakness.[95,96] Turning the head to the weaker side serves to narrow the pharynx by closing off the lateral channel and piriform sinus on that side. This sends the bolus down the presumably stronger side of the pharynx, which can propel it with more force and result in less residue. It should also bring the stronger vocal fold closer to the weaker one (a technique used in voice therapy for unilateral vocal fold weakness) and help achieve closure at the level of the vocal folds. *Bolus modifications* (e.g., thickeners, bolus size) may also be used to compensate for decreased closure at the level of the vocal folds.

## Reduced Closure at the Entrance to the Airway

Closure at the entrance to the airway serves to keep the bolus from penetrating the upper laryngeal vestibule, which then might be aspirated during or after the swallow. The super-supraglottic maneuver[94] adds effort to the supraglottic maneuver, which results in the anterior tipping of the arytenoids and subsequent folding in of the aryepiglottic folds to fill the vestibule. So while the supraglottic seems indicated for aspiration during the swallow due to reduced closure of the vocal folds, the super-supraglottic might afford protection against penetration and aspiration before and/or during the swallow by closing the laryngeal vestibule.

The chin tuck maneuver may also compensate for reduced closure at the entrance to the airway by changing the position of the larynx so the entrance to the airway is more protected, reducing penetration or aspiration before the swallow. The position should be tried during the instrumental study; Ra et al[91] found that the posture was successful for less than 20% of the subjects who aspirated. The compensatory strategies of other bolus modifications or texture change (see Chapter 9) can also be tried.

## Reduced Hyolaryngeal Complex Excursion (Reduced Hyolaryngeal Elevation/Superior Movement and Reduced Hyolaryngeal Anterior Movement)

Hyolaryngeal elevation (superior) and forward movement (anterior) are grouped together since the upward and forward movement typically occurs as one fluid movement. These movements bring the complex into a safer position so that the airway is protected. There are instances when a PWD will have adequate elevation but reduced anterior movement, but the strategies that address one typically address the other.

The Mendelsohn maneuver maintains the hyolaryngeal complex in the elevated and forward position. Some studies have shown that the PES remains open longer,[86] that the lateral walls maintain the squeeze longer,[85] and that there are increased pharyngeal peak contractions[24] as well as increased effort and duration of the submental muscle group.[97] Picture a trash can that has a pedal you step on to open the lid. A typical swallow might be compared to a quick step on the pedal, with quick opening/closing of the lid with little time to toss in the trash. If the trash can had an opening at the bottom, that would be the PES of the trash can. A swallow utilizing the Mendelsohn maneuver would have the pedal held down and the lid remain open, offering plenty of time to throw in the trash. The Mendelsohn essentially keeps the "lid" (the hyolaryngeal complex) up and forward as well as the PES open for a longer period of time. This protects the airway while reducing piriform sinus residue because the bolus has more time to make its way through the PES.

The maneuver can be used in a compensatory way during meals to reduce the residue that might then be aspirated,[5,87] but the clinician must remember the fatiguing effect this might have on the PWD. Several studies have reported long-term functional gains (thus rehabilitative) with the use of the technique.[87,98] To help PWDs learn to perform the maneuver and improve their swallow, several studies report the use of *surface electromyography (sEMG)* as a biofeedback tool. Crary used a technique similar to the Mendelsohn maneuver that he called sustained pharyngeal contraction with patients with chronic dysphagia in an intensive therapy program to get them back to eating by mouth.[1,6] Huckabee and colleagues also experienced success in using the technique with sEMG.[5]

The *effortful swallow* has also been shown to modify hyoid bone movement and increase the activation of the submental muscle group when compared with a normal swallow task.[4,6,97] This increased movement of the submental muscles should then improve anterior and superior movement of the hyolaryngeal complex. sEMG has also been used with the effortful swallow.[6]

Clinicians have used a technique called *falsetto* for years, hypothesizing that the elevation of the larynx for falsetto was similar to the elevation during swallowing.[70] A recent study with healthy adults demonstrated the similarity between what they call *effortful pitch glide* and these movements for swallowing: anterior hyoid, hyolaryngeal approximation, laryngeal elevation, and lateral pharyngeal wall medialization. Only superior hyoid movement was greater during swallowing. This initial study supports that, theoretically, this technique might work to improve the movements for swallowing.[99]

The *head lift (Shaker)* exercise is rehabilitative only. That is, it cannot be used during swallowing. There is both an isometric (sustained) and isotonic (repetitive lifts) portion to the exercise. It is designed to increase the superior and anterior movement of the hyolaryngeal complex by strengthening the suprahyoid[100,101] (and probably the infrahyoid)[102,103] muscles. This heightened up and forward motion of the hyolaryngeal complex then pulls open the PES, which would help to reduce residue, especially in the piriform sinuses.

Another exercise, *tongue press*, was studied by Yoshida et al in healthy adults who were asked to push the tongue hard against the palate and maintain that position. The sustained posture (isometric) yielded higher muscle activity in the submental muscles.[104] Presumably, this would yield better elevation and anterior movement of the hyolaryngeal complex.

Sapienza and colleagues have conducted many studies on the use of a pressure threshold resistance device called the *Expiratory Muscle Strength Trainer* (EMST150, Aspire, LLC).[105,106,107] The device requires that the PWD blow against a preset level of resistance in order to open the spring-loaded valve.[108] This forceful blowing increases the activity of the submental muscles, resulting in an increase in hyolaryngeal excursion. It uses the principles of intensity, repetition, and time because it utilizes a training regimen with multiple repetitions over many treatment sessions and requires the muscles to work harder than they usually do. The use of this rehabilitative strategy has been demonstrated to reduce penetration and aspiration in PWD with Parkinson's disease.[109] An interesting related finding is that it increases the strength of the cough, an important protective function.

Research in dysphagia treatment often presents new strategies or modifications of currently used strategies. An example of that is *chin tuck against resistance (CTAR)*, designed by Yoon et al[110] in which the patient presses the chin down against a small ball held between the chin and the chest. The initial study revealed an increase in submental muscle activity with the use of CTAR in healthy adults. Kraaijenga et al[111] conducted a feasibility study with healthy adults on CTAR, a related strategy called *jaw opening against resistance (JOAR)* and using a *swallow exercise aid* to practice both of those movements, each of which included isometric and isotonic components. The results indicate healthy adults could increase muscle strength and volume by using the exercise aid.

The tongue press, CTAR, JOAR, and/or use of EMST might be good alternatives for improving hyolaryngeal excursion when the PWD cannot complete the head lift maneuver. The head lift maneuver can be difficult for PWDs who have problems with their neck, cannot lie flat, or fatigue easily.

The super-supraglottic swallow might help with laryngeal elevation because it has been observed to result in a higher position of the hyoid bone at the onset of the swallow and overall increased hyoid movement during the swallow.[66]

### 11.7.3 Movement Impairments That Affect Efficient Flow of Bolus for Clearance

The movements just described are needed for a safe swallow. Impaired movements also have an impact on the efficiency of the swallow.

### Reduced Hyolaryngeal Excursion

Hyolaryngeal excursion (upward and forward movement) is important not only for airway protection but also for helping the bolus move efficiently through the pharynx. Lacking adequate movement, the PWD is often left with residue in the pharynx, particularly in the piriform sinuses. It is logical, then, that some of the strategies described in the previous section to address impaired movements related to airway protection before and during the swallow also address impaired movements that impact the PWD's ability to clear the bolus from the hypopharynx efficiently and completely. This is important so that no residue remains that might fall into the airway and be aspirated after the swallow. When the hyolaryngeal complex moves up and forward as it should, it opens the PES, which allows the bolus to flow more freely into the esophagus. Thus there is no residue to put the PWD at risk for aspiration of the residue after the swallow. The rehabilitative strategies for reduced hyolaryngeal excursion (elevation and anterior movement) (e.g., Mendelsohn maneuver, head lift, effortful swallow) and the compensatory strategies (e.g., multiple swallows, liquid wash) should be considered if the PWD has difficulty clearing the bolus through the pharynx (**Table 11.1**).

### Reduced Tongue Base and Pharyngeal Walls Pressure

The driving force to propel the bolus through the hypopharynx comes from the posterior movement of the tongue base and the forward and inward movement of the pharyngeal walls. As these structures come together, they exert force on the bolus. If enough force is generated (and the movements of the hyolaryngeal complex are adequate), the bolus moves through the hypopharynx and into the esophagus with no residue. When these driving forces are reduced, residue can remain in the vallecula, on the pharyngeal walls, and in the piriform sinuses, and there is then a risk that the material will be aspirated after the swallow.

The *effortful swallow* occurs when the PWD swallows with increased force, or effort. Recent studies have indicated that the instruction to patients should have them focus on pushing hard with the tongue.[112,113] This results in increased pressures not only with the tongue to the hard palate but also in the pharynx. Though there are some studies with PWDs,[4,69] as in the research on many techniques the effortful swallow has mostly been conducted with healthy volunteers. However, clinicians can use this information, paired with understanding of physiology and principles of motor movement and learning, to apply the technique to PWDs. The technique does help to clear residue in the laryngopharynx, particularly from the vallecula, when used in a compensatory fashion during meals. Regarding long-term gains (rehabilitative), Crary[1] and Carnaby-Mann and Crary[2] reported significant clinical improvements when using sEMG with the technique.

To specifically address tongue base movement, two strategies have been described: *tongue retraction against resistance* and *tongue hold*. The tongue-hold maneuver, sometimes called the *Masako*,[114] was discovered in PWDs who had had surgical anchoring of the tongue, and thus the tongue base could not move posteriorly to meet the pharyngeal walls. It was noted that the posterior wall began to bulge, as if in an effort to make up the distance between the wall and the tongue base. The exercise was then developed whereby the PWD who had not had surgery artificially anchored the tongue by biting on the tip of the tongue and keeping the tongue in that position during the swallow. Obviously the maneuver is completed only on saliva swallows because the anchored position of the tongue leaves the airway vulnerable. Lazarus et al demonstrated increased contact pressure between the base of the tongue and pharyngeal walls in a small number of subjects.[4] As is so characteristic of research on treatment methods in dysphagia, later research by Doeltgen et al provided more information that requires careful thought about when to use the technique.[115] That study showed conflicting results (lower peak pressures), potential other benefits (possible increased activity of extrinsic tongue muscles), possible negative side effects (increased pharyngeal constrictor strength may have negative implications for hyoid anterior movement, so the maneuver may potentially be contraindicated for individuals with generally decreased anterior hyoid movement), and the need for more information on all aspects of physiological change with use of the maneuver (e.g., what are the lateral pharyngeal walls doing?).

*Tongue retraction against resistance* involves the clinician holding the tip of the tongue with a gauze pad while the PWD pulls the back and base of the tongue posteriorly toward the back wall of the throat and sustains this position for several seconds (an isotonic movement). No studies exist to support this strategy, but Veis et al[116] did investigate tongue retraction without resistance.

Veis et al explored the effects of three different maneuvers on maximum retraction of the tongue base: *tongue pull-back, yawn, gargle*.[116] The gargle task was the most successful in eliciting most tongue base retraction for the group of subjects, although not in every subject. Gargle also resulted in greater tongue base movement than swallow more often than the other two voluntary tasks. The authors suggest that, if the PWD needs to improve posterior movement of the tongue base, each maneuver be tried under videofluoroscopy to determine which is most effective for that person.

The effect of *head rotation (head turn)* is increased opening of the PES[96] as well as the increased swallowing pressures on the side toward which the head is turned and keeping the PES open longer.[117] So this strategy could be applied for PWDs who do not clear the bolus well due to reduced movements in the pharynx that result in residue, particularly in the piriform sinuses. The head rotation should be tried during the instrumental exam to determine whether benefit will be gained. Logemann also indicated that, inexplicably, it sometimes helps to turn the head toward the unaffected side. This is also worth testing during the instrumental exam. Compensations to help clear residue might include multiple swallows, bolus size and texture changes, and, if found to be safe on instrumental exam, liquid wash to help clear residue.

## 11.8 Evaluating New Strategies

*Neuromuscular electrical stimulation (NMES)*, commonly called e-stim or neuromuscular e-stim, has been used by physical therapists for years but was first described as a treatment for pharyngeal dysphagia in 1996, by Freed et al, who introduced and described a method of NMES with electrodes applied to the front of the neck to improve swallowing.[118] The intent is to improve contraction of muscles in the pharynx in PWDs who have intact peripheral nerves. A full discussion of NMES is beyond the scope of the chapter, and because research continues to be conducted into the technique's application, information summarized here may become quickly outdated. This should be considered an introductory overview of the technique, which involves placement of electrodes on the neck, through which an electrical stimulation is provided at different levels of intensity. NMES is not the same as sEMG. The latter is measuring electrical activity in a muscle, whereas NMES is supplying electrical stimulation to the muscle.

Some studies have shown functional improvement in swallowing ability,[2,118,119,120,121,122,123,124] whereas others have shown no significant difference when comparing therapy with and without the use of NMES.[125,126] The most consistent criticism of the studies showing benefit is that no controls were used and that the benefits gained may have been a result of the intensive training schedule (often completed at least daily with multiple swallows per session). The training schedule typically followed the principles of use it and improve it, repetition matters, intensity matters, time matters, and salience matters. Until these factors are controlled for in well-designed studies, a fully informed conclusion about the effectiveness of the technique cannot be made.

Clinicians choosing to apply the technique should have a complete understanding of the anatomy of the neck because the surface placement of the electrodes necessitates the electrical signal travel through layers of muscles (some of which pull the hyoid down) before reaching the intended target muscle (e.g., thyrohyoid) to pull the hyoid up. In fact, Humbert et al reported laryngeal and hyoid descent at rest and reduced hyolaryngeal elevation during swallowing with NMES in healthy adults.[127] Could this mean that using the technique on PWDs who already have airway protection issues due to reduced hyolaryngeal movement would put them more at risk? As a result of another study, Ludlow et al[128] suggested that, for PWDs who have at least some ability to elevate the hyoid, the lowering caused by the electrical stimulation might actually serve as providing resistance for the hyolaryngeal complex, perhaps serving an important role in strengthening these muscles.

An excellent article by Humbert and colleagues[129] provides background information about the use of electrical stimulation, implications when applying the treatment for swallowing, and a discussion of limitations of the current studies that have been done using the modality. A thoughtful point–counterpoint article on the pros and cons of using electrical stimulation was published in 2012 and provides food for thought for the reader.[130]

## 11.9 Questions

1. This chapter describes three types of strategies that can be used to manage dysphagia: compensatory, postural, and rehabilitative. The clinician is explaining the use of these different types of strategies to the family of a person with dysphagia (PWD). Which of the following best describes the correct application of these strategies?

A. Compensatory strategies are always used with a PWD before trying postural strategies.

B. Any combination of the three types of strategies can be used at any point in the course of treatment. There are many factors that a clinician must consider when selecting which types of strategies will be appropriate for a particular PWD.

C. Compensatory and postural strategies can be used together, but rehabilitative strategies should not be used with those strategies.

D. All three types of strategies are used with every PWD.

E. Patients who cannot perform any rehabilitative strategies will not be able to perform compensatory strategies either.

2. A clinician is establishing a schedule for a PWD to practice rehabilitation strategies at home between therapy sessions. In order to use the principle of intensity, and not violate other principles of neural plasticity, which instruction should the clinician provide?

A. Schedule practice sessions for swallowing three or four times each day and complete two or three effortful swallows each time.

B. Use the effortful swallow on the first sip of liquid at each of your three meals/day.

C. To improve your ability to keep liquids in your mouth, practice blowing bubbles for 2 minutes each day.

D. Complete the effortful swallow technique enough times in each session that you feel like you can't possibly complete one more.

E. Practice the effortful swallow by doing two effortful swallows during a morning and an afternoon practice session for 3 days.

3. An adolescent who has suffered a head injury has anterior loss of liquids from the left side of his lips and is unable to close his lips on a spoon. When food is placed in his mouth, he has a hard time keeping it on his tongue, and residue is formed in his left cheek. Which combination of postural and compensatory strategies might be recommended to help him eat more efficiently?

A. Head tilt to the right with external pressure to the left side of the lips and left cheek

B. Head tilt to the left with external pressure on the left cheek

C. Head tilt to the right and chin tuck

D. Head rotation to the left with food placed on the left

E. Placing food onto the right side and having the patient practice pushing the lateral borders of the tongue against a tongue depressor between meals.

4. A videofluoroscopic swallow study (VFSS) is completed on a PWD and reveals reduced hyolaryngeal excursion with significant residue of all consistencies in the piriform sinuses bilaterally. This residue is then aspirated after the swallow. Which combination of rehabilitative strategies might be indicated to work on improved excursion?

A. Mendelsohn maneuver and chin tuck

B. Supraglottic and effortful swallow

C. Mendelsohn maneuver, head lift, and effortful pitch glide

D. Pretend to gargle and pretend to yawn

E. Tongue hold, supraglottic swallow, and breath hold

5. You attend a seminar that describes a new rehabilitative strategy to address pharyngeal dysphagia. There is no published evidence yet on this new strategy. What is a reasonable action for a clinician to take when determining whether to use the new technique?

A. Refuse to use the technique because it has no evidence.

B. Use it if one of your colleagues tells you she tried it on one patient and it worked.

C. Try it on each of the PWDs in your current caseload and see what results you get.

D. Use it if the technique is easy to teach because what is the harm in that?

E. Use it if it makes theoretical sense and if what it is intended to improve matches the need your PWD has.

## 11.10 Answers and Explanations

**1. Correct: Any combination of the three types of strategies can be used at any point in the course of treatment. There are many factors that a clinician must consider when selecting which types of strategies will be appropriate for a particular PWD (B).**
(A) Decisions need to be made based on the individual PWD's needs and abilities. For some PWDs, postural strategies might be the first (or only) thing used. (C) Rehabilitative strategies can be used with any of the other strategy types. (D) Some PWDs are not able to perform the rehabilitative strategies and so might only use compensatory or postural strategies. Still other PWDs might need only one type of strategy. (E) Some compensatory strategies (e.g., using a specific type of utensil) don't require the PWD to "perform" anything.

**2. Correct: Complete the effortful swallow technique enough times in each session that you feel like you can't possibly complete one more (D).**
The principle of intensity indicates you should work the body part past the point of typical activity. (A) These instructions violate the principle of repetition. Although we don't know how many is enough, two or three surely aren't enough. (B) This would not push the body part past the point of typical activity. (C) There is no intensity specified; in addition, this exercise violates the principle of specificity because rounding the lips and blowing are not parts of drinking.

**3. Correct: Head tilt to the right with external pressure to the left side of the lips and left cheek (A).**
Tilting the head to the right keeps the food on the strong side, and using external pressure on the lips will help prevent anterior loss, whereas pressure on the cheek on the weak side may lead to reduced residue pocketing on that side. (B) You don't want to tilt the head to the weak side, though pressure on the cheek might be helpful. (C) Head tilt to this side is appropriate, but a chin tuck is likely to cause more anterior loss. (D) Head rotation is effective to address pharyngeal residue, but it does not impact residue in the oral cavity. (E) It is a good idea to put food on the right side, but pushing on a tongue depressor is not compensatory.

**4. Correct: Mendelsohn maneuver, head lift, and effortful pitch glide (C).**
Each of these strategies works on superior and anterior movement of the hyolaryngeal complex. (A) The Mendelsohn maneuver is a good strategy, but the chin tuck is postural (not rehabilitative) and would not help with aspiration after the swallow. (B) The supraglottic swallow might help with closure and timing, but not elevation. The effortful swallow

would address excursion. (**D**) These address the tongue base and pharyngeal wall squeeze which would be used to reduce vallecular residue rather than piriform residue. (**E**) The tongue hold addresses pharyngeal wall movement, whereas the supraglottic swallow addresses timing and airway closure and breath hold addresses airway closure.

5. **Correct: Use if it makes theoretical sense and what it is intended to improve matches the need your PWD has (E).** The clinician should use an understanding of related principles (e.g., neural plasticity, motor learning) and match the technique to the impaired physiology. (**A**) Rosenbek states that a lack of evidence does not mean a technique doesn't work. Many strategies have been initiated before solid evidence exists to support their use. (**B**) This is anecdotal evidence only. Your colleague's patient might not be anything like yours. (**C**) Applying a strategy without consideration for what specific physiological deficit each PWD has is not good treatment planning. (**D**) Some techniques might actually cause harm, and the PWD may learn a maladaptive compensation (e.g., interference).

# References

[1] Crary MA. A direct intervention program for chronic neurogenic dysphagia secondary to brainstem stroke. *Dysphagia* 1995;10(1):6–18

[2] Carnaby-Mann GD, Crary MA. Adjunctive neuromuscular electrical stimulation for treatment-refractory dysphagia. *Ann Otol Rhinol Laryngol* 2008;117(4):279–287

[3] Hind JA, Nicosia MA, Roecker EB, Carnes ML, Robbins J. Comparison of effortful and noneffortful swallows in healthy middle-aged and older adults. *Arch Phys Med Rehabil* 2001;82(12):1661–1665

[4] Lazarus C, Logemann JA, Song CW, Rademaker AW, Kahrilas PJ. Effects of voluntary maneuvers on tongue base function for swallowing. *Folia Phoniatr Logop* 2002;54(4):171–176

[5] Huckabee M-L, Butler SG, Barclay M, Jit S. Submental surface electromyographic measurement and pharyngeal pressures during normal and effortful swallowing. *Arch Phys Med Rehabil* 2005;86(11):2144–2149

[6] Crary MA, Carnaby Mann GD, Groher ME, Helseth E. Functional benefits of dysphagia therapy using adjunctive sEMG biofeedback. *Dysphagia* 2004;19(3):160–164

[7] Buonomano DV, Merzenich MM. Cortical plasticity: from synapses to maps. *Annu Rev Neurosci* 1998;21(1):149–186

[8] Cohen LG, Ziemann U, Chen R, et al. Studies of neuroplasticity with transcranial magnetic stimulation. *J Clin Neurophysiol* 1998;15(4):305–324

[9] Martin RE. Neuroplasticity and swallowing. *Dysphagia* 2009;24(2):218–229

[10] Robbins J, Butler SG, Daniels SK, et al. Swallowing and dysphagia rehabilitation: translating principles of neural plasticity into clinically oriented evidence. *J Speech Lang Hear Res* 2008;51(1):S276–S300

[11] Kleim JA, Jones TA. Principles of experience-dependent neural plasticity: implications for rehabilitation after brain damage. *J Speech Lang Hear Res* 2008;51(1):S225–S239

[12] Clark HM. Specificity of training in the lingual musculature. *J Speech Lang Hear Res* 2012;55(2):657–667

[13] Pollock M, Gaesser G, Butcher J, et al. American College of Sports Medicine Position Stand. The recommended quantity and quality of exercise for developing and maintaining cardiorespiratory and muscular fitness, and flexibility in healthy adults. *Med Sci Sports Exerc* 1998;30(6):975–991

[14] Burkhead LM, Sapienza CM, Rosenbek JC. Strength-training exercise in dysphagia rehabilitation: principles, procedures, and directions for future research. *Dysphagia* 2007;22(3):251–265

[15] Fisher BE, Sullivan KJ. Activity-dependent factors affecting poststroke functional outcomes. *Top Stroke Rehabil* 2001;8(3):31–44

[16] Morgen K, Kadom N, Sawaki L, et al. Training-dependent plasticity in patients with multiple sclerosis. *Brain* 2004;127(Pt 11):2506–2517

[17] Remple MS, Bruneau RM, VandenBerg PM, Goertzen C, Kleim JA. Sensitivity of cortical movement representations to motor experience: evidence that skill learning but not strength training induces cortical reorganization. *Behav Brain Res* 2001;123(2):133–141

[18] Kramer AF, Bherer L, Colcombe SJ, Dong W, Greenough WT. Environmental influences on cognitive and brain plasticity during aging. *J Gerontol A Biol Sci Med Sci* 2004;59(9):M940–M957

[19] Sawaki L, Yaseen Z, Kopylev L, Cohen LG. Age-dependent changes in the ability to encode a novel elementary motor memory. *Ann Neurol* 2003;53(4):521–524

[20] Gonzalez Rothi LJ, Musson N, Rosenbek JC, Sapienza CM. Neuroplasticity and rehabilitation research for speech, language, and swallowing disorders. *J Speech Lang Hear Res* 2008;51(1):S222–S224

[21] Humbert IA, German RZ. New directions for understanding neural control in swallowing: the potential and promise of motor learning. *Dysphagia* 2013;28(1):1–10

[22] Martin BJ, Logemann JA, Shaker R, Dodds WJ. Normal laryngeal valving patterns during three breath-hold maneuvers: a pilot investigation. *Dysphagia* 1993;8(1):11–20

[23] Bodén K, Hallgren A, Witt Hedström H. Effects of three different swallow maneuvers analyzed by videomanometry. *Acta Radiol* 2006;47(7):628–633

[24] Kern MK, Jaradeh S, Arndorfer RC, Shaker R. Cerebral cortical representation of reflexive and volitional swallowing in humans. *Am J Physiol Gastrointest Liver Physiol* 2001;280(3):G354–G360

[25] Babaei A, Kern M, Antonik S, et al. Enhancing effects of flavored nutritive stimuli on cortical swallowing network activity. *Am J Physiol Gastrointest Liver Physiol* 2010;299(2):G422–G429

[26] Humbert IA, Joel S. Tactile, gustatory, and visual biofeedback stimuli modulate neural substrates of deglutition. *Neuroimage* 2012;59(2):1485–1490

[27] Ertekin C. Voluntary versus spontaneous swallowing in man. *Dysphagia* 2011;26(2):183–192

[28] Latash ML. Neurophysiological Basis of Movement. 2d ed. Champaign, IL: Human Kinetics; 2008

[29] Shadmehr R, Mussa-Ivaldi FA. Adaptive representation of dynamics during learning of a motor task. *J Neurosci* 1994;14(5 Pt 2):3208–3224

[30] Clark HM. Neuromuscular treatments for speech and swallowing: a tutorial. *Am J Speech Lang Pathol* 2003;12(4):400–415

[31] Clark HM, Henson PA, Barber WD, Stierwalt JA, Sherrill M. Relationships among subjective and objective measures of tongue strength and oral phase swallowing impairments. *Am J Speech Lang Pathol* 2003;12(1):40–50

[32] Stierwalt JA, Youmans SR. Tongue measures in individuals with normal and impaired swallowing. *Am J Speech Lang Pathol* 2007;16(2):148–156

[33] Yoshida M, Kikutani T, Tsuga K, Utanohara Y, Hayashi R, Akagawa Y. Decreased tongue pressure reflects symptom of dysphagia. *Dysphagia* 2006;21(1):61–65

[34] Love RJ, Hagerman EL, Taimi EG. Speech performance, dysphagia and oral reflexes in cerebral palsy. *J Speech Hear Disord* 1980;45(1):59–75

[35] Miller AJ, Bowman JP. Precentral cortical modulation of mastication and swallowing. *J Dent Res* 1977;56(10):1154–1154

[36] Yorkston KM, Miller RM, Strand EA. Management of Speech and Swallowing in Degenerative Diseases. Tucson, AZ: Communication Skill Builders; 1995

[37] Sheppard JJ. Using motor learning approaches for treating swallowing and feeding disorders: a review. *Lang Speech Hear Serv Sch* 2008;39(2):227–236

[38] Frymark T, Schooling T, Mullen R, et al. Evidence-based systematic review: Oropharyngeal dysphagia behavioral treatments. Part I--background and methodology. *J Rehabil Res Dev* 2009;46(2):175–183

[39] Wheeler-Hegland K, Ashford J, Frymark T, et al. Evidence-based systematic review: Oropharyngeal dysphagia behavioral treatments. Part II—impact of dysphagia treatment on normal swallow function. *J Rehabil Res Dev* 2009;46(2):185–194

[40] Ashford J, McCabe D, Wheeler-Hegland K, et al. Evidence-based systematic review: Oropharyngeal dysphagia behavioral treatments. Part III—impact of dysphagia treatments on populations with neurological disorders. *J Rehabil Res Dev* 2009;46(2):195–204

[41] McCabe D, Ashford J, Wheeler-Hegland K, et al. Evidence-based systematic review: Oropharyngeal dysphagia behavioral treatments. Part IV—impact of dysphagia treatment on individuals' postcancer treatments. *J Rehabil Res Dev* 2009;46(2):205–214

[42] Speyer R, Baijens L, Heijnen M, Zwijnenberg I. Effects of therapy in oropharyngeal dysphagia by speech and language therapists: a systematic review. *Dysphagia* 2010;25(1):40–65

[43] Rosenbek JC. Efficacy in dysphagia. *Dysphagia* 1995;10(4):263–267

[44] American Speech-Language-Hearing Association. http://www.asha.org/NOMS/. National Outcomes Measurement System.

[45] Arvedson J, Clark H, Lazarus C, Schooling T, Frymark T. The effects of oral-motor exercises on swallowing in children: an evidence-based systematic review. *Dev Med Child Neurol* 2010;*52*(11):1000–1013

[46] Hägg M, Anniko M. Lip muscle training in stroke patients with dysphagia. *Acta Otolaryngol* 2008;*128*(9):1027–1033

[47] Shelton NL. Resistance Straws and the Effortful Swallow Technique, Appalachian State University; 2011

[48] IOPI Medical. http://www.iopimedical.com/

[49] Therasip Swallowing Treatment. http://www.therasip.com/

[50] Ora-Light. Kapitex. http://www.kapitex.com/dysphagia/therapy/ora-light

[51] Steele CM, Van Lieshout PH. The dynamics of lingual-mandibular coordination during liquid swallowing. *Dysphagia* 2008;*23*(1):33–46

[52] Tzakis MG, Kiliaridis S, Carlsson GE. Effect of chewing training on masticatory efficiency. *Acta Odontol Scand* 1989;*47*(6):355–360

[53] Kiliaridis S, Tzakis MG, Carlsson GE. Effects of fatigue and chewing training on maximal bite force and endurance. *Am J Orthod Dentofacial Orthop* 1995;*107*(4):372–378

[54] Clark HM, O'Brien K, Calleja A, Corrie SN. Effects of directional exercise on lingual strength. *J Speech Lang Hear Res* 2009;*52*(4):1034–1047

[55] Matsuo K et al. Cyclic motion of the soft palate in feeding. *JDR* 2005; *84*(1): 39–42

[56] Robbins J, Gangnon RE, Theis SM, Kays SA, Hewitt AL, Hind JA. The effects of lingual exercise on swallowing in older adults. *J Am Geriatr Soc* 2005;*53*(9):1483–1489

[57] Robbins J, Kays SA, Gangnon RE, et al. The effects of lingual exercise in stroke patients with dysphagia. *Arch Phys Med Rehabil* 2007;*88*(2):150–158

[58] Yeates EM, Molfenter SM, Steele CM. Improvements in tongue strength and pressure-generation precision following a tongue-pressure training protocol in older individuals with dysphagia: three case reports. *Clin Interv Aging* 2008;*3*(4):735–747

[59] SwallowSTRONG Device. Swallow Solutions. http://www.swallowsolutions.com/product-information/swallowstrong-device

[60] Juan J, Hind J, Jones C, McCulloch T, Gangnon R, Robbins J. Case study: application of isometric progressive resistance oropharyngeal therapy using the Madison Oral Strengthening Therapeutic device. *Top Stroke Rehabil* 2013;*20*(5):450–470 doi: 10.1310/tsr2005-1450

[61] Pelletier CA, Dhanaraj GE. The effect of taste and palatability on lingual swallowing pressure. *Dysphagia* 2006;*21*(2):121–128

[62] Miyaoka Y, Haishima K, Takagi M, Haishima H, Asari J, Yamada Y. Influences of thermal and gustatory characteristics on sensory and motor aspects of swallowing. *Dysphagia* 2006;*21*(1):38–48

[63] Castell JA, Castell DO, Schultz AR, Georgeson S. Effect of head position on the dynamics of the upper esophageal sphincter and pharynx. *Dysphagia* 1993;*8*(1):1–6

[64] Dozier TS, Brodsky MB, Michel Y, Walters BC Jr, Martin-Harris B. Coordination of swallowing and respiration in normal sequential cup swallows. *Laryngoscope* 2006;*116*(8):1489–1493

[65] Ohmae Y, Logemann JA, Kaiser P, Hanson DG, Kahrilas PJ. Effects of two breath-holding maneuvers on oropharyngeal swallow. *Ann Otol Rhinol Laryngol* 1996;*105*(2):123–131

[66] Logemann JA, Pauloski BR, Rademaker AW, Colangelo LA. Super-supraglottic swallow in irradiated head and neck cancer patients. *Head Neck* 1997;*19*(6):535–540

[67] Hiss SG, Huckabee ML. Timing of pharyngeal and upper esophageal sphincter pressures as a function of normal and effortful swallowing in young healthy adults. *Dysphagia* 2005;*20*(2):149–156

[68] Bülow M, Olsson R, Ekberg O. Videomanometric analysis of supraglottic swallow, effortful swallow, and chin tuck in healthy volunteers. *Dysphagia* 1999;*14*(2):67–72

[69] Bülow M, Olsson R, Ekberg O. Supraglottic swallow, effortful swallow, and chin tuck did not alter hypopharyngeal intrabolus pressure in patients with pharyngeal dysfunction. *Dysphagia* 2002;*17*(3):197–201

[70] Swigert NB. The source for dysphagia. Austin, TX: LinguiSystems; 1996, 2000, 2007, 2019

[71] Greenslade W. A beginning list of dysphagia exercises that have evidence base. https://medicalspeechpathology.wordpress.com/swallowing/dysphagia-exercises

[72] National Foundation of Swallowing Disorders. https://swallowingdisorderfoundation.com/

[73] Logemann JA, Evaluation and Treatment of Swallowing Disorders. Evanston, IL: Northwestern University Press; 1983

[74] de Lama Lazzara G, Lazarus C, Logemann JA. Impact of thermal stimulation on the triggering of the swallowing reflex. *Dysphagia* 1986;*1*(2):73–77

[75] Rosenbek JC, Robbins J, Fishback B, Levine RL. Effects of thermal application on dysphagia after stroke. *J Speech Hear Res* 1991;*34*(6):1257–1268

[76] Rosenbek JC, Roecker EB, Wood JL, Robbins J. Thermal application reduces the duration of stage transition in dysphagia after stroke. *Dysphagia* 1996;*11*(4):225–233

[77] Rosenbek JC, Robbins J, Willford WO, et al. Comparing treatment intensities of tactile-thermal application. *Dysphagia* 1998;*13*(1):1–9

[78] Kaatzke-McDonald MN, Post E, Davis PJ. The effects of cold, touch, and chemical stimulation of the anterior faucial pillar on human swallowing. *Dysphagia* 1996;*11*(3):198–206

[79] Sciortino K, Liss JM, Case JL, Gerritsen KG, Katz RC. Effects of mechanical, cold, gustatory, and combined stimulation to the human anterior faucial pillars. *Dysphagia* 2003;*18*(1):16–26

[80] Logemann JA, Pauloski BR, Colangelo L, Lazarus C, Fujiu M, Kahrilas PJ. Effects of a sour bolus on oropharyngeal swallowing measures in patients with neurogenic dysphagia. *J Speech Hear Res* 1995;*38*(3):556–563

[81] Sdravou K, Walshe M, Dagdilelis L. Effects of carbonated liquids on oropharyngeal swallowing measures in people with neurogenic dysphagia. *Dysphagia* 2012;*27*(2):240–250

[82] Rasley A, Logemann JA, Kahrilas PJ, Rademaker AW, Pauloski BR, Dodds WJ. Prevention of barium aspiration during videofluoroscopic swallowing studies: value of change in posture. *AJR Am J Roentgenol* 1993;*160*(5):1005–1009

[83] Lewin JS, Hebert TM, Putnam JB Jr, DuBrow RA. Experience with the chin tuck maneuver in postesophagectomy aspirators. *Dysphagia* 2001;*16*(3):216–219

[84] Logemann JA, Gensler G, Robbins J, et al. A randomized study of three interventions for aspiration of thin liquids in patients with dementia or Parkinson's disease. *J Speech Lang Hear Res* 2008;*51*(1):173–183

[85] Miller JL, Watkin KL. Lateral pharyngeal wall motion during swallowing using real time ultrasound. *Dysphagia* 1997;*12*(3):125–132

[86] Kahrilas PJ, Logemann JA, Krugler C, Flanagan E. Volitional augmentation of upper esophageal sphincter opening during swallowing. *Am J Physiol* 1991;*260*(3 Pt 1):G450–G456

[87] Lazarus C, Logemann JA, Gibbons P. Effects of maneuvers on swallowing function in a dysphagic oral cancer patient. *Head Neck* 1993;*15*(5):419–424

[88] Langmore S. Endoscopic Evaluation and Treatment of Swallowing Disorders. New York, NY: Thieme; 2011

[89] Ekberg O. Posture of the head and pharyngeal swallowing. *Acta Radiol Diagn (Stockh)* 1986;*27*(6):691–696

[90] Welch MV, Logemann JA, Rademaker AW, Kahrilas PJ. Changes in pharyngeal dimensions effected by chin tuck. *Arch Phys Med Rehabil* 1993;*74*(2):178–181

[91] Ra JY, Hyun JK, Ko KR, Lee SJ. Chin tuck for prevention of aspiration: effectiveness and appropriate posture. *Dysphagia* 2014;*29*(5):603–609

[92] Hung D, Sejdić E, Steele CM, Chau T. Extraction of average neck flexion angle during swallowing in neutral and chin-tuck positions. *Biomed Eng Online* 2009;*8*(1):25

[93] Mendelsohn MS, Martin RE. Airway protection during breath-holding. *Ann Otol Rhinol Laryngol* 1993;*102*(12):941–944

[94] Donzelli J, Brady S. The effects of breath-holding on vocal fold adduction: implications for safe swallowing. *Arch Otolaryngol Head Neck Surg* 2004;*130*(2):208–210

[95] Kirchner JA. Pharyngeal and esophageal dysfunction: the diagnosis. *Minn Med* 1967;*50*(6):921–924

[96] Logemann JA, Kahrilas PJ, Kobara M, Vakil NB. The benefit of head rotation on pharyngoesophageal dysphagia. *Arch Phys Med Rehabil* 1989;*70*(10):767–771

[97] Ding R, Larson CR, Logemann JA, Rademaker AW. Surface electromyographic and electroglottographic studies in normal subjects under two swallow conditions: normal and during the Mendelsohn manuever. *Dysphagia* 2002;*17*(1):1–12

[98] Neumann S, Bartolome G, Buchholz D, Prosiegel M. Swallowing therapy of neurologic patients: correlation of outcome with pretreatment variables and therapeutic methods. *Dysphagia* 1995;*10*(1):1–5

[99] Miloro KV, Pearson WG Jr, Langmore SE. Effortful pitch glide: a potential new exercise evaluated by dynamic MRI. *J Speech Lang Hear Res* 2014;*57*(4):1243–1250

[100] Shaker R, Kern M, Bardan E, et al. Augmentation of deglutitive upper esophageal sphincter opening in the elderly by exercise. *Am J Physiol* 1997;*272*(6 Pt 1):G1518–G1522

[101] Shaker R, Easterling C, Kern M, et al. Rehabilitation of swallowing by exercise in tube-fed patients with pharyngeal dysphagia secondary to abnormal UES opening. *Gastroenterology* 2002;*122*(5):1314–1321

[102] Ferdjallah M, Wertsch JJ, Shaker R. Spectral analysis of surface electromyography (EMG) of upper esophageal sphincter-opening muscles during head lift exercise. *J Rehabil Res Dev* 2000;*37*(3):335–340

[103] White KT, Easterling C, Roberts N, Wertsch J, Shaker R. Fatigue analysis before and after Shaker exercise: physiologic tool for exercise design. *Dysphagia* 2008;*23*(4):385–391

[104] Yoshida M, Groher ME, Crary MA, Mann GC, Akagawa Y. Comparison of surface electromyographic (sEMG) activity of submental muscles between the head lift and tongue press exercises as a therapeutic exercise for pharyngeal dysphagia. *Gerodontology* 2007;*24*(2):111–116

[105] Baker S, Davenport P, Sapienza C. Examination of strength training and detraining effects in expiratory muscles. *J Speech Lang Hear Res* 2005;*48*(6):1325–1333

[106] Kim J, Sapienza CM. Implications of expiratory muscle strength training for rehabilitation of the elderly: tutorial. *J Rehabil Res Dev* 2005;*42*(2):211–224

[107] Saleem AF, Sapienza CM, Okun MS. Respiratory muscle strength training: treatment and response duration in a patient with early idiopathic Parkinson's disease. *NeuroRehabilitation* 2005;*20*(4):323–333

[108] Aspire, LLC. EMST 150 Device. Expiratory muscle strength trainer. https://emst150.com/

[109] Troche MS, Okun MS, Rosenbek JC, et al. Aspiration and swallowing in Parkinson disease and rehabilitation with EMST: a randomized trial. *Neurology* 2010;*75*(21):1912–1919

[110] Yoon WL, Khoo JKP, Rickard Liow SJ. Chin tuck against resistance (CTAR): new method for enhancing suprahyoid muscle activity using a Shaker-type exercise. *Dysphagia* 2014;*29*(2):243–248

[111] Kraaijenga SA, van der Molen L, Stuiver MM, Teertstra HJ, Hilgers FJ, van den Brekel MW. Effects of strengthening exercises on swallowing musculature and function in senior healthy subjects: a prospective effectiveness and feasibility study. *Dysphagia* 2015;*30*(4):392–403

[112] Huckabee M-L, Steele CM. An analysis of lingual contribution to submental surface electromyographic measures and pharyngeal pressure during effortful swallow. *Arch Phys Med Rehabil* 2006;*87*(8):1067–1072

[113] Steele CM, Huckabee ML. The influence of orolingual pressure on the timing of pharyngeal pressure events. *Dysphagia* 2007;*22*(1):30–36

[114] Fujiu M, Logemann JA, Pauloski BR. Increased postoperative posterior pharyngeal wall movement in patients with anterior oral cancer: preliminary findings and possible implications for treatment. *Am J Speech Lang Pathol* 1995;*4*(2):24–30

[115] Doeltgen SH, Witte U, Gumbley F, Huckabee M-L. Evaluation of manometric measures during tongue-hold swallows. *Am J Speech Lang Pathol* 2009;*18*(1):65–73

[116] Veis S, Logemann JA, Colangelo L. Effects of three techniques on maximum posterior movement of the tongue base. *Dysphagia* 2000;*15*(3):142–145

[117] Ohmae Y, Ogura M, Kitahara S, Karaho T, Inouye T. Effects of head rotation on pharyngeal function during normal swallow. *Ann Otol Rhinol Laryngol* 1998;*107*(4):344–348

[118] Freed ML, Freed L, Chatburn RL, Christian M. Electrical stimulation for swallowing disorders caused by stroke. *Respir Care* 2001;*46*(5):466–474

[119] Leelamanit V, Limsakul C, Geater A. Synchronized electrical stimulation in treating pharyngeal dysphagia. *Laryngoscope* 2002;*112*(12):2204–2210

[120] Blumenfeld L, Hahn Y, Lepage A, Leonard R, Belafsky PC. Transcutaneous electrical stimulation versus traditional dysphagia therapy: a nonconcurrent cohort study. *Otolaryngol Head Neck Surg* 2006;*135*(5):754–757

[121] Shaw GY, Sechtem PR, Searl J, Keller K, Rawi TA, Dowdy E. Transcutaneous neuromuscular electrical stimulation (VitalStim) curative therapy for severe dysphagia: myth or reality? *Ann Otol Rhinol Laryngol* 2007;*116*(1):36–44

[122] Oh B-M, Kim D-Y, Paik N-J. Recovery of swallowing function is accompanied by the expansion of the cortical map. *Int J Neurosci* 2007;*117*(9):1215–1227

[123] Baijens LW, Speyer R, Roodenburg N, Manni JJ. The effects of neuromuscular electrical stimulation for dysphagia in opercular syndrome: a case study. *Eur Arch Otorhinolaryngol* 2008;*265*(7):825–830

[124] Ryu JS, Kang JY, Park JY, et al. The effect of electrical stimulation therapy on dysphagia following treatment for head and neck cancer. *Oral Oncol* 2009;*45*(8):665–668

[125] Kiger M, Brown CS, Watkins L. Dysphagia management: an analysis of patient outcomes using VitalStim therapy compared to traditional swallow therapy. *Dysphagia* 2006;*21*(4):243–253

[126] Bülow M, Speyer R, Baijens L, Woisard V, Ekberg O. Neuromuscular electrical stimulation (NMES) in stroke patients with oral and pharyngeal dysfunction. *Dysphagia* 2008;*23*(3):302–309

[127] Humbert IA, Poletto CJ, Saxon KG, et al. The effect of surface electrical stimulation on hyolaryngeal movement in normal individuals at rest and during swallowing. *J Appl Physiol (1985)* 2006;*101*(6):1657–1663

[128] Ludlow CL, Humbert I, Saxon K, Poletto C, Sonies B, Crujido L. Effects of surface electrical stimulation both at rest and during swallowing in chronic pharyngeal Dysphagia. *Dysphagia* 2007;*22*(1):1–10

[129] Humbert IA, Michou E, MacRae PR, Crujido L. Electrical stimulation and swallowing: how much do we know? *Semin Speech Lang* 2012;*33*(3):203–216

[130] Carter J, Humbert IA. E-stim for dysphagia: yes or no? https://leader.pubs.asha.org/article.aspx?articleid=2280201

# 12 Bolus Modifications

*Jane Mertz Garcia and Edgar Chambers IV*

## Summary

Bolus modifications (changing the texture of a beverage and/or food consistency) are prescribed commonly in dysphagia management to help maintain safe oral nutrition. They involve a texture change to help achieve a bolus consistency that more closely matches capabilities for safe swallowing. Thickening a thin liquid (such as water) and blending or chopping regular foods (such as meat) represent compensations to maintain safe oral nutrition and minimize the health risk for medical complications, such as aspiration pneumonia or malnutrition. This chapter addresses the complex issues surrounding the use of bolus modifications in the clinical management of dysphagia and provides the reader foundational knowledge important to clinical decision making in nutrition care. One aspect is helping readers understand the science of thickening, including differences that relate to thickening agents and base composition of liquids to appreciate the importance of these factors in their clinical recommendations. Foods also have different texture properties, and modifications have implications for ease of bolus preparation, oral control, and efficient transit during swallowing. It is imperative for clinicians to understand their roles and responsibilities in service delivery, including staff instruction and patient/family education. The overall effectiveness and safe implementation of bolus modifications require multidisciplinary planning and careful clinical decision making for the health and well-being of both children and adults with dysphagia.

## Keywords

diet modifications, thickened liquids, bolus, food, texture, nutrition, prethickened, swallowing, dysphagia

### Learning Objectives
- Indicate reasons for making changes to foods or beverages and the challenges associated with making those changes
- Describe characteristics of thickening products important to making clinical decisions about the use of thickened liquids
- Describe important texture properties of foods and types of food modification
- Understand the impact of service delivery challenges for individuals who are prescribed liquid or food modified diets
- Identify ways to improve accountability in the use of liquid or food modifications for children or adults in different care environments

## 12.1 Introduction

Bolus modifications (changing the texture of foods or beverages) are prescribed commonly in dysphagia management. Modifying the texture of thin liquids such as water and/or regular foods represents a compensation strategy to maintain oral intake while minimizing health risk for medical complications, such as aspiration pneumonia, asphyxiation, or malnutrition.[1,2,3,4] The intended goal is to achieve a bolus consistency (beverage and/or food texture) that more closely matches a patient's capabilities for safe swallowing. For example, the addition of a thickening agent to a thin liquid slows its transit, which may be an important compensation for a patient with a pharyngeal swallow response that is slow to protect the airway. Many solid foods are typically modified by softening, blending, or chopping them to a consistency that requires less chewing effort and is easier to control in the mouth. The degree of texture modification typically becomes less or more restrictive related to a patient's improvement or decline in swallowing status.

The use of bolus modifications highlights the multidisciplinary aspect of dysphagia management. Although speech-language pathologists (SLPs) typically assess patients' swallowing status and make recommendations to physicians about bolus modifications, it is often the registered dietitian who ensures that nutritional needs (caloric and nutrition content) are balanced with recommendations for safe swallowing. Nursing personnel coordinate the overall care plan, including safe intake of solids and oral fluids to meet hydration and nutritional needs.

The overall effectiveness of bolus modifications and their safe implementation in care requires careful clinical decision making for the health and well-being of both children and adults with dysphagia. For example, knowledge about the science of thickening thin liquids (interaction of thickening agents with beverage content) provides a foundation for making informed decisions about products. Kitchen recipes for modifying foods must reflect consistent textural properties important for safe swallowing (e.g., mechanically altered meats that are finely chopped and mixed with a binding agent for appropriate cohesiveness). We know that changes to oral nutrition have social and psychological consequences that impact quality of life.[5] Although bolus modifications may result in food or drink that is clinically safer to swallow, our patients may not view the benefits positively. Swan and colleagues[6] concluded that many patients tend to associate bolus modifications with a poorer quality of life, emphasizing the importance of balancing clinical decisions about safe oral intake with perceptions of well-being, especially for patients with chronic dysphagia.

Unfortunately, there is not one agreed-upon dysphagia diet because the specific labels applied to liquid and food modifications are numerous and often vary from one care setting to another. The National Dysphagia Diet[7] labels and descriptions for levels of modification have not been readily adopted across practice settings.[8] A more recent proposal of the International Dysphagia Diet Standardization Initiative (IDDSI) seeks to standardize terminology globally in an effort to enhance communication across health care providers, industry partners, and researchers who document treatment outcomes.[2] Given current challenges in standardization, this chapter focuses on core concepts about bolus modifications and service delivery while encouraging readers to further advance their knowledge about past and current initiatives to standardize practices (**Box 12.1**).

## Box 12.1

**The Dysphagia Diet Task Force**

The Dysphagia Diet Task Force, comprising dietitians, the food service industry, and speech-language pathologists, collaborated in the development of the National Dysphagia Diet (2002). The first edition was previously available through the Academy of Nutrition and Dietetics (formerly the American Dietetic Association), but is no longer in publication. Information about the International Dysphagia Diet Standardization Initiative (IDDSI), which began in 2012, is available at their website (https://iddsi.org/). Proposed guidelines became available for review in 2015; the implementation phase of the IDDSI framework started in 2016.[9]

## 12.2 Texture Modifications to Beverages

Adequate intake of liquids is essential for our health and well-being. Texture changes to liquids represent a compensatory strategy to ensure that patients receive adequate hydration and nutrition.

### 12.2.1 Importance of Liquids in Nutrition Care

Our bodies need water to function for life.[10] Water can be taken in as liquids (typically the greatest source of water), in foods, and intravenously (as a result of other medical issues). Because many liquids, such as milk and some juices, contain nutrients, they also provide a common method of obtaining many vitamins and minerals (e.g., vitamins C and D, calcium, and phosphorus). Proteins, carbohydrates (sugars), and even limited amounts of fats are consumed in many beverages and liquid meal replacements.

Safe oral consumption and swallowing of thin liquids, such as water, can be challenging for many patients with dysphagia. Other examples of thin liquids include fruit juices, milk, coffee, hot chocolate, sodas, and alcoholic beverages. Although quite different in taste and composition, they are similar to one another in terms of having a low viscosity (thickness) whether or not they are served cold, hot, or at room temperature. Modifying the texture of thin liquids is a cornerstone of dysphagia management, with SLPs reporting their use for one-fourth to three-fourths of primarily adult patients with dysphagia in medical settings.[11] A survey of registered dietitians indicated that thickened water was an option for residents in 92% of skilled nursing facilities.[12]

Both SLPs and registered dietitians perceive texture-modified liquids to be an effective management strategy for many of their patients.[8,11] Commonly identified reasons for thickening relate to patients' compromised oral control or changes in the timing of their pharyngeal swallow response.[11] In these cases, the fast movement of a regular (thin) liquid, such as water or juice, and the inability to contain it in the mouth might result in aspirating a portion into the lungs, heightening the risk of pulmonary complications related to aspiration pneumonia. Studies that have examined effectiveness have primarily focused on adults, showing decreases in instances of penetration and aspiration with texture-modified liquids in comparison to thin liquids.[13,14,15] Gosa and colleagues[16] raised concerns about the insufficiency of similar evidence for children with dysphagia.

Although current evidence indicates positive benefits for the use of thickened liquids with adults, there appear to be tradeoffs to other aspects of swallowing.[17,18] For example, the consistency of a thickened liquid starts changing (thinning) when mixed with saliva and in response to body temperature.[19,20] This highlights the importance of recognizing other patient conditions (e.g., apraxia of swallow or lengthy oral transit) that might contribute to a prolonged dwell time in the oral cavity that significantly alters a target level of modification. Another consideration for thickened liquids is an increase in postswallow residue in the pharynx, particularly for thicker modifications.[18]

### 12.2.2 Rheology and Thickened Liquids

The use of bolus modifications, including thickened liquids, introduces clinicians to a new area of study. Rheology focuses on the deformation and flow of matter.[21] As applied to thickened liquids, important rheological characteristics include viscosity, density, and yield stress.[22,23]

The absorption of a thickening agent into a liquid causes a swelling process (thickening) that changes viscosity, which can be physically quantified in laboratory settings with the use of viscometers and rheometers. Viscosity is defined as "the internal friction of a fluid or its tendency to resist flow"[21] (**Box 12.2**). For example, water has little resistance and is fast moving (low viscosity), whereas modified liquids have more resistance (slow moving) depending on their degree of thickness. Fluids are further distinguished as Newtonian versus non-Newtonian.[21] Examples of Newtonian fluids include water, milk, edible oils, and filtered juices.[21] A common characteristic of each is that it has a constant, predictable viscosity and flow pattern (i.e., applying a force/stress that changes its speed of movement has no appreciable effect on viscosity). Many other beverages, including thickened liquids, are considered non-Newtonian, which simply means that they have a less constant flow (viscosity) in response to different forces or stresses. Thickened liquids are a type of non-Newtonian fluid that is "shear thinning," which means that viscosity decreases (there is less resistance) as the rate of flow increases (**Box 12.3**).[24,25]

## Box 12.2

**The Physical Measure of Viscosity**

The physical measurement of viscosity is typically reported in one of two ways in the dysphagia literature.[23] One is expressed in units of centipoise (cP) and the other is as millipascal-seconds (mPa s). The conversion is roughly equal in that 1 cP = 1 mPa s.

The shear-thinning characteristics of thickened liquids have practical consequences in relation to swallowing. Because bolus thickness can change in response to muscular forces applied to its speed of movement through the oral and pharyngeal cavities, it is difficult to know which shear rate(s) are most important for describing healthy versus disordered swallowing in light of a person's age (infant/young child vs. older adult) and associated conditions.[23,24,26] It also emphasizes the importance of knowing the reported shear rate if one is reading literature about thickening products because viscosity may vary at different measurement points (shear rates). For example, the National Dysphagia Diet identified a shear rate of 50 (average shear rate to represent normal swallowing) for the viscosity ranges of thin (1–50 cP), nectar (51–50 cP), honey (51–350 cP), and spoon-thick consistency (> 1,750 cP). Studies that have replicated their measurement procedures highlight differences between commercial products and within product lines when thickening a variety of beverages.[27,28] The International Dysphagia Diet Standardization Initiative provides narrative descriptions and texture/flow characteristics of various modifications. Instead of specifying ranges of viscosity, the IDDSI includes a gravity flow test for determining levels of liquid consistency.[9]

Other important rheological characteristics of thickened liquids include density and yield stress.[22,23] Density is a general reference to heaviness or bolus weight. Although thin liquids such as water and juice are generally similar to one another in density,[26,29] barium is considered denser.[23] The clinical implication is that the density of barium may provide different sensory information than other liquids during swallowing and changes the amount of force needed to move it through the mouth.[22,23] Yield stress reflects the amount of effort it takes for a liquid to start to flow. For example, water pours easily from a bottle (low yield stress), whereas ketchup often requires an additional "push" to initiate flow (high-yield stress). The yield stress of modified liquids may enhance sensory awareness of the bolus and

its manipulation for swallowing[26]; however, the combination of these factors (density and yield stress) raise additional considerations for infants and young children who are bottle fed. Cichero and colleagues[30] reported that higher-yield stress and density of barium-impregnated liquids in comparison to infant formula may complicate bolus flow characteristics through a nipple and the necessary pressure on a nipple for an infant to initiate and maintain bolus flow.

## 12.2.3 Thickening Products

Knowing that a person consumes "thickened liquids" simply means that the consistency of a beverage has been altered with the use of a thickening agent; it does not specify the type of thickening agent or the degree of adjustment. An early report (1983) of thickening described the addition of a "clear gelatin" to beverages.[31] Commercial thickening products, such as Thick It and Thick & Easy were introduced in the late 1980s. These are instant powder (granular), starch-based thickeners (**Fig. 12.1**) that are stirred into a beverage to achieve a target modification using product label guidelines for its preparation.

The number and type of commercial thickening products have increased substantially since that time. Products are now broadly distinguished as those that require preparation and products that are available for purchase in a ready-to-serve form (known as "prethickened") (**Fig. 12.2**). In addition to starch-based products, there are gum-based (also called hydrocolloid) thickening agents, such as the gel-form of Simply Thick (Simply Thick, LLC, St. Louis, MO) introduced in 2001, and the more recent introduction of gum thickeners in granular form (e.g., ThickenUp Clear [Nestlé]

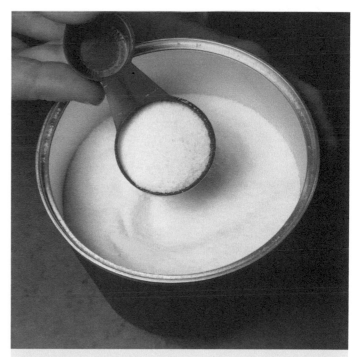

**Fig. 12.1** Instant thickening agent.

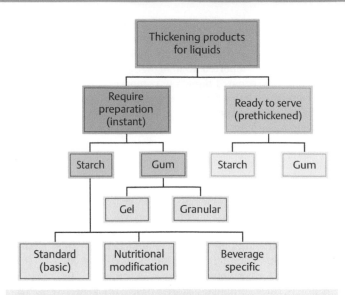

**Fig. 12.2** Types of thickening products for liquids.

## 12.2.4 The Science of Thickening

Because of the diversity of commercial thickening products and frequency of application in dysphagia management, it is essential for clinicians to have basic knowledge about thickening processes to promote effective decision making about liquid modifications. Although it seems simplistic (thickening agent mixed with fluid), the resulting modifications can be quite variable, especially related to the type of thickening agent (gum vs. starch) and composition of the base liquid (e.g., amount of acidity, sugars, fats, minerals). The property of human saliva provides another factor to consider in terms of how it affects viscosity.[19]

Starch-based agents used in thickening products for dysphagia are usually based on cornstarch that has been modified to make it mix without lumps and thicken quickly; they typically list "modified food starch" or "modified cornstarch" as the primary ingredient (**Box 12.4**). This is similar to the starch used in instant pudding mixes commonly found in supermarkets.

---

### Box 12.4

**The Science of Thickening**

Although the primary ingredient for starch thickening typically uses a modified cornstarch (maize starch), the label information does not include any details about the modification. This helps explain why starch-based products often vary from one another in thickening characteristics because companies apply different manufacturing processes that modify the starches differently. Some starch products also list maltodextrin, which is an ingredient that provides bulk and contributes to a smooth mouth feel.[33]

---

in 2012). Prethickened products (starch-thickened when initially offered) are now available for purchase in both starch- and gum-based forms. For example, Thick-It AquaCareH2O (Kent Precision Foods Group, Inc.) is a xanthan gum–based, ready-to-drink thickened water introduced in 2008. Although a greater variety of prethickened products are available for purchase (e.g., water, juices, and dairy drinks), there is limited information about them. Initial reports raise awareness about possible variability. For example, comparisons of prethickened water products reflected different ranges of thickness and patterns of liking (taste, texture, appearance).[32]

Practice patterns continue to suggest that a substantial percentage of care settings continue to rely totally or partly on thickening products that require some type of preparation, such as mixing an instant powder or gel with a beverage to achieve a prescribed consistency.[8,9] The labels applied to different levels of modification also vary as illustrated in the guidelines of the National Dysphagia Diet (NDD)[7] in comparison to the IDDSI[9] (**Table 12.1**). Although commercially available thickening products in the United States tend to reflect the nomenclature of the NDD, as of 2017, that is likely to change with implementation of the IDDSI Framework.

A starch is a carbohydrate or polysaccharide made up of long chains of various sugar molecules. Although the liquid may seem very thin when the starch granules are initially stirred into the beverage, it gradually begins to "swell" (analogous to a balloon being slowly filled with air) as fluid begins to enter the starch granules. The gradual swelling process also explains why some liquid modifications continue to thicken 10 or 20 minutes after their initial preparation.[27,34,35] This phenomenon may also affect starch-based prethickened products because when measured they have been shown to be thicker than their instant counterparts, suggesting that hydration (thickening) may continue as part of the packaging process.[36]

Gum-based thickening agents also thicken beverages but in a slightly different way. The most common types used in dysphagia products are xanthan and carrageenan gums. Both are polysaccharides, but their structures differ somewhat from those of starches. Polysaccharides also differ structurally from each other; they contain different sugar groups and different compounds, such as sulfur. In the scientific literature they are called hydrocolloid from "hydro" meaning water and "colloid" referring to a microscopic substance. A main difference in starch- and gum-based thickeners is the way in which they trap liquid. When the hydrocolloid is mixed with a liquid, it begins to spread its "chains" or "arms" in a manner that causes masses of strands to separate, tangle, and cling to each other (analogous to wading through water filled with long strands of weeds that trap and create resistance to

**Table 12.1** Labels to describe levels of liquid modification

| National Dysphagia Diet (2002) | International Dysphagia Diet Standardization Initiative[a] |
|---|---|
| Thin | Thin |
|  | Slightly thick |
| Nectar | Mildly thick |
| Honey | Moderately thick and liquidized |
| Spoon-thick | Extremely thick and pureed |

[a] The International Dysphagia Diet Standardization Initiative 2016 (https://iddsi.org/framework/).

movement). Gum products and starch-based products are also prepared differently; gums typically need more vigorous mixing to separate and dislodge the long ends of the strands from the particles to start binding the liquid together. Many gum thickeners must be vigorously shaken or mixed with a whisk in order for the gum thickening agent to mix appropriately with the liquid. Because various starches and various gums differ in terms of chemical structure, it is essential to read package directions and follow them for the given product because the instructions have been optimized for the thickener that the product contains.

Thickeners are often mischaracterized as promoting dehydration because they actually "bind" the water so tightly that they prevent its release in the body. This is incorrect. Starch is broken down during digestion, and the liquid is released just as it is in any food or beverage that is consumed. With gum-based thickeners, the actual physiological action is much more complex and dependent on the actual hydrocolloid and its concentration, but all the thickening agents used in these products do release the water at some point during digestion in the small intestine, large intestine, or colon.[37]

Infant cereals such as rice or oat cereal mixes are sometimes used as a natural thickening agent for infants.[38] They thicken similarly to starch-based thickeners, because the main thickening agent in rice and oats is starch, although a small amount of the hydrocolloid β-glucan is also found in oats. The effectiveness of starch as a thickening agent may be further impacted by whether it is mixed with infant formula or human breastmilk. For example, the presence of amylase (a digestive enzyme) in human breast milk causes the breakdown of starch, which highlights the preparation and timing of an infant feeding as clinically important because a modification may continue to thin[39,40] (**Box 12.5**).

## Box 12.5

### The Composition of Breastmilk

The composition of breastmilk varies depending on the individual mother, the period of lactation, and even during a single feeding or pumping of the breast. It contains proteins (including enzymes), lipids, carbohydrates, vitamins, minerals, and bacteria. Thickening agents such as instant rice or oat cereals for infants or starch-based thickening agents can be used (gum-based agents are not recommended in the first year), but must be carefully planned. First, the thickener chosen should be finely ground and well mixed to ensure that it does not result in lumps or particles. Because of enzymes and bacteria in the milk and the starchy components of the cereals or thickeners, the thickeners should be added and mixed shortly before serving to the infant and generally should not be stored, which could result in changes in thickness, separation, or potential spoilage.

Gums are less reactive to the amylase in human milk.[39,41] However, the use of some gum thickening agents has been discouraged for young children, particularly for premature infants or children under 1 year of age. The U.S. Food and Drug Administration (FDA) issued a consumer warning for the use of Simply Thick (xanthan gum) with premature infants in 2011 due to its possible association with necrotizing enterocolitis (**Box 12.6**). The concern is that the immature digestive system of an infant is unable to handle the transit of hydrocolloids, increasing the possible risk of necrotizing enterocolitis and resulting death. Although this risk was originally associated with prematurity, it has also been documented in a full-term birth.[42] This has resulted in changes to product labels to include a manufacturer warning about its intended use and changes to practice patterns for infants in some pediatric care settings.[43] Findings further highlight the importance of caution and careful clinical decision making about the use of thickeners with infants and young children due to fragile systems and complex medical conditions.[16]

## Box 12.6

### Thickening Agents

The U.S. Food and Drug Administration is an important resource for keeping up to date on any consumer warnings about thickening agents, including concerns for infants and young children. Simply Thick includes a warning to consult with a healthcare professional before using its product with infants and children under 12 years of age: https://www.simplythick.com/Safety.

The multitude of liquids that care providers thicken vary in their base composition, such as level of fat, sugar, or acidity (**Table 12.2**). The composition is important to the thickening process because of how it may interact with a thickening agent (**Table 12.3**). For example, some liquids, such as orange juice, contain pulp and acid content, both of which promote a high degree of initial thickening (bonding) of the starch and water complex. However, over time, the acid in products such as orange juice can cause the starch bonds to break, resulting in thinning of the thickened liquid. The thickening pattern for orange juice may be quite different in comparison to liquids that contain higher levels of fat (milk), carbonation (soda), or soluble solids (coffee).

Generally speaking, starches are considered *less* stable because they react more to acid, temperature, and thickening time, which contributes to more variable thickening patterns when they are

**Table 12.2** Sample beverages and base composition

| Liquid | Composition (primary content) |
| --- | --- |
| Barium | Heavy metal salt in liquid with high density |
| Water | Water, a few minerals |
| Apple, grape, pear juice | Water, sugars, vitamins, minerals, acid, pectin (a naturally occurring gum), maybe other starch or gum-based stabilizers |
| Orange juice | Water, sugars, vitamins, minerals, acid, fiber (pulp), maybe other stabilizers |
| Milk | Water, fat, vitamins, sugars, minerals (enzymes—breastmilk) |
| Nutritional drinks/meal replacements (e.g., Ensure) | Water, sugars, vitamins, many minerals, some starches or other stabilizers |
| Coffee | Water, a few minerals, tannins (temperature issues) |
| Power beverages | Water, sugars, acid, and sometimes minerals, stabilizers, and other ingredients |

**Table 12.3** Examples of beverage content interactions with thickening agents

| Composition | Possible interactions (specific products should be tested) |
|---|---|
| Barium | Interacts differently with starch and gum (see minerals below) |
| Sugar | Typically increases viscosity in thin liquids, can decrease viscosity of thicker liquids by keeping water in solution |
| Protein | Usually little impact unless heated, which can cause thickening or thinning after curdling |
| Fat | Provides low levels of thickening by itself, but can coat starch or gum particles and keep them from absorbing, water resulting in less thickness |
| Acid | Little or no impact on gum-based thickeners. Acid can impact starch-based thickeners by breaking starch bonds, which can initially increase viscosity slightly by making the starch absorb more quickly. However, over time, acid will continue to break the bonds and likely reduce viscosity. Differences in pH (the amount of acid in the liquid or food) can also impact other ingredients, such as the interaction with minerals. |
| Minerals | Can interact with gums and to some extent with starches causing clumping or various changes in viscosity (increases or decreases) depending on the specific minerals and gum. Divalent and trivalent mineral salts (calcium, magnesium, barium, aluminum, iron) are most likely to cause these changes depending on pH. |
| Vitamins | Usually none. Most vitamins have little impact because they are present in such small amounts. However, if present in large amounts, some produce weak acid reactions. |
| Other gums and stabilizers | Variable. Many other gums and stabilizers are used to promote a positive mouth feel in products, to help pulpiness or cloudiness in products, such as apple cider and grapefruit juice. These can interact in unexpected ways with both starches and gums and often result in clumping, increased thickening, gelling (forming a semisolid like gelatin over time), or cause solids to precipitate or fall to the bottom. |

mixed with different liquid compositions.[27] Gum-based thickening agents are known for their stabilization of food products for patients with dysphagia[7] and seem to be less impacted by the base fluid at lower levels[35]; however, Cho and Yoo[44] showed that at higher thickness levels (i.e., pudding-thick) there was clear interaction with base beverage components and xanthan gum–based thickeners, which produced different consistencies among different types of beverages. One finding in studies is that many modified liquids that are mixed or prethickened with a gum agent are less viscous in comparison to similar liquids that are thickened with starch.[32,35]

Some modified liquids may continue to change as they mix with saliva in the mouth or when saliva enters the glass containing a thickened drink. Saliva also contains amylase, which has been shown to reduce the viscosity of some modifications.[45,46] Although Hanson and colleagues[19] reported a decrease in the viscosity of thickened water, the added saliva had no appreciable effect on the thickness of modified orange juice. Their findings suggest that the amylase enzyme may be neutralized by the pH content of orange juice, further highlighting the importance of liquid composition to the thickening process.

## 12.2.5 Challenges in Clinical Application and Service Delivery

One immediate challenge is the lack of standardization in test materials (ready-mixed barium or manually prepared barium stimuli). Barium stimuli are typically more viscous than the modifications that patients actually consume.[47,48] The mismatch may be more pronounced for honey-like modifications in comparison to nectar-like consistencies.[49] Concerns about thickened barium are not limited to test stimuli for adults; they are also concerns about barium-impregnated liquids for infants because they also are more viscous than regular (unthickened) or thickened infant formula.[30,38] Another consideration is the procedure for preparing barium stimuli. For example, adding barium powder into an already thickened liquid causes the sample to thicken further, which changes its viscosity.[50] Conversely, if the barium product is diluted, its viscosity will decrease depending on the change to its concentration.[50] Test results may also be influenced by the use of gum versus starch-thickened barium.[51] These findings highlight the importance of developing specific recipes and protocols in the use of barium test stimuli to more closely represent the mealtime modifications consumed by children or adults.[49,50]

Current literature emphasizes the importance of recommending the least viscous modification that can be swallowed safely.[18,52] Although clinicians report that nectar-like consistency is their most common level of modification, a substantial number of patients routinely receive more viscous modifications.[8,11] Leder and colleagues[14] studied inpatients in a hospital who aspirated thin liquids but swallowed both nectar- and honey-like consistencies safely during instrumental assessment. Patients were then closely monitored over the next 24 hours for any signs of aspiration or health changes during and after meals. All of their 84 patients successfully ingested both levels of modification, leading the authors to conclude that "nectar is enough" (p. 58) in terms of assessing and providing the least viscous modification that is safe to consume.

The level of modification that provides optimal benefit to young children is unclear.[16] Variability in thickness is one concern in that thickened infant formula measures 12 to 70 times thicker than thickened human milk.[39] This adds to challenges that relate to the nutrient density of thickened formula and thickened human milk because young infants may have difficulty consuming adequate volumes to meet caloric and nutrient needs.[41] Starch-thickened modifications add calories that increase their energy density but reduce the volume available to obtain other nutrients; gum thickeners add volume without calories or other nutrients for infants.[41]

Clinicians must be knowledgeable about service delivery for any level of bolus modification, including reasons for product selection and modification practices to ensure that staff and/or family prepare liquids in an accurate and consistent manner. The dietitian, in comparison to the SLP, is more likely to know facility-based factors that influence the purchase of thickening products (e.g., cost considerations or food service contracts).[8] Because thickening agents are different from one another, it is essential that SLPs collaborate with dietitians about facility practices and decision making about thickening products selected for their care settings. Because the nutrient content of products also varies (e.g., sodium content), it is critical that SLPs collaborate with nutrition specialists to assure fluid and caloric needs are patient specific.[53]

Although dietitians and SLPs contribute in significant ways in dysphagia management, neither profession reports a high level of ongoing involvement in terms of personally preparing thickened liquids for their patients.[8,11] Day-to-day preparation is typically the responsibility of other staff, including dietary/food service assistants, certified nursing assistants, and other administrative and support staff. Research findings suggest that only about half of those who make the modifications receive formal instruction about how to mix or prepare them[11,54] even though the SLP is typically viewed as the responsible professional for this process.[8]

An ongoing concern is that individuals with dysphagia may be given modifications to consume that are different than their prescribed level of thickness (often too thick). Inaccuracies in preparation were shown in a study of thickened liquids prepared by health care providers in that a substantial percentage were unable to modify samples to measure within nectar- or honey-like ranges of thickness.[54] Many caregivers overthickened both levels of modification, which seemed consistent with the belief or myth that it is better to overthicken versus underthicken when preparing modified liquids (the concept that "thicker is better").[8] Because the added thickening agent suppresses the flavor of the base liquid and changes its texture,[55,56] creating overly thickened liquids results in less palatable drinks and negatively contributes to patients' acceptance. In addition, it may increase risk of health complications if aspirated because a more viscous substance may be more difficult for some patients (such as frail elders) to clear from their airway.[57]

Staff education is crucial to ensure that liquids are modified in accordance with product guidelines to achieve the prescribed level of thickness. There is a risk that care providers who have learned to prepare thickened liquids by spoon to stir a starch-based thickening agent into a liquid may inaccurately apply that same procedure to gum-based products, which may require very different mixing procedures.[54] Lack of compliance in some cases might reflect the staff's belief systems and their perception that the recommendations are a "hassle.[58,59,60] In addition to staff education, service delivery includes recognition of facility practices in bolus modifications. For example, liquids that are thickened and then refrigerated for later serving may also overthicken because of the manner in which temperature and setting time interact, especially with starch thickeners.[35] As a general rule, thickened liquids that are cold tend to be more viscous than those consumed at room temperature. The amount of storage time may even result in different rheological properties for gum-based thickening products, especially when these products are held for over 1 hour.[44]

It is important to recognize that opinions and beliefs about thickened liquids may directly or indirectly influence aspects of clinical practice. Clinicians perceive that their patients dislike thickened liquids.[11] This may contribute to another commonly held belief that thickened liquids cause dehydration, which is not an accurate statement. As mentioned, it has been shown that the addition of a thickening agent does not affect water absorportion by the body once it is ingested.[61] It is reasonable to think that modifications make thickened drinks less desirable (e.g., suppression of base liquid, additional off-flavors, or grainy texture), which might impact a patient's desire to consume them. In addition, the nutrient content of thickening agents and physiological changes in oral processing while drinking them may further contribute to feelings of fullness and drinking less as a result.[52] Cichero concluded that the "literature on satiety suggests that dehydration may be due to physiological expectation that thick fluids will make them feel full." [52] The combination of some or all of these factors may result in patients who have less motivation to drink thickened liquids, leading them to consume less fluid, which heightens their risk of dehydration.

Thickened liquids represent one important type of bolus modification in dysphagia management. Clinicians who recommend thickened liquids must be responsible for what patients consume regardless of the care setting. In addition to knowledge about the science of thickening, it is important for clinicians to understand their roles and responsibilities in service delivery, including the importance of staff instruction about their preparation and use. Inclusion of simple measurement tools provides objective information about levels of texture modification and visual feedback to staff and family members during instruction about preparation.[9,29,62] These are important components of professional accountability in patients' nutritional care when thickened liquids are a prescribed bolus modification.

## 12.2.6 Free Water Protocols

The use of thickened liquids is not without potential adverse consequences for patients. As stated previously, clinicians perceive that many patients do not find thickened liquids palatable, and nonadherence to recommendations for consuming thickened liquids is common.[11] Patients who do not have easy access to thin liquids and who do not wish to consume thickened liquids often limit their liquid intake. Thus dehydration becomes a concern. In addition, because many patients do not like thickened liquids, the use of modified liquids can negatively affect quality of life. There is also empirical evidence indicating a higher incidence of aspiration pneumonia in individuals who aspirate thicker (honey-thick) liquids compared to those who aspirate thin liquids, such as water.[57]

In response to these issues, clinicians at Frazier Rehabilitation Hospital in Louisville, Kentucky, developed a protocol, now known as the Frazier Free Water Protocol, in which individuals admitted to their facility who, following an instrumental assessment of swallowing, are recommended thickened liquids or individuals who are recommended a nonoral diet are allowed to consume water.[63] Those who are taking an oral diet are allowed water between meals; those who are on nonoral means of nutrition are allowed water as desired. A strict oral hygiene program is a key part of the protocol, and oral care must be administered each time prior to the patient consuming water. This is to ensure removal of any potentially harmful bacteria contained within the patient's mouth. Exclusion criteria for the protocol include impulsivity or excessive coughing and discomfort when consuming water.[63]

Rationale for development of the Frazier Free Water protocol, and other similar water protocols that have followed, is based on the argument that aspiration of water is safer than aspiration of other liquids because water is a naturally occurring fluid in the body.[64] Additionally, small amounts of water are absorbed easily through small, specialized proteins called aquaporins.[65] However, it remains unclear how much water can be aspirated before there are negative consequences, such as aspiration pneumonia.

Proponents of free water protocols report improved hydration and patient quality of life when patients are allowed to take water between meals. However, evidence in the research literature is equivocal. Some studies[66] have reported no increase in aspiration pneumonia incidence in patients on free water protocols compared to those who were restricted to thickened liquids, whereas others have found increased rates of aspiration pneumonia in individuals on free water protocols.[67,68]

Clinicians are urged to use caution, examine the literature, and carefully weigh risks versus benefits to patients when making decisions regarding whether to adopt a free water protocol. Decision making should be a shared process and include the SLP, the patient or the patient's health care proxy, and the care team. It appears that patient medical status, risk factors for development of aspiration pneumonia,[69] and availability of facility resources necessary to implement a stringent oral hygiene program and ensure proper implementation of a water protocol are all critical factors to consider.[63] Readers are encouraged to read Langmore et al[68] for a review of risk factors for aspiration pneumonia. At present, there is insufficient empirical evidence to suggest that the use of a free water protocol is safe for most patients.

## 12.3 Texture Modification to Food Consistencies

The nutrients from food (water, protein, carbohydrate, fat, vitamins, and minerals) provide essential elements that enhance our energy and health and how we function.

### 12.3.1 Importance of Food for Health and Well-Being

One of the primary concerns of the health care team for persons with dysphagia is malnutrition.[70] Decreased food intake from the consequences of dysphagia (e.g., dislike of modified foods, difficulty in oral or pharyngeal movement) or from the consequences of comorbid conditions (e.g., muscle weakness, physical modification, medications) is real and can lead to major nutritional problems that lead to other health issues.[71] This is particularly true after the acute phase of a condition, such as stroke, has progressed to the rehabilitation phase.[72] A key issue is that modified diets often reduce patient intake of energy (calories), with reductions of greater than 50% seen in many patients.[73] This is an alarming statistic because energy is a critical need both physiologically and psychologically during illness, rehabilitation, and maintenance.

Part of the challenge is that oral nutrition of a semisolid or solid consistency in normal swallowing requires proficiency in bolus preparation and control, and also for its propulsion through the oral cavity. Texture-modified foods are altered in some manner (e.g., softened, minced, mashed, blended, ground, or chopped). Clinical recommendations to modify regular (semisolid/solid) foods often result from anatomical or physiological changes that impact chewing and oral preparation/transit for swallowing. Additional factors that may contribute to their use include poor dentition, slow eating, and self-feeding difficulties.[74] Foods that are altered typically require less chewing effort and are easier to control in the mouth, while reducing a patient's risk of choking and lessening difficulty while eating.[2] The frequency of texture-modified foods varies greatly, ranging from 15 to more than 45% of individuals in some care settings.[74,75,76,77,78]

### 12.3.2 Texture Properties and Levels of Modification

The texture of any food item represents a group of physical properties that are derived from its structure.[21] Food properties identified as having more significance in management of dysphagia include adhesiveness, cohesiveness, firmness, fracturability, hardness, springiness, viscosity, and yield stress.[7] For example, an adhesive food is one that is more attracted to another surface (e.g., peanut butter, which "sticks" to the roof of the hard palate because its high adhesiveness requires more lingual effort to remove it). Even items of a similar food type (e.g., cookies) vary greatly in their textural properties, creating challenges for individuals with impaired swallowing. For example, a ginger snap cookie has a hard texture that takes force in order for it to deform (break). It fractures into parts, in contrast to a shortbread cookie, which often requires less force to break or compress and more easily forms a cohesive bolus when mixed with saliva. The relative importance of food properties is further magnified by factors such as bite strength and adequacy of dentition.[2]

Efforts for standardization are represented in the different grades of modification as identified by the NDD and IDDSI (**Table 12.4**). The level or degree of food texture modification generally represents the integrity of oral motor control and oral preparatory skills. For example, a pureed diet (sometimes described as pudding-like) provides food textures that require no or minimal chewing effort because they are presented in the mouth as a smooth, cohesive bolus. The "blended" or pureed bolus compensates for highly compromised oral motor skills for preparation (mastication and bolus control) and propulsion through the oral cavity. Subsequent levels gradually introduce textures that

**Table 12.4** Levels of food texture modification

| National Dysphagia Diet (2002) | International Dysphagia Diet Standardization Initiative[a] |
|---|---|
| | 3—Liquidized |
| Level 1: Dysphagia pureed | 4—Extremely thick and pureed |
| Level 2: Dysphagia mechanically altered | 5—Minced and moist |
| Level 3: Dysphagia advanced | 6—Soft |
| Level 4: Regular | 7—Regular |

[a] The International Dysphagia Diet Standardization Initiative 2016 (https://iddsi.org/framework/).

require more chewing effort and oral management. Foods that are difficult to chew, such as meats, must be mechanically altered (e.g., ground, chopped, blended, or minced) to compensate for compromised mastication. Because the alteration results in many small fragments or finely chopped pieces, a binding agent or carrier is important to promote cohesion and mouth control. Thick, but not sticky, gravy might work well as a carrier for many meats by binding the fragmented parts together for a cohesive bite. More advanced diet levels require functional oral motor skills for chewing and bolus control. For example, patients may receive modifications that include soft, moist foods (e.g., well-cooked vegetables that can be fork mashed), with more difficult food consistencies (e.g., popcorn, crusty bread) eliminated from their diet. Advancement to a "regular" diet simply means that that patient does not have any restriction with regard to solid food textures, which conveys safe management of any food texture. It is important to realize that a so-called regular diet can vary tremendously between individuals and cultures; patients and caregivers should be cautioned that not every food, particularly those with unusual textures, may work. For example, hard candies, particularly sticky, gummy pastes found in some cultures, may not be appropriate for some patients.

### 12.3.3 Challenges with Modified Food Textures

Changes in texture can affect the moisture and cohesiveness of foods, which can potentially affect their caloric and nutritional content. Patients are at risk for deficiency in protein intake and overall energy in comparison to those receiving a regular diet.[73] For example, the gravy added to a chopped meat may be high in starch and fat content. The added fluid can further dilute its nutritional content, unless the patient compensates by consuming a larger volume.[74] The imbalance of nutrients may contribute to protein-energy malnutrition, which can lead to life-threatening conditions, such as pneumonia, chronic heart failure, chronic obstructive pulmonary disease, altered gastrointestinal function, and infections related to decreased immune function.[70,79]

An incorrect food modification could have other consequences, including risk of choking and/or asphyxiation. Berzlanovich and colleagues[1] reported that asphyxiation from food is a concern for complex boluses (e.g., sandwiches) and modified foods (e.g., mashed fruit), indicating the importance of regular evaluation and careful monitoring as part of a patient's nutritional care plan. A difficult food texture is also a risk factor for asphyxiation for infants and children, along with inadequate dentition, accompanying neurological conditions, and the amount of supervision needed while the patient is eating.[2]

Systematic reevaluation is important to assure that improved capabilities result in dietary advancement to a less restrictive level of modification. Groher and McKaig[77] found that many nursing home residents did not have systematic reevaluation of their status, remaining at a more restrictive level of modification than necessary. Texture changes (particularly pureed textures) may simply contribute to a lack of eating interest influenced by diminished sensory characteristics of blended consistencies (e.g., taste, temperature, and mouth feel). Changes also may make foods less visually appealing, which may be a contributing factor

to lack of acceptance. Menus that offer expanded options (e.g., reformed meats) and food choices may be one way to balance these concerns.[76,80]

Although substantial attention has been focused on practice patterns involving thickened liquids, there has been less attention with regard to texture-modified foods. Standardization extends beyond labels and food texture descriptions to include the use of standardized recipes and preparation practices to ensure that foods are modified in a consistent manner.[7,81] Lack of standardized recipes might result in textural properties ranging from an appropriate target level of cohesiveness to excessive firmness and adhesiveness (i.e., dry and sticky) from one meal to the next.

Quality control extends to the food production staff involved in its preparation, who may not always follow the specific recipe for a texture-modified food, which can alter its nutritional and texture benefits.[82] Other influencing factors include attitudes and beliefs, amount of managerial supervision, inadequate knowledge about modifications.[74,82] **Fig. 12.3** illustrates a lack of consistency in one or more aspects of food production in a hospital setting for a pureed diet of breakfast foods (eggs and ham) across a 2-day period. On the first day, the pureed eggs and ham (**Fig. 12.3a,b**) reflected limited moisture and a pasty consistency when fork mashed. The appearance of the eggs before mashing (**Fig. 12.3a**) actually indicates they had been overscrambled, frozen, and thawed before serving, a process that results in the moisture separating from the eggs. On day 2, the family requested white gravy to use as a binding agent. A very thin gravy accompanied bowls of watery ham with scrambled eggs (**Fig. 12.3c**). The ham particles quickly separated from the fluid. The scrambled eggs appeared to be freshly scrambled and noncohesive (less representative of a puree consistency). The reader is encouraged to learn more about methods for assessing the texture of modified foods at IDDSI 2016 (http://iddsi.org/framework/).[9]

## 12.4 Clinical Decision Making about Liquid and Food Modifications

Clinicians who recommend dietary changes must carefully evaluate the potential consequences for their patients because bolus modifications pose special challenges that require consideration in nutritional care. Although simple in concept (modifying the texture of a liquid or solid consistency), it is one of the most complex interventions to execute successfully. We know that thickening agents are *not* the same, and some food textures are simply less safe than others for patients with impaired swallowing to tolerate (e.g., "sticky" foods, or mixed consistencies like fruit cocktail in which the liquid and solid easily separate in the mouth).

The roles and responsibilities of SLPs in the use of bolus modifications are numerous. Recommendations must be patient specific and reflect collaborative decision making with nutrition specialists and other health care professionals because modifications may have unintended consequences for other aspects of a patient's health (e.g., changes in energy and protein intake). Because other staff and care providers typically execute recommendations, it is incumbent that SLPs provide ongoing education and instruction to ensure that bolus modifications consistently reflect product guidelines (liquids) and target levels of food

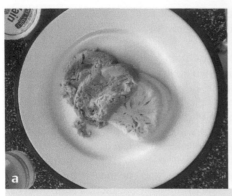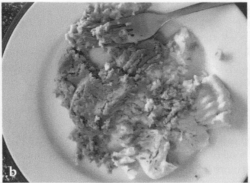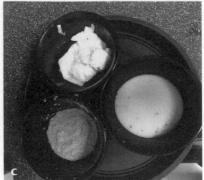

**Fig. 12.3** Illustration of inconsistency in texture-modified diet (puree consistency) served to patient in hospital across 2-day period. **(a)** Day 1, pureed ham and eggs. **(b)** Eggs and ham, subsequently, forked mashed shows lack of moisture and cohesion. **(c)** Day 2, pureed, watery ham with thin white gravy as binding agent and scrambled eggs.

texture. SLPs also serve a vital role of advocacy to ensure that the dietary needs of patients are systematically reevaluated and adjusted to best address nutritional needs and quality of life. This includes ensuring that dietary recommendations remain part of nutrition plans during patient transitions to new care environments because information about dietary changes is frequently omitted.[83] Clinicians must be accountable in balancing decisions about safe swallowing with a patient's well-being as part of continuity in nutritional care.

## 12.5 Questions

1. It is common to observe mealtimes at your facility as part of dysphagia management. Over the past weeks, you have made frequent observations about inconsistent levels of beverage thickness for patients prescribed similar levels of modification. An important factor that may be contributing to the variability of thickened liquids at your facility includes which of the following?

A. Thickening product and type of thickening agent
B. Composition of beverages that are typically thickened
C. Amount of setting time before a modified liquid is consumed
D. Opinions and beliefs of care providers who prepare modifications
E. All of the above are important factors

2. The addition of a thickening agent causes a swelling process that changes the viscosity of a liquid. The two main types of thickening agents are _____ and _____.

A. Infant cereals and starch based
B. Starch and gum
C. Prethickened and instant
D. Powder (granular) and gel
E. Hydrocolloid and gum
F. Xanthan and carrageenan

3. Thickened liquids are considered non-Newtonian fluids that are shear thinning. This means that

A. A thickened liquid has a constant, predictable viscosity that is independent of an applied shear stress.
B. Muscular forces that change the speed of liquid flow during swallowing have no appreciable impact on viscosity.
C. Thickened liquids may have a less constant flow (viscosity) in response to the muscular forces applied during swallowing.
D. Non-Newtonian fluids are primarily characterized by their heaviness or bolus weight.
E. The amount of effort needed for the liquid to flow is an important characteristics that distinguishes Newtonian from non-Newtonian fluids.

4. What is an important clinical consideration in recommending modified food textures for children and adults?

A. Changes to food texture may alter caloric and nutritional content.
B. The timing of a patient's pharyngeal swallow response is a frequently identified reason for modifying food textures.
C. Food properties such as adhesiveness and hardness have little impact on oral preparatory skills.
D. A and B only
E. A and C only

5. Which of the following reflects an accurate statement about the use of bolus modifications in dysphagia management for children and/or adults?

A. There are highly standardized practice guidelines about the implementation of liquid and food modifications across care settings.
B. Patients who consume thickened liquids become dehydrated because the thickening agent limits the amount of water absorption by the body.
C. Modified liquid and food diets are prescribed in an effort to restore swallow function.

D. Clinicians must be considerate of "mismatches" in the thickness of test barium and mealtime preparations of thickened liquids for both children and adults.

E. Both starch- and gum-based thickening agents mix similarly with human breastmilk.

## 12.6 Answers and Explanations

**1. Correct: All of the above are important factors (E).**

All are important considerations. Thickening patterns can be quite different in relation to the type and amount of thickening agent (gum vs. starch) (**A**), composition of the base liquid (**B**) (e.g., acidity of orange juice vs. fats of milk), and storage or setting time before modifications are consumed (**C**). Starches are considered *less* stable because they react more to the base content of a liquid, its temperature, and thickening time. For example, the pulp and acidity of orange juice promote a high degree of initial bonding (thickening) with starch molecules, which can cause orange juice to thicken quite differently compared to other beverages like water. Opinions and beliefs of care providers who prepare modifications (**D**) may be a contributing factor to inaccuracies in preparation and the commonly held belief that it is better to overthicken versus underthicken when preparing modified liquids. The lack of staff instruction and education about thickened liquids contributes to all of these problems by not providing adequate training about preparation and by not dispelling myths.

**2. Correct: Starch and gum (B).**

Starch-based thickeners were introduced in the late 1980s, and gum thickening agents were introduced after 2000. Infant cereals and starch-based thickeners (**A**) thicken in a similar way because starch is the main thickening agent. (**C**) describes commercially available products but does not clarify the type of thickening agent. For example, gum thickening agents are now available in both gel and granular (instant powder) forms. (**E**) and (**F**) are terms associated with gum thickening agents. *Hydrocolloid* means gum; xanthan and carrageenan are types of gums.

**3. Correct: Thickened liquids may have a less constant flow (viscosity) in response to the muscular forces applied during swallowing (C).**

The viscosity of a thickened liquid decreases with an increasing shear rate. This is important because bolus thickness can change in response to muscular forces applied during its movement through the oral/pharyngeal cavities. Choices (**A**) and (**B**) reflect statements associated with Newtonian fluids. Rheology focuses on the deformation and flow of matter, which includes viscosity, density, and yield stress. (**D**) is a general reference to denseness (e.g., barium is denser than water). (**E**) describes yield stress.

**4. Correct: Changes to food texture may alter caloric and nutritional content (A).**

Patients are at risk for deficiency in caloric and protein intake, which may result in the need to consume a larger volume to compensate for diluted nutritional content. The timing of the patient's pharyngeal swallow response (**B**) is a commonly identified reason for modifying the texture of *liquids* (not foods); recommendations to modify foods often result from anatomical or physiological changes that impact chewing and oral preparation/transit. Adhesiveness and hardness are important food properties (**C**) in dysphagia management. A hard texture takes more force to break it and may fracture in parts that are difficult to control in the mouth. An adhesive food is one that is more attracted to another surface and requires more muscular control to clear, such as peanut butter adhering to the hard palate.

**5. Correct: Clinicians must be considerate of "mismatches" in the thickness of test barium and mealtime preparations of thickened liquids for both children and adults (D).**

The viscosity of barium stimuli is typically more viscous than the modifications that are actually consumed by children and adults. Standardization is an ongoing challenge (**A**). Although the National Dysphagia Diet (NDD) and International Dysphagia Diet Standardization Initiative (IDDSI) provide labels and descriptions for different levels of modifications, guidelines have yet to be readily adopted across practice settings or by manufacturers. It is a common misconception that thickening agents cause dehydration (**B**). The addition of a thickening agent does not affect water absorption by the body once ingested. It is more reasonable to think that patients drink less because the thickened liquid is unpalatable (the thickening agent negatively impacts taste and texture) and the added thickening agent contributes to feelings of fullness. Modifying the texture of a liquid and or food represents a compensation strategy to maintain oral intake (**C**). The intended goal is to achieve a bolus consistency that more closely matches capabilities for safe swallowing. The presence of amylase (a digestive enzyme) in human breastmilk causes the breakdown of starch (**E**). Although gums are less reactive to the amylase in human milk, there are other safety issues. The U.S. Food and Drug Administration issued a consumer warning due to the possible association of gum thickening agents with necrotizing enterocolitis.

## References

[1] Berzlanovich AM, Fazeny-Dorner B, Waldhoer T, Fashing P, Keil W. Foreign body asphyxia: a preventable cause of death in the elderly. Am J Prev Med 2005;28(1):65–69

[2] Cichero JAY, Steele C, Duivestein J, et al. The need for international terminology and definitions for texture-modified foods and thickened liquid used in dysphagia management: foundations of a global initiative. Curr Phys Med Rehabil Rep 2013;1(4):280–291. doi: 10.1007/s40141-013-0024-z

[3] Chang CC, Roberts BL. Feeding difficulty in older adults with dementia. J Clin Nurs 2008;17(17):2266–2274. doi: 10.1111/j.1365-2702.2007.02275.x

[4] Doggett DL, Tappe KA, Mitchell MD, Chapell VC, Turkelson CM. Prevention of pneumonia in elderly stroke patients by systematic diagnosis and treatment of dysphagia: an evidence-based comprehensive analysis of the literature. Dysphagia. 2001;16(4):279–295. doi: 10.1007/s00455-001-0087-3

[5] Ekberg O, Hamdy S, Woisard V, Wuttge-Hannig A, Ortega P. Social and psychological burden of dysphagia: Its impact on diagnosis and treatment. Dysphagia. 2002;17(2):139–146. doi: 10.1007/s00455-001-0113-5

[6] Swan K, Speyer R, Heijnen BJ, Wagg B, Cordier R. Living with oropharyngeal dysphagia: effects of bolus modification on health-related quality of life—a systematic review. Qual Life Res 2015;24(10):2447–2456. doi: 10.1007/s11136-015-0990-y

[7] National Dysphagia Diet Task Force. National Dysphagia Diet: Standardization for Optimal Care. Chicago, IL: American Dietetic Association; 2002

[8] Garcia JM, Chambers E IV. Perspectives of registered dietitians about thickened beverages in nutrition management of dysphagia. Top Clin Nutr 2012;27(2):105–113. doi: 10.1097/TIN.0b013e3182542117

[9] Cichero JAY, Lam P, Steele CM, et al. Development of international terminology and definitions for texture-modified foods and thickened fluids used in dysphagia management: the IDDSI framework. Dysphagia 2017;32:293–314. doi: 10.1007/s00455-016-9758-y

[10] Popkin BM, D'Anci KE, Rosenberg IH. Water, hydration, and health. Nutr Rev 2010;68(8):439–458. doi: 10.1111/j.1753-4887.2010.00304.x

[11] Garcia JM, Chambers E IV, Molander M. Thickened liquids: practice patterns of speech-language pathologists. Am J Speech Lang Pathol 2005;14(1):4–13. doi: 10.1044/1058-0360(2005/003)

[12] Castellanos VH, Butler E, Gluch L, Burke B. Use of thickened liquids in skilled nursing facilities. J Am Diet Assoc 2004;104(8):1222–1226. doi: 10.1016/j.jada.2004.05.203

[13] Kuhlemeier KV, Palmer JB, Rosenberg D. Effect of liquid bolus consistency and delivery method on aspiration and pharyngeal retention in dysphagia patients. Dysphagia 2001;16(2):119–122. doi: 10.1007/s004550011003

[14] Leder SB, Judson BL, Sliwinski E, Madson L. Promoting safe swallowing when puree is swallowed without aspiration but this liquid is aspirated: nectar is enough. Dysphagia 2013;28(1):58–62. doi: 10.1007/s00455-012-9412-2

[15] Logemann JA, Gensler G, Robbins J, et al. A randomized study of three interventions for aspiration of thin liquids in patients with dementia or Parkinson's disease. J Speech Lang Hear Res 2008;51(1):173–183. doi: 10.1044/1092-4388(2008/013)

[16] Gosa M, Schooling T, Coleman J. Thickened liquids as a treatment for children with dysphagia and associated adverse effects: A systematic review. Infant Child Adolesc Nutr 2011;3(6):344–350. doi: 10.1177/1941406411407664

[17] Newman R, Vilardell N, Clave P, Speyer R. Effect of bolus viscosity on the safety and efficacy of swallowing and the kinematics of the swallow response in patients with oropharyngeal dysphagia: white paper by the European Society for Swallowing Disorders. Dysphagia. 2016;31:232–249. doi: 10.1007/s00455-016-9696-8

[18] Steele CM, Alasanei, WA, Ayanikalath S, et al. The influence of food texture and liquid consistency modification on swallowing physiology and function: a systematic review. Dysphagia. 2015;30:2–26. doi: 0.1007/s00455-014-9578-x

[19] Hanson B, O'Leary MT, Smith CH. The effect of saliva on the viscosity of thickened drinks. Dysphagia 2012;27(1):10–19. doi: 10.1007/s00455-011-9330-8

[20] Suiter DM, Gosa MM, Leder SB. Intraoral dwell time results in increased bolus temperature and decreased bolus viscosity for thickened liquids. Top Clin Nutr 2013;28(1),3–7. doi: 10.1097/TIN.0b013e31827df962

[21] Bourne MC. Food Texture and Viscosity: Concept and Measurement. 2nd ed. San Diego, CA: Academic; 2002

[22] Steele CM, Cichero JAY. A question of rheological control. Dysphagia 2008;23(2):193–203. doi: 10.1007/s00455-007-9105-4

[23] Cichero JAY, Lam P. Thickened liquids for children and adults with oropharyngeal dysphagia: the complexity of rheological considerations. J Gastroenterol Hepatol 2014;3(5):1073–1079. doi: 10.6051/j.issn.2224-3992.2014.03.408-13

[24] O'Leary M, Hanson B, Smith C. Viscosity and non-Newtonian features of thickened fluids used for dysphagia therapy. J Food Sci 2010;75. doi: 10.1111/j.1750-3841.2010.01673.x

[25] Viswanath DS, Ghosh TK, Prasad DL, Dutt NVK, Rani KY. Viscosity of Liquids: Theory, Estimation, Experiment, and Data. New York, NY: Springer; 2007.

[26] Vickers Z, Damodhar H, Grummer C, et al. Relationships among rheological sensory texture, and swallowing pressure measurements of hydrocolloid thickened fluids. Dysphagia 2015; 30(6):702–713: doi: 10.1007/s00455-015-9647-9

[27] Garcia JM, Chambers E IV, Matta Z, Clark M. Viscosity measurements of nectar and honey thick liquids: product, liquid, and time comparisons. Dysphagia 2005;20(4):325–335. doi: 10.1007/s00455-005-0034-9

[28] Payne C, Methven L, Fairfield C, Bell A. Consistently inconsistent: commercially available starch-based dysphagia products. Dysphagia 2011;26(1):27–33. doi: 10.1007/s00455-009-9263-7

[29] Lund AM, Garcia JM, Chambers E IV. Line spread as a visual clinical tool for thickened liquids. Am J Speech Lang Pathol 2013;22(3):566–571. doi: 10.1044/1058-0360(2013/12-0044)

[30] Cichero JAY, Nicholson TM, Dodrill P. Liquid barium is not representative of infant formula: characterisation of rheological and material properties. Dysphagia 2011;26(3):264–271. doi: 10.1007/s00455-010-9303-3

[31] Winstein CJ. Neurogenic dysphagia: frequency, progression, and outcome in adults following head injury. Phys Ther 1983;63(12):1992–1997

[32] Garcia JM, Chambers E IV, Chacon C, Di Donfrancesco B. Consumer acceptance testing of prethickened water products: implications for nutrition care. Top Clin Nutr 2015;30(3):264–275. doi: 10.1097/TIN.0000000000000039

[33] Akoh CC. Fat replacers. Food Tech 1998;52(3):47–53

[34] Dewar R, Joyce MJ. Time-dependent rheology of starch thickeners and the clinical implications for dysphagia therapy. Dysphagia 2006;21(4):264–269. doi: 10.1007/s00455-006-9050-7

[35] Garcia JM, Chambers E IV, Matta Z, Clark M. Serving temperature viscosity comparisons of nectar and honey-thick liquids. Dysphagia 2008;23(1):65–75. doi: 10.1007/s00455-007-9098-z

[36] Adeleye B, Rachal C. Comparison of the rheological properties of ready-to-serve and powdered instant food-thickened beverages at different temperatures for dysphagic patients. J Am Diet Assoc 2007;107(7):1176–1182. doi: 10.1016/j.jada.2007.04.011

[37] Edwards CA, Garcia AL. The health aspects of hyrocolloids. In: Phillips GO, Williams PA, eds. Handbook of Hydrocolloids. 2nd ed. Cambridge, UK: Woodhead; 2009:50–81.

[38] Stuart S, Motz JM. Viscosity in infant dysphagia management: comparison of viscosity of thickened liquids used in assessment and thickened liquids used in treatment. Dysphagia 2009;24(4):412–422. doi: 10.1007/s00455-009-9219-y

[39] Cichero JAY, Nicholson TM, September C. Thickened milk for the management of feeding and swallowing issues in infants: a call for interdisciplinary professional guidelines. J Hum Lact 2013;29(2):132–135.

[40] de Almeida MB, de Almedia JAG, Moreira MEL, Novak FR. Adequacy of human milk viscosity to respond to infants with dysphagia: experimental study. J Appl Oral Sci 2011;19(6):554–559. doi: 10.1590/S1678-77572011000600003

[41] McCallum S. Addressing nutrient density in the context of the use of thickened liquids in dysphagia treatment. Infant Child Adolesc Nutr 2011;3(6):351–360. doi: 10.1177/1941406411427442

[42] Beal J, Silverman B, Bellant J, Young T, Klontz K. Late onset necrotizing enterocolitis in infants following use of a xanthan gum-containing thickening agent. J Pediatr 2012;161(2):354–356. doi: dx.doi.org/10.1016/j.jpeds.2012.03.054

[43] Dion S, Duivestein JA, St. Pierre A, Harris SR. Use of thickened liquids to manage feeding difficulties in infants: a pilot survey of practice patterns in Canadian pediatric centers. Dysphagia 2015;30(4):457–472. doi: 10.1007/s00455-015-9625-2

[44] Cho HM, Yoo B. Rheological characteristics of cold thickened beverages containing xanthan gum-based food thickeners used for dysphagia diets. J Acad Nutr Diet 2015;115(1):106–111. doi: 10.1016/j.jand.2014.08.028

[45] Hanson, B. Management of swallowing disorders using thickened drinks. Complete Nutr 2013;13(1):33–35

[46] Newman R, Vilardell N, Claave P, Speyer R. Effect of bolus viscosity of the safety and efficacy of swallowing and the kinematics of the swallow response in patients with oropharyngeal dysphagia: white paper by the European Society for swallowing disorders (ESSD). Dysphagia 2016;31(2):232–249. doi: 10.1007/s00455-016-9696-8

[47] Cichero JAY, Jackson O, Halley P, Murdoch B. How thick is it? Multicenter study of the rheological and material property characteristic of mealtime fluids and videofluoroscopy fluids. Dysphagia 2000;15(4):188–200. doi: 10.1007/s004550000027

[48] Strowd L, Kyzima J, Pillsbury D, Valley T, Rubin BR. Dysphagia dietary guidelines and the rheology of nutritional feeds and barium test feeds. Chest 2008;33:1397–1401. doi: 10.1378/chest.08-0255

[49] Nita SP, Murith M, Chisholm H, Engmann J. Matching the rheological properties of videofluoroscopic contrast agents and thickened liquid prescriptions. Dysphagia 2013;28(2):245–252. doi: 10.1007/s00455-012-9441-x

[50] Steele CM, Molfenter SM, Peladeau-Pigeon M, Stokely S. Challenges in preparing contrast media for videofluoroscopy. Dysphagia 2013;28(3):464–467. doi: 10.1007/s00455-013-9476-7

[51] Leonard RJ, White C, McKenzie S, Belafsky PC. Effects of bolus rheology on aspiration in patients with dysphagia. J Acad Nutr Diet 2014;114(4):590–594. doi: 10.1016/j.jand.2013.07.037

[52] Cichero JAY. Thickening agents used for dysphagia management: effect of bioavailability of water, medication and feelings of satiety. Nutr J 2013;12(54):1–8. doi: 10.1186/1475-2891-12-54

[53] Joyce A, Robbins J, Hind J. Nutrient intake from thickened beverages and patient-specific implications for care. Nutr Clin Pract 2014;30(3):440–445

[54] Garcia JM, Chambers E IV, Clark M, Helverson J, Matta Z. Quality of care issues for dysphagia: modifications involving oral fluids. J Clin Nurs 2010;19(11–12):1618–1624. doi: 10.1111/j.1365-2702.2009.03009.x

[55] Lotong V, Chun SS, Chambers E IV, Garcia JM. Texture and flavor characteristics of beverages containing commercial thickening agents for dysphagia diets. J Food Sci 2003;68(4):1537–1521. doi: 10.1111/j.1365-2621.2003.tb09680.x

[56] Matta Z, Chambers E IV, Garcia JM, Helverson JM. Sensory characteristics of beverages prepared with commercial thickeners used for dysphagia diets. J Am Diet Assoc 2006;106(7):1049–1054. doi: 10.1016/j.jada.2006.04.022

[57] Robbins J, Gensler G, Hind J, et al. Comparison of two interventions for liquid aspiration on pneumonia incidence. Ann Intern Med 2008;148(7):509–518. doi: 10.7326/0003-4819-148-7-200804010-00007

[58] Colodny N. Construction and validation of the mealtime and dysphagia questionnaire: an instrument designed to assess nursing staff reasons for noncompliance with SLP dysphagia and feeding recommendations. Dysphagia. 2001;16(4):263–271. doi: 10.1007/s00455-001-0085-5

[59] Pelletier CA. Feeding beliefs of certified nurse assistants in the nursing home: a factor influencing practice. J Gerontol Nurs 2005;31(7):5–10. doi: 10.3928/0098-9134-20050701-04

[60] Pelletier CA. What do certified nurse assistants actually know about dysphagia and feeding nursing home residents? Am J Speech Lang Pathol 2004;13(2):99–113. doi: 10.1044/1058-0360(2004/012)

[61] Sharpe K, Ward L, Cichero J, Sopade P, Halley P. Thickened fluids and water absorption in rats and humans. Dysphagia 2007;22(3):193–203. doi:10.1007/s00455-006-9072-1

[62] Garcia JM, Chambers IV E, Cook K. Visualizing the consistency of thickened liquids with simple tools: Implications for clinical practice. Am J Speech Lang Pathol 2017;27(1);270–277. doi: 10.1044/2017_AJSLP-16-0160

[63] Panther KM. The Frazier Free Water Protocol. Perspectives on Swallowing and Swallowing Disorders (Dysphagia) 2005;14(1):4–9. doi:10.1044/sasd14.1.4

[64] Carlaw C, Finlayson H, Beggs K, et al. Outcomes of a pilot water protocol project in a rehabilitation setting. Dysphagia 2012;27(3):297–306

[65] Coyle JL. Water, water everywhere, but why? Argument against free water protocols. Perspectives on Swallowing and Swallowing Disorders (Dysphagia) 2011;20(4):109–115. doi: 10.1044/sasd20.4.109

[66] Becker DL, Tews LK, Lemke JH. An oral water protocol for rehabilitation patients with dysphagia for liquids. Presented at American Speech-Language Hearing Association Convention, Chicago, Il, 2008. https://www.google.com/url?sa=t&rct=j&q=&esrc=s&source=web&cd=2&ved=2ahUKEwjcz9CJ7IbfAh-VFAqwKHe_WDz8QFjABegQICBAB&url=http%3A%2F%2Fwww.asha.org%2FEvents%2Fconvention%2Fhandouts%2F2008%2F1877_Tews_Lisa.htm&usg=AOvVaw21KhC_8w7stOnk4CM0bnHX

[67] Karagiannis MJ, Chivers L, Karagiannis TC. Effects of oral intake of water in patients with oropharyngeal dysphagia. BMC Geriatr 2011;11(1):9

[68] Langmore SE, Terpenning MS, Schork A, et al. Predictors of aspiration pneumonia: how important is dysphagia? Dysphagia 1998;13(2):69–81

[69] Gillman A, Winkler R, Taylor NF. Implementing the Free Water Protocol does not result in aspiration pneumonia in carefully selected patients with dysphagia: a systematic review. Dysphagia 2016; 32(3):345–361. doi: 10.1007/s00455-016-9761-3

[70] Yarrow L, Garcia JM. Malnutrition: risks and concerns in dysphagia management. Perspectives on Swallowing and Swallowing Disorders (Dysphagia) 2010;19(4):115–120. doi: 10.1044/sasd19.4.115

[71] Sura L, Madhavan A, Carnaby G, Crary MA. Dysphagia in the elderly: management and nutritional considerations. Clin Interv Aging 2012;7:287–298. doi: 10.2147/CIA.S23404

[72] Finestone HM, Foley NC, Woodbury MG, Greene-Finestone L. Quantifying fluid intake in dysphagic stroke patients: a preliminary comparison of oral and nonoral strategies. Arch Phys Med Rehabil 2001;82(12):1744–1746. doi: dx.doi.org/10.1053/apmr.2001.27379

[73] Wright L, Cotter D, Hickson M, Frost G. Comparison of energy and protein intakes of older people consuming a texture modified diet with a normal hospital diet. J Hum Nutr Diet 2005;18(3):213–219. doi: 10.1111/j.1365-277X.2005.00605.x

[74] Keller H, Chambers L, Niezgoda H, Duizer L. Issues associated with the use of modified texture foods. J Nutr Health Aging 2012;16(3):195–200. doi: 10.1007/s12603-011-0160-z

[75] ADA. Position of the American Dietetic Association: liberalization of the diet prescription improves quality of life for older adults in long-term care. J Am Diet Assoc 2005;105:1955–1965. doi: 10.1016/j.jada.2005.10.004

[76] Germain I, Dufresne T, Gray-Donald K. A novel dysphagia diet improves the nutrient intake of institutionalized elders. J Am Diet Assoc 2006;106:1614–1623. doi: 10.1016/j.jada.2006.07.008

[77] Groher ME, McKaig TN. Dysphagia and dietary levels in skills nursing facilities. J Am Geriatr Soc 1995;43(5):528–532. doi: 10.1111/j.1532-5415.1995.tb06100.x

[78] Steele CM, Greenwood C, Ens I, Robertson C, Seidman-Carlson R. Mealtime difficulties in a home for the aged: not just dysphagia. Dysphagia 1997;12(1):45–50. doi: 10.1007/PL00009517

[79] Akner G, Cederholm T. Treatment of protein-energy malnutrition in chronic nonmalignant disorders. Am J Clin Nutr 2001;74(1):6–24

[80] Farrer O, Olsen C, Mousley K, Teo E. Does presentation of smooth pureed meals improve patients consumption in an acute care setting: a pilot study. Nutr Diet 2016;73(5):405–409

[81] Niezgoda H, Miville A, Chambers LW, Keller H. Issues and challenges of modified-texture foods in long-term care: a workshop report. Ann Longterm Care 2012:20(7):22–27

[82] Ilhamto N, Anciado K, Keller HH, Duizer LM. In-house pureed food production in long-term care: perspectives of dietary staff and implications for improvement. J Nutr Gerontol Geriatr 2014;33(3):210–228. doi: 10.1080/21551197.2014.927306

[83] Kind A, Anderson P, Hind J, Robbins J, Smith M. Omission of dysphagia therapies in hospital discharge communications. Dysphagia 2011;26(1):49–61. doi: 10.1007/s00455-009-9266-4

## Suggested Reading

[1] Cichero JAY. Thickening agents used for dysphagia management: effect of bioavailability of water, medication and feelings of satiety. Nutr J 2013;12(54):1–8. doi: 10.1186/1475-2891-12-54

[2] Cichero JAY, Lam P. Thickened Liquids for children and adults with oropharyngeal dysphagia: the complexity of rheological considerations. J Gastroenterol Hepatol 2014;3(5):1073–1079. doi: 10.6051/j.issn.2224-3992.2014.03.408-13

[3] Cichero JAY, Lam P, Steele CM, et al. Development of international terminology and definitions for texture-modified foods and thickened fluids used in dysphagia management: the IDDSI framework. Dysphagia 2017;32:293–314. doi: 10.1007/s00455-016-9758-y

[4] Cichero JAY, Nicholson TM, September C. Thickened milk for the management of feeding and swallowing issues in infants: a call for interdisciplinary professional guidelines. J Hum Lact 2013;29(2):132–135

[5] Garcia JM, Chambers E IV. Managing dysphagia through diet modifications. Am J Nurs 2010;110(11):26–33. doi: 10.1097/01.NAJ.0000390519.83887.02

[6] Garcia JM, Chambers E IV. Perspectives of registered dietitians about thickened beverages in nutrition management of dysphagia. Top Clin Nutr 2012;27(2):105–113. doi: 10.1097/TIN.0b013e3182542117

[7] Garcia JM, Chambers E IV, Molander M. Thickened liquids: practice patterns of speech-language pathologists. Am J Speech Lang Pathol 2005;14(1):4–13. doi: 10.1044/1058-0360(2005/003)

[8] Gosa M, Schooling T, Coleman J. Thickened liquids as a treatment for children with dysphagia and associated adverse effects: a systematic review. Infant Child Adolesc Nutr 2011;3(6):344–350. doi: 10.1177/1941406411407664

[9] McCallum S. Addressing nutrient density in the context of the use of thickened liquids in dysphagia treatment. Infant Child Adolesc Nutr 2011;3(6):351–360. doi: 10.1177/1941406411427442

[10] Robbins J, Gensler G, Hind J, et al. Comparison of two interventions for liquid aspiration on pneumonia incidence: a randomized trial. Ann Intern Med 2008;148(7),509–518

[11] Steele CM, Alasanei WA, Ayanikalath S, et al. The influence of food texture and liquid consistency modification on swallowing physiology and function: a systematic review. Dysphagia 2015;30(1):2–26. doi: 0.1007/s00455-014-9578-x

# 13 Tube Feeding

Mark R. Corkins and Kelly Green Corkins

## Summary

Children and adults with dysphagia often have other, primarily neurologic, medical difficulties. These individuals have associated gastrointestinal (GI) tract difficulties that are probably related to the neurologic control of many GI tract functions. They often present with gastroesophageal reflux, which can be primary or secondary or both. The secondary reflux is often due to dysmotility of the GI tract. Because of the numerous medical issues these patients often require feeding assistance by a nasogastric (NG) tube or other feeding device.

A complete evaluation of the patient is important when one is making decisions related to tube feedings. The type of device, whether temporary or semipermanent, depends on the medical condition and realistic treatment goals. The next decision is related to the appropriate site for placement in the GI tract. Once the device is placed, the medical team needs to decide which feeding delivery method and enteral formulation are most appropriate for the patient. A variety of nutritional substances can be given via a feeding tube with particular effects on the GI tract that influence feeding tolerance. Each member of the medical team plays a role in the overall nutrition care plan.

### Keywords

blenderized tube feeding, dysmotility, enteral formula, feeding delivery, feeding tube, formula, gastroesophageal reflux, nutrition, nutrition assessment

### Learning Objectives

- Understand the associated changes in the gastrointestinal (GI) tract function in children with dysphagia
- Have a working knowledge of the various feeding access devices and the indications for using them
- Have a basic understanding of the differences among enteral feedings and their effects on GI tract function
- Have a basic understanding of the types/categories of enteral formulations available

## 13.1 Introduction

Enteral nutrition is the provision of nutrients to the gastrointestinal (GI) tract. This can be accomplished orally or via a feeding tube. There are clearly times when swallowing issues lead to the need for an alternative route for providing the patient with nutrition. For some patients, the swallow is so unsafe that no oral feedings are appropriate. There are other patients where breathing or fatigue may limit the amount of oral intake. In these situations, it is necessary to use a feeding tube to ensure that a patient receives the nutrition required for growth and recovery from an injury or disease.

There are contraindications to enteral feeding (either oral or via feeding tube). Some contraindications include bowel obstruction, severe malabsorption, high-output fistulas, decreased blood pressure resulting in decreased gut perfusion, and use of certain medications.[1] Once the decision is made to provide tube feedings, a complete nutrition assessment is important to determine the type of feeding tube needed, its placement in the GI tract, and the type of enteral formulation to use.

## 13.2 Background

The presence of dysphagia may indicate that the patient has some sort of neurologic difficulty. The nervous system has many effects on GI tract function as well.[2] Some of the basic controls of GI tract function may be altered and not functioning appropriately. This can manifest in many ways and can affect the type and method of feedings.

Children with neurologic impairment have a much higher rate of gastroesophageal reflux (often referred to simply as reflux).[2,3] Despite what many parents report, the North American Society for Pediatric Gastroenterology, Hepatology, and Nutrition and the European Society for Pediatric Gastroenterology, Hepatology, and Nutrition joint recommendations found after an extensive literature review that there are no symptoms or clusters of symptoms that can reliably predict reflux issues in infants.[3] Classic gastroesophageal reflux is due to dysfunction of the lower esophageal sphincter (LES). The LES is controlled by the nervous system and should have a tonic signal to remain closed. When there is dysfunction of the nervous system, the control of the LES may be altered. This is thought of as primary reflux.

Some reflux is due to other issues and is considered secondary reflux. The leading cause of secondary reflux is dysmotility.[2] One of the functions of the GI tract is the movement by coordinated muscle contractions of ingested nutrition from the mouth to the anus. This process is called peristalsis or motility. Children with neurologic problems often have disordered peristalsis, with poor stomach emptying. If the stomach does not empty, it will create feeding intolerance and vomiting. The patients can become distended and uncomfortable with feedings or have vomiting due to the secondary reflux.

Dysmotility can be short term or long term depending on the cause. Some short-term causes of dysmotility include medications, such as anesthetics or pain medications. Postsurgical patients are most likely to have short-term dysmotility related to these medications. Some disease states, particularly the neuromuscular diseases, may result in long-term dysmotility or progressive dysmotility. Reflux and dysmotility must always be considered when determining type and placement of the feeding tube, enteral formulation, and feeding regimen. If reflux and motility continue, changes in medical therapy or in the feeding plan are necessary.

# 13.3 Temporary Tubes

Once it is determined that a feeding tube is necessary, the next important question becomes what type of tube. A nasogastric (NG) tube is a temporary feeding tube that is placed through a nostril and advanced into the stomach. There has been a concern that an NG tube might increase reflux by acting as a "wick" for the reflux. Studies have not supported this theory. Placement of an NG tube has the risk of accidental placement into a site other than the GI tract. The primary concern would be placement into the lungs where formula infusion could be fatal. An X-ray study is the only certain way to determine that the feeding tube is properly placed in the GI tract.[4] In children, there is always a concern about radiation exposure, but there is no acceptable alternative. Once the NG is in place, most patients will be able to safely consume foods and fluids orally as determined by the speech-language pathologist. However, a small number of children refuse to speak or attempt to swallow while an NG tube is in place.

For patients with delayed gastric emptying (a component of dysmotility) and known reflux with aspiration of gastric contents, small bowel feedings beyond the pylorus of the stomach are indicated.[4] A nasojejunal (NJ) tube can be placed at the bedside, by fluoroscopy or by endoscopy. Placement of the tube must be verified with an X-ray before the feeding tube is used.

One issue with the temporary feedings devices is that they are easily displaced. In fact, NG displacement is a major cause of decreased formula intake in patients on NG feedings.[5] Once any kind of feeding tube is in place and in use, it is recommended to mark the exit site on the tube.[4] If this mark is not in place it means the tube may no longer be in the correct location.

# 13.4 Semipermanent Tubes

One of the difficult decisions is when to consider placement of a semipermanent feeding tube. This is a crucial step for many families because it indicates that the process is not temporary and is another indicator that the patient is medically dependent. The American Society for Parenteral and Enteral Nutrition recommends placement of a semipermanent feeding device if the need for a feeding tube exceeds 4 weeks.[4] A study of long-term feeding device placement in children with cerebral palsy found that 28% of the families cited stresses by having a tube, but 86% felt the tube feedings had a positive impact on the child's care.[6] Although patients think of these tubes as permanent, they can actually be removed with a very small "spot" scar in the left upper quadrant of the abdomen.

Gastrostomy tubes (G-tubes) can be placed by endoscopic, laparoscopic, fluoroscopic, or open surgical methods. Some health care professionals believe that having a G-tube leads to a greater risk of having reflux. A child who has a neurologic difficulty has a greater incidence of postprocedure reflux.[7] This is most likely due to the neurologic issue, not the G-tube placement. A study found that, in children, a pH probe prior to feeding tube placement could be used to predict who would develop reflux.[8] Those with elevated reflux values before the feeding tube placement were most likely to have problems with reflux afterward.

For those patients with delayed gastric emptying (stomach dysmotility) and known reflux with aspiration of gastric contents, small bowel feedings bypassing the stomach are recommended.

Nasojejunal (NJ) tubes are very long and hard to maintain, with frequent clogging and displacement. A G-tube can be converted by fluoroscopy or endoscopy to a gastrojejunal tube (G-J tube). G-J tubes have a high rate of complications, and long-term patients often eventually require placement of a jejunal feeding tube.[9] In adults, there are techniques for endoscopic placement of jejunal feeding devices. Currently, there are no such devices available for children, leaving the G-J tube as the best option.

An important factor to remember with jejunal feedings is that there is no longer the reservoir function of the stomach. The small intestine is limited in size; therefore the feedings cannot be given in large, quick boluses. Small intestine feedings require slower infusion that is spread over a longer time span, and they usually require a pump.

# 13.5 Feeding Delivery Method

Once a feeding device is in place, the feeding delivery method most appropriate for the patient must be selected. Tube feedings can be administered as continuous feedings, cyclic feedings, or intermittent/bolus feedings. The type of feeding device, placement in the gastrointestinal tract, the medical condition of the patient, gastrointestinal motility, and the patient's goals all require careful consideration when one is deciding on the feeding delivery method.[10] When one is working to advance to oral feedings, intermittent/bolus feedings or cyclic night feedings may be preferred, but they may not be appropriate.

Continuous feedings are given via a pump. They are indicated if the tube terminates in the small bowel (postpyloric) because the feedings are bypassing the stomach, which serves as a reservoir.[11] Continuous feedings may be indicated even if the feedings are going into the stomach, such as when there is poor glycemic control or the patient has poor motility.

Cyclic feedings are a modification of continuous feedings. Cyclic feedings can be given over a period of time with feeding breaks, or they may be given only at night to allow the patient to take oral feedings during the day.[11] In dysmotility, cyclic feedings can be beneficial and allow time for the stomach to empty a bit before more feeding is infused. Also, cyclic feedings allow some time off the pump. Though the pumps available for home tube feedings are portable and easy to use, it is nice for the patient to have an hour or two to bathe or run errands without having to bring the pump along.

Intermittent/bolus feedings can be given over a short period of time with a pump or be given by gravity. For gravity bolus feedings, the formula is in a bag or a syringe and the rate of infusion is controlled by how high the formula container is held.[10] Larger-volume intermittent/bolus feedings are given into the stomach. Intermittent/bolus feedings are more "normal." Physiologically they mimic the pattern of normal meals and are more convenient for families.[2] When trying to advance to oral intake, foods can be offered prior to the bolus feeding.

Transitional feedings are used when the goal is to increase oral intake. The tube feeding is held and an oral diet is offered. The percentage of the oral diet not consumed is then given as a tube feeding. A dietitian will calculate what formula and what amount represent the percentage of the meal not eaten. Another option is to offer an oral diet throughout the day and give a night tube feeding over 8 to 10 hours to provide a percentage of estimated needs.[10],[11] Usually once a patient is taking two-thirds to three-fourths of the estimated needs orally the tube feeding can be stopped. If the tube is a temporary tube, then it can be removed. If the feeding tube was surgically placed, it will be left in until the patient can meet certain goals as outlined by the medical team. Usually a semipermanent tube is not removed until the patient has not used the tube for 6 months and is maintaining a normal weight for adults or is demonstrating adequate weight gain and linear growth velocity for children.

## 13.6 Enteral Formulations

Prior to one year of age, expressed breastmilk or infant formulas are given via the feeding tube. Enteral formulas for both adult and pediatric patients fall under the category of medical foods, defined as "a food which is formulated to be consumed or administered enterally under the supervision of a physician and which is intended for the specific dietary management of a disease or condition for which distinctive nutritional requirements, based on recognized scientific principles, are established by medical evaluation."[12] Infant formulas are subject to more rigorous regulations applying to quality control, labeling, nutrient requirements, formula recall, and notification for new products. Some infant formulas are "exempt" from meeting a particular regulation because they are instead formulated to meet a specific medical need (e.g., a formula with lower than the regulated level of minerals for a patient with renal disease). This does not mean they are exempt from the same rigorous regulations for quality control, labeling, and so forth. Medical foods are regulated minimally with only application of Good Manufacturing Practices for conventional foods. Thus, medical professionals need to interpret the content and health claims of enteral formulas with caution.[4]

There are more than 200 enteral products available to meet the needs of patients from 1 year old to the elderly.[13] The composition of each enteral formulation differs in both macronutrients (carbohydrate, protein, and fat) and micronutrients (vitamins, minerals, and electrolytes). Each is formulated either to meet general nutrition needs or to meet the nutrition needs for more specialized disease states.[14] See **Table 13.1** for a general description of available enteral products and their composition. In addition, modular products are available to modify enteral formulas further to meet more individualized needs of a specific patient.

Carbohydrates include starch polymers (e.g., maltodextrin, modified cornstarch) and simple sugars (e.g., sucrose or dextrose).[14] Many formulas intended for both oral and tube feeding contain a higher amount of sucrose for taste. Sucrose and other simple sugars add to osmolality, so formulas intended only for tube feeding contain more maltodextrin and modified cornstarch as the carbohydrate source to lessen their impact on osmolality. Osmolality is important for formula tolerance, particularly if the patient is taking a high percentage of nutrition by tube feedings.

Protein in enteral formulations is provided from milk protein (casein and whey), soy protein, or amino acids (building blocks of protein).[14] The protein can be hydrolyzed, or broken down for better tolerance or absorption. When a person has an allergic reaction, it is to the protein in the food. The more the protein is broken down, the less allergenic the protein is. Amino acids are nonallergenic. As with carbohydrates, the smaller the particle, the more impact on osmolality. Manufacturers will balance an amino acid formula with a longer-chain carbohydrate, such as modified cornstarch, to maintain a moderate osmolality for the product.

Fat is provided as long- and medium-chain triglycerides from various oils.[14] Long-chain triglycerides require bile salts for absorption through the gut lymph. Medium-chain triglycerides are absorbed through the portal system. This is an important differentiation when one is choosing a formulation for certain disease states. Medium-chain triglycerides promote gastric emptying and intestinal motility and can be used in patients with motility issues.

Modular products are available as protein (intact or extensively hydrolyzed), carbohydrate (modified starch), fat (medium- or long-chain triglycerides), or combinations of macronutrients. Modular macronutrients will not increase the concentration of micronutrients, but they will alter macronutrient distribution of the product and can be used to increase the caloric concentration of ready-to-use products. Protein and carbohydrate modulars may significantly alter osmolarity of the formula and may result in intolerance.

## 13.7 Blenderized or Pureed Diets through Feeding Tubes

Blenderized (or pureed) tube feedings are simply a variety of foods pureed in a blender to be fed through a gastrostomy tube. This concept is not new; the first attempts at tube feedings in the 1800s were mixtures of foods.[17],[19] Even with the wide variety of products available for many different diseases and conditions, there is a renewed interest in blenderized tube feedings. The renewed interest may be due to the changing health care environment. An increasing number of insurance companies are not paying for tube-feeding formulas because they are considered food. The manufactured tube-feeding products are more expensive than preparing meals for someone. Another reason caregivers may desire to use a blenderized diet may be that food is nurturing, and caregivers want to be involved with their loved one's care.[19] Whatever the reason, careful consideration must be given before initiating the blenderized tube feeding with a patient because this type of feeding is not appropriate for all patients. Contraindications to the blenderized tube feeding include continuous feedings, jejunal feedings, tube size less than a no. 10 French, inadequate refrigeration, and lack of knowledge or motivation of the caregiver.[19]

Benefits of the blenderized tube feeding may be improved regulation of bowel movements; decreased gagging, retching, and vomiting; and decreased food refusal.[13],[18] Potential complications of the blenderized tube feeding include nutrient deficiencies, electrolyte disturbances, increased wear on the gastrostomy tube, and foodborne illness related to improper preparation or handling of foods.[18]

Open communication between the caregiver and the health care professionals, especially a registered dietitian, must be established before considering a blenderized tube feeding for a patient. This communication is key to preventing the potential complications of the feeding.[19]

**Table 13.1**  Enteral formulations[13,14,15]

| Category | Subcategory | General description | Use |
|---|---|---|---|
| Standard polymeric oral or enteral | Adult<br>* With or without fiber<br>*1 cal/mL, 1.5 cal/mL, 2 cal/mL | Lactose free, usually milk-based protein, but some are soy protein<br><br>Meets the recommended needs of the general population | Most patients will use one of these products.<br><br>General population who needs supplemental tube feeding or is transitioning to oral feeding |
| | Pediatric<br>*With or without fiber<br>*1 cal/mL, 1.5 cal/mL | May come in a variety of flavors<br><br>Variety of calorie densities to meet needs in lower volumes<br><br>Intact macronutrients | |
| Semi-elemental/peptide based | Adult<br>*With or without fiber<br>*1 cal/mL, 1.2 cal/mL, 1.5 cal/mL | Lactose free, usually milk-based protein<br><br>Meets the recommended needs of the general population<br><br>Some are made to be taken orally so are flavored | Designed for malabsorption and other gastrointestinal disorders including pancreatic insufficiency and dysmotility |
| | Pediatric<br>*With or without fiber<br>*1 cal/mL, 1.5 cal/mL | Variety of calorie densities to meet needs in lower volumes<br><br>Protein is hydrolyzed and a percentage of the fat is from medium-chain triglycerides | |
| Elemental/amino acid based | Adult<br>*Some are powder that can be concentrated | Amino acid based<br><br>Meets the recommended needs of the general population<br><br>Standard dilution is 1 cal/mL Usually a powder that must be reconstituted, so the caloric concentration can be varied | Malabsorption, pancreatic insufficiency, dysmotility, allergies |
| | Pediatric<br>*May contain prebiotic fiber<br>*Powder—standard dilution 1 cal/mL | | |
| Specialized/disease specific | Adult (use in pediatric patients) | Most are polymeric with modifications specific to a condition | For use with the disease specified in the subcategory |
| | *Renal | Usually lower protein, potassium, magnesium, and phosphorus | |
| | *Pulmonary | Higher fat and lower carbohydrate to lower $CO_2$ production | |
| | *Diabetes | Lower carbohydrate and more complex carbohydrates, including fiber | |
| | *Hepatic | Higher branched chain amino acids and lower aromatic amino acids | |
| | *Bariatric | Higher protein and contains omega-3 fatty acids | |

# 13.8 Questions

1. A developmentally delayed infant is found to have aspiration with all textures. The child tolerates nasogastric (NG) tube feedings well. On follow-up study a month later the aspiration persists at the same level. The indicated intervention at this time frame is

A. Continued ng feedings
B. Placement of a semipermanent gastrostomy
C. Placement of a gastrojejunal tube
D. Selection of an elemental formula
E. Selection of a thickened formula

2. A pediatric patient is found to have delayed gastric emptying and has a gastrojejunal tube in place for feedings. The feedings must be

A. With an elemental formula
B. Rapid bolus infusion

C. Slow bolus infusion
D. With a blenderized diet feeding
E. Continuous drip feeding

3. During transitioning of a child's enteral formula from an extensively hydrolyzed infant formula to a peptide-based pediatric formula, the child has a classic allergic reaction. What component of the formula is the child reacting to?

A. Lactose
B. Fat
C. Protein
D. Vitamin mixture
E. Mineral mixture

4. A caregiver comes to you requesting information on the blenderized tube feeding. What is a contraindication for this diet?

A. Jejunal tube feedings
B. Bolus feedings

C. Constipation

D. Gastroesophageal reflux

E. Taking some food orally

**5.** An infant with developmental delay has chronic dysphagia, and a gastrostomy is being planned. The best way to determine the risk of reflux is

A. The infant's symptoms

B. A barium swallow study

C. The formula used for feedings

D. The infant's developmental level

E. A pH probe study

# 13.9 Answers and Explanations

**1. Correct: placement of a semipermanent gastrostomy (B).**
(**A**) The patient has now been on NG tube feedings for at least 4 weeks. The history indicates this is going to be a persistent issue and it is time to place a safer and more stable feeding device. (**C**) Because the patient is tolerating gastric feedings, there is no need to proceed to jejunal feedings. (**D**) The patient does not appear to have any dysmotility, so an elemental formula is not indicated. (**E**) The patient aspirates all textures, so thickening will not help.

**2. Correct: continuous drip feeding (E).**
The small intestine does not have the reservoir function of the stomach, so the feedings must be infused over a time span. (**A**) The formula initially does not have to be elemental unless there is evidence of small bowel dysmotility. (**B, C**) Neither rapid nor slow boluses will be tolerated because of the need for infusion over time. (**D**) Because the feedings are continuous, the nonsterile blenderized diet is at high risk for bacterial growth.

**3. Correct: protein (C).**
Allergies are a reaction to protein. The extensively hydrolyzed protein in the infant formula is less allergenic than the less-broken-down protein in the form of peptides in the peptide-based pediatric formula. (**A**) Lactose is a carbohydrate, and although people can have an intolerance to lactose, it is not an allergic reaction. (**B**) Fats may be malabsorbed, but it is not an allergic reaction. (**D**) Vitamins and (**E**) minerals are needed for metabolism and are not protein based and so do not induce an allergic reaction.

**4. Correct: jejunal tube feedings (A).**
Jejunal feedings must be given continuously. Due to the risk of foodborne illness and that the tube feeding is bypassing the acid stomach, a blenderized tube feeding should not be given through a jejunal tube. (**B**) Bolus feedings < 2 hours are appropriate and decrease the potential for bacterial growth. (**C**) Constipation can be managed using the blenderized tube feeding. (**D**) Liquids reflux more than solids, and the blenderized tube feeding in case studies has been shown to improve reflux symptoms. (**E**) The diet has also been shown to improve oral intake, so taking foods orally is appropriate with this tube feeding.

**5. Correct: a pH probe study (E).**
The studies indicate only a pH probe study that actually measures and records reflux events over a period of time predicts the risk of reflux. (**A**) As indicated in the chapter, studies have shown that symptoms do not accurately predict reflux. (**B**) A barium swallow study of the upper gastrointestinal tract is a good way to look at the structures of the GI tract, but it is a single snapshot in time and does not predict overall reflux. (**C**) The formula used can have different levels of emptying depending on content but can be changed if needed. (**D**) The developmental level may correlate with the patient's neurologic status and thus correlate with a risk for reflux, but this is imprecise at best.

# References

[1] ASPEN Board of Directors and the Clinical Guidelines Task Force. Guidelines for the use of parenteral and enteral nutrition in adult and pediatric patients. *JPEN J Parenter Enteral Nutr* 2002;*26*(1 Suppl):1SA–138SA

[2] Marchand V, Motil KJ; NASPGHAN Committee on Nutrition. Nutrition support for neurologically impaired children: a clinical report of the North American Society for Pediatric Gastroenterology, Hepatology, and Nutrition. *J Pediatr Gastroenterol Nutr* 2006;*43*(1):123–135

[3] Vandenplas Y, Rudolph CD, Di Lorenzo C, et al; North American Society for Pediatric Gastroenterology Hepatology and Nutrition; European Society for Pediatric Gastroenterology Hepatology and Nutrition. Pediatric gastroesophageal reflux clinical practice guidelines: joint recommendations of the North American Society for Pediatric Gastroenterology, Hepatology, and Nutrition (NASPGHAN) and the European Society for Pediatric Gastroenterology, Hepatology, and Nutrition (ESPGHAN). *J Pediatr Gastroenterol Nutr* 2009;*49*(4):498–547

[4] Bankhead R, Boullata J, Brantley S, et al; A.S.P.E.N. Board of Directors. Enteral nutrition practice recommendations. *JPEN J Parenter Enteral Nutr* 2009;*33*(2):122–167

[5] Whelan K, Hill L, Preedy VR, Judd PA, Taylor MA. Formula delivery in patients receiving enteral tube feeding on general hospital wards: the impact of nasogastric extubation and diarrhea. *Nutrition* 2006;*22*(10):1025–1031

[6] Smith SW, Camfield C, Camfield P. Living with cerebral palsy and tube feeding: A population-based follow-up study. *J Pediatr* 1999;*135*(3):307–310

[7] Isch JA, Rescorla FJ, Scherer LRT III, West KW, Grosfeld JL. The development of gastroesophageal reflux after percutaneous endoscopic gastrostomy. *J Pediatr Surg* 1997;*32*(2):321–322, discussion 322–323

[8] Sulaeman E, Udall JN Jr, Brown RF, et al. Gastroesophageal reflux and Nissen fundoplication following percutaneous endoscopic gastrostomy in children. *J Pediatr Gastroenterol Nutr* 1998;*26*(3):269–273

[9] Raval MV, Phillips JD. Optimal enteral feeding in children with gastric dysfunction: surgical jejunostomy vs image-guided gastrojejunal tube placement. *J Pediatr Surg* 2006;*41*(10):1679–1682

[10] Brantley SL, Mills ME. Overview of enteral nutrition. In: Mueller CM, ed. *The A.S.P.E.N. Adult Nutrition Support Core Curriculum.* 2nd ed. Silver Spring, MD: ASPEN; 2012

[11] Axelrod D, Kazmerski K, Iyer K. Pediatric enteral nutrition. *JPEN J Parenter Enteral Nutr* 2006;*30*(1, Suppl):S21–S26

[12] Grants and contracts for development of drugs for rare diseases and condition. 21 USC §360ee(b)(3)

[13] Johnson TW, Spurlock A, Galloway P. Blenderized formula by gastrostomy tube, a case presentation and review of literature. *Top Clin Nutr* 2013;*28*(1):84–92

[14] Brown B, Roehl K, Betz M. Enteral nutrition formula selection: current evidence and implications for practice. *Nutr Clin Pract* 2015;*30*(1):72–85

[15] Chen Y, Peterson SJ. Enteral nutrition formulas: which formula is right for your adult patient? *Nutr Clin Pract* 2009;*24*(3):344–355

[16] Cresci G, Lefton J, Esper DH. Enteral formulations. In: Mueller CM, ed. *The A.S.P.E.N. Adult Nutrition Support Core Curriculum.* 2nd ed. Silver Spring, MD: ASPEN; 2012

[17] Harkness L. The history of enteral nutrition therapy: from raw eggs and nasal tubes to purified amino acids and early postoperative jejunal delivery. *J Am Diet Assoc* 2002;*102*(3):399–404

[18] Pentiuk S, O'Flaherty T, Santoro K, Willging P, Kaul A. Pureed by gastrostomy tube diet improves gagging and retching in children with fundoplication. *JPEN J Parenter Enteral Nutr* 2011;*35*(3):375–379

[19] Bobo E. Reemergence of blenderized tube feedings: Exploring the evidence. *Nutr Clin Pract* 2016;*31*(6):730–735

# 14 Dysphagia Assessment and Treatment in the Neonatal Intensive Care Unit

*Pamela Dodrill and Saima Aftab*

## Summary

In the United States, approximately 1 in 10 babies are born prematurely each year, which equates to approximately 400,000 preterm infants entering the population annually. Infants require adequate energy balance to allow them to thrive and grow in the ex utero environment. Many preterm infants are born with inadequate energy stores, and they continue to struggle obtaining sufficient energy. Adequate energy and nutrition intake is essential during this very critical period of neonatal brain growth. If their energy and nutritional intake is less than their requirements, infants will display a negative energy balance and growth faltering, as well as potential increased risk for developmental delay and impaired cognitive outcomes. For many preterm infants, the major barrier to attaining full oral feeding is immaturity of suck–swallow–breathe coordination. Any intervention applied to assist the infant in achieving oral feeding success must consider physiological stability of the infant during feeds, efficiency of oral feeding, and gestational age at achievement of full oral feeding. There are varying levels of evidence to support different intervention strategies, and most are based on small sample sizes and short follow-up periods. As with all special populations, in the absence of high-quality scientific evidence to guide practice, any intervention used should be guided by individualized assessment, evaluated for efficacy, and discontinued or modified if not effective in achieving the documented outcome. Speech-language pathologists, and other disciplines with specialty training in the care of infants born prematurely, play an essential role in supporting safe and adequate oral intake.

## Keywords

preterm, premature, newborn, infant, Neonatal Intensive Care Unit), feeding, ebreastfeeding, bottle feeding, dysphagia

### Learning Objectives

- Describe, in detail, at least three etiologies of feeding difficulties in the neonatal intensive care unit (NICU)
- Explain how respiratory disorders common in the NICU can impact feeding development
- Explain the synactive theory of development and how it can impact oral feeding expectations of infants in the NICU
- Define the concept of suck–swallow–breathe coordination
- List the three main outcomes of interest for any feeding intervention implemented in the NICU environment
- Describe the different elements of a clinical swallowing and feeding assessment in the NICU

## 14.1 Introduction

Infants born following a term gestation are born between 37 and 42 weeks gestational age. Those infants born prior to 37 weeks gestational age are classified as premature. Prior to discharge, infants born prematurely must demonstrate physiological stability and have adequate nutritional intake. Successful infant feeding requires intact oral anatomy, intact neurophysiological responses, and coordination of those neurophysiological responses for safe and adequate oral intake. Premature infants are known to have swallowing and feeding difficulties due to system immaturity; comorbid conditions, especially those involving the respiratory and gastrointestinal systems; environmental causes; and iatrogenic causes. This chapter explores the many causes of feeding and swallowing problems for infants in the neonatal intensive care unit (NICU) and also describes the various treatment options available to best support adequate nutritional intake for infants born prematurely.

## 14.2 Case Presentation

### 14.2.1 Case History

You receive a referral to see a patient named Gerard.

- Gerard was born at 26/40 weeks' gestational age (GA) and is now aged 37/40 weeks. His birth weight was 750 g (26th percentile), and his Apgar scores were 5 at 1 minute and 8 at 5 minutes.
- You obtain the following case history from a brief review of his medical records:
  - Gerard was intubated soon after birth and received mechanical ventilation until day of life 3. At that point he was able to be switched to continuous positive airway pressure (CPAP) via mask, which he remained on for 6 weeks. He was then able to be switched to high-flow therapy via nasal cannula (HFNC), which he was on from 32/20 to 35/40 weeks. He remains on supplemental oxygen ($O_2$) therapy. He was trialed on room air at 36/40 weeks but was unable to maintain adequate oxygen saturation ($SpO_2$), so was returned to supplemental $O_2$ (25%).
  - Gerard has a history of patent ductus arteriosus (PDA). He also presented with apnea of prematurity and required caffeine treatment until 36/40 weeks. Gerard was in an isolette until 32/40 weeks and is now in an open crib. He displayed jaundice and required phototherapy for 2 weeks. He also displayed anemia and required three blood transfusions, and he continues on iron supplementation.
  - Gerard initially received parenteral nutrition from birth until 2 weeks of age. He began enteral gavage feeds at day of life 2, starting off with continuous nasogastric (NG) feeds,

then moving to bolus NG feeds within 24 hours. He displays some signs consistent with gastroesophageal reflux (GER) but is not receiving any active medical treatment. Gerard is receiving a combination of expressed breastmilk and formula.

- ○ Gerard was first offered oral feeds at 35/40 weeks, but he had been showing little interest until today.
- Describe how three factors in Gerard's respiratory history may potentially affect oral feeding.
- Describe how three factors in Gerard's gastrointestinal history may potentially affect oral feeding.
- Describe how three other factors in Gerard's medical history may potentially impact on oral feeding.
- In addition to the information provided, list three other pieces of information you would want to obtain from Gerard's medical record, medical team, or mother to help inform your feeding assessment.

## 14.2.2 Assessment

- Describe how you would explain the role of the feeding therapist to Gerard's mother.
- After obtaining a case history, describe the first steps in a feeding assessment.
- Knowing that Gerard's mother intends to offer some bottle feeds, describe how you would offer the first bottle feed (equipment, positioning, any other strategies).

If you assessed that Gerard was physiologically unstable during the feed assessment, and at risk of aspiration or apnea during feeds, describe how you would explain theses findings to his mother.

## 14.2.3 Management

- Describe how you would explain the role of milk flow in influencing suck—swallow—breath coordination to other staff and Gerard's mother.
- Describe how you would explain external pacing to other staff and Gerard's mother.
- In addition to the information obtained from the basic case history, you find out the additional information below:
  - ○ Gerard was a twin. His twin brother passed away shortly after birth due to complications associated with intestinal perforation.
  - ○ Gerard's mother miscarried her first pregnancy and underwent four cycles of fertility treatment prior to this pregnancy.
- Explain how this may affect his mother and how it would affect your interaction with her.
- Describe how you would explain to other staff the potential role of the feeding therapist in working with infants in the NICU prior to the commencement of oral feeding.

## 14.3 Epidemiology of Prematurity

### 14.3.1 Background

Typical human gestation is around 40 weeks, with a range of 37 to 42 weeks. Preterm birth is defined as birth prior to 37/40 weeks gestational age.[1] **Table 14.1** provides a breakdown of prematurity based on gestational age (GA) and birth weight.

**Table 14.1** Degrees of prematurity, based on gestational age and birth weight

|  | Extremely low | Very low | Low | Term |
|---|---|---|---|---|
| Gestational age | < 28;0 weeks | 28;0–31;6 weeks | 32;0–36;6 weeks | 37;0–41;6 weeks |
| Birth weight | < 1,000 g | < 1,500 g | 32;0–36;6 weeks | 3,500 g (average) |

### 14.3.2 Incidence

The current incidence rate of preterm birth in the United States is 9.6%, or 1 in 10 babies.[2,3] This equates to approximately 400,000 preterm infants entering the population each year. The rate of prematurity rate rose by 36% over 25 years (1981–2006),[2] due to factors such as increasing maternal age and increased use of assistive reproduction, as well as increased survival in this population. The incidence of preterm birth had recently been greater than 12%, but now has been slowly declining[2,3] due to factors such as improvements in antenatal care. Risk factors for preterm delivery include low or advanced maternal age, infection, a history of prior preterm birth, multiple births, high blood pressure during pregnancy, stress, tobacco and alcohol use, substance abuse, late prenatal care, and low maternal income or socioeconomic status.[3]

**Table 14.2** provides a list of common terms used to describe preterm infants and their care facilities.

## 14.4 Etiology of Feeding Difficulties in the NICU

### 14.4.1 Effects of Prematurity and Associated Illness on Feeding

In utero, oxygen and nutrients are provided for the fetus via the placenta. In the ex utero environment, infants are forced to breathe and feed for themselves, before their respiratory, gut, and neurologic body systems have fully matured. Many preterm infants are unable to complete these tasks without assistance. In addition to their prematurity, many preterm infants present with severe illnesses. Both prematurity and illness, as well as the interventions required to manage them (e.g., intubation, tube feeding, surgery, medications), have the potential to interrupt feeding development further in these infants.[4]

Infants require adequate energy balance to allow them to thrive and grow in the ex utero environment. Adequate energy and nutritional intake are also essential for this very critical period of neonatal brain growth. Unfortunately, many preterm infants are born with inadequate energy stores and then continue to struggle obtaining sufficient energy. If their energy and nutritional intake is less than their requirements, infants will display a negative energy balance and growth faltering, as well as potential increased risk for developmental delay and impaired cognitive outcomes.

There are three main contributors to negative energy balance that are common in the preterm population:

1. **Increased energy requirements:** The physiological demands of breathing, feeding, and thermoregulation with immature body systems result in increased energy demand for preterm infants. Medical conditions, including respiratory disease, hypotension, infection, and surgery, which are common in this population, also increase metabolic energy requirements and, thus, energy needs.

2. **Increased energy losses:** Immaturity of the gastrointestinal tract, including decreased gastrointestinal motility and reduced intestinal enzyme activity, and therapies such as corticosteroids (which are often used for chronic lung disease), can adversely affect digestion and growth. There can also be loss of feeds due to emesis (e.g., GER), which is relatively common in this population.

3. **Reduced energy intake:** Many preterm infants display immature and inefficient feeding skills, which result in reduced intake by mouth. In addition, many preterm infants display reduced stamina for the work of oral feeding due to poor energy reserves and illness. Some medical treatments necessary in this population (e.g., intubation and ventilation) can also have an impact on the ability to feed by mouth.

Prolonged hospitalization can affect the family's ability to interact and bond with their infant, which can have an impact on feeding interactions. Hospitalization can have other effects as well:

- Illness and physiological instability can affect the infant's ability to tolerate handling.
- Motor delays/disorders can affect the infant's ability to interact normally to stimulation.
- Immature state control (i.e., level of alertness) can result in the infant spending large amounts of time either sleeping or in an irritable state, and not in a state suitable for feeding or other interaction.
- Noxious environmental stimuli (bright lights, loud hospital noises, painful procedures) can cause the preterm infant's developing sensory system to react and show signs of distress or go into shutdown.

Infant feeding difficulties can add to parental feelings of guilt, inadequacy, or failure, which are common in the NICU environment, contributing toward an incredible amount of stress. Hence it is essential that parents are provided with support and training in how best to assist their infant.

It is important to remember that in infancy, relative to other times in life, there is never a time when nutrition is more important, there is never a time when the brain is more plastic, and there is never a time when an individual is more dependent on others for meeting nutritional and developmental needs.

**Table 14.2** Common terms used in relation to preterm infants

| | |
|---|---|
| Postmenstrual age (PMA) | Age of infant based on time since the date at start of the mother's last menstrual cycle.<br>This is the most common method for estimating the age of a fetus and calculating estimated due date (estimated due date = 280 days [40 weeks] from date at start of the mother's last menstrual cycle). |
| Postconceptional age (PCA) | Age of infant based on time since known conception date.<br>PCA is generally 14 days less than PMA. |
| Gestational age (GA) | Often used interchangeably with PMA.<br>*GA at birth* is age based on the time between date at start of the mother's last menstrual cycle and birth.<br>*Corrected GA* is an infant's current age calculated from date of mother's last menstrual cycle (e.g., a child who was born at 28 weeks GA, who is now 4 weeks old, would be 32 weeks CGA).<br>An infant's "due date" is 40 weeks GA. Thus GA is often written in the format of:<br>• 34/40 or 34;0 to signify 34 weeks GA<br>• 34⁴/40 or 34;4 to signify 34 weeks and 4 days GA |
| Chronological age | Age of infant based on time since birth.<br>Chronological age does not take into consideration degree of prematurity. |
| Corrected age (CA) | The age of the infant relative to the expected delivery date (due date)<br>(e.g., a child who was born 8 weeks early at 32/40 weeks, who is now 10 weeks old, would be 2 weeks CA). |
| Small for GA (SGA) | An infant born smaller than would be expected for his or her GA (generally defined as BW < 10%ile for GA). |
| Intrauterine growth restriction/retardation (IUGR) | This term describes a fetus that has not reached its growth potential because of genetic or environmental factors in utero (also known as pathological SGA). |
| Neonatal intensive care unit (NICU) | Intensive care unit for medically unstable infants who require life-sustaining treatments (e.g., mechanical ventilation) and/or surgery. Generally 1:1 or 1:2 nurse to patient ratio. |
| Special care nursery (SCN) | Step-down unit for infants who require medical supervision and/or interventions, such as tube feeds, but who are generally medically stable. SCNs have fewer nurses to patients than NICUs. |

*Note:* Different regions use different systems to define the various levels (and sublevels) of care for high-risk infants. *NICU* and *SCN* are two of the more common terms used to describe the two main levels, but these terms are not used universally.

## 14.4.2 Synactive Theory of Development

The synactive theory of development[5] was developed by Heidelise Als, who is widely considered the founder of modern developmental care in the NICU environment. The theory describes the infant's four subsystems of functioning, and their continuous interaction with each other and with the environment across time.

1. **Physiological (autonomic) subsystem:** Expressed in the pattern of respiration (e.g., fast, slow, pauses), cardiovascular functioning and color changes (e.g., pink, red, pale, blue), neurologic indicators (e.g., seizures, tremulousness), and visceral or gut signals (e.g., bowel movements, gagging, and hiccupping) observed at rest and during activity.

2. **Motor subsystem:** Observable through the tone, posture, and movement patterns of the infant, and through the infant's tolerance of handling and ability to achieve a supportive flexed position.

3. **State and attention/interaction subsystem:** Expressed via the range of states available to the infant (i.e., deep sleep, light sleep, drowsy, alert, hyperalert, and crying), how clear it is to observably differentiate one state from the other, and the patterns of transitions from one state to another (e.g., smooth, well-differentiated state transitions vs. abrupt, unorganized state transitions). The infant uses the alert, attentive state to take in information from the environment; hence the amount of time the infant spends in this state is indicative of his or her learning ability.

4. **Regulatory subsystem:** Behaviorally represented via (a) self-regulation—the observable strategies the infant uses to achieve stability or for self-recovery, and (b) coregulation—the type and amount of support required from the caregiver (e.g., supporting a tucked, flexed position of the infant's arms and legs) or the environment (e.g., dimming the lights in the nursery). Coregulation may be necessary to help the infant's return to balance in situations when his or her own self-regulatory capacities are exceeded.

The graphic representation of the synactive theory (**Fig. 14.1**) depicts the developing infant in constant interaction with the environment from within the in utero to the ex utero environment. This theory gives NICU clinicians the framework and tools with which to identify the infant's strengths, challenges, and accomplishments. The synactive theory is the foundation of both:

- **The Assessment of Preterm Infants' Behavior**[6]: a standardized assessment of newborn behavior and functioning
- **The Newborn Individualized Developmental Care and Assessment Program**[7]: a care and intervention approach that focuses on each infant's behavioral cues in order to support

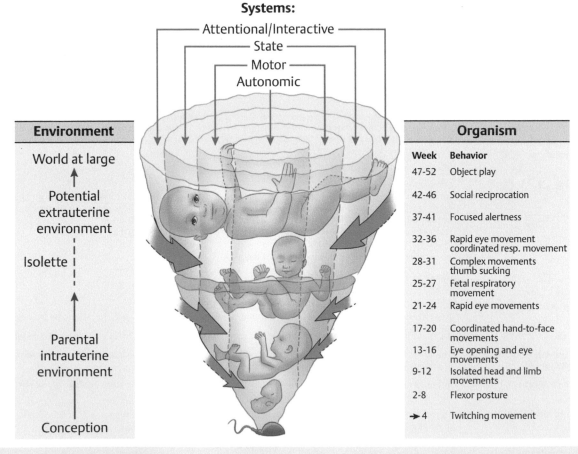

**Fig. 14.1** The synactive theory of development.[5]

the infant's strengths and reduce his or her vulnerabilities (also known as cue-based care, individualized care, or developmentally supportive care). The infant's family is viewed as the infant's most important nurturer and is integrated in all care throughout the infant's hospitalization (often referred to as family-centered care).

### 14.4.3 Development and Illness in Major Body Systems in the NICU Population

#### Neurological Development
The central nervous system matures in a bottom-up sequence.

- During the first trimester of gestation, early synapses begin forming in a fetus's spinal cord.[8,9,10]
- In the second trimester, the brainstem begins to mature.[8,9,10]
  - Brainstem-mediated reflexes, such as breathing movements and primitive sucking and swallowing, begin to emerge.
  - By the end of the second trimester, the brainstem provides autonomic function (control of other basic life functions, such as heart rate, blood pressure, digestion, and sleep), which enables some infants to become capable of survival in the ex utero environment.
- In the third trimester, the cerebral volume and surface area increase markedly.[8,9,10]
  - The cerebral cortex is responsible for most of what we think of as functional life (voluntary actions, thinking, remembering).
  - Preterm infants show only very basic electrical activity in primary motor regions and in the primary sensory regions of the cerebral cortex (those areas that perceive touch, hearing, and vision),[9] because these areas have not developed well by the time of birth.

### 14.4.4 Neurological Disorders and Related Conditions Common in the NICU Population That Can Have an Impact on Feeding

- **Intraventricular hemorrhage** (IVH) is bleeding into the fluid-filled areas (ventricles) of the brain. It commonly occurs in preterm infants born less than 34/40 weeks GA[8] due to vulnerability of the blood vessels of the germinal matrix in the floor of the lateral ventricles. IVH is graded into four categories:
  - **Grade I:** Bleeding occurs only in the germinal matrix.
  - **Grade II:** Bleeding occurs inside the ventricles, but they are not enlarged.
  - **Grade III:** Ventricles are enlarged by accumulated blood.
  - **Grade IV:** Bleeding extends into the brain tissue around the ventricles.
  - IVH grades I and II are most common, and usually resolve without permanent complications.[8]
  - IVH grades III and IV are the most serious and may result in long-term brain injury to the infant.[8,9,10] After a grade III or IV IVH, blood clots may form, which can block the flow of cerebrospinal fluid (CSF), leading to increased fluid in the brain (posthemorrhagic hydrocephalus).
- **Hydrocephalus** is a condition in which there is an abnormal accumulation of CSF in the ventricles of the brain. This may cause increased intracranial pressure inside the skull and progressive enlargement of the head. Hydrocephalus can also cause seizures, intellectual impairment, or death, as a result of damage to brain structures from compression. Management of hydrocephalus often involves inserting a shunt to allow drainage of CSF.
- **Periventricular leukomalacia** is a brain injury characterized by the death of white matter (leuko = white, malacia = soft) near the lateral ventricles. Preterm infants are at the greatest risk of this condition.[8] Because of the location of the injury, affected individuals may exhibit motor control problems and other developmental delays, and they often develop cerebral palsy or epilepsy.[8,9,10]
- **Hypoxic ischemic encephalopathy (HIE)** results from hypoxia and/or ischemia to the cerebral circulation. It can occur during birth (birth asphyxia) or in the perinatal period, and it results in variable inflammation, injury, or death of neural tissues of the brain (other organs may also be affected). Many children with HIE will develop intellectual impairment or learning difficulties, and some develop sensory and motor impairments, such as cerebral palsy.[10] The only treatment that has been shown to reduce the symptoms of HIE is the use of therapeutic hypothermia (a deliberate reduction of the core body temperature, typically to around 32° to 34°C [89.6° to 93.2°F], with the intention of reducing metabolic rate). Therapeutic hypothermia for 3 days postbirth has been shown to reduce brain damage and lead to improved survival and reduced disability.[11]

### 14.4.5 Gut Development

Anatomical development of the fetal gut is essentially complete by 20/40 weeks GA.[8,9,10] However, maturation of physiological function does not occur until later in gestation, and extends throughout the early postnatal period.[8,9,10] Gastrointestinal function that is immature at birth increases the risk of malabsorption (failure to fully absorb nutrients ingested), specific gut disease (e.g., necrotizing enterocolitis, see following description), and malnutrition. Functional and anatomical maturation is evidenced by improvements in esophageal motility, function of the lower esophageal sphincter (which acts to control GER), gastric emptying, intestinal motility, and development of the absorptive surface area of the gut.

### 14.4.6 Gastrointestinal and Related Conditions Common in the NICU Population That Can Have an Impact on Feeding

- **Necrotizing enterocolitis (NEC)** is a condition where portions of the bowel undergo inflammation and necrosis (tissue death).

NEC occurs most frequently in very preterm infants (< 32/40 weeks GA).[8] Surgical correction usually requires removing a section of the bowel, which results in a shortening of the gut length and reduced absorptive area (short gut syndrome). The baby may present with belly distension, abdominal tenderness, poor tolerance of feeds, and bloody stools. Early radiological signs of NEC may include bowel dilation, air bubbles in the bowel wall (pneumatosis intestinalis), and, in more severe cases, signs of perforation with free air in the abdomen.

- **Gastroesophageal reflux (GER)** is the return of stomach contents into the esophagus (and sometimes the pharynx and mouth). GER is usually caused by low tone in the lower esophageal sphincter (LES), which normally holds the top of the stomach closed, reduced gastric emptying, and/or abnormal pressure in the abdomen.

- **Gastroesophageal reflux disease** (GERD) is a chronic symptom of mucosal damage caused by stomach acid in the esophagus. Treatment may consist of the following:

  o Feed manipulations (e.g., smaller, more frequent feeds, slow bolus feeds into the stomach, continuous feeds into the stomach or into the small intestines—also known as transpyloric/postpyloric feeds, which may be duodenal or jejunal feeds).

  o Positioning changes (e.g., elevated bed, left side down). These should only be used when the child is in a supervised environment. They should not be used during sleep at home, if the child is not in direct view of an attentive adult (see sudden infant death syndrome [SIDS] guidelines for safe sleep).

  o Specialty formula (e.g., semielemental or elemental feeds) if protein allergy or intolerance is thought to be contributing to reflux or otherwise causing gastrointestinal distress.

  o Thickened feeds are sometimes used as part of GER management in older children.[12] However, due to the risk of poor digestion and gut damage, they should not be used in infants prior to term age,[13] or in those at risk with gut disease or cardiac conditions that can lead to poor gut perfusion, because this may increase the risk of NEC.

  o Pharmacological treatment, such as proton pump inhibitors or histamine receptor antagonists, may be considered if GERD symptoms persist after other treatment options are applied. However, potential side effects of these medications must be considered.

  o Surgery (e.g., fundoplication) is occasionally considered in those whose GER does not improve with other interventions.

- **Jaundice** (or hyperbilirubinemia or icterus) is a yellowing of the skin and other tissues (e.g., sclera of eyes) caused by increased levels of bilirubin. In neonates, a bilirubin level of more than 85 $\mu$mol/L manifests as clinical jaundice.[8,9,10] In most cases, jaundice is benign and will resolve within 2 to 3 weeks after birth, or sooner with light treatment (phototherapy). Adverse symptoms to be alert for include if the infant appears lethargic, is feeding poorly, or is making high-pitched (irritable) cries. Prolonged high levels of bilirubin can put a baby at risk for neurologic injury (kernicterus).[8,9,10]

- **Diabetes** is a group of metabolic diseases in which there are high blood glucose levels over a prolonged period. Diabetes is caused by either the pancreas not producing enough insulin or the cells of the body not responding properly to the insulin produced (insulin resistance). Increased health risk has been found for infants of mothers with gestational diabetes (a temporary form of diabetes caused by hormonal changes during pregnancy), as well as those of mothers with prepregnancy type 1 (insulin-dependent) and type 2 (non-insulin-dependent/insulin-resistant) diabetes.[8,9,10] The main risks to infants of diabetic mothers are fetal obesity (macrosomia) and low blood sugar levels (leading to lethargy, irritability, and potential neurologic injury).[8,9,10] Infants of diabetic mothers are also at increased risk of respiratory distress syndrome (due to reduced surfactant production), hyperbilirubinemia, and mild neurological deficits.[8,9,10] Given their larger size they are also more prone to injury during the birthing process. This may be in the form of head trauma, with or without bleeding in the skull or brain, fractures, or nerve palsies.

## 14.4.7 Gastrointestinal Management in the NICU Population

There are a number of terms used to describe feeding options used in the NICU to ensure that infants receive the appropriate amounts of fluid, energy, nutrition, and medications. These are summarized below:

- **PO** (per os): by mouth
- **NPO** (nil per os): nothing by mouth
- **PG** (per gavage): by gavage tube into the gut through various routes:
  o **NG** (nasogastric) tube: a feeding tube inserted via the nose into the stomach; often left indwelling; can be used to deliver bolus or continuous feeds
  o **OG** (orogastric) tube: a feeding tube inserted via the mouth into the stomach; sometimes inserted intermittently for feeds and removed afterward; sometimes left indwelling and used when the nostrils are occluded (e.g., by CPAP prongs)
  o **NJ** (nasojejunal) tube: a feeding tube inserted via the mouth into the intestines; also known as transpyloric/postpyloric feeds; generally used when there are concerns for complications from GER; feeds are delivered continuously
  o **G** (gastrostomy) tube: a feeding tube inserted directly into the stomach surgically; can be used to deliver bolus or continuous feeds
  o **GJ** (gastrojejunal) tube: a feeding tube inserted directly into the stomach surgically with extension into the intestines; feeds are delivered continuously
  o **J** (jejunostomy) tube: a feeding tube inserted directly into the intestines surgically; feeds are delivered continuously
- **Parenteral nutrition:** by peripheral intravenous line or central line into bloodstream

## 14.4.8 Cardiac Development

There are a number of changes to the cardiovascular system around birth, summarized as follows:

- **In utero** the placenta performs the function of gas exchange (providing oxygen and removing carbon dioxide), which means the placenta does the "breathing" for the fetus instead of the lungs. As a result, only a small amount of the blood (approximately 10% of the cardiac output) needs to pass through the lungs.[8] Most of the remaining blood is bypassed (shunted) away from the lungs, traveling from the pulmonary artery to the aorta through an opening known as the ductus arteriosus.

- **Ex utero** deoxygenated (blue) blood flows into the right side of the heart from the superior and inferior vena cava veins. It travels through the right atrium and ventricle of the heart, and then travels via the pulmonary artery to the lungs, where it is reoxygenated. This oxygenated (red) blood travels through the pulmonary veins to the left side of the heart. It then travels through the left atrium and ventricle and leaves the heart via the aorta.

- **At birth** the newborn needs to transition from the fluid-filled environment of the amniotic sac to the outside air-filled environment and to commence spontaneous breathing. Normally, the ductus arteriosus starts closing over within the first hours after birth, directing the majority of blood entering the heart to pass through the lungs before returning to the heart. Once breathing is established, pulmonary pressures also start to drop, which also facilitates increased blood flow to the lungs.

## 14.4.9 Cardiac and Hematological Disorders Common in the NICU Population That Can Have an Impact on Feeding

- **Patent ductus arteriosus** (PDA) is a condition in which the ductus arteriosus remains patent (i.e., does not close over), as would normally occur following birth. This can cause pulmonary overcirculation and heart failure. Sometimes the PDA will close spontaneously with time. In cases where this does not occur and is causing pulmonary overcirculation, treatment may be required. This may include pharmacological treatment (indomethacin or ibuprofen) or surgical treatment (via catheter or ligation). Injury to the left recurrent laryngeal nerve may occur during surgical ligation of a PDA, potentially resulting in left vocal cord paralysis and increased risk for **aspiration** with oral feeds.[14,15]

- **Persistent pulmonary hypertension of the newborn** (PPHN) is caused by failure of the normal circulatory transition that occurs after birth. The pulmonary vascular resistance remains high, leading to right-to-left shunting of blood within the heart at the level of a PDA and/or a patent foramen ovale (PFO). This results in increased work for the lungs and hypoxemia.

- **Acyanotic heart defects** are a group of heart conditions where there is overcirculation and left-to-right shunting of blood within the heart. These conditions are typically not associated with cyanosis, but they do place stress on the heart, which has to pump more oxygenated blood through to keep up with any losses.

- **Cyanotic heart defects** are a group of heart conditions that present with low oxygen saturation and cyanosis. This either results from insufficient pulmonary blood flow or abnormal vascular connections. They are usually caused by structural defects of the heart that allow right-to-left shunting.

- **Extracorporeal membrane oxygenation** (ECMO) is a form of heart–lung bypass that is used when the heart and lungs are unable to perform adequate gas exchange. ECMO works by removing blood from the body, oxygenating red blood cells (RBCs), and removing carbon dioxide from the blood through a membrane. ECMO is typically used either as a bridge to surgery or to allow the heart to recover from temporary diseases, such as pulmonary hypertension.

- **Anemia of prematurity** is a condition in which blood lacks enough hemoglobin (healthy RBCs). During the first weeks of life, all infants experience a decline in circulating RBC volume. However, preterm infants experience increased RBC decline due to immaturity of organs involved in RBC production, blood loss from bleeding and blood testing, and nutritional deficiencies. Hemoglobin binds oxygen; hence, when the hemoglobin level is low, the cells in the body will not receive enough oxygen. Anemia often presents as pallor and lethargy and can contribute to respiratory symptoms, such as tachycardia and tachypnea. Treatment may involve iron supplementation ($FeSO_4$, erythropoietin) and a possible need for blood transfusion.

## 14.4.10 Lung Development

The lungs are among the latest organ systems to reach an ex utero survival threshold:

- **By 23/40 weeks GA,** some primitive alveoli are present and are vascularized enough that the respiratory system is able to perform basic gas exchange and ex utero respiration is possible.[8,9,10] This is part of the reason that 23 weeks GA is considered the limit of viability for premature neonates.

- **By 28/40 weeks GA,** more alveoli are present, and vascularization is better developed, allowing for greater gas exchange. Type I alveolar cells, which secrete surfactant (see next section), begin to appear.[8,9,10]

  o Surfactant acts to increase pulmonary compliance (ease of expansion of the lungs) and prevent atelectasis (collapse of part(s) of the lung).

  o Neonates with insufficient surfactant often require exogenous (transplanted) surfactant treatment until endogenous (self-developed) production is established.

- **By 32 to 34/40 weeks GA,** alveolar development reaches a structural and functional stage where respiration is generally more efficient. Gas exchange may be developed sufficiently that well neonates at this age are not likely to require any mechanical ventilatory assistance.

- **By 37/40 weeks GA,** immature alveoli have developed and surfactant production is generally sufficient for normal respiration.

- **Alveoli numbers** continue to develop over the first 2 years of life.

## 14.4.11 Respiratory Disorders Common in the NICU Population That Can Have an Impact on Feeding

- **Respiratory distress syndrome** (RDS), also known as hyaline membrane disease, is a condition caused by insufficient surfactant production. Surfactant is a lipid–protein compound that decreases surface tension of the alveoli and helps prevent collapse during exhalation. RDS often occurs as a consequence of premature birth.

- **Bronchopulmonary dysplasia** (BPD), also known as chronic neonatal lung disease, is a chronic lung condition characterized by inflammation and scarring in the lungs. BPD is most common among those who received prolonged assisted ventilation to treat RDS.[8] Barotrauma, oxygen-related injury, and infection are the main causes of BPD.[8]
  - **Mild:** Need for supplemental oxygen for ≥ 28 days, but not at 36/40 weeks GA or discharge
  - **Moderate:** Need for supplemental oxygen for ≥ 28 days plus treatment with < 30% $O_2$ at 36/40 weeks GA
  - **Severe:** Need for supplemental oxygen for ≥ 28 days plus treatment with ≥ 30% $O_2$ and/or positive pressure ventilation at 36/40 weeks GA[8]

- **Atelectasis** is the collapse of one of more lung segments, preventing gas exchange in that area.

- **Pneumothorax** is the collapse of one of more lung segments, accompanied by air escape from the lung. The escaped air builds up in the pleural space between the lung and chest wall, putting pressure on the lung from the outside, causing collapse of the lung and making breathing more difficult. In severe cases, these infants may experience cardiorespiratory arrest.

- **Stridor** is a high-pitched breath sound resulting from turbulent air flow in the airway at or below the level of the larynx.

- **Laryngo-/tracheo-/bronchomalacia** is a condition where the larynx (and/or trachea and bronchi) are softer and less rigid than usual (*malacia* means soft tissue). Laryngomalacia is the most common cause of inspiratory stridor in early infancy,[8,10] due to the soft cartilage of the airway collapsing inward during inhalation, causing upper airway obstruction. Tracheomalacia or bronchomalacia is mostly associated with expiratory stridor.

- **Pulmonary hypoplasia** is incomplete development of the lungs, resulting in a reduced number of bronchopulmonary segments and/or alveoli. It most often occurs secondary to other fetal abnormalities that interfere with normal development of the lungs. It may be seen in the setting of severe oligohydroamnios, congenital diaphragmatic hernias, and severe chest wall deformities.

- **Apnea of the newborn**, or apnea of prematurity, is defined as cessation of breathing that lasts for more than 20 seconds and/or more than 10 seconds if accompanied by hypoxia or bradycardia.[16] **Apnea** is traditionally classified as either central, obstructive, or mixed.
  - **Central apnea** occurs when there is a lack of respiratory effort. This may result from central nervous system immaturity or from the effects of medications or illness. Respiratory drive is primarily dependent on response to increased levels of carbon dioxide ($CO_2$) (hypercapnia) and acid in the blood (acidosis). A secondary stimulus is low levels of oxygen in the blood (hypoxemia). Responses to these stimuli are impaired in premature infants due to immaturity in regions of the brainstem that sense these changes. Caffeine therapy is often used to assist in managing central apnea.
  - **Obstructive apnea** can occur due to low pharyngeal muscle tone or to inflammation of the soft tissues, which can block the flow of air though the pharynx and larynx. It may also occur when the infant's neck is hyperflexed or hyperextended.
  - **Mixed apnea** arises when episodes of apnea of prematurity that start as either central or obstructive change to involve elements of both and thus become *mixed* in nature.
  - **Apnea can also be induced** in premature infants who have an exaggerated response to laryngeal stimulation. Touch-pressure receptors within the pharynx can be stimulated by the presence of NG tubes. Stretch receptors may be stimulated by a large fluid bolus. Chemoreceptors can be stimulated by aspiration of food or by reflux of gastric content.

## 14.4.12 Respiratory Management in the NICU Population

- Mechanical ventilation is used to provide respiratory support to a patient with ineffective or absent spontaneous breathing. Spontaneous breathing can be affected by neurological, anatomical, or physiological abnormalities. Many extremely and very preterm infants are initially unable to breathe spontaneously, as they lack respiratory drive due to immaturity of their brainstem.

**Table 14.3** Types of non-invasive ventilation support

| | |
|---|---|
| Supplemental $O_2$ therapy | Additional $O_2$ mixed with room air (of potentially varying concentrations) usually applied via mask or nasal cannula (note: $O_2$ supplementation can also be used on top of mechanical ventilation, CPAP, or HFNC). If applied via mask or traditional nasal cannual, the flow delivered is considered 'low-flow'. |
| Heated-humidified high-flow therapy | 'High-flow' therapy (also known as transnasal insufflation) consists of room air (+/- additional $O_2$) that is heated and humidified to allow higher flow rates than can be delivered via traditional nasal cannula. This can allow the delivery of flow rates that meet or exceed the patient's inspiratory flow rate (i.e. usually some degree of positive pressure is achieved). |
| CPAP | Positive airway pressure (+/- additional $O_2$) applied throughout the respiratory cycle to a patient who is spontaneously breathing. Usually applied via mask, but can be delivered by a special nasal cannula. Conventional CPAP systems allow measurement of received airway pressure and can automatically correct for leak. Other systems (e.g. bubble CPAP) only allow measurement of delivered pressure vs received airway pressure, and do not automatically correct for leak. |

- In patients who have respiratory drive and are spontaneously breathing, but are unable to ventilate sufficiently (e.g. due to immature lung development), other forms of ventilatory support can be used. These include continuous positive airway pressure (CPAP), heated-humidified high-flow therapy, and supplemental oxygen therapy (O2).

- Ventilatory support is considered to be delivering positive pressure if it delivers air and/or O2 flow that meets or exceeds the patient's inspiratory flow demands. Positive pressure stents open the patient's airway, which can increase lung volume, reduce the risk of obstructive apnea and atelectasis, and reduce work of breathing.

- The aim of any ventilatory support measure is to achieve adequate airflow volume and O2 supply to the lungs with the lowest possible airway pressure (high pressure at the level of the alveoli can cause lung damage – e.g. pneumothorax, bronchopulmonary dysplasia) and lowest possible amount of supplemental O2 (oxygen toxicity can cause damage to fragile blood vessels and associated complications - e.g. retinopathy of prematurity from oxygen toxicity to the immature retinal blood vessels).

- Ventilation is deemed invasive if it is delivered directly into the lower airway via endotracheal tube (ETT) or tracheostomy, and noninvasive if delivered into the upper airway via an interface, such as a nasal mask or nasal prongs/ cannula.

- Common forms of noninvasive ventilatory support used in the NICU include nasal CPAP (nCPAP) delivered via mask or nasal cannula, high-flow therapy via nasal cannula (HFNC), low-flow O2 therapy via nasal canula (LFNC), and blow-by O2 via mask (BBO2).

- Clinicians have to weigh the relative benefits and risks of different interfaces. Ideally, interfaces should have minimal leak (i.e. minimal escape of gas, so that received airflow pressure and O2 volume is similar to what is delivered), while causing the minimal trauma to the face (particularly the nose), pharynx, larynx, and lower airway.

- Extracorporeal membrane oxygenation (ECMO) is a form of cardiopulmonary bypass used for infants who cannot be oxygenated adequately or ventilated with conventional ventilation support measures. Blood is cycled out of the body, through a membrane oxygenator that acts as an artificial lung by removing CO2 and adding O2, before the blood is cycled back through the body.

# 14.5 Pathophysiology of Feeding Difficulties in the NICU

## 14.5.1 Sucking

### Development of Structures and Functions Necessary for Sucking

Oral reflexes and feeding-like behaviors begin to emerge in utero and continue to mature throughout the period up to term age and beyond. In clinical practice, most feeding assessments will commence with an examination of the oral region and an assessment of oral reflexes (see Chapter 5). However, on their own, intact oral reflexes, such as sucking, do not necessarily indicate that the infant is ready for oral feeds.[17,18,19] Hence factors other than those assessed in a basic oral examination must also be considered when one is deciding whether an infant is ready to commence oral feeding.

### Development of Nonnutritive Sucking

Nonnutritive sucking is the type of sucking seen when an infant is not feeding. To elicit nonnutritive sucking, a gloved finger or pacifier is generally placed in the infant's mouth. In preterm infants, this type of sucking is generally seen as a precursor to nutritive sucking, and some degree of nonnutritive sucking can often be elicited weeks before nutritive sucking emerges.[20,21] Nonnutritive sucking generally becomes more rhythmic and stronger with maturity,[22,23] and the literature suggests that 34 weeks GA represents an important milestone in the maturation process, with significant improvements in number of sucks and intensity of sucking pressures.[24,25]

### Development of Nutritive Sucking

Nutritive sucking is the type of sucking seen when an infant is feeding. It results in infants drawing milk into their mouth from the breast or bottle. Greater displacement of the tongue is required during nutritive sucking compared with nonnutritive sucking.[26] Nutritive sucking is also characterized by slower, more rhythmic sucking movements, with regular breaks required for swallowing and breathing.[26]

Numerous studies indicate that, like nonnutritive sucking, nutritive sucking skills generally improve with maturity[27,28,29,30] as well as with practice.[31,32] Lau et al[24] developed a classification scale (**Fig. 14.2**) for sucking skills, consisting of five primary stages, based on the presence/absence of suction and the rhythmicity of the two components of sucking: positive pressure (i.e., expression/ compression) and negative pressure (i.e., suction). The authors reported that significant positive correlations are observed between GA, the five stages of sucking, feeding performance during feeds, and the number of daily oral feedings. The authors also reported that overall milk transfer and rate of transfer (i.e., feeding efficiency) are enhanced when infants reach the more mature stages of sucking.

Palmer et al[33] developed the Neonatal Oral Motor Assessment Scale (NOMAS), which categorizes oral skills involved in sucking as normal, dysfunctional, or disorganized. Studies using this tool have shown improvement in NOMAS scores for preterm infants with increasing GA,[30,34] and moderate correlations have been reported between scores on the NOMAS and feeding performance up to 36 weeks GA.[35]

More recently, Thoyre et al[36] developed the Early Feeding Skills (EFS) Assessment, which categorizes necessary oral skills involved in sucking as being present none, some, most, or all of the time, in recognition of the fact that preterm infants generally become more consistent with their oral skills with advancing age. In addition to rating sucking skills, this tool can also be used to rate coordination of sucking and swallowing, physiological stability, and engagement in feeding.

| Stage | Sample Tracings | | Suction/Expression Amplitude Range of Tracing (mm Hg) | Description |
|---|---|---|---|---|
| **1A** and **1B** | Suction 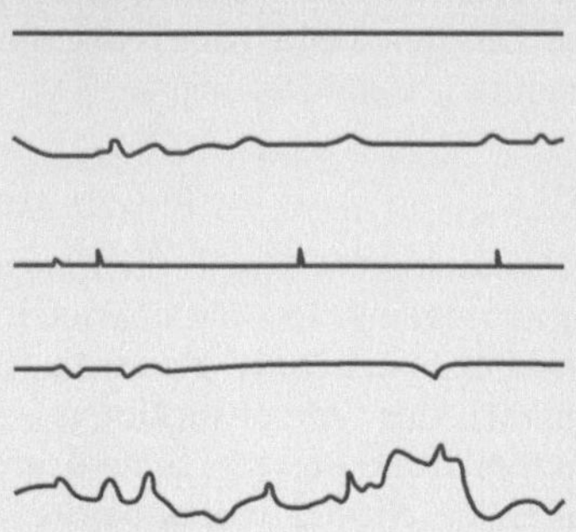 | | Absent | No suction |
| | Expression | | +0.5 to +1.0 mm Hg | Arrhythmic expression |
| | Time (sec) | | | and |
| | Suction | | −2.5 to −12.5 mm Hg | Arrhythmic alternation suction/expression |
| | Expression | | +0.5 to +1.0 mm Hg | |
| **2A** and **2B** | Suction 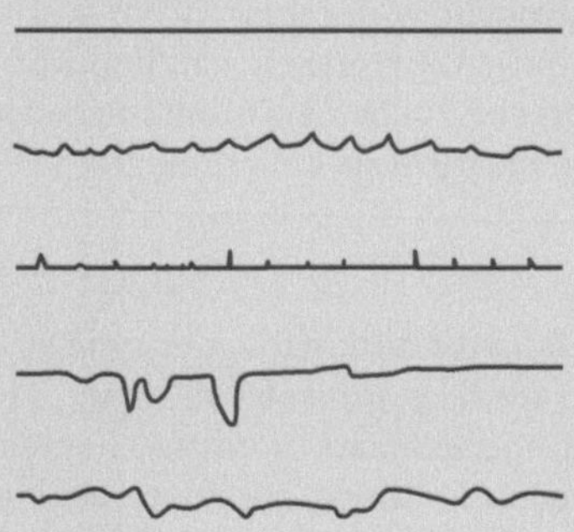 | | Absent | No suction |
| | Expression | | +0.2 to +0.4 mm Hg | Rhythmic expression |
| | Time (sec) | | | and |
| | Suction | | −7.5 to −15.0 mm Hg | Arrhythmic alternation of suction/expression presence of sucking bursts |
| | Expression | | +0.2 mm Hg | |
| **3A** and **3B** | Suction 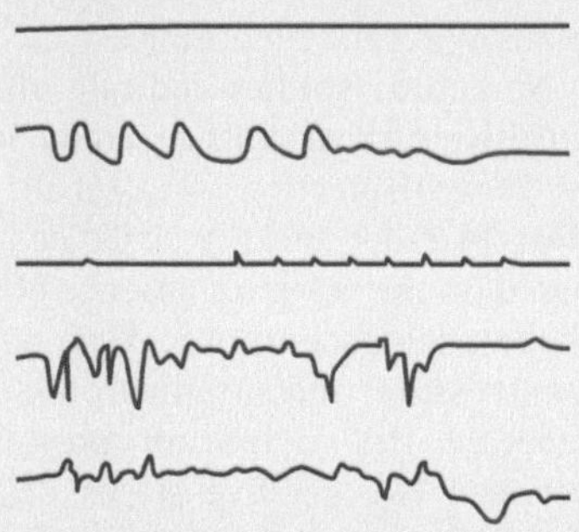 | | Absent | No suction |
| | Expression | | +0.8 to +1.0 mm Hg | Rhythmic expression and |
| | Time (sec) | | | Rhythmic suction/expression: |
| | Suction | | −15 to −75 mm Hg | - Suction amplitude - Wild amplitude range |
| | Expression | | +0.5 to +0.7 mm Hg | - Prolonged sucking bursts |
| **4** | Suction 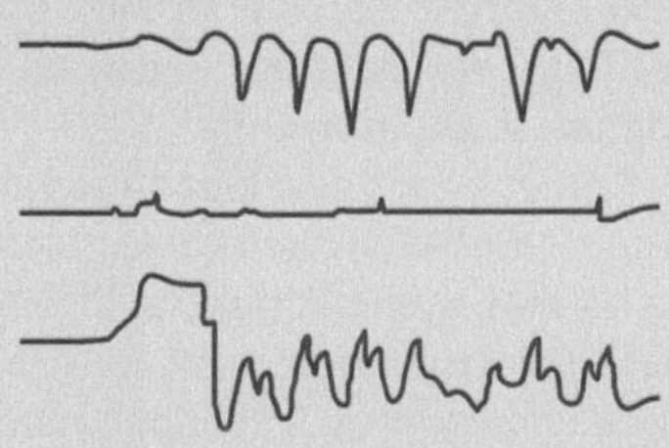 | | −50 to −75 mm Hg | Rhythmic suction/expression: - Suction well defined - Decreased amplitude range |
| | Time (sec) | | | |
| | Expression | | +0.4 to +1.0 mm Hg | |
| **5** | Suction 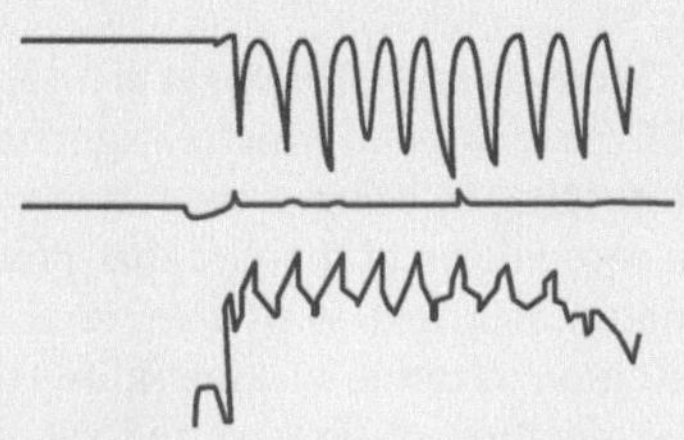 | | −110 to −160 mm Hg | Rhythmic/well defined suction/expression: - Suction amplitude increase - Sucking pattern similar to that of full-term infant |
| | Time (sec) | | | |
| | Expression | | +0.6 to +0.75 mm Hg | |

**Fig. 14.2** Characterization of the developmental stages of sucking in preterm infants during bottle feeding, by Lau et al.[24]

Once preterm infants approach term age, it is often assumed that their nutritive feeding skills will match those of full-term infants. However, numerous research studies indicate that the sucking patterns of preterm infants often remain significantly less coordinated and less efficient than those of full-term infants at term age and beyond.[25,29,37,38,39,40,41] In addition, preterm infants born small for GA can take even longer to develop a fully efficient sucking pattern than preterm infants born at an appropriate size for GA.[29] Besides potentially prolonging the need for tube feeding and delaying discharge to home, ongoing sucking problems in preterm infants at or around term age have been reported to be are predictive of poorer developmental outcomes later in infanthood.[42,43,44]

## 14.5.2 Suck—Swallow—Breath Coordination

### Suck—Swallow—Breath Cycle

Within the pharynx, swallowing and breathing utilize a common space; hence difficulties are often observed when sucking, swallowing, and breathing are not well coordinated. Suck—swallow—breath (SSB) coordination is more important during nutritive sucking than during nonnutritive sucking, which means that an infant who displays coordinated sucking on a finger or pacifier may not necessarily display coordinated sucking during oral feeds.[45] Research has shown that components of sucking, swallowing, and breathing and their coordinated activity mature at different times and rates in preterm infants.[46] Several studies have also reported that preterm infants often swallow preferentially at different phases of respiration than do their full-term counterparts,[47,48,49] which puts them at increased risk of aspiration and apnea events during feeds.

### Respiratory Support during Sucking

Preterm infants generally develop improved respiratory support for oral feeding as they mature. Research has shown that deglutition apnea times (the normal brief cessation in breathing that occurs during swallowing) reduce as neonates mature and swallowing becomes more efficient.[50] Studies have also shown that the number and length of episodes of multiple-swallow deglutition apnea reduce with maturation.[51,52] Consequently, with advancing GA, preterm neonates generally experience fewer drops in ventilation during feeds and recover more quickly.[53] However, even at term age, some preterm neonates continue to display oxygen desaturation events during feeding.[54]

Clinicians involved in feeding preterm infants need to monitor the infant for drops in respiratory rate and ventilation during feeds, as well as apnea events, because any of these problems may indicate immaturity or dysfunction in SSB coordination. Research has shown that even healthy, term infants who have previously been feeding well display altered sucking during feeding (poor SSB coordination, irregular sucking pattern, weak lip seal, less efficient intake) when they have respiratory illness.[55]

### Sucking in Infants with Respiratory Morbidity

Preterm infants with respiratory disease[56,57,58,59,60,61,62,63,64,65,66,67,68] and immature cardiorespiratory control[69,70] display particular difficulty with SSB coordination and feeding efficiency and should be considered a "high-risk" group for early feeding difficulties. Research has shown that infants with active cardiorespiratory disease don't suck as well as those without disease—both in relation to nonnutritive sucking[60,61,62] and in relation to nutritive sucking.[56,57,58,59] This is reflective of the fact that if infants are having difficulty breathing, it is often difficult for them to coordinate sucking, swallowing, and breathing.

## 14.5.3 Transition from Starting Oral Feeds to Reaching Full Oral Feeds

Once an infant starts some oral feeding, there is often a lot of focus on how long it will take the child to reach full oral feeding because this can ultimately affect length of stay in the NICU.

A number of studies have specifically investigated the transition time from commencement of oral feeds to the attainment of full oral feeding in preterm infants. This research suggests the following:

- GA at birth is negatively associated with transition time.[35,71,72,73,74]
- Morbidity is positively associated with transition time.[35,73,74,75,76,77]

Stated another way, preterm infants who are less mature at birth and those who display a greater degree of illness take longer to transition from starting oral feeds to achieving full oral feeding and are more mature at attainment of full oral feeding. See **Table 14.4**, **Fig. 14.3**, and **Fig. 14.4**.

Infants with respiratory and cardiac morbidities are at particular risk of prolonged transition time and delayed attainment of full oral feeding.[74,76,78,79,80] Immature state control and neurobehavioral functioning can also prolong transition time.[81]

## 14.5.4 Effects of Illness, Interventions, and Hospitalization on Feeding

Given their initial difficulties with oral feeding, most preterm infants will require some degree of tube feeding until they are mature enough and stable enough to feed fully by mouth. However, while necessary to supply nutrition to the gut while oral feeding is being established, it has been shown that the presence of gavage feeding tubes may hinder oral feeding attempts. Studies have shown that the presence of an NG feeding tube in preterm infants can have an impact on respiratory support for breathing,[82,83] as well as SSB coordination.[83] It has also been shown that NG feeds, which obstruct the nose, have the potential to alter breathing, whereas orogastric feeds, which obstruct the oral cavity, have the potential to alter oral reflexes.[84] Research also suggests that gavage tube feeding can induce increased GER in preterm infants,[85] and that premature infants who are fed by gavage tube display reduced upper esophageal sphincter tone compared to those who are not tube fed, as well as a reduction in swallow frequency, swallow propagation, and adaptive peristaltic reflexes.[86]

**Table 14.5** summarizes possible interruptions to oral feeding development associated with illness and medical treatment in the NICU population.[87]

**Table 14.4** Relationships between gestational age (GA) at birth and age at commencement and full oral feeds[72]

| GA at birth (weeks) | N | Duration of artificial feeds (weeks; days) | Chronological age at commencement of suckle-feeds (weeks; days) | Chronological age at attainment of exclusive suckle-feeding (weeks; days) | GA at commencement of suckle-feeds (weeks; days) | GA at attainment of exclusive suckle-feeding (weeks; days) | Transition time: Commencement of suckle-feeds to exclusive suckle-feeding (weeks; days) |
|---|---|---|---|---|---|---|---|
| | | M (SD) | M (SD) | M (SD) | M (SD) | M (SD) | M (SD) |
| ≤ 25 | 19 | 15;3 (3;3) | 11;1 (2;0) | 13;4 (4;0) | 34;6 (2;2) | 39;6 (4;2) | 4;6 (1;0) |
| 26 | 15 | 14;6 (5;3) | 9;4 (1;4) | 14;1 (2;2) | 35;0 (1;5) | 39;1 (2;3) | 4;1 (2;1) |
| 27 | 14 | 8;6 (3;1) | 6;3 (1;5) | 9;2 (2;4) | 34;6 (1;6) | 38;4 (2;6) | 3;6 (1;2) |
| 28 | 17 | 8;0 (2;2) | 5;2 (1;6) | 7;6 (0;8) | 33;4 (1;6) | 37;4 (1;6) | 3;5 (1;4) |
| 29 | 25 | 6;0 (4;6) | 5;0 (3;1) | 8;1 (5;2) | 33;6 (3;1) | 37;2 (3;2) | 3;3 (3;2) |
| 30 | 34 | 5;1 (3;2) | 3;3 (1;3) | 6;6 (2;2) | 33;5 (1;4) | 37;1 (2;4) | 3;2 (1;3) |
| 31 | 42 | 3;5 (2;1) | 2;3 (1;4) | 4;6 (1;1) | 33;4 (1;2) | 36;1 (1;2) | 2;6 (1;4) |
| 32 | 41 | 2;4 (1;4) | 1;3 (0;6) | 4;1 (1;1) | 33;3 (0;6) | 36;2 (1;1) | 2;4 (1;3) |
| 33 | 44 | 2;1 (1;1) | 1;0 (0;5) | 2;6 (0;9) | 34;1 (0;6) | 36;0 (0;6) | 1;6 (0;5) |
| 34 | 62 | 1;2 (1;2) | 0;3 (0;6) | 1;3 (1;2) | 34;5 (0;4) | 35;6 (1;2) | 1;0 (0;6) |
| 35 | 68 | 0;6 (0;6) | 0;3 (0;3) | 0;6 (0;8) | 35;7 (0;4) | 36;1 (0;6) | 0;4 (0;4) |
| 36 | 91 | 0;3 (0;8) | 0;1 (0;3) | 0;3 (0;6) | 36;5 (0;5) | 36;6 (0;2) | 0;2 (0;4) |

*Abbreviations:* M, mean; SD, standard deviation.

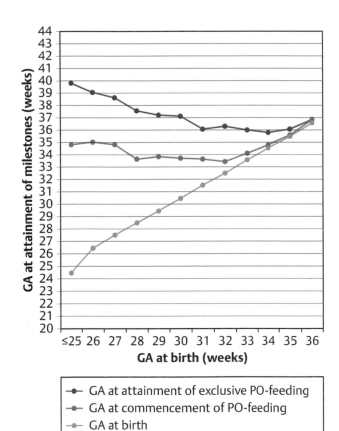

**Fig. 14.3** Relationships between gestational age at birth and age at starting and attaining full oral feeds.[72]

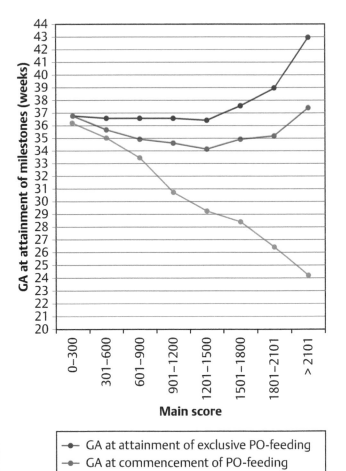

**Fig. 14.4** Relationships between degree of illness and age at starting and attaining full oral feeds.[72]

## 14.5.5 Influence of Caregivers on Feeding in the NICU Population

All newborns rely on their caregivers to feed them, but preterm infants are particularly dependent on their caregivers to provide them with adequate support and assistance during feeds, and to recognize any distress cues when feeding becomes problematic. Several studies have investigated the influence of parenting style on feeding outcomes in preterm infants, as well as parental concerns related to preterm neonatal feeding patterns. These studies suggest that feeding interactions do not just reflect neonatal feeding ability, they also reflect the feeder's skills,[88,89] and that a mother's attunement to her infant's behaviors is important for optimal feeding interaction in preterm infants.[90,91] Other research has also highlighted the strong association between neonatal feeding patterns and maternal stress/concern.[92,93,94]

## 14.5.6 Breastfeeding in the NICU Population

Breastfeeding is the natural method for feeding infants. However, establishing successful breastfeeding may be a challenge for many preterm infants and their mother, due to both neonatal feeding issues and maternal lactation issues associated with preterm delivery, as well as maternal–neonatal separation while the infant is in the NICU.[95,96,97,98,99]

Despite these potential challenges, if breastfeeding is successful, research has shown that preterm infants are generally more physiologically stable during breastfeeds than bottle-feeds,[100,101,102] which is a clearly desirable outcome. This may relate to milk flow rate, neonatal positioning, maternal attunement to neonatal cues, or other factors that may differ between breastfeeding and bottle-feeding situations.

Benefits of breastmilk and breastfeeding include the following:

- Breastmilk contains the optimal mixture of energy for growth, nutrients for development, and immune factors for health. Infant formula attempts to replicate breastmilk and, although many improvements have been made to infant formula to make it similar to breastmilk, no formula contains all of the many benefits of breastmilk.

- Breastfeeding/breastmilk feeding has been associated with reduced fat mass proportion and a reduced risk of allergies and intolerances, gastroenteritis, respiratory infections, otitis media, sudden infant death syndrome, and type 2 diabetes later in life.[103]

- For mothers, breastfeeding/breastmilk feeding has been associated with reduced risk of type 2 diabetes, ovarian cancer, and breast cancer.[103] Breastfeeding is also associated with improved postpregnancy weight loss and control of fertility.[103]

- Breastfeeding is convenient and economical. Bottle-feeding requires the purchase of feeding equipment (bottles and artificial nipples, as well as formula if expressed breastmilk is not used), thorough cleaning and decontamination of feeding equipment for each use, and safe storage and preparation of feeds (formula and/or expressed breastmilk).

- Breastfeeding allows infants to self-regulate their appetite. Infants who are breastfed tend to feed on demand, taking feeds when they are hungry and only feeding until they are full. In contrast, infants who are bottle-fed are often fed on a schedule (e.g., every 3 hours) and tend to be encouraged to feed until the bottle is finished. Learning to self-regulate appetite is important for healthy lifelong eating patterns.

**Table 14.5** Possible interruptions to oral feeding development associated with illness and medical treatment[87]

| Primary condition | Intervention | Outcomes |
|---|---|---|
| *Prematurity* | *Artificial feeding* | *Primary condition persists to some degree* |
| Premature:<br>• Anatomical and physiological development (cardiac, respiratory, gastrointestinal systems)<br>• Neurological development (reflexes, tone, coordination) | Parenteral nutrition (PN)<br>Enteral nutrition (gavage feeds, PG):<br>• Orogastric (OG)<br>• Nasogastric (NG)<br>• Nasojejunal (NJ)<br>• Gastrostomy (G)<br>• Gastrojejunal (GJ)<br>• Jejunostomy (J) | • Ongoing morbidity<br>• Energy imbalance |
| *Illness/morbidity* | *Other interventions* | *Effects of interventions* |
| Impairment of:<br>• Swallowing mechanism (oral region, pharynx, larynx, esophagus)<br>• Major body systems (neurologic, cardiac, respiratory, gastrointestinal systems) | Intubation, positive pressure respiratory support, and suctioning:<br>• Orotracheal<br>• Nasotracheal<br>• Via nasopharyngeal (NP) airway<br>• Via tracheostomy | Immediate:<br>• Local irritation of swallowing mechanism<br>• Obstruction of swallowing mechanism<br>• Injury to swallow mechanism<br>• Altered breathing<br>Delayed:<br>• Disuse of muscles involved in swallowing<br>• Altered sensitivity in swallowing mechanism |
| *Other issues* | *Variables* | *Interrupted development for infants* |
| Physiological instability:<br>• Altered alertness/state<br>• Poor endurance | • Age when intervention started | Possible developmental delays |

## 14.5.7 Monitoring Nutrition and Growth in the NICU

Dietitians have specialized knowledge and skills in assessing individual energy, nutrient, and fluid requirements and in making individualized recommendations and diet plans to meet growth and developmental needs. Referral to a pediatric dietitian should be made whenever there are concerns regarding intake or growth. However, all health professionals associated with infant feeding should have a general awareness of issues related to infant nutrition and growth.

### Infant Feeding Guidelines

Health professionals working in the area of pediatric feeding/ dysphagia management should be familiar with current feeding and nutrition guidelines for infants, which cover topics such as recommended duration of breastfeeding, the use of infant formula, and the recommended age for introduction of solids. Check the websites of government and leading nongovernmental organizations for up-to-date information, including the following:

- World Health Organization
- American Academy of Pediatrics
- North American Society for Pediatric Hepatology, Gastroenterology and Nutrition
- European Society for Paediatric Hepatology, Gastroenterology and Nutrition

### Energy

In general, energy requirements are provided as the amount of energy required per day per unit of body weight of the child (usually kcal/kg/d).

- Breastmilk and standard formulas are 20 kcal/oz or 67 kcal/100 mL.
- At discharge, the minimum energy intake for healthy full-term infants is 90 to 100 kcal/kg/d[8,9,10] (which equates to approximately 120 to 150 mL of breastmilk or standard formula per kilogram of body weight per day).
- Preterm infants, infants with medical complications (e.g., cardiac, respiratory, neurologic), and those who are born with intrauterine growth restriction/retardation, generally have increased energy requirements (e.g., 120–150 kcal/kg/d).[8,9,10]
- Many of these infants receive fortified breastmilk or concentrated formula (e.g., 22–30 kcal/oz, 87 kcal/100 mL) to reduce the total volume of fluid that must be ingested to obtain the energy they require. This can be achieved by adding extra formula, fortifiers, or other nutritional supplements (e.g., fats) to breastmilk or formula.

### Fluid

Fluid intake and losses need to be closely monitored in preterm infants. Changes in fluid volume can affect electrolyte balance. In addition, too much fluid can cause complications for the lungs, whereas too little can affect kidney function.

- The minimum fluid target for most preterm infants is 120 mL/ kg/d.[8,9,10]
- Signs that a child is not getting enough fluid can include the presence of dry eyes, mouth, or skin, infrequent urination/wet diapers, urine that has a strong color or smell, constipation, lethargy, and irritability.

### Nutrients

In healthy term infants, breastmilk and formula meet the recommended intake for macronutrients (protein, fat, carbohydrate: the main sources of energy in the diet) and micronutrients (essential vitamins and minerals, including iron, calcium, zinc, and fiber, among others). Most preterm infants require supplementation for iron (due to anemia), vitamin D (for adequate bone development), and protein (to enhance growth and brain development).[8,9,10]

### Preterm and Infant Growth Charts

Prior to term age, preterm infant growth is plotted on specific preterm growth charts.[8,9,10] Beyond term age, preterm infants' growth is plotted on regular growth charts (e.g., those from the Centers for Disease Control and Prevention and the World Health Organization), with adjustment made for the corrected GA up until 2 years of age.

- Growth charts can be used to estimate a child's growth percentile relative to a normative sample of typical children.
- Most growth series include charts for weight and height (or length in children under 2 years of age), as well as for head circumference.
- Most paper growth charts provide growth percentiles for the 3rd, 5th, 10th, 25th, 50th, 75th, 90th, 95th, and 97th percentiles, whereas electronic growth charts can be used to calculate exact percentiles and z-scores.
- In general, growth patterns are more important than single growth measurements in monitoring a child's health and development. Hence several growth measurements are generally required to determine whether children are moving away from their growth trajectory.
- On average, infants should gain approximately an ounce for every pound of body weight per day (15–20 g/kg/d), though infants who are born small for gestational age may be encouraged to gain more, which is often referred to as catch-up growth.

## 14.6 Feeding Assessment in the NICU

### 14.6.1 Case History

Prior to direct assessment of an infant's feeding skills, case history information should be collected from the infant's medical record, as well as from discussion with the infant's medical team, nurse, and parents. Key information that should be collected from a case history is listed in **Box 14.1.** Case history information assists feeding therapists in planning their assessment.

---

**Box 14.1**

**Summary of Key Information to Be Collected from a Case History**
- GA at birth
- Current GA
- Birth weight and birth weight percentile
- Apgar scores
- Medical conditions present
- Medical interventions required
- Mother's intention to breastfeed
- Multiple birth status

---

## 14.6.2 Feeding Readiness

The first step in a feeding assessment is to establish the infant's readiness to feed.

- Observations are first made across the four areas of functioning, as outlined in the synactive theory[5] (physiological stability, motor organization, state control and attention, and self-regulation), both at rest and during activity, such as handling. See **Box 14.2** and **Box 14.3** for indicators of stress across different areas of functioning, as well as common physiological descriptors.
- Next an assessment is made of the of the infant's oral structures and function, including nonnutritive sucking (lip seal, tongue cupping, sucking strength and rhythm). See Chapter 5 for further information.

---

**Box 14.2**

**Indicators of Stress across Different Areas of Functioning**
- **Physiological/autonomic stability:** changes in heart rate, respiratory rate, $SpO_2$; yawning, hiccupping, coughing, gagging; color changes (e.g., red, pale, or blue)
- **Motor organization:** extension patterns (arching, finger splaying), increase or decrease in tone
- **State control and attention/interaction:** extremes of state—hypervigilance, irritability, or shut down—or rapid changes in state
- **Self-regulation:** inability to calm, requiring high levels of coregulation

---

**Box 14.3**

**Common Terms Related to Physiological Functioning**
- **Bradycardia:** reduced heart rate (HR)
- **Tachycardia:** increased HR
- **Tachypnea:** increased respiratory rate (RR)
- **Apnea:** cessation of breathing. An apnea event is the cessation of breathing for > 20 seconds or > 10 seconds with oxygen desaturation or bradycardia.
- **Typical vital signs in neonates and young infants**
  - RR: 30 to 50 breaths per minute
  - HR: 110 to 160 beats per minute
- **Hypoxemia:** reduced oxygen ($O_2$) in the blood
  - Usually, hypoxemia is defined as an $O_2$ saturation < 95%.
  - In preterm infants < 34/40 weeks GA, who are usually anemic, an $O_2$ saturation < 90% is generally considered to indicate hypoxemia.[8]
  - Note: Refer to your local unit guidelines for optimal target saturation levels
  - Oxygen saturation is generally written as SpO2.
- **Cyanosis:** blue tinge to skin or mucous membranes associated with hypoxemia
- **Increased work of breathing:** physical presentation of respiratory distress that includes signs such as nostril flaring, neck extension, head bobbing, tracheal tug, subcostal recession, accessory chest muscle use, and grunting
- **Stridor:** high-pitched sound originating in the larynx, trachea, or bronchi, caused by a narrow or obstructed airway; can be inspiratory, expiratory, or biphasic
- **Stertor:** coarse sound originating in the pharynx and caused by a narrow or obstructed airway
- **Fremitus:** vibration caused by partial airway obstruction (often secretions) that can be felt from outside the body

---

## 14.6.3 Direct Feeding Assessment

If an infant is showing readiness to feed, the infant undergoes a direct feeding assessment of the infant's nutritive sucking and SSB coordination.

In general, an assessment of feeding in the NICU setting will provide a description of how the infant was fed (feeder, infant position, equipment used, and any strategies used), as well as a rating of the following:

- **Sucking:** lip seal, tongue cupping, sucking strength, sucking rhythm
- **SSB coordination:** beginner/ intermediate/ mature pattern, see **Box 14.4**
- **Physiological status:** any changes in HR, RR, $SPO_2$, or work of breathing during feed
- **Stress cues:** any changes in motor organization, state control, and attention/interaction, as well as self-regulation ability to return to an optimal state of functioning after a stressful event

## Box 14.4

**Stages of Preterm Suck–Swallow–Breath Coordination**

- **Beginner:** bursts of multiple suck–swallows without a break to catch breath; the feeder needs to assist the infant to take breaks to catch breath and thus prevent an adverse event ($SpO_2$ desaturation, apnea, bradycardia event, or aspiration)
- **Intermediate:** bursts of multiple suck–swallows followed by a self-imposed break to catch breath
- **Mature:** integrated SSB pattern

Infants may also be rated on a scale of feeding ability (**Table 14.6**). **Appendix 14.1** provides an example of a template for reporting assessment findings in a patient's medical record.

Ideally, formal feeding assessments should be performed at standard time points (e.g., 36/40 and 40/40 weeks GA) to allow comparison of infants' progress against others at the same gestational age. The following are examples of published, formal feeding development tools:

- Neonatal Oral Motor Assessment (NOMAS)[33]
- Early Feeding Skills (EFS) Assessment[36]

Formal feeding assessments should be performed by developmental therapists or registered nurses (RNs) trained in using these tools. Results should be recorded in the infant's medical record. Results may also be used to track outcomes across the unit, or for research studies, with Institutional Review Board (IRB) approval.

Separately from rating the infant's feeding skill, parental competence and confidence in feeding the infant should be assessed to help determine whether they are able to help their infant to feed safely and efficiently; the assessment can then be used to guide any training needs.

## 14.7 Feeding Interventions in the NICU

A range of feeding therapy interventions are used in the NICU to assist with infant feeding. Varying levels of evidence support different intervention strategies, though most of the published studies in this area are based on small sample sizes and short follow-up periods (to be discussed). In the absence of high-quality scientific evidence to guide practice, any intervention used should be guided by individualized assessment, evaluated for efficacy, and discontinued or modified if not effective in achieving the intended outcome.

**Box 14.5** presents a summary of the literature on feeding interventions. In general, feeding interventions in the NICU seek the following outcomes:

- Physiological stability during feeds (and reduction of aspiration risk)
- Efficiency of oral feeding
- GA at full oral feeds

For many preterm infants, the major barrier to attaining full oral feeds is immaturity of SSB coordination. SSB coordination is

**Table 14.6** Boston Infant Feeding Scale

| Overall PO feeding status: | |
|---|---|
| 1 | Competent feeder |
| 2 | Functional feeder with therapeutic compensations (any or all of the following): <br> • Slower-flowing bottle nipple (i.e., slower than a standard newborn bottle nipple, level 1) <br> • Altered positioning (e.g., side-lying position with horizontal milk flow) <br> • External pacing (i.e., tipping the bottle down and/or removing from the infant's mouth to slow milk flow and impose break in sucking for infant to catch a breath) |
| 3 | Struggling/beginner feeder despite compensations |
| 4 | Not ready for PO feeds |
| Current route for feeds: | |
| A | PO |
| B | PO with close monitoring |
| C | PO with PG top-up as required |
| D | NPO (all PG) with conservative PO trials |
| E | NPO (all PG) |

*Abbreviations:* NPO, nil per os (nothing by mouth); PG, per gavage (by feeding tube); PO, per os (by mouth).

easier to attain with no milk flow or slower milk flow, and harder to attain with faster milk flow.

## Box 14.5

**Summary of Outcomes Reported in the Literature for Different Feeding Interventions Used in the NICU**

*Preparation for Oral Feeds*

- **Kangaroo care** (skin to skin contact) has been shown to be associated with a longer duration of breastfeeding and improved physiological stability.[104]
- **Nonnutritive sucking (NNS)** during tube feeds appears to improve the rate of intake during later oral feeding and has been reported to shorten the transition time to full oral feeding.[105,106,107,108,109,110,111,112]
- **NNS for 5 to 10 minutes before oral feeds** appears to improve state control for feeding, physiological stability during feeds, and volume consumed during feeds.[113,114,115,116,117,118,119] It is not clear from the existing literature whether offering kangaroo care or NNS opportunities has an impact on later oral feeding efficiency or GA at full oral feeding.

*Interventions Aimed at Improving Sucking*

- **Suck training** is reported to increase the percentage of oral intake between 34 and 38/40 weeks GA,[120,121] though it is not clear from the existing literature whether it ultimately affects physiological stability during oral feeding, efficiency of oral feeding, or GA at full oral feeding.
- **Oral tactile stimulation** programs are reported to improve the frequency of sucking and rate of intake[122,123,124,125,126,127,128,129,130,131,132,133] during oral feeds. However, based on the existing literature, it is not clear whether these programs have any

effect on physiological stability during oral feeding, or GA at full oral feeding.[122,123,124,125,126,127,128,129,130,131,132,133]

- **Oral support during oral feeds** has been reported to reduce pauses in sucking, increase rate of intake, and increase volume of intake during feeds.[130,134,135] It remains unclear whether it has an impact on physiological stability during oral feeds or ultimately affects GA at full oral feeding.

### Interventions Aimed at Improving SSB Coordination

- **Slower-flowing nipples** over faster-flowing nipples have been shown to improve physiological stability during feeds for preterm infants who are bottle fed.[136,137,138] However, the existing literature does not evaluate the impact that the use of slow-flowing nipples has on efficiency of oral feeding or GA at attainment of full oral feeding.
- **Side-lying position** for feeds has been reported to improve physiological stability during feeding and increased volume taken in a feed.[139,140]
- **Externally paced feeding** (i.e., where the feeder intermittently tips the bottle down to slow milk flow or imposes a break in sucking) is also associated with improved physiological stability during feeding.[141]
- **Combining the side-lying position and externally paced feeding** (coregulation approach) is associated with improved physiological stability during feeding.[142]

The existing literature has not evaluated the impact of these approaches on the efficiency of oral feeding or on GA at attainment of full oral feeding. These techniques are discussed in greater detail in the next section.

When an infant is developing SSB coordination, and milk flow exceeds the infant's coordination ability, there are a number of possible outcomes, which are listed here and summarized in **Fig. 14.5**:

1. **The infant applies strategies to control milk flow:** An infant may potentially slow the milk flow by taking intermittent breaks in sucking, by using a slower sucking pattern, or by using a weaker sucking pattern. If an infant displays the ability to display a fast, firm, rhythmic suck on a pacifier or finger but not when drinking at the breast or bottle, this is not a sucking problem; it is an SSB coordination problem.

2. **The infant is unable to control milk flow:** An infant who is unable to slow the milk flow may have an adverse respiratory event:

   a. An infant who is unable to protect the airway may experience aspiration.

   b. If an infant protects the airway through prolonged airway closure, apnea may result (with or without bradycardia).

3. **The feeder assists the infant to control milk flow:** If an infant is unable to slow the milk flow, the feeder may be able to slow the milk flow (coregulation) by using strategies such as those listed in **Fig. 14.6,** and described further in the next sections.

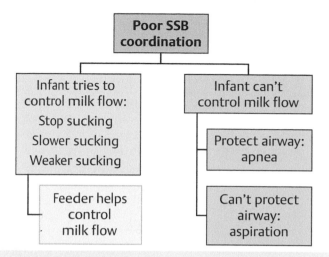

**Fig. 14.5** Possible consequences of immature or dysfunctional suck–swallow–breath coordination.

## 14.8 Suggested Approach to Feeding in the NICU

### 14.8.1 Promoting Breastfeeding

Feeding therapists should support and promote breastfeeding as the natural and ideal way to feed babies. Feeding therapists should be aware of the principles set out in the Baby Friendly Hospital Initiative,[143] and, wherever possible, practices should be guided by the World Health Organization and UNICEF document, "10 Steps to Successful Breastfeeding"[144] (**Box 14.6**).

### Box 14.6

**10 Steps to Successful Breastfeeding**[146]

1. Have a written breastfeeding policy that is routinely communicated to all health care staff.
2. Train all health care staff in the skills necessary to implement this policy.
3. Inform all pregnant women about the benefits and management of breastfeeding.
4. Help mothers initiate breastfeeding within 1 hour of birth.
5. Show mothers how to breastfeed and how to maintain lactation, even if they are separated from their infant.
6. Give infants no food or drink other than breastmilk, unless medically indicated.
7. Practice rooming in—allow mothers and infants to remain together 24 hours a day.
8. Encourage breastfeeding on demand.
9. Give no pacifiers or artificial nipples to breastfeeding infants.
10. Foster the establishment of breastfeeding support groups, and refer mothers to them on discharge from the hospital or birth center.

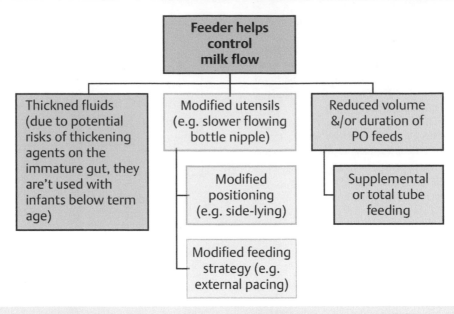

**Fig. 14.6** Possible strategies the feeder can use to assist in managing suck—swallow—breath incoordination.

It is widely acknowledged that breastfeeding success in the NICU environment may be affected by factors such as infant prematurity and illness, maternal illness, and separation of mother and infant. As a result, a modified version of the "10 Steps" for the NICU environment has been proposed by an international group of experts[147] (**Box 14.7**). All feeding therapists working in the NICU should be familiar with these guidelines. In particular, any staff involved in supporting infant feeding (nursing, medical, allied health) should make themselves aware of each mother's intention to breastfeed and preferences regarding any bottle feeding and formula feeding.

## Box 14.7

**Modified 10 Steps to Successful Breastfeeding for the NICU[145]**

*Guiding Principles*

- The staff attitude toward the mother must focus on the individual mother and her situation.
- The faculty must provide family-centered care, supported by the environment.
- The health care system must ensure continuity of care, that is, continuity of pre-, peri-, and postnatal care and postdischarge care.

1. Have a written breastfeeding policy that is routinely communicated to all health care staff.
2. Educate and train all staff in the specific knowledge and skills necessary to implement this policy.
3. Inform all hospitalized pregnant women at risk for preterm delivery of birth of a sick infant about the management of lactation and breastfeeding and benefits of breastfeeding.
4. Encourage early, continuous, and prolonger mother–infant skin-to-skin contact (kangaroo mother care) without unjustified restrictions. Place babies in skin-to-skin contact with their mothers immediately following birth for at east an hour. Encourage mothers to recognize when their babies are ready to breastfeed, and offer help if needed.
5. Show mothers how to initiate and maintain lactation and establish early breastfeeding with infant stability the only criterion.
6. Give newborn infants no food or drink other than breastmilk, unless medically indicated.
7. Enable mothers and infants to remain together 24 hours a day.
8. Encourage demand feeding or, when needed, semidemand feeding.
9. Use alternatives to bottle feeding at least until breastfeeding is well established, and use pacifiers and nipple shields only for justifiable reasons.
10. Prepare parents for continued breastfeeding and ensure access to support services/groups after hospital discharge.

In general, infant feeding plans should be guided by the following principles[143]:

1. Provide sufficient fluid and nutrition to meet the infant's requirements for health, growth, and development.
2. Protect the mother's milk supply (teach methods for expressing and storing milk, if breastfeeding at the breast is not possible at that time).
3. Work to address any obstacles to breastfeeding and/or breast milk feeding.
4. Where possible, provide support to have the infant feed at the mother's breast.
5. Where breastfeeding isn't possible, support the infant to receive breastmilk where possible (own mother's milk is the first preference; with parental consent, donor milk is the next preference; formula is the last preference).

However, while breastfeeding is generally the best method for infants to feed, all mothers and infants should be supported by NICU staff regardless of their choice or ability to breastfeed.

### Nutritive Sucking

Wherever possible, offer breastfeeding as the first oral feed.

### Nonnutritive Sucking

NNS while the infant is on tube feeds has been shown to have benefits for the infant, such as improved transition from tube to oral feeds and better oral feeding performance.[111] NNS on a fully emptied breast may be an option for some infants while they are on tube feeds. Mothers intending to use this technique should be taught to recognize the following:

- **Signs of a fully emptied breast:** inability to pump any additional milk, soft breast
- **Signs of an additional let down:** because sucking stimulation often triggers more milk production
- **Indicators that the infant is not managing any flow:** such as change in physiological status, coughing, or stress cues

For all infants whose mother intends to breastfeed, a referral to a lactation consultant should ideally be made within 24 hours of birth. Education provided by the lactation consultant includes the following:

- Education for pumping strategies to initiate and maintain milk supply
- Education to help facilitate appropriate positioning and effective latch
- Use of breastfeeding equipment, such as breast pumps, nipple shields, supplemental nursing systems (line feeders), and safe use of an oral syringe to deliver small volumes of breastmilk when nursing at the breast isn't possible

Other education that is provided by the lactation consultant, in association with other members of staff includes the following:

- Education regarding kangaroo care (skin-to-skin contact). RNs and feeding therapists often assist in providing this information and training.
- Education for assessing infant feeding readiness cues. RNs and feeding therapists often assist in providing this information and training also.
- Discussion regarding offering an "empty" breast for NNS practice during gavage feeding. This decision should involve medical and feeding therapy staff, in addition to lactation (LC) and RN staff, if concerns regarding aspiration or apnea exist.
- Discussion of the potential need for supplementation, with test weights and feeding assessment. This decision should involve medical and nutrition staff, in addition to LC and RN staff, if there are concerns regarding growth.
- Discussion regarding number of breastfeeds per day versus bottles in infants who need to be supplemented. This decision should also involve medical and nutrition staff, in addition to LC and RN staff, if there are concerns regarding growth.

## 14.8.2 General Bottle Feeding Approach in Low-Risk Infants

For the general preterm population, staff may consider offering the first bottle feed with a standard newborn bottle nipple (level 1) and holding the infant in a standard feeding position (i.e., traditional cradle hold). Then, if needed (i.e., if the infant shows any decline in physiological stability or engagement), staff should implement the following compensations[147,148], ideally in the following order, until a suitable option is found:

- **Slower-flowing bottle nipple:** slower than a standard newborn level 1 bottle nipple
- **Horizontal milk flow:** bottle horizontal, parallel to floor; this is easiest achieved in either a side-lying or semi-upright position (avoid holding the infant in a reclined/supine position):
  - **Side-lying position:** as when being nursed, with the infant on her side, with her ear, shoulder, and hip facing up toward the ceiling
  - **Semi-upright position:** supported upright position, with the infant's head above his chest and hips, and with the infant's neck supported, such as by the inside of the feeder's elbow
- **External pacing;** tipping the bottle down to slow milk flow or removing the bottle from the infant's mouth to impose a break in sucking

Note: The rationale for the order of changes is based on gradually increasing demands on the feeder. Changing the bottle nipple puts the least amount of burden on the feeder, whereas implementing horizontal milk flow (and associated positioning changes) and external pacing require more effort, skill, and critical thinking from the feeder, and there is a greater potential for variation between feeders.

## 14.8.3 Feeding Infants at High Risk of Adverse Respiratory Events during Feeds

Some preterm infants (such as those listed in **Box 14.8**) are at increased risk of apnea or aspiration during feeds.[149] Aspiration often presents as "silent aspiration" in this group (i.e., no overt clinical signs of aspiration (e.g., coughing[149,150]). Often suspicion is raised via subtle cues (e.g., changes in state) or by symptoms (i.e., otherwise unexplained worsening of respiratory condition, failure to wean from supplemental $O_2$).

### Box 14.8

**Infants at High Risk of Swallowing Difficulties and Impaired Airway Protection during Oral Feeds**

- Bronchopulmonary dysplasia
- Congenital heart disease, including patent ductus arteriosus (PDA)
- Airway malformation (e.g., laryngomalacia, laryngeal cleft)
- Neurologic injury or altered neurologic state (e.g., IVH 3 or 4, HIE, seizures; those on antiepileptic drugs or sedatives)

For these infants, given the high risk of aspiration (which can contribute to or prolong recovery from lung disease, as well as prolonging transition to full oral feeds and length of stay) or apnea events during oral feeds (which are potentially life threatening), a conservative approach to the introduction of oral feeds is encouraged as described here:

- Commencement of any oral feeding with full compensations:
  - **Slow milk flow** (half-emptied breast or slowest-flowing bottle nipple)
  - **Side-lying position** and **horizontal milk flow**
  - **External pacing** as required
- Breastfeeding only if possible:
  - Flow of milk from the breast is generally more responsive to the infant's sucking than milk flow from the bottle, which generally occurs passively whether the infant is actively sucking or not.
  - In addition, breastfeeding is infant driven, unlike bottle feeding, which can be feeder driven if the infant is "encouraged" to feed by holding the bottle nipple in the infant's mouth, twisting or jiggling the bottle nipple to stimulate sucking, or holding the infant's mouth closed around the nipple in the form of chin and cheek support.

There should be a low threshold for discontinuation of oral feeds in this population if any concerns regarding airway protection arise (e.g., change in physiological stability and vital signs, cough, choke, transmitted airway sounds, increased work of breathing, changes in state or motor functioning).

If oral feeds are slow to progress, respiratory support needs to increase, or the patient is unable to wean from respiratory support, an instrumental assessment of swallowing (e.g., modified barium swallow study or fiberoptic endoscopic evaluation of feeding) may be warranted to objectively evaluate swallow function and determine aspiration risk. Some patients who are unable to feed safely with one feeding plan may be able to feed safely with other plans (i.e., change of feeding equipment, position, or external pacing).

While, in general, the feeding therapist should encourage and support cue-based feeding, if there is a concern regarding silent aspiration during feeding (i.e., aspiration with no overt clinical signs), staff must use a very conservative approach. In these cases, staff should work to provide developmental and bonding opportunities through other means (e.g., NNS, swaddling, and holding during tube feeds). In addition to safety issues, staff should actively work to avoid adverse patient experiences, which are likely to cause long-term feed aversion.

## Feeding an Infant on Nasal CPAP/HFNC Therapy via Nasal Cannula

Given the potential for adverse respiratory events related to the underlying respiratory disease, as well as from the effect of positive pressure flow delivered through the pharynx and larynx,[151] many NICUs use the following guidelines:

- Infants will not be fed orally while on CPAP or HFNC.
- For infants with chronic respiratory support needs on low-flow $O_2$ therapy via nasal cannula (LFNC), the infant should be stable on this flow for ≥ 12 hours prior to any initiation of oral feeding.

Note:
- Oral feeding includes any fluids given by mouth that are swallowed (e.g., medication, breastmilk, formula, sucrose solutions).
- Oral cares (< 1 mL liquid used to moisten and clean the mouth) and gels applied to the oral mucosa may be used with caution, as needed.

## Feeding Infants Who Demonstrate Increased Work of Breathing or Tachypnea, Regardless of Degree of Respiratory Support

Given the potential for adverse respiratory events related to the underlying respiratory disease, as well as from the effect of mistiming of swallows during inspiration, many NICUs use the following guidelines:

- Infants who display increased work of breathing (e.g., nostril flaring, head bobbing, subcostal retractions, tracheal tug) or who are tachypneic (RR > 70 breaths per minute) should not be fed orally at that time.

## Infants with Severe Neurologic Impairment or Altered Neurologic State

Infants who display an altered neurologic state should not be fed orally at that time due to increased risk of aspiration. Infants with severe IVH (grade 3 or 4) or HIE (including those who have received therapeutic hypothermia) should also be considered at risk of silent aspiration, and any oral intake should proceed with caution.

Any staff involved in feeding patients at risk of adverse respiratory events during oral feeding should be alert for signs and symptoms suggestive of swallowing incoordination (**Box 14.9**).

### Box 14.9

**Signs and Symptoms Suggestive of Possible Swallowing Incoordination**[154]
- Apnea (with or without bradycardia) during oral feeds
- $SpO_2$ desaturation events during oral feeds
- Increased work of breathing during or after oral feeds
- Coughing during or after oral feeds
- Increased congestion during or after oral feeds
- Unexplained respiratory infection
- Unexplained inability to wean from $O_2$ support
- Delayed oral feeding milestones
- Requiring compensations during oral feeds (e.g., modified feeding equipment, modified positioning, or external pacing)

## 14.8.4 Therapeutic Feeding Compensations

### Therapeutic Feeding Positioning

Given that fluids flow more slowly when a bottle is held horizontally rather than vertically, horizontal milk flow may be used to help the infant regulate milk flow (reducing bolus size) and assist with SSB coordination.

- It is easiest to achieve horizontal milk flow if the infant is positioned in a supported upright position or in a side-lying position for oral feeds. Avoid feeding infants in a reclined/ supine position.
- The transition to standard cradle hold (semireclined) position should be made when tolerated by the infant.

In addition, given that most infants are held in a horizontal position when breastfeeding, the use of a side-lying position when bottle feeding may assist with the transition to breastfeeding (**Fig. 14.7**).

Regardless of the position the infant is held in (cradle hold, side-lying, upright), many preterm infants benefit from being firmly swaddled during oral feeds. Because many preterm infants have altered tone, swaddling and containment can assist them to obtain a flexed position, which is most conducive to effective sucking, and can make handling easier for the feeder and less stressful for the infant.

## Therapeutic Feeding Strategies

External pacing is a strategy that may be used if an infant is having difficulty self-coordinating sucking, swallowing, and breathing. External pacing involves either or both of the following:

- Tipping the bottle down, to reduce the amount of milk in the nipple and slow the milk flow
- Removing the nipple from the infant's mouth, to impose a break in sucking to allow the infant to catch a breath.

External pacing may be performed on a schedule (e.g., every three sucks) or on demand (i.e., cue based).

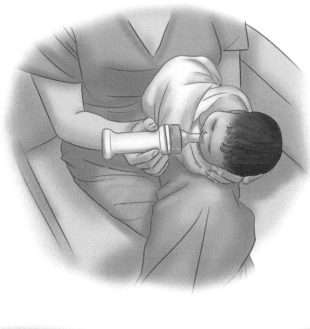

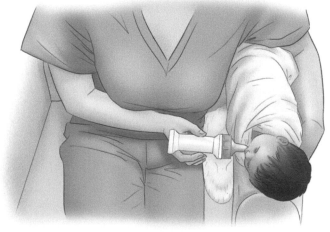

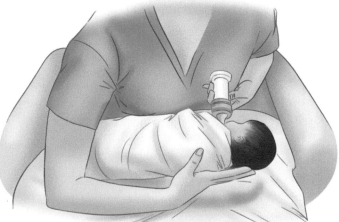

**Fig. 14.7** Side-lying positioning for feeding.

## Therapeutic Feeding Equipment

Slower-flow bottle nipples (nipples that are slower than a standard newborn level 1 bottle nipple, such as very slow flow and ultra slow flow nipples) may be used to help the infant regulate milk flow and assist with SSB coordination. In addition, given that milk flow from the breast is generally not as fast as from many bottle nipples, the use of slower-flowing bottle nipples when bottle feeding may assist with transition to breastfeeding.

The following list provides a summary of information from a recent study by Pados et al[153]:

### Disposable Bottle Nipples Labeled "Slow Flow"

- On average, these nipples are equivalent to a standard newborn nipple (level 1).
- There is often variable flow rate between nipples (poor quality control).
- These nipples are made to be single use.

### Commercial Bottle Nipples Labeled "Preemie" or "Ultra Preemie"

- These nipples are considered *very* slow flow or *ultra* slow flow.
- They have a more consistent flow rate than disposable nipples (due to stricter quality control).
- These nipples are made to be reusable (**Box 14.10**).

---

### Box 14.10

**Discussion Point**

Is there any role for fast-flowing nipples in the NICU?

- Many NICUs stock fast-flowing bottle nipples, with the thought that faster milk flow may make sucking easier.
- In infants with poor SSB coordination, it is known that faster milk flow generally does not help and can make feeding harder. Concerns include airway compromise (aspiration, apnea, increased work of breathing), reduced patient enjoyment of feeding (reduced engagement with feeder and potential development of aversion to feeds), and possible flow confusion if moving between breastfeeds and bottle feeds.
- Infants who may benefit from a somewhat faster flow include those with true oral-phase feeding difficulties (vs. pharyngeal phase), such as infants with cleft lip or palate. In these cases, an assessment must be made to determine the flow rate that is fast enough to assist with effective milk transfer, without being so fast as to interfere with swallowing safety.

---

### Rationale and Considerations When Recommending a Bottle Nipple with a Slower Flow Rate

#### Suck–Swallow–Breathe Coordination

Difficulty with SSB coordination often presents as follows:

- Physiological changes, such as apnea, bradycardia, $SpO_2$ desaturations
- Anterior milk spillage
- A change to weaker or slower sucking patterns, or an NNS pattern
- Frequent rest breaks, requiring frequent burp breaks as a form of pacing
- Requiring external pacing throughout feeding

If slower flow rate is effective, there should be fewer of these events.

### Time to Finish Feedings

Typical infant feeding lasts 20 to 25 minutes.[154] A slower flow rate may have the potential to extend feeding times. However, in clinical practice, slower flow often does not push infant feeding times outside normal limits because the slower flow generally improves SSB coordination, so the infant spends less time pulling away from the nipple or requiring breaks to catch a breath. It should be noted that infants do not need to complete feedings in 10 to 15 minutes. That is not normal, and it may contribute to reflux or a preference for bottle feeding over breastfeeding.

### For All Therapeutic Feeding Compensations

If a staff member (RN or feeding therapist) assesses that therapeutic compensation is useful for an infant, this should be documented in the infant's medical record. Other staff members should continue use of therapeutic compensation unless they assess that this is no longer useful. If so, the reason for this change should be documented in the infant's medical record. Parent training will be required when therapeutic compensations are used because these are special strategies that are often not intuitive to parents or other caregivers who may be feeding the infant. Feeding therapists and RNs may be involved in performing parent training.

## 14.8.5 Logistics of Managing Therapeutic Feeding Equipment

### Who Recommends Feeding Equipment and How Is It Supplied?

Some NICUs are not currently funded to supply reusable feeding equipment to all infants. Hence an assessment of clinical need is required to support use, and a record of demand and supply should be kept. In many NICUs, feeding therapists will supply therapeutic feeding equipment, as required, based on assessment. If required, several sets of necessary equipment should be supplied to allow time between cleaning.

### When to Discontinue Therapeutic Feeding Equipment

Slower-flowing bottle nipples are often used as infants are establishing SSB coordination. Collaboration is needed between the feeding therapist and RN in determining an infant's readiness to transition to a faster flow. It should be noted that some infants will require therapeutic feeding equipment beyond discharge. An infant who is managing with a level 1 nipple will often be able to manage with a standard newborn level 1 nipple from most commercial brands.

## Family Preference for Feeding Equipment

In preparation for home, once the discharge date has been identified, staff should recommend the family brings the in-home bottle system at least 3 days before the identified date to ensure the nipple flow is appropriate:

- Disposable feeding equipment available in the NICU for inpatient use is manufactured to be single use. These items are not suitable to reuse and should not be given to parents to take home. They are generally not available in the community.

- If the reusable system brought by the infant's family is not appropriate, staff should provide guidance on this (this usually applies to nipple flow rate, and a slower-flowing nipple for the same bottle may be available).

- If a specialized bottle system is required, the family should ideally be provided with at least two full sets to take home, and be guided on where and how to obtain additional sets.

## Cleaning Feeding Equipment

All NICUs should have a guideline for cleaning special reusable feeding equipment that complies with state and hospital infection management policies. Appropriate cleaning involves washing (with water and detergent), as well as sanitizing (with heat, such as a microwave or dishwasher).

## 14.8.6 Feeding Progression

A doctor's order (from an MD) is generally required for all feeding types (parenteral nutrition, per gavage, oral). Feeding therapists and other staff should be aware of orders that are in place, and discuss them with the MD if you believe a patient is ready to commence oral feeding, or if your assessment suggests they should remain nonoral.

## Commencing Oral Feeds

An order to start oral feeds should be placed only when the infant is physiologically stable (e.g., not requiring positive pressure respiratory support, tachypneic, or displaying increased work of breathing) and presenting with feeding-readiness cues (i.e., alert, sucking on a pacifier, waking for feeds).

## Feeding Progression for Low-Risk Infants

Research shows most healthy preterm infants follow a feeding progression, typically achieving full oral feedings between 36 and 37/40 weeks GA.[72] Many infants present with feeding readiness cues around 34/40 weeks GA (i.e., NNS, waking for feeds).[72] Most NICUs do not promote bottle feeding trials earlier than this time point. Some safe breastfeeding may be possible from as early as 30/40 weeks GA,[155] though volume is unlikely to be large.

## Feeding Progression for High-Risk Infants

It should be acknowledged from the onset that infants who are at risk for feeding and swallowing difficulties may require a longer amount of time to show feeding readiness and to progress to full oral feeding.

## In General

- The literature suggests that progressing oral feeds based on a cue-based approach may shorten the transition time to full oral feeding by up to a week.[156,157]

- **Cue-based feeding** involves the following:
  - Offering oral feeds when the infant displays engagement cues (e.g., physiological stability, flexed position, quiet alert state)
  - Discontinuing oral feeds when the infant displays disengagement cues (e.g., physiological stability, extension patterns, sleepy or irritable state)

- **Semidemand feeding** involves offering the infant the opportunity to oral feed on a schedule (e.g., every 3 hours). An assigned volume is provided at each feed (whatever is not taken orally is given by gavage). An oral feed progresses only when the infant shows feeding-readiness cues before the feed and engagement cues during the feed, and it is discontinued based on disengagement cues. Progression of the number of oral feeds and the amount offered is determined by the infant's cues and physiological stability.

- **Demand (ad lib) feeding** involves offering oral feeds based entirely on the infant's cues. Infants are fed orally as much (or as little) as they want, and as often as they demand, provided they meet minimal daily fluid and energy quotas.

- **Cautions** regarding the transition to demand feeding are as follows:
  - A discussion regarding an infant's suitability to transition to demand feeding is required between medical, nutrition, nursing, and feeding therapy staff.
  - When an infant is transitioned to demand feeds, a minimum amount of daily fluid and energy intake needs to be agreed on by the team (usually 120 mL/kg/d or 100 kcal/kg/d as a minimum).[8,9,10]
  - A gavage tube will generally need to remain in situ until the patient has achieved oral intake equivalent to 75% of the total energy goal, but not less than 120 mL/kg/d.[8,9,10]
  - Close management is required by all disciplines to ensure the infant is medically stable and obtaining all fluids, energy, and nutrients required for appropriate growth and development.
  - Infants should not go more than 5 hours (and not more than once in a 24-hour period) between feedings. There should continue to be close monitoring of hydration status, weight gain, and blood glucose.
  - In general, the length of a demand feeding trial should be no longer than 48 hours. If an infant is not meeting the fluid and energy minimums, the infant should be transitioned back to a semidemand schedule (which often involves reinsertion of a gavage tube).

## 14.8.7 Documentation in Electronic Medical Records

Ideally, feeding assessment and therapy templates should be available to allow consistent reporting. Other efforts should also be made between the various health professionals involved in infant feeding to facilitate consistent reporting.

At a minimum, infants should be rated as being one of the following:

- Competent feeder
- Functional feeder with compensations
- Beginner feeder/struggling feeder despite compensations

Any compensations required (e.g., slower-flowing bottle nipple, side-lying, and external pacing) should be documented. In addition, the occurrence of, and reason for, any deviations from the agreed-upon plan should also be documented.

## 14.8.8 When to Refer to Feeding Therapy

Some NICUs have feeding therapists on staff and have full coverage throughout the week. Other NICUs have feeding therapists that provide a drop-in (consult) service. Depending on the amount of therapy coverage available, feeding therapists may be able to work with all infants throughout the NICU, or they may have to prioritize their time with those infants most in need of therapy input.

Priority should be given to the following populations:

- All infants who fall in the high-risk category for aspiration/apnea during oral feeds
- Infants born < 28/40 weeks GA, because they are at high risk for these conditions
- Infants with any of the following:
  - Craniofacial malformation (e.g., cleft lip/palate, Pierre Robin sequence)
  - Syndromes (e.g., trisomy 21)
  - GERD
  - GA at birth < 28/40 weeks
- Any infant where there is a concern regarding aspiration or apnea during oral feeds
- Infants 36/40 weeks GA who do not show readiness to feed orally
- Infants 40/40 weeks GA who are not fully oral feeding
- If physiological instability is observed with oral feeding despite compensation strategies (therapeutic feeding equipment, positioning, strategies)

## 14.8.9 Subspecialty Consults and Specialized Assessments Relative to Feeding

NICU attendees may consider referral to the following subspecialties, as needed:

- **Pediatric gastroenterology (GI)**
  - In cases of presumed GERD or milk intolerance

  - For infants with prolonged NG/NJ tube feedings, and anticipated need for long-term gavage or surgical tube feedings (G or GJ) upon discharge to home
- **Pediatric otorhinolaryngology (ORL)**
  - Where these is concern for palate or airway anomalies
  - In cases of presumed vocal cord dysfunction
- **Radiology for modified barium swallow assessment**
  - Where there is concern regarding aspiration during swallowing
  - Eligible infants should ideally be assessed by NICU feeding therapist first, who will make a recommendation and facilitate the study.
  - Studies may need to be conducted at an outside facility that has access to fluoroscopy. Ideally, the NICU feeding therapist and RN should attend the study, so that findings can be integrated into the care plan.

## 14.8.10 When to Consider Frenotomy

Effective milk transfer from the breast or bottle requires infants to use their tongue to express milk from the breast or bottle nipple. For fully functional suckling, the tongue tip should be able to extend beyond the lower gum line and be able to move backward along the roof of the mouth in a stripping action. A lingual frenulum that attaches close to the tip of the tongue, or that is thick and immobile, may prevent normal tongue movement during sucking.[160]

### Criteria for Frenotomy

1. Infant beginning to oral feed
2. Tongue-tie (ankyloglossia) noted on clinical exam
3. Clinical signs of tongue-tie noted:
   - Difficulty latching effectively at the breast
   - Painful breastfeeding (e.g., blisters, other nipple trauma, mastitis)
   - Poor extraction of fluids from a bottle

### Steps to Follow

1. The LC and the feeding therapist have a consultation.
2. If it is assessed that an infant meets any of the foregoing criteria, and the MD agrees, ORL is consulted to perform the procedure.
3. Parental consent is obtained for frenotomy.
4. The frenotomy is performed.
5. The LC and speech-language pathologist reevaluate feeding.

## 14.8.11 Growth, Development, and Discharge Planning Meetings

Ideally, there should be a weekly encounter of allied health disciplines (developmental therapy—physical therapy, occupational therapy, speech-language pathologist, as well as nutrition, social work, case coordination) along with the MD and RN staff to assess neurodevelopmental progress and review readiness for discharge. Goals should include (1) to flag active neurodevelopmental and growth issues and (2) to identify infants likely to be discharged home in the next 1 to 2 weeks in order to allow sufficient time for coordination of outpatient follow-up care. Following the meeting, a multidisciplinary team note should be placed in the infant's medical record.

### 14.8.12 Discharge on Enteral Tube Feeds or Supplemental Oxygen

Discharge from the NICU is dependent on physiological stability and adequate growth. Historically many NICUs would not consider discharging infants who continued to require enteral tube feeds or supplemental oxygen to meet their nutritional and respiratory requirements. However, more recently, an increasing number of NICUs have begun to allow infants to be discharged with a feeding tube in situ or with a nasal cannula, provided that (1) the infant is physiologically stable, (2) the parents are willing and trained in how to use these support systems, and (3) appropriate follow-up is in place.

With regard to enteral tube feeds, a decision often has to be made prior to discharge regarding whether to continue with a temporary gavage tube (e.g., NG tube) or whether to transition to a surgical feeding tube (e.g., gastrostomy). Different facilities use different guidelines to determine when to transition to a surgical feeding tube, but many consider the expected need for tube feeding for greater than 3 months post term age to justify transitioning to a surgical feeding tube.

### 14.8.13 When to Refer for Postdischarge Follow-Up

Most infants with ongoing feeding difficulties at term age would benefit from monitoring beyond discharge. NICU attendees may consider referral to the following health professionals:

- **Feeding therapist:** if the infant has demonstrated difficulties achieving full oral feeds, aspiration risk, and/or feeding aversive behaviors at any point during the hospital stay, or if the infant is discharged home on special feeding equipment (e.g., ultra preemie nipple), special feeds (e.g., thickened feeds), or tube feeds
- **Dietitian:** If the infant has demonstrated difficulties gaining weight, and is discharged home on (1) tube feeds, (2) preterm feedings, or (3) ≥ 50% of feeds fortified with additional calories, or is discharged home at less than the 10th percentile for weight
- **Gastroenterology specialist:** If the infant has severe GERD requiring intervention at the time of discharge, growth faltering, or a need for any kind of tube feedings
- **Pulmonology specialist:** if the infant has a history of severe lung disease or is on any supplemental oxygen therapy at discharge
- **Otorhinolaryngology specialist:** if the infant has suspected or confirmed vocal fold dysfunction, or any structural airway issues

Of note, infants may be referred separately to nutrition, feeding, or medical programs. However, for medically complex babies with multiple challenges, a multidisciplinary clinic (where available) is likely to best meet their needs and provide a comprehensive and consistent plan for the family. For all eligible babies, referrals to other outpatient programs (e.g., infant developmental follow-up) should be made in addition, as clinically indicated.

## 14.9 Questions

1. What is the incidence rate of preterm birth in the United States?

A. 9.6%
B. 1.2%
C. 5.9%
D. 7.1%
E. 12.5%

2. When do most healthy preterm infants typically achieve full oral feedings?

A. 28/30 weeks GA
B. 30/32 weeks GA
C. 36–37/40 weeks GA
D. 34/40 weeks GA
E. 28/32 weeks GA

3. Infants who display increased work of breathing or who are tachypneic should not be fed orally at that time. What respiratory rate (RR) is indicative of tachypnea?

A. RR > 30 breaths per minute
B. RR > 70 breaths per minute
C. RR > 50 breaths per minute
D. RR > 20 breaths per minute
E. RR > 10 breaths per minute

4. How long does a typical infant feeding last?

A. 5–7 minutes
B. 10–12 minutes
C. Less than 10 minutes
D. 15–20 minutes
E. 20–25 minutes

5. What is the minimum energy intake most infants at NICU discharge?

A. 50–75 kcal/kg/d
B. 20–30 kcal/kg/d
C. 40–50 kcal/kg/d
D. 90–100 kcal/kg/d
E. 100–120 kcal/kg/d

# 14.10 Answers and Explanations

**1. Correct: 9.6% One in 10 babies (A).**[2,3]
The other choices are not accurate representations of the current incidence rate of preterm birth in the United States.

**2. Correct: 36–37/40 weeks GA (C).**
Research shows most healthy preterm infants follow a feeding progression, typically achieving full oral feedings between 36 and 37/40 weeks GA.[72] Many infants present with feeding-readiness cues around 34/40 weeks GA (i.e., nonnutritive sucking, waking for feeds).[72] Most NICUs do not promote bottle feeding trials earlier than this time point. Some safe breastfeeding may be possible from as early as 30/40 weeks GA,[157] though volume is unlikely to be large.

**3. Correct: RR > 70 breaths per minute (B).**
Tachypnea is abnormally rapid breathing. Typical respiratory rate for infants from birth to six months of age is 30 to 60 breaths per minute. Infants who display increased work of breathing and/or tachypnea (respiratory rate of > 70 breaths per minute) should not be fed by mouth until those symptoms resolve.

**4. Correct: 20–25 minutes (E).**
Typical infant feeding lasts 20 to 25 minutes.[156] Using a bottle with a significantly slower flow rate may have the potential to extend feeding times. However, in clinical practice, slower flow often does not push infant feed times outside normal limits because the slower flow generally improves suck—swallow—breathe coordination, so the infant spends less time pulling away from the nipple or requiring breaks to catch a breath. It should be noted that infants do not need to complete feedings in 10 to 15 minutes. That is not normal, and may possibly contribute to reflux or a preference for bottle feeding over breastfeeding.

**5. Correct: 90–100 kcal/kg/d (D).**
At discharge, the minimum energy intake for healthy term infants is 90 to 100 kcal/kg/d[8,9,10] (which equates to approximately 120 to 150 mL of breastmilk or standard formula per kilogram of body weight per day). Preterm infants, infants with medical complications (e.g., cardiac, respiratory, neurologic) and those who are born with intrauterine growth restriction/retardation generally have increased energy requirements.[8,9,10]

# Appendix 14.1 Clinical Feeding Evaluation Template

- Patient is a male/female infant born at 00/40 weeks GA, currently aged 00/40 weeks corrected GA, who was referred to Feeding Therapy Services for assessment.

- Patient is a male/female infant born at 00/40 weeks GA, currently aged 00/40 weeks corrected GA, who is being followed by Feeding Therapy Services.

## Medical History

- Respiratory:
- Gastrointestinal:
- Neurological:
- Other:

## Feeding History

- PO feeding started:
- Current %PO:
- Last adverse event with PO feeding:

## Assessment/Session

- Oral ax: Oral structures were/were not intact; range of motion is within normal limits/restricted; and there was/was not apparent ankyloglossia
- Non-nutritive sucking on pacifier/gloved finger: weak/strong, rhythmical/uncoordinated.

**Table 14.7** Assessment/session

| Subsystems of functioning | Goal | Baseline | During PO feeding |
|---|---|---|---|
| Physiological | Within normal limits, stable | | |
| Motor | Appropriate tone and movement | | |
| State/interaction | Able to achieve and maintain a quiet, alert state | | |
| Regulation | Able to self-regulate/soothe | | |

- Patient was offered PO feed by Mom/RN/therapist under the following conditions:
  - Bottle nipple: Standard newborn bottle nipple (level 1); very slow flow bottle nipple; ultra slow flow bottle nipple
  - Position: Cradle hold; side-lying with horizontal milk flow; semi-upright with horizontal milk flow
  - Strategies: External pacing as required, per infant cues
- Patient willingly latched to bottle nipple/Patient latched to bottle nipple after some prompting.
- Sucking was weak and ineffective/Sucking was rhythmical, firm, and effective.

- Patient displayed mature/immature SSB coordination (see below):

**Table 14.8** Mature/immature suck–swallow–breathe coordination

| Mature | Integrated suck—swallow—breath pattern |
|---|---|
| Intermediate | Bursts of multiple suck—swallows followed by a self-imposed break to catch breath |
| Beginner | Bursts of multiple suck—swallows without a break to catch breath; the feeder needs to assist the infant to take breaks to catch their breath, or an adverse event (SpO2 desaturation, apnea, bradycardia event, or aspiration) may occur. |

- Patient's vital signs were stable/unstable thoughout the feed.
- No/mild/moderate increase in work of breathing was apparent throughout the feed (e.g. increased RR, nostril flaring, head bobbing).
- No/mild/moderate stress cues were apparent during the feed (e.g. hyper-vigilance, staring, forehead furrowing, reddened eyes/eyebrows, finger splaying).
- Cue-based external pacing was/was not required throughout the feed (i.e. bottle was tipped to slow flow when Patient displayed stress cues – this generally occurred after 5-6 sucks).
- Patient demonstrated benefit from upright/side-lying positioning with horizontal milk flow to assist Patient to control milk delivery.
- The feed was stopped after 00 mins due to increasing Patient fatigue/refusal (e.g. pulling away from nipple, letting milk flow from mouth, gagging). Approximately 00mL was taken during this time.
- Clinical signs suggestive of aspiration were observed (i.e. cough, wet breath sounds, increased congestion, SpO2 desaturation, apnea, RR, HR)/There were no overt signs suggestive of aspiration/airway compromise observed (e.g. cough, wet breath sounds, apnea, SpO2 desaturation). However, multiple compensation strategies were used to minimize Patient risk.

## Impressions

- Patient is a male/female infant born at 00/40 weeks GA, currently aged 00/40 weeks corrected GA who is being followed by Feeding Therapy Services.
- Diagnosis code: Dysphagia (oropharyngeal/oral/pharyngeal); Feeding Difficulties

## Overall PO Feeding Status

- Competent feeder
- Functional feeder with therapeutic compensations (any or all of the following):
  - Slower flowing bottle nipple (i.e. slower than a standard newborn bottle nipple, level 1)

- Altered positioning (e.g. side-lying position with horizontal milk flow)
- External pacing (i.e. tipping the bottle down and/or removing from the infant's mouth to slow milk flow and impose break in sucking for them to catch breath)
- Struggling/beginner feeder despite compensations
- Not ready for PO feeds

## Current Route for Feeds

- PO
- PO with close monitoring
- PO with PG top-up as required
- NPO with conservative PO trials
- NPO

## Recommendations—to Be Implemented with Physician Approval

To assist with physiological stability and engagement during PO feeds, and advancement of PO feeding skills, it is suggested that Patient is fed with the following therapeutic compensations in place:

- Encourage breastfeeding, where possible
- Offer any bottle feeds with a ** flow nipple
- Utilize horizontal milk flow to assist Patient to control liquid flow and support improved SSB coordination (Note: It is easiest to achieve horizontal milk flow if Patient is positioned upright or in a side-lying position for PO feeds. Avoid feeding Patient in a reclined/supine position).
- Offer external pacing as required (i.e. tip bottle down to slow milk flow and/or impose break in sucking to allow Patient to catch breath).
- If Patient displays stress cues during PO feeds (e.g. hyper-vigilance, staring, forehead furrowing, reddened eyes/eyebrows, finger splaying), please allow break to recover and consider discontinuing feed if cues continue.
- If any signs suggestive of aspiration/airway compromise are observed during PO feeds (e.g. cough, wet breath sounds, increased congestion, SpO2 desaturation, apnea), please discontinue feed and document observations.
- To avoid aversion, please do not force feeds if Patient is gagging or distressed.
- To avoid fatigue, PO feeds should last no more than 30 minutes. If feeds consistently take longer than this, ongoing PG supplementation will likely be required.
- Given clinical signs suggestive of possible aspiration/airway compromise during PO feeds, an MBS (modified barium swallow) study is warranted to objectively evaluate swallow function and determine aspiration risk (Note: MD/NP orders are required to proceed).

- NICU Feeding Therapy Services to continue to provide support/guidance for Patient and family during stay, in association with nursing and medical staff.
- If required, outpatient feeding review/support can be arranged. To schedule, please call or email ***.

## References

[1] World Health Organization (WHO). Preterm birth. 2015. http://www.who.int/mediacentre/factsheets/fs363/en/

[2] March of Dimes. 2015 premature birth report card. 2016. http://www.marchofdimes.org/materials/premature-birth-report-card-united-states.pdf

[3] Centers for Disease Control and Prevention. Birth weight and gestation. 2015. http://www.cdc.gov/nchs/fastats/birthweight.htm

[4] Dodrill P. Feeding and swallowing development in infants and children. In: Groher M, Crary M, eds. Dysphagia: Clinical Management in Adults and Children. St. Louis, MO: Mosby; 2015

[5] Als H. Toward a synactive theory of development: Promise for the assessment of infant individuality. Infant Ment Health J 1982; (3):229–243

[6] Als H, Lester BM, Tronick EZ, Brazelton TB. Manual for the Assessment of Preterm Infants' Behavior (APIB). In: Fitzgerald HE, Lester BM, Yogman MW, eds. Theory and Research in Behavioral Pediatrics. New York, NY: Plenum; 1982:65–132

[7] Als H. Program Guide—Newborn Individualized Developmental Care and Assessment Program (NIDCAP): An Education and Training Program for Health Care Professionals. Unpublished manuscript, 11th revision. Boston, MA: Children's Medical Center Corporation; 2002

[8] Gardner S, Merenstein G. Handbook of Neonatal Intensive Care. St. Louis, MO: Mosby; 2002

[9] Kenner C, McGrath JM, eds. Developmental Care of Newborns and Infants: A Guide for Health Professionals. 2nd ed. St Louis, MO: Mosby; 2010

[10] Kliegman R, Stanton R, Geme J, Schor N, Behrman R. Nelson Textbook of Pediatrics. 19th ed. Philadelphia, PA: Elesiver Saunders; 2011

[11] Jacobs SE, Berg M, Hunt R, Tarnow-Mordi WO, Inder TE, Davis PG. Cooling for newborns with hypoxic ischaemic encephalopathy. Cochrane Database Syst Rev 2013;1(1):CD003311

[12] Vandenplas Y, Rudolph CD, Di Lorenzo C, et al; North American Society for Pediatric Gastroenterology Hepatology and Nutrition; European Society for Pediatric Gastroenterology Hepatology and Nutrition. Pediatric gastroesophageal reflux clinical practice guidelines: joint recommendations of the North American Society for Pediatric Gastroenterology, Hepatology, and Nutrition (NASPGHAN) and the European Society for Pediatric Gastroenterology, Hepatology, and Nutrition (ESPGHAN). J Pediatr Gastroenterol Nutr 2009;49(4):498–547

[13] U.S. Food and Drug Administration. FDA Expands Caution about SimplyThick 2015. http://www.fda.gov/ForConsumers/ConsumerUpdates/ucm256250.htm

[14] Smith ME, King JD, Elsherif A, Muntz HR, Park AH, Kouretas PC. Should all newborns who undergo patent ductus arteriosus ligation be examined for vocal fold mobility? Laryngoscope 2009;119(8):1606–1609

[15] Zbar RI, Chen AH, Behrendt DM, Bell EF, Smith RJ. Incidence of vocal fold paralysis in infants undergoing ligation of patent ductus arteriosus. Ann Thorac Surg 1996;61(3):814–816

[16] Committee on Fetus and Newborn. American Academy of Pediatrics. Apnea, sudden infant death syndrome, and home monitoring. Pediatrics 2003;111(4 Pt 1):914–917

[17] Dodrill P. Feeding difficulties in preterm neonates. Infant Child Adolesc Nutr 2011;3(6):324–331

[18] Burns Y, Rogers Y, Neil M, et al. Development of oral function in pre-term infants. Physiother Prac 1987;3:168–178

[19] Miller JL, Sonies BC, Macedonia C. Emergence of oropharyngeal, laryngeal and swallowing activity in the developing fetal upper aerodigestive tract: an ultrasound evaluation. Early Hum Dev 2003;71(1):61–87

[20] Hack M, Estabrook MM, Robertson SS. Development of sucking rhythm in preterm infants. Early Hum Dev 1985;11(2):133–140

[21] Hafström M, Kjellmer I. Non-nutritive sucking in sick preterm infants. Early Hum Dev 2001;63(1):37–52

[22] Lundqvist C, Hafström M. Non-nutritive sucking in full-term and preterm infants studied at term conceptional age. Acta Paediatr 1999;88(11):1287–1289

[23] Neiva FC, Leone C, Leone CR. Non-nutritive sucking scoring system for preterm newborns. Acta Paediatr 2008;97(10):1370–1375

[24] Lau C, Alagugurusamy R, Schanler RJ, Smith EO, Shulman RJ. Characterization of the developmental stages of sucking in preterm infants during bottle feeding. Acta Paediatr 2000;89(7):846–852

[25] Medoff-Cooper B. Changes in nutritive sucking patterns with increasing gestational age. Nurs Res 1991;40(4):245–247

[26] Miller JL, Kang SM. Preliminary ultrasound observation of lingual movement patterns during nutritive versus non-nutritive sucking in a premature infant. Dysphagia 2007;22(2):150–160

[27] Wrotniak BH, Stettler N, Medoff-Cooper B. The relationship between birth weight and feeding maturation in preterm infants. Acta Paediatr 2009;98(2):286–290

[28] Cunha M, Barreiros J, Gonçalves I, Figueiredo H. Nutritive sucking pattern—from very low birth weight preterm to term newborn. Early Hum Dev 2009;85(2):125–130

[29] da Costa SP, van der Schans CP, Zweens MJ, et al. The development of sucking patterns in preterm, small-for-gestational age infants. J Pediatr 2010;157(4):603–609, 609.e1–609.e3

[30] da Costa SP, van der Schans CP. The reliability of the Neonatal Oral-Motor Assessment Scale. Acta Paediatr 2008;97(1):21–26

[31] Pickler RH, Chiaranai C, Reyna BA. Relationship of the first suck burst to feeding outcomes in preterm infants. J Perinat Neonatal Nurs 2006;20(2):157–162

[32] Pickler RH, Best AM, Reyna BA, Gutcher G, Wetzel PA. Predictors of nutritive sucking in preterm infants. J Perinatol 2006;26(11):693–699

[33] Palmer MM, Crawley K, Blanco IA. Neonatal Oral-Motor Assessment scale: a reliability study. J Perinatol 1993;13(1):28–35

[34] Howe TH, Sheu CF, Hsieh YW, Hsieh CL. Psychometric characteristics of the Neonatal Oral-Motor Assessment Scale in healthy preterm infants. Dev Med Child Neurol 2007;49(12):915–919

[35] Howe TH, Sheu CF, Hinojosa J, Lin J, Holzman IR. Multiple factors related to bottle-feeding performance in preterm infants. Nurs Res 2007;56(5):307–311

[36] Thoyre SM, Shaker CS, Pridham KF. The early feeding skills assessment for preterm infants. Neonatal Netw 2005;24(3):7–16

[37] Medoff-Cooper B, McGrath JM, Bilker W. Nutritive sucking and neurobehavioral development in preterm infants from 34 weeks PCA to term. MCN Am J Matern Child Nurs 2000;25(2):64–70

[38] Medoff-Cooper B, McGrath JM, Shults J. Feeding patterns of full-term and preterm infants at forty weeks postconceptional age. J Dev Behav Pediatr 2002;23(4):231–236

[39] Medoff-Cooper B, Weininger S, Zukowsky K. Neonatal sucking as a clinical assessment tool: preliminary findings. Nurs Res 1989;38(3):162–165

[40] Jain L, Sivieri E, Abbasi S, Bhutani VK. Energetics and mechanics of nutritive sucking in the preterm and term neonate. J Pediatr 1987;111(6 Pt 1):894–898

[41] Iwayama K, Eishima M. [Sucking behavior of normal full-term and low-risk preterm infants]. No To Hattatsu 1995;27(5):363–369

[42] Tsai SW, Chen CH, Lin MC. Prediction for developmental delay on Neonatal Oral Motor Assessment Scale in preterm infants without brain lesion. Pediatr Int 2010;52(1):65–68

[43] Medoff-Cooper B, Shults J, Kaplan J. Sucking behavior of preterm neonates as a predictor of developmental outcomes. J Dev Behav Pediatr 2009;30(1):16–22

[44] de Castro AG, Lima MdeC, de Aquino RR, Eickmann SH. [Sensory oral motor and global motor development of preterm infants]. Pro Fono 2007;19(1):29–38

[45] Daniëls H, Devlieger H, Casaer P, Callens M, Eggermont E. Nutritive and non-nutritive sucking in preterm infants. J Dev Physiol 1986;8(2):117–121

[46] Amaizu N, Shulman R, Schanler R, Lau C. Maturation of oral feeding skills in preterm infants. Acta Paediatr 2008;97(1):61–67

[47] Mizuno K, Ueda A. The maturation and coordination of sucking, swallowing, and respiration in preterm infants. J Pediatr 2003;142(1):36–40

[48] Lau C, Smith EO, Schanler RJ. Coordination of suck-swallow and swallow respiration in preterm infants. Acta Paediatr 2003;92(6):721–727

[49] Vice FL, Gewolb IH. Respiratory patterns and strategies during feeding in preterm infants. Dev Med Child Neurol 2008;50(6):467–472

[50] Reynolds EW, Grider D, Caldwell R, et al. Swallow-breath interaction and phase of respiration with swallow during nonnutritive suck among low-risk preterm infants. Am J Perinatol 2010;27(10):831–840

[51] Hanlon MB, Tripp JH, Ellis RE, Flack FC, Selley WG, Shoesmith HJ. Deglutition apnoea as indicator of maturation of suckle feeding in bottle-fed preterm infants. Dev Med Child Neurol 1997;39(8):534–542

[52] Gewolb IH, Vice FL. Maturational changes in the rhythms, patterning, and coordination of respiration and swallow during feeding in preterm and term infants. Dev Med Child Neurol 2006;48(7):589–594

[53] Shivpuri CR, Martin RJ, Carlo WA, Fanaroff AA. Decreased ventilation in preterm infants during oral feeding. J Pediatr 1983;103(2):285–289

[54] Thoyre SM, Carlson J. Occurrence of oxygen desaturation events during preterm infant bottle feeding near discharge. *Early Hum Dev* 2003;72(1):25–36

[55] Conway AE. Young infants' feeding patterns when sick and well. *Matern Child Nurs J* 1989;18(4):1–353

[56] Craig CM, Lee DN, Freer YN, Laing IA. Modulations in breathing patterns during intermittent feeding in term infants and preterm infants with bronchopulmonary dysplasia. *Dev Med Child Neurol* 1999;41(9):616–624

[57] Garg M, Kurzner SI, Bautista DB, Keens TG. Clinically unsuspected hypoxia during sleep and feeding in infants with bronchopulmonary dysplasia. *Pediatrics* 1988;81(5):635–642

[58] Gewolb IH, Bosma JF, Taciak VL, Vice FL. Abnormal developmental patterns of suck and swallow rhythms during feeding in preterm infants with bronchopulmonary dysplasia. *Dev Med Child Neurol* 2001;43(7):454–459

[59] Gewolb IH, Bosma JF, Reynolds EW, Vice FL. Integration of suck and swallow rhythms during feeding in preterm infants with and without bronchopulmonary dysplasia. *Dev Med Child Neurol* 2003;45(5):344–348

[60] Stumm S, Barlow SM, Estep M, et al. Respiratory distress syndrome degrades the fine structure of the non-nutritive suck in preterm infants. *J Neonatal Nurs* 2008;14(1):9–16

[61] Estep M, Barlow SM, Vantipalli R, Finan D, Lee J. Non-nutritive suck parameter in preterm infants with RDS. *J Neonatal Nurs* 2008;14(1):28–34

[62] Poore M, Barlow SM, Wang J, Estep M, Lee J. Respiratory treatment history predicts suck pattern stability in preterm infants. *J Neonatal Nurs* 2008;14(6):185–192

[63] Howe TH, Sheu CF, Holzman IR. Bottle-feeding behaviors in preterm infants with and without bronchopulmonary dysplasia. *Am J Occup Ther* 2007;61(4):378–383

[64] Mizuno K, Nishida Y, Taki M, et al. Infants with bronchopulmonary dysplasia suckle with weak pressures to maintain breathing during feeding. *Pediatrics* 2007;120(4):e1035–e1042

[65] Wang LY, Luo HJ, Hsieh WS, et al. Severity of bronchopulmonary dysplasia and increased risk of feeding desaturation and growth delay in very low birth weight preterm infants. *Pediatr Pulmonol* 2010;45(2):165–173

[66] Gewolb IH, Vice FL. Abnormalities in the coordination of respiration and swallow in preterm infants with bronchopulmonary dysplasia. *Dev Med Child Neurol* 2006;48(7):595–599

[67] Daniels H, Devlieger H, Casaer P, Ramaekers V, van den Broeck J, Eggermont E. Feeding, behavioural state and cardiorespiratory control. *Acta Paediatr Scand* 1988;77(3):369–373

[68] Daniels H, Devlieger H, Minami T, Eggermont E, Casaer P. Infant feeding and cardiorespiratory maturation. *Neuropediatrics* 1990;21(1):9–10

[69] Eichenwald EC, Blackwell M, Lloyd JS, Tran T, Wilker RE, Richardson DK. Inter-neonatal intensive care unit variation in discharge timing: influence of apnea and feeding management. *Pediatrics* 2001;108(4):928–933

[70] Dodrill P, Donovan T, Cleghorn G, McMahon S, Davies PS. Attainment of early feeding milestones in preterm neonates. *J Perinatol* 2008;28(8):549–555

[71] Bingham PM, Ashikaga T, Abbasi S. Prospective study of non-nutritive sucking and feeding skills in premature infants. *Arch Dis Child Fetal Neonatal Ed* 2010;95(3):F194–F200

[72] Jadcherla SR, Wang M, Vijayapal AS, Leuthner SR. Impact of prematurity and co-morbidities on feeding milestones in neonates: a retrospective study. *J Perinatol* 2010;30(3):201–208

[73] Pickler RH, Mauck AG, Geldmaker B. Bottle-feeding histories of preterm infants. *J Obstet Gynecol Neonatal Nurs* 1997;26(4):414–420

[74] Bühler KE, Limongi SC. [Factors associated to oral feeding transition in preterm infants]. *Pro Fono* 2004;16(3):301–310

[75] Pickler RH, Best A, Crosson D. The effect of feeding experience on clinical outcomes in preterm infants. *J Perinatol* 2009;29(2):124–129

[76] Pridham KF, Sondel S, Chang A, Green C. Nipple feeding for preterm infants with bronchopulmonary dysplasia. *J Obstet Gynecol Neonatal Nurs* 1993;22(2):147–155

[77] Mandich MB, Ritchie SK, Mullett M. Transition times to oral feeding in premature infants with and without apnea. *J Obstet Gynecol Neonatal Nurs* 1996;25(9):771–776

[78] Hawdon JM, Beauregard N, Slattery J, Kennedy G. Identification of neonates at risk of developing feeding problems in infancy. *Dev Med Child Neurol* 2000;42(4):235–239

[79] McCain GC. Behavioral state activity during nipple feedings for preterm infants. *Neonatal Netw* 1997;16(5):43–47

[80] White-Traut RC, Berbaum ML, Lessen B, McFarlin B, Cardenas L. Feeding readiness in preterm infants: the relationship between preterm behavioral state and feeding readiness behaviors and efficiency during transition from gavage to oral feeding. *MCN Am J Matern Child Nurs* 2005;30(1):52–59

[81] Silberstein D, Geva R, Feldman R, et al. The transition to oral feeding in low-risk premature infants: relation to infant neurobehavioral functioning and mother-infant feeding interaction. *Early Hum Dev* 2009;85(3):157–162

[82] Shiao SY, Brooker J, DiFiore T. Desaturation events during oral feedings with and without a nasogastric tube in very low birth weight infants. *Heart Lung* 1996;25(3):236–245

[83] Shiao SY, Youngblut JM, Anderson GC, DiFiore JM, Martin RJ. Nasogastric tube placement: effects on breathing and sucking in very-low-birth-weight infants. *Nurs Res* 1995;44(2):82–88

[84] Daga SR, Lunkad NG, Daga AS, Ahuja VK. Orogastric versus nasogastric feeding of newborn babies. *Trop Doct* 1999;29(4):242–243

[85] Peter CS, Wiechers C, Bohnhorst B, Silny J, Poets CF. Influence of nasogastric tubes on gastroesophageal reflux in preterm infants: a multiple intraluminal impedance study. *J Pediatr* 2002;141(2):277–279

[86] Jadcherla SR, Stoner E, Gupta A, et al. Evaluation and management of neonatal dysphagia: impact of pharyngoesophageal motility studies and multidisciplinary feeding strategy. *J Pediatr Gastroenterol Nutr* 2009;48(2):186–192

[87] Dodrill P. Medical conditions impacting on feeding and swallowing development in infants and children. In: Groher M, Crary M, eds. Dysphagia: Clinical Management in Adults and Children. St. Louis, MO: Mosby; 2015

[88] Pierrehumbert B, Nicole A, Muller-Nix C, Forcada-Guex M, Ansermet F. Parental post-traumatic reactions after premature birth: implications for sleeping and eating problems in the infant. *Arch Dis Child Fetal Neonatal Ed* 2003;88(5):F400–F404

[89] Thoyre SM. Mothers' ideas about their role in feeding their high-risk infants. *J Obstet Gynecol Neonatal Nurs* 2000;29(6):613–624

[90] Thoyre SM, Brown RL. Factors contributing to preterm infant engagement during bottle-feeding. *Nurs Res* 2004;53(5):304–313

[91] Pridham KF, Schroeder M, Brown R, Clark R. The relationship of a mother's working model of feeding to her feeding behaviour. *J Adv Nurs* 2001;35(5):741–750

[92] Thoyre SM. Challenges mothers identify in bottle feeding their preterm infants. *Neonatal Netw* 2001;20(1):41–50

[93] Pridham KF, Martin R, Sondel S, Tluczek A. Parental issues in feeding young children with bronchopulmonary dysplasia. *J Pediatr Nurs* 1989;4(3):177–185

[94] Swift MC, Scholten I. Not feeding, not coming home: parental experiences of infant feeding difficulties and family relationships in a neonatal unit. *J Clin Nurs* 2010;19(1 2):249–258

[95] Hill PD, Hanson KS, Mefford AL. Mothers of low birthweight infants: breastfeeding patterns and problems. *J Hum Lact* 1994;10(3):169 176

[96] Kavanaugh K, Mead L, Meier P, Mangurten HH. Getting enough: mothers' concerns about breastfeeding a preterm infant after discharge. *J Obstet Gynecol Neonatal Nurs* 1995;24(1):23–32

[97] Kavanaugh K, Meier P, Zimmermann B, Mead L. The rewards outweigh the efforts: breastfeeding outcomes for mothers of preterm infants. *J Hum Lact* 1997;13(1):15–21

[98] Dowling DA, Madigan E, Anthony MK, Abou Elfettoh A, Graham G. Reliability and validity of the Preterm Infant Feeding Survey: instrument development and testing. *J Nurs Meas* 2009;17(3):171–182

[99] Dowling DA, Shapiro J, Burant CJ, Elfettoh AA. Factors influencing feeding decisions of black and white mothers of preterm infants. *J Obstet Gynecol Neonatal Nurs* 2009;38(3):300–309

[100] Meier P. Bottle- and breast-feeding: effects on transcutaneous oxygen pressure and temperature in preterm infants. *Nurs Res* 1988;37(1):36–41

[101] Dowling DA. Physiological responses of preterm infants to breast-feeding and bottle-feeding with the orthodontic nipple. *Nurs Res* 1999;48(2):78–85

[102] Chen CH, Wang TM, Chang HM, Chi CS. The effect of breast- and bottle-feeding on oxygen saturation and body temperature in preterm infants. *J Hum Lact* 2000;16(1):21–27

[103] American Academy of Pediatrics. Breastfeeding and the use of human milk. 2012. http://pediatrics.aappublications.org/content/pediatrics/129/3/e827.full.pdf

[104] Conde-Agudelo A, Díaz-Rossello JL. Kangaroo mother care to reduce morbidity and mortality in low birthweight infants. *Cochrane Database Syst Rev* 2014;4(4):CD002771

[105] Measel CP, Anderson GC. Nonnutritive sucking during tube feedings: effect on clinical course in premature infants. *JOGN Nurs* 1979;8(5):265–272

[106] Bernbaum JC, Pereira GR, Watkins JB, Peckham GJ. Nonnutritive sucking during gavage feeding enhances growth and maturation in premature infants. *Pediatrics* 1983;71(1):41–45

[107] Field T, Ignatoff E, Stringer S, et al. Nonnutritive sucking during tube feedings: effects on preterm neonates in an intensive care unit. *Pediatrics* 1982;70(3):381–384

[108] Sehgal SK, Prakash O, Gupta A, Mohan M, Anand NK. Evaluation of beneficial effects of nonnutritive sucking in preterm infants. *Indian Pediatr* 1990;27(3):263–266

[109] Pinelli J, Symington A. How rewarding can a pacifier be? A systematic review of nonnutritive sucking in preterm infants. *Neonatal Netw* 2000;19(8):41–48

[110] Pinelli J, Symington A, Ciliska D. Nonnutritive sucking in high-risk infants: benign intervention or legitimate therapy? *J Obstet Gynecol Neonatal Nurs* 2002;31(5):582–591

[111] Pinelli J, Symington A. Non-nutritive sucking for promoting physiologic stability and nutrition in preterm infants. *Cochrane Database Syst Rev* 2005; (4):CD001071

[112] Schwartz R, Moody L, Yarandi H, Anderson GC. A meta-analysis of critical outcome variables in nonnutritive sucking in preterm infants. *Nurs Res* 1987;36(5):292–295

[113] Pickler RH, Frankel HB, Walsh KM, Thompson NM. Effects of nonnutritive sucking on behavioral organization and feeding performance in preterm infants. *Nurs Res* 1996;45(3):132–135

[114] Pickler RH, Higgins KE, Crummette BD. The effect of nonnutritive sucking on bottle-feeding stress in preterm infants. *J Obstet Gynecol Neonatal Nurs* 1993;22(3):230–234

[115] Pickler RH, Reyna BA. Effects of non-nutritive sucking on nutritive sucking, breathing, and behavior during bottle feedings of preterm infants. *Adv Neonatal Care* 2004;4(4):226–234

[116] Gill NE, Behnke M, Conlon M, Anderson GC. Nonnutritive sucking modulates behavioral state for preterm infants before feeding. *Scand J Caring Sci* 1992;6(1):3–7

[117] Gill NE, Behnke M, Conlon M, McNeely JB, Anderson GC. Effect of nonnutritive sucking on behavioral state in preterm infants before feeding. *Nurs Res* 1988;37(6):347–350

[118] McCain GC. Promotion of preterm infant nipple feeding with nonnutritive sucking. *J Pediatr Nurs* 1995;10(1):3–8

[119] McCain GC. Facilitating inactive awake states in preterm infants: a study of three interventions. *Nurs Res* 1992;41(3):157–160

[120] Barlow SM, Finan DS, Lee J, Chu S. Synthetic orocutaneous stimulation entrains preterm infants with feeding difficulties to suck. *J Perinatol* 2008;28(8):541–548

[121] Poore M, Zimmerman E, Barlow SM, Wang J, Gu F. Patterned orocutaneous therapy improves sucking and oral feeding in preterm infants. *Acta Paediatr* 2008;97(7):920–927

[122] Fucile S, Gisel E, Lau C. Oral stimulation accelerates the transition from tube to oral feeding in preterm infants. *J Pediatr* 2002;141(2):230–236

[123] Fucile S, Gisel EG, Lau C. Effect of an oral stimulation program on sucking skill maturation of preterm infants. *Dev Med Child Neurol* 2005;47(3):158–162

[124] Gaebler CP, Hanzlik JR. The effects of a prefeeding stimulation program on preterm infants. *Am J Occup Ther* 1996;50(3):184–192

[125] Leonard EL, Trykowski LE, Kirkpatrick BV. Nutritive sucking in high-risk neonates after perioral stimulation. *Phys Ther* 1980;60(3):299–302

[126] Case-Smith J. An efficacy study of occupational therapy with high-risk neonates. *Am J Occup Ther* 1988;42(8):499–506

[127] Rausch PB. Effects of tactile and kinesthetic stimulation on premature infants. *J Obstet Gynecol Neonatal Nurs* 1981;10(1):34–37

[128] White JL, Labarba RC. The effects of tactile and kinesthetic stimulation on neonatal development in the premature infant. *Dev Psychobiol* 1976;9(6):569–577

[129] Hill AS, Kurkowski TB, Garcia J. Oral support measures used in feeding the preterm infant. *Nurs Res* 2000;49(1):2–10

[130] Boiron M, Da Nobrega L, Roux S, Henrot A, Saliba E. Effects of oral stimulation and oral support on non-nutritive sucking and feeding performance in preterm infants. *Dev Med Child Neurol* 2007;49(6):439–444

[131] Hwang YS, Vergara E, Lin CH, Coster WJ, Bigsby R, Tsai WH. Effects of prefeeding oral stimulation on feeding performance of preterm infants. *Indian J Pediatr* 2010;77(8):869–873

[132] Bragelien R, Røkke W, Markestad T. Stimulation of sucking and swallowing to promote oral feeding in premature infants. *Acta Paediatr* 2007;96(10):1430–1432

[133] Pimenta HP, Moreira ME, Rocha AD, Gomes SC Jr, Pinto LW, Lucena SL. Effects of non-nutritive sucking and oral stimulation on breastfeeding rates for preterm, low birth weight infants: a randomized clinical trial. *J Pediatr (Rio J)* 2008;84(5):423–427

[134] Einarsson-Backes LM, Deitz J, Price R, Glass R, Hays R. The effect of oral support on sucking efficiency in preterm infants. *Am J Occup Ther* 1994;48(6):490–498

[135] Hwang YS, Lin CH, Coster WJ, Bigsby R, Vergara E. Effectiveness of cheek and jaw support to improve feeding performance of preterm infants. *Am J Occup Ther* 2010;64(6):886–894

[136] Chang YJ, Lin CP, Lin YJ, Lin CH. Effects of single-hole and cross-cut nipple units on feeding efficiency and physiological parameters in premature infants. *J Nurs Res* 2007;15(3):215–223

[137] Mathew OP. Breathing patterns of preterm infants during bottle feeding: role of milk flow. *J Pediatr* 1991;119(6):960–965

[138] Fucile S, Gisel E, Schanler RJ, Lau C. A controlled-flow vacuum-free bottle system enhances preterm infants' nutritive sucking skills. *Dysphagia* 2009;24(2):145–151

[139] Park J, Thoyre S, Knafl GJ, Hodges EA, Nix WB. Efficacy of semielevated side-lying positioning during bottle-feeding of very preterm infants: a pilot study. *J Perinat Neonatal Nurs* 2014;28(1):69–79

[140] Dawson JA, Myers LR, Moorhead A, et al. A randomised trial of two techniques for bottle feeding preterm infants. *J Paediatr Child Health* 2013;49(6):462–466

[141] Law-Morstatt L, Judd DM, Snyder P, Baier RJ, Dhanireddy R. Pacing as a treatment technique for transitional sucking patterns. *J Perinatol* 2003;23(6):483–488

[142] Thoyre SM, Holditch-Davis D, Schwartz TA, Melendez Roman CR, Nix W. Coregulated approach to feeding preterm infants with lung disease: effects during feeding. *Nurs Res* 2012;61(4):242–251

[143] World Health Organization (WHO). Baby Friendly Hospital Initiative. 2009. http://www.who.int/nutrition/publications/infantfeeding/bfhi_trainingcourse/en/

[144] United Nations Children's Fund (UNICEF). 10 Steps to successful breastfeeding. http://www.unicef.org/programme/breastfeeding/baby.htm

[145] Nyqvist KH, Häggkvist AP, Hansen MN, et al; Baby-Friendly Hospital Initiative Expert Group. Expansion of the baby-friendly hospital initiative ten steps to successful breastfeeding into neonatal intensive care: expert group recommendations. *J Hum Lact* 2013;29(3):300–309

[146] Pinelli J, Symington A. Non-nutritive sucking for promoting physiologic stability and nutrition in preterm infants. *Cochrane Database Syst Rev* 2005;(4):CD001071

[147] Ross ES, Philbin MK. Supporting oral feeding in fragile infants: an evidence-based method for quality bottle-feedings of preterm, ill, and fragile infants. *J Perinat Neonatal Nurs* 2011;25(4):349–357, quiz 358–359

[148] Philbin MK, Ross ES. The SOFFI Reference Guide: text, algorithms, and appendices: a manualized method for quality bottle-feedings. *J Perinat Neonatal Nurs* 2011;25(4):360–380

[149] Arvedson J, Rogers B, Buck G, Smart P, Msall M. Silent aspiration prominent in children with dysphagia. *Int J Pediatr Otorhinolaryngol* 1994;28(2-3):173–181

[150] Weir KA, McMahon S, Taylor S, Chang AB. Oropharyngeal aspiration and silent aspiration in children. *Chest* 2011;140(3):589–597

[151] Ferrara L, Bidiwala A, Sher I, et al. Effect of nasal continuous positive airway pressure on the pharyngeal swallow in neonates. *J Perinatol* 2017;37(4):398–403. doi: 10.1038/jp.2016.229

[152] Weir K, McMahon S, Barry L, Masters IB, Chang AB. Clinical signs and symptoms of oropharyngeal aspiration and dysphagia in children. *Eur Respir J* 2009;33(3):604–611

[153] Pados BF, Park J, Thoyre SM, Estrem H, Nix WB. Milk flow rates from bottle nipples used for feeding infants who are hospitalized. *Am J Speech Lang Pathol* 2015;24(4):671–679

[154] Reau NR, Senturia YD, Lebailly SA, Christoffel KK; Pediatric Practice Research Group. Infant and toddler feeding patterns and problems: normative data and a new direction. *J Dev Behav Pediatr* 1996;17(3):149–153

[155] Nyqvist KH. Lack of knowledge persists about early breastfeeding competence in preterm infants. *J Hum Lact* 2013;29(3):296–299

[156] Simpson C, Schanler RJ, Lau C. Early introduction of oral feeding in preterm infants. *Pediatrics* 2002;110(3):517–522

[157] Kirk AT, Alder SC, King JD. Cue-based oral feeding clinical pathway results in earlier attainment of full oral feeding in premature infants. *J Perinatol* 2007;27(9):572–578

[158] NICE. Division of ankyloglossia (tongue-tie) for breastfeeding. Interventional procedures guidance [IPG 149]. December 2005. http://www.nice.org.uk/Guidance/IPG149

## Suggested Reading

[1] Arvedson J, Clark H, Lazarus C, Schooling T, Frymark T. Evidence-based systematic review: effects of oral motor interventions on feeding and swallowing in preterm infants. *Am J Speech Lang Pathol* 2010;19(4):321–340

[2] Dodrill P. Feeding difficulties in preterm infants. *Inf Child Adolesc Nutr.* 2011;3(6):324–331

[3] Pados BF, Park J, Thoyre SM, Estrem H, Nix WB. Milk flow rates from bottle nipples used for feeding infants who are hospitalized. *Am J Speech Lang Pathol* 2015;24(4):671–679

[4] Pados BF, Park J, Estrem H, Awotwi A. Assessment tools for evaluation of oral feeding in infants younger than 6 months. *Adv Neonatal Care* 2016;16(2):143–150

[5] Shaker CS. Infant-guided, co-regulated feeding in the neonatal intensive care unit. Part I: theoretical underpinnings for neuroprotection and safety. *Semin Speech Lang* 2017;38(2):96–105

# 15 Dysphagia in Craniofacial Syndromes

*Scott Dailey*

## Summary

Infants and children with cleft and craniofacial syndromes are at risk for feeding and swallowing disorders. The difficulties may be related to anatomical defects, such as clefts, or to neuromotor disorders associated with some syndromic diagnoses. An interdisciplinary team that includes caregivers as members of the care team is best suited for the management of feeding and swallowing difficulties. Growth, development, and overall health are the goals of team management.

## Keywords

cleft palate, feeding, syndrome, sequence, orofacial, craniofacial, submucous

## Learning Objectives

- Describe the differences between syndrome, sequence, and association
- Define craniofacial disorder
- Explain the impact of a cleft lip with or without cleft palate on nipple feeding
- Describe the various nipple considerations that may impact feeding success
- List the orofacial regions impacted by orofacial clefts

## 15.1 Introduction

Feeding is one of the first bonding opportunities for families and their newborns. When an infant is born with a **craniofacial** disorder, the time following birth can be stressful, with many concerns and questions, as families work with a team of multidisciplinary professionals to determine the best way to feed their newborn. Caregivers need support and education about how to feed their infant with a craniofacial disorder, and they need to understand the plan for long-term care of their newborn. Speech-language pathologists are part of the multidisciplinary craniofacial team that will partner with families during their child's lifetime and are frequently the first professionals to assist caregivers with successfully feeding their infant.

## 15.2 Clefts as Part of Syndromes, Sequences, and Associations

*Craniofacial disorder* is a broad description applied to any abnormality of the face or head. Craniofacial disorders are congenital, meaning they are present at birth, and range in severity from mild to severe. Craniofacial disorders may include **craniosynostosis**, **hemifacial microsomia**, **submucous cleft palate**, **velopharyngeal insufficiency**, and **clefts** of the lip or palate. Recall from previous discussion in Chapter 2 that facial development begins approximately 3 weeks after conception. Facial development is a multidimensional process (**Fig. 15.1**), and students may find it helpful to reference video examples of facial development to fully conceptualize what is happening in the rapidly changing fetus (https://www.youtube.com/watch?v=oz1kJexvEFE), in addition to reviewing embryological development discussed in Chapter 2. Clefts occur early in facial development when developing structures do not completely fuse together. Clefts can affect the lip, hard palate, and soft palate (**Fig. 15.2**). A cleft lip may be unilateral, affecting only one side, or bilateral, affecting both sides. A cleft of the lip may be complete, extending from the **vermilion** into the base of the nose, or may be incomplete and extend only partially superior from the vermilion. **Fig. 15.3** provides a view of typical infant orofacial features for review. A cleft lip may be associated with clefting of more posterior structures, including the alveolus and hard and soft palate. A cleft of the palate may involve all or only part of the palate. For a video discussion of the types of clefts and the typical schedule for repair, please see https://www.youtube.com/watch?v=luYZ-mBHs30, produced by Boston Children's Hospital. A submucous cleft is a cleft of the underlying structures of the palate (bone and muscle), whereas the overlying **mucosa** appears intact or nearly intact. Classic signs of a submucous cleft include a **bifid uvula**; **zona pellucida**, which is a blue/white midline appearance of the posterior palate; a **V**-shaped notch in the hard palate on palpation; and velar tenting on elevation (**Fig. 15.4**).

Parker and colleagues of the National Birth Defects Prevention Network, in an analysis from 2004 to 2006, reported that 2,650 babies are born with a cleft palate, and 4,440 babies are born with a cleft lip with or without a cleft palate.[1] Clefts that occur with no other birth defect (isolated **orofacial** clefts) are one of the most common types of birth defects in the United States.[1] Clefts of the lip and/or palate also occur as part of other genetic syndromes. More than 200 different syndromes have cleft lip or palate as an associated feature.[2]

*Syndrome* refers to a pattern of features and symptoms that occur together consistently with a common known or suspected cause that can usually be traced to a single genetic **malformation**.[3] Individuals with craniofacial syndromes share similar, often recognizable, facial features, such as individuals with Down syndrome (trisomy 21). In contrast to a syndrome, the term *sequence* describes anomalies that occur due to one primary defect that causes additional secondary anomalies. A sequence may have multiple causes, in contrast to syndromes. Pierre Robin sequence is arguably one of the best known and recognized examples of a sequence. A nonrandom pattern of multiple anomalies in two or more individuals that do not meet the definition of *syndrome* or *sequence* is referred to as an

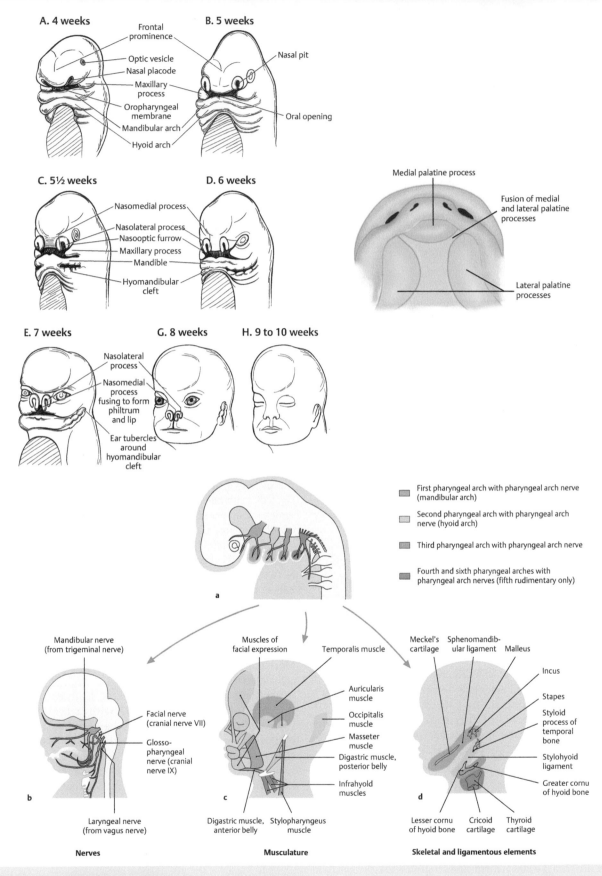

**Fig. 15.1** Typical facial development in utero.

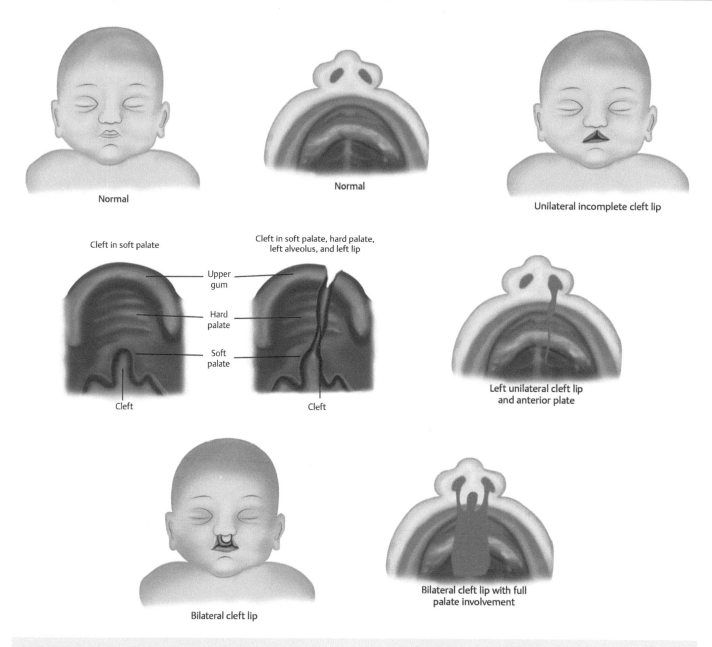

Normal

Normal

Unilateral incomplete cleft lip

Cleft in soft palate

Cleft in soft palate, hard palate, left alveolus, and left lip

Upper gum

Hard palate

Soft palate

Cleft

Cleft

Left unilateral cleft lip and anterior plate

Bilateral cleft lip

Bilateral cleft lip with full palate involvement

**Fig. 15.2** Types of clefts.

*association.*[3] With an association, the genetic etiology cannot be determined, and the pathogenesis is not known. VACTERL or VATER association consists of the occurrence of three or more of the following anomalies co-occurring in an individual: V—verte-brae, A—imperforate anus or anal atresia, C—cardiac anomalies, TE—tracheoesophageal fistula, R—renal (kidney) anomalies, L—limb anomalies. It is important to distinguish between syndromes, sequences, and associations for medical management and genetic counseling. Infants and children with syndromes, sequences, and associations that have craniofacial disorders with or without clefts of the lip and/or palate often have feeding and swallowing difficulty related to the craniofacial disorder and the resulting impact on airway patency.

## 15.3 Swallowing and Feeding Concerns in Syndromes

Pierre Robin sequence (PRS) (**Fig. 15.5**) features multiple craniofacial anomalies, including **micrognathia** (small mandible, also known as hypoplastic, or underdeveloped, mandible), **retrognathia** (posteriorly displaced mandible), and **glossoptosis** (posterior positioning of the tongue) and may include a **U**-shaped cleft palate.[4,5] PRS has been associated with several syndromes, including **Stickler syndrome**, **Treacher Collins syndrome**, **22q11.2 deletion syndrome**, and **craniofacial microsomia** (**Fig. 15.6**).[4,5] Glossoptosis is associated with airway obstruction

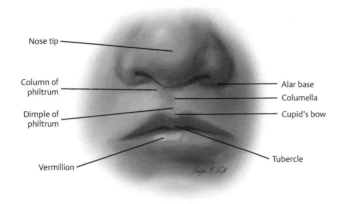

**Fig. 15.3** Surface anatomy of the infant face.

Nose tip
Column of philtrum
Dimple of philtrum
Vermillion
Alar base
Columella
Cupid's bow
Tubercle

adequate oral intake. **Nasopharyngeal tubes**, which stent the pharyngeal airway, have also been used (**Fig. 15.7**).[8,9,10] Surgical intervention is typically the last option when other less invasive options have failed. The surgical procedures used for airway management vary among institutions and surgeons but include **lip-tongue adhesion, tracheostomy**, and **mandibular distraction** (**Fig. 15.8**).[4,5,9,10] Airway management does not always result in improved feeding.[11]

In addition, some infants with PRS have neuromotor differences that may impact feeding.[11,12,13,14,15] Disorganization of the tongue, pharynx, and esophagus has been identified in some infants with PRS by electromyography and manometry.[11,12,13,14,15] Infants with these identified neuromotor difficulties are more likely to have long-term respiratory obstruction and feeding difficulties.[11,12,13,14,15] Therefore, the feeding difficulties of some infants with PRS may not be the result of just the physical difference; they may also be related to neurologic differences.

22q11.2 deletion syndrome includes **DiGeorge syndrome, velocardiofacial syndrome**, and **conotruncal anomaly face syndrome**.[16,17,18,19,20] Common features of 22q11.2 deletion syndrome include cleft lip and palate, other palatal anomalies (e.g., submucous cleft or noncleft velopharyngeal incompetence), PRS, and feeding difficulties.[16,17,18,19,20] Other anomalies associated with 22q11.2 deletion syndrome may impact infant feeding and swallowing as well and include congenital cardiac disease,

from the base of the tongue, choking, and aspiration of liquids.[6] Primary medical management is concerned with airway management before feeding management.[7] Airway management usually starts with conservative and noninvasive options, including positioning. Typically prone position allows gravity to maintain a tongue-forward position.[4,8,9,10] The use of prone positioning has provided variable success in promoting safe and

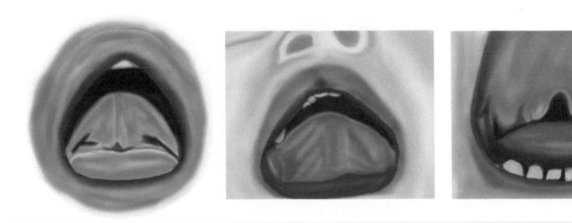

**Fig. 15.4** Features of a submucous cleft.

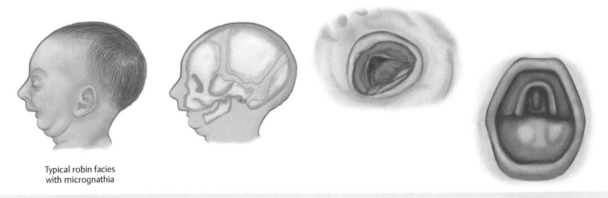

Typical robin facies with micrognathia

**Fig. 15.5** Pierre Robin sequence.

immunodeficiency, hypocalcemia, hypotonia, and gastrointestinal issues.[19] Other associated characteristics may affect feeding at later ages, including cognitive dysfunction, behavioral disorders, and psychiatric disorders.[19]

Feeding difficulties associated with 22q11.2 deletion syndrome may include those associated with cleft lip or palate if present.

However, feeding difficulties may be present in the absence of a cleft and can include nasopharyngeal regurgitation, pharyngeal hypotonia, hyperdynamic pharyngeal constrictor, cricopharyngeal prominence, prolonged feeding times, fatigue with feeding, disorganized suck–swallow–breathe sequence, gagging, and choking.[19] Tracheolaryngeal anomalies, such as laryngeal web,

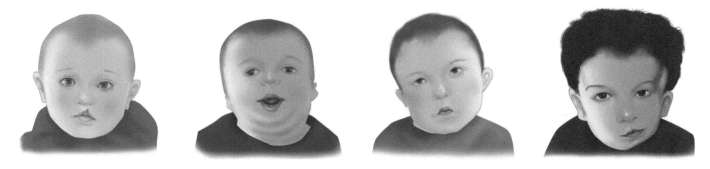

Fig. 15.6 Syndromes with co-occurring Pierre Robin sequence.

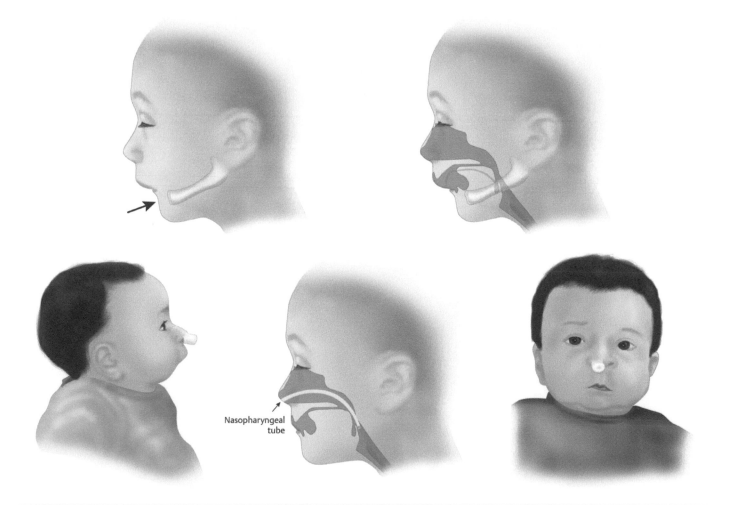

Nasopharyngeal tube

Fig. 15.7 Micrognathia, glossoptosis, and nasopharyngeal tubes.

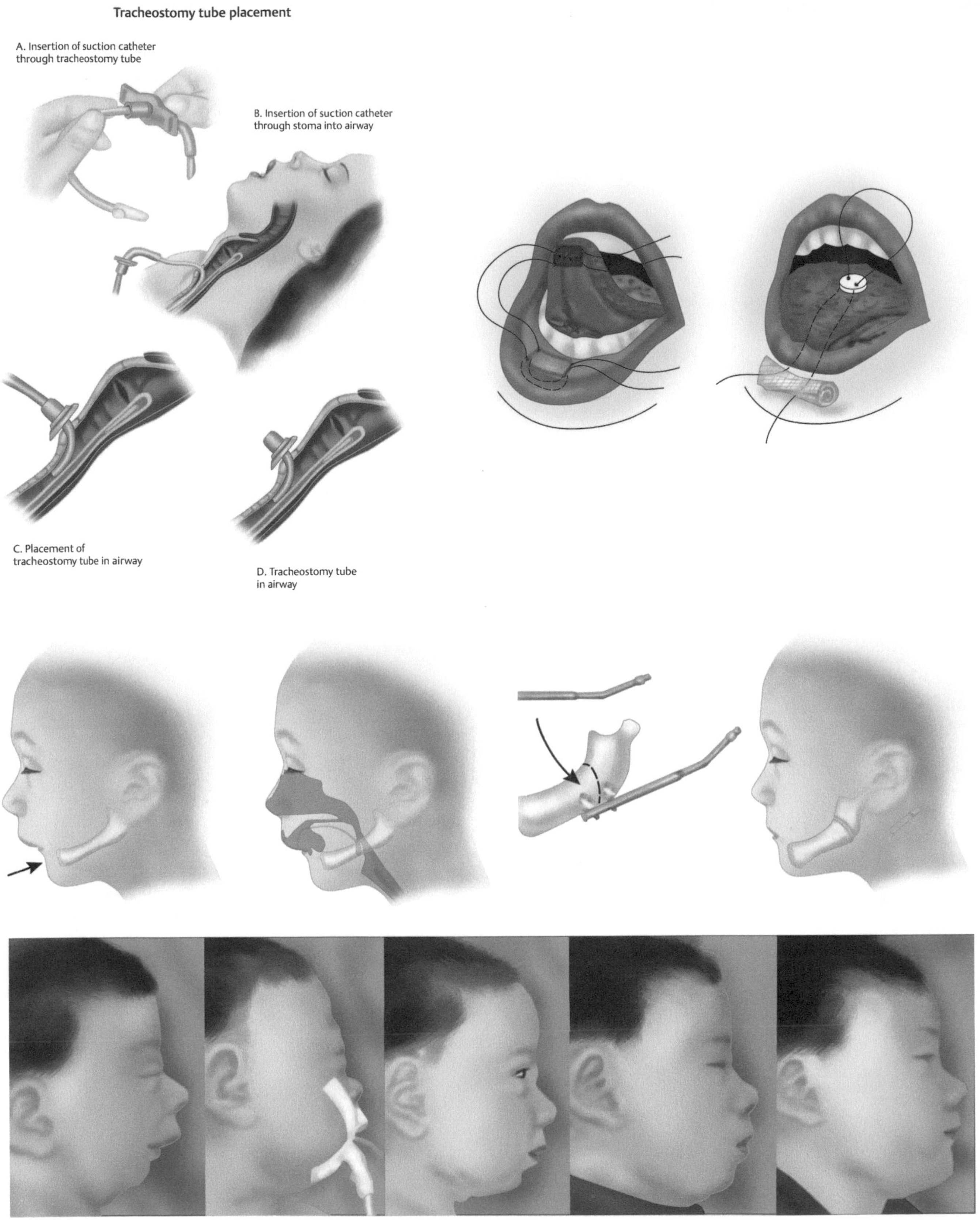

Tracheostomy tube placement

A. Insertion of suction catheter
through tracheostomy tube

B. Insertion of suction catheter
through stoma into airway

C. Placement of
tracheostomy tube in airway

D. Tracheostomy tube
in airway

**Fig. 15.8** Surgical procedures to alleviate airway obstruction.

**laryngeal paralysis**, **laryngeal cleft**, or **vascular rings** (**Fig. 15.9**) may also worsen feeding difficulties.[19,20] Feeding difficulties, such as intolerance for increased volume of feeding and difficulty advancing textures, may persist into childhood. Many individuals with 22q11.2 deletion syndrome need supplemental feeding or alternative feeding via gastrostomy tubes to have adequate growth.[19] Conditions that contribute to airway compromise, like those already reviewed, interfere with suck—swallow—breathe coordination, but of all the congenital anomalies that impact swallowing and feeding, cleft of the lip and/or palate is the most common.

## 15.4 Swallowing and Feeding Concerns Due to Cleft Lip and/or Palate

Feeding difficulties are common in infants with clefts, particularly if there is a cleft of the palate, even when they occur as an isolated anomaly (not part of a syndrome, sequence, or association). Some infants with cleft lip and/or palate may have only mild difficulties, and other infants may have more severe feeding difficulties.[21] In addition, infants with a cleft as part

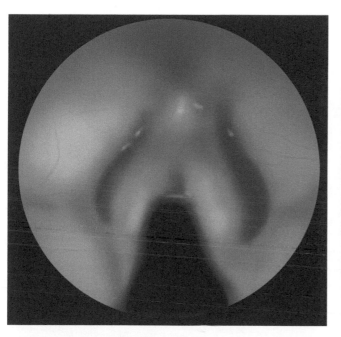
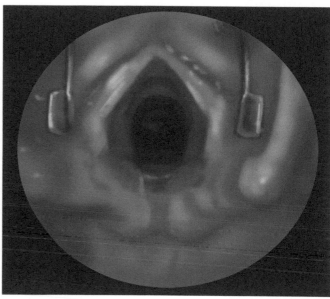
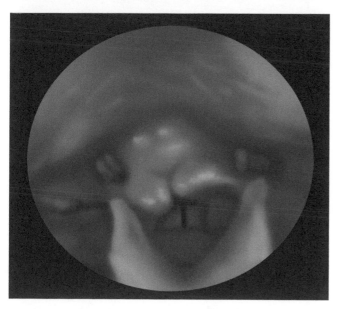
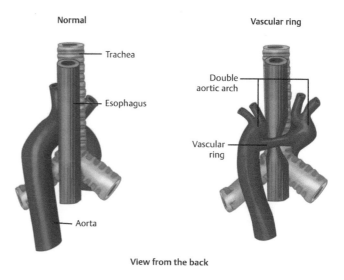

**Fig. 15.9** Tracheolaryngeal anomalies that contribute to feeding difficulties.

of a syndrome may have additional feeding and swallowing difficulties.[7] Feeding difficulties can lead to poor growth.[22] Due to the feeding difficulties, compensations and modifications are necessary.

The feeding difficulties in infants with clefts are directly related to anatomical defects. Recall from the discussion of typical nipple feeding in Chapter 3, that sucking on a nipple (bottle or breast) requires an intact lip, alveolus, and palate to create positive pressure during compression with the jaw and tongue.[23] Negative intraoral pressure is created as the lips and tongue are sealed around the nipple and the tongue retracts and the jaw lowers. This negative intraoral pressure, or suction, draws fluid from the nipple.[23] The fluid is deposited from the nipple onto the midtongue and moved posteriorly toward the pharynx as the tongue elevates from anterior to posterior against the palate.[23] As the infant swallows, the soft palate rises to seal the nasopharynx from the oropharynx to prevent nasal regurgitation and provide a superior sealed pharynx.[23] These are the events that are most likely impacted during feeding when a cleft is present.[21]

Common feeding difficulties associated with clefts and craniofacial anomalies are presented in **Box 15.1**. Reduced ability to draw the nipple into the mouth and difficulty expressing fluid from the nipple are observed frequently.[23,24] Infants with cleft palate have been found to have faster sucking rates and higher mean suck–swallow ratios when using regular nipples; these are likely a compensation for inefficiency by the infant to try to draw more from the nipple.[21] The ability to create negative and positive pressure during sucking varies based on the type of cleft.[25] Infants with cleft lip only generate positive pressure and negative pressure, but infants with cleft lip and palate or cleft palate only create similar positive pressure but less negative pressure.[25] Smaller clefts are associated with better levels of compression and expression.[25] Feeding efficiency was directly related to the ability to create negative and positive pressures.[25]

## Box 15.1

**Common Feeding Difficulties for Infants with Cleft Plate**
- Difficulty drawing the nipple into the mouth
- Difficulty creating negative pressure (suction)
- Difficulty with expression of fluid from the nipple
- Nasal regurgitation
- Greater ingestion of air
- Fatigue with feeding
- Poor growth and intake

Breastfeeding can be significantly difficult, especially if there is a cleft lip and palate or cleft palate due to the difficulties with drawing in of the nipple, latching adequately, and producing adequate pressures for expression of milk.[23,26,27] Infants with cleft lip only may breastfeed with minimal difficulties or with only minor support needed.[26,27]

Infants with clefts may ingest excess air due to the lack of ability to seal adequately on the nipple.[23,24] This may lead to bloating, choking, gagging, or fatigue with feeding and contributes to spitting up and emesis.[23,24] The lack of separation between the oral and nasal cavities in cleft palate may prevent the infant from completely clearing material from the mouth, nasopharynx, and oropharynx and may also result in nasal regurgitation with feeding.[7,24]

The feeding difficulties associated with clefts can result in feeding inefficiency and can impact growth.[22] Infants with clefts have been found to have birth weights similar to those of noncleft infants, but growth concerns were noted after birth prior to palate repair. Close monitoring of growth and development with strategies to facilitate successful feeding (**Fig. 15.10**) are needed to optimize growth.[28] Feeding and swallowing difficulties associated with clefts should be managed by a cleft–craniofacial team.[29,30] A cleft–craniofacial team consists of physicians, speech pathologists, nurses, orthodontists, audiologists, psychologists, and other medical professionals to provide coordinated care for the multiple health concerns of a child with a cleft/craniofacial disorder who may experience feeding and swallowing difficulties (**Box 15.2**).[30,31] For a video review of the role of the speech pathologist in the care and treatment of feeding concerns for infants with cleft of lip and/or palate, the reader is referred to https://www.youtube.com/watch?v=y0-b6e_pweg produced by Foundations for Faces of Children (info@facesofchildren.org).

## Box 15.2

**Members of a Cleft—Craniofacial Team**
The American Cleft Palate–Craniofacial Association recommends that coordinated care for infants and children with craniofacial anomalies be provided by a team of professionals from the following fields:
- Plastic surgery
- Orthodontics
- Speech-language pathology
- Audiology
- Otolaryngology
- Pediatrics
- Dentistry
- Oral surgery

A listing of cleft palate–craniofacial teams that meet the American Cleft Palate–Craniofacial Association standards is available on their website (http://www.acpa-cpf.org/team_care/).

## 15.5 Evaluating Swallowing and Feeding Difficulties

Interdisciplinary evaluation is necessary for proper management of feeding and swallowing difficulties associated with craniofacial disorders.[30] Evaluation and management are best completed by a cleft–craniofacial team (**Box 15.2**). Evaluation should include a review of medical information, an interview with caregivers, and examination and evaluation of the infant. The infant should be clinically evaluated during one or more oral feedings.[7] Clinical evaluation should include assessment of breathing in different positions, including nearly upright,

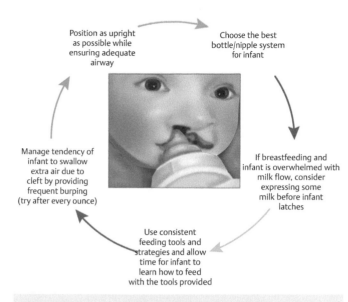

Position as upright as possible while ensuring adequate airway → Choose the best bottle/nipple system for infant → If breastfeeding and infant is overwhelmed with milk flow, consider expressing some milk before infant latches → Use consistent feeding tools and strategies and allow time for infant to learn how to feed with the tools provided → Manage tendency of infant to swallow extra air due to cleft by providing frequent burping (try after every ounce) →

**Fig. 15.10** General considerations to promote successful feeding.

side-lying, and prone.[7,24] Feeding should be attempted in the positions where the infant is most comfortable breathing. Specialty bottles/nipples should be selected based on the observations of the infant's difficulties, consideration of flow from the nipple, and parental preferences (**Table 15.1**).[7,24] The evaluation should include the use of one or more specialty feeding systems so that the infant and feeder responses can be evaluated, caregivers can be guided, and appropriate additional compensations can be implemented.

For infants with concern for pharyngeal dysphagia, airway issues, and/or aspiration, a videofluorographic swallow study is warranted if the infant has coughing, choking, desaturations, or increased lung congestion with feeding.[7] For infants with airway/breathing positioning constraints, a videofluorographic swallow evaluation should be completed only if the positioning optimal airway management may be maintained during the study.[7]

## 15.6 Management of Feeding and Swallowing Difficulties in Craniofacial Disorders

Management of feeding and swallowing difficulties in infants with cleft or craniofacial disorders is based on the results of interdisciplinary assessment.[7,24] Several specialty bottles and nipples have been developed and marketed for the feeding difficulties of infants with clefts. The specialty bottles and nipples are designed to compensate for the feeding inefficiency, including the reduced ability to create negative pressure and some reduced ability to create compression to express fluid from the nipple/bottle.[7,27,32] The Dr. Brown's Specialty Feeding System (Handi-Craft Company), the Medela SpecialNeeds Feeder, and the Pigeon Bottle with Cleft Palate Nipple all have highly pliable nipples of varying shapes with a valve at the base (valves differ by brand). The valve allows fluid to flow into the nipple but prevents flow back into the bottle when tongue/jaw movement compresses the nipple upward so the nipple is compressed against the **alveolar ridge** and/or the **vomer**. With the soft nipple and the valve, the infant compresses the nipple to express fluid. Negative pressure or suction is not required for fluid to flow from the nipple. Dr. Brown's Specialty Feeding System can be used with Dr. Brown's nipples of different flow rate based on the infant's need (the flow rate is determined by hole type and size). The Pigeon Bottle with Cleft Palate Nipple has a regular nipple and a small nipple. Both nipples have a **Y**-cut configuration and feature a stiff side that is positioned against the cleft and a more pliable side that makes contact with the tongue to encourage compression. The Medela SpecialNeeds Feeder nipple has a slit, and the nipple may be turned to adjust the orientation of the slit to the alveolar ridge to modify the flow from the nipple when it is compressed (**Fig. 15.11**).

Other options include soft, squeezable bottles, such as the Mead Johnson Cleft Lip/Palate Nurser.[7,27,32] The feeder compresses the bottle in sync with the infant's sucking motions (jaw and tongue). The feeder squeezes the milk into the infant's mouth with each sucking motion. The nipple is cross cut. The Medela SpecialNeeds

**Table 15.1** Nipple considerations

| Characteristic | Consideration for feeding infant with cleft lip and/or palate |
| --- | --- |
| Pliability: quality of being easily bent or flexible | The nipple should be pliable enough to allow milk flow with little compression (positive pressure from tongue-to-palate contact) and no suction. |
| Shape | The nipple should be of appropriate shape to provide contact between the nipple and the tongue to allow sufficient compression to express milk or formula.<br>For infants with isolated clefts of the lip, an orthodontically shaped nipple is desirable because it often forms to the cleft and assists in preventing the air leakage during feeding. |
| Size | Nipples come in various sizes with relation to the length between the tip to the base; the strength of the infant's suck must be considered as well as the ability of the infant to close the lips around the nipple and maintain an effective position of the nipple in the mouth for efficient feeding. |
| Hole type and size | The size and type of nipple hole affect flow rate of the milk or formula.<br>Most nipples feature a standard hole(s) or a cross-cut/**Y**-cut configuration.<br>The size of the hole typically correlates with flow rate and should be modified as necessary to help the infant coordinate sucking–swallowing–breathing.<br>Cross-cut nipples typically allow the infant to control flow rate primarily through compression and are typically advantageous to infants with cleft lip and/or palate. |

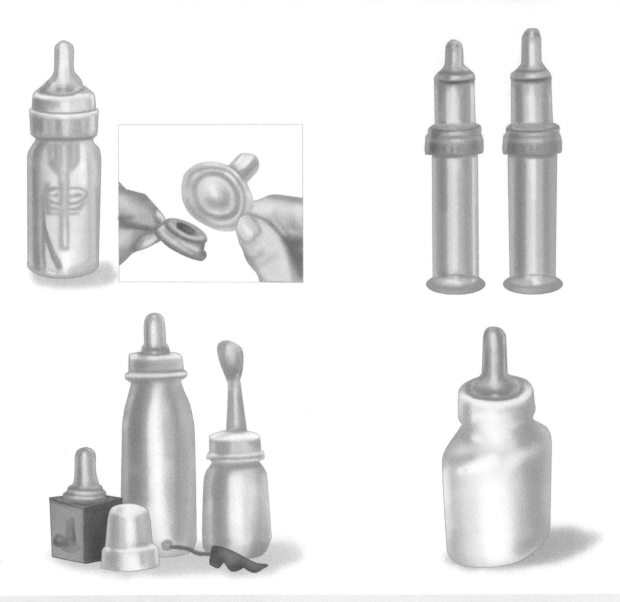

**Fig. 15.11** Specialty feeding equipment.

Feeder's nipple is soft and large enough that the feeder may also provide some compression of the nipple to assist with expression of fluid. Other soft bottles or feeding systems with bags may also be used with compression to express fluid into the infant's mouth.

A review of feeding interventions for breastfeeding infants with clefts indicates that supplemental nursing systems that enable the infant to attempt breastfeeding and also receive expressed breastmilk through a small tube have been successful for some mothers and infants.[32] However, there has been no literature evaluating the success of complementary/supplementary feeding with breastfeeding. Some centers use palatal obturators to assist with breastfeeding.[27] Similarly, there is limited evidence of the benefit of obturators to improve breastfeeding in infants with cleft lip and palate or cleft palate.[32]

Other feeding compensations and modifications have also been recommended for infants with cleft or craniofacial anomalies.

The infant should be well supported in a midline orientation and positioned so that breathing and airway are optimal.[7] For an infant with an isolated cleft and no airway concerns, a more upright or slightly reclined position is usually recommended to minimize entry of the fluid into the nasal cavity and eustachian tubes during feeding. For infants with airway issues, side-lying or a slightly prone position may be used to compensate for glossoptosis.[7,24] The feeder also needs to be comfortable during the feeding, and different options for positioning on the feeder's lap may need to be explored to find what is optimal for infant and feeder. Due to increased air ingestion, infants should be burped frequently during the feeding.[7,24] For the known risk of growth concerns, the intake and growth of infants with clefts and craniofacial disorders should be monitored closely with weights taken once or twice per week after discharge from the hospital. Many infants require fortification of breastmilk or formula for adequate intake and growth.[7,24]

Infants with anomalies in addition to a cleft, such as those with a syndrome, may need additional evaluation, including videofluorographic evaluation of swallowing. As noted previously, airway management does not necessarily remediate all feeding difficulties in infants with PRS. Infants with PRS may need more positioning considerations, such as side-lying or slightly prone. A longer nipple may be needed to allow placement on the tongue in infants with micrognathia.[7,24] Compression of the nipple may be reduced with a discrepancy between upper and lower alveolar ridges, and a system that allows the feeder to compress the nipple/bottle for expression of milk may be needed.

For individuals with 22q11.2 deletion syndrome with feeding difficulties, assessment and management should also be completed by an interdisciplinary team familiar with the continuum of feeding difficulties within the syndrome. The interdisciplinary team members should include medical specialties due to the possible involvement of multiple systems. Speech-language pathologists provide assessment of oral motor skills and of coordination of swallowing with respiration. They also perform videofluorographic swallow studies.[7,24] The speech-language pathologist will provide recommendations for feeding and swallowing management and therapy goals and activities if necessary. Pediatric gastroenterologists may be needed for management of gastrointestinal symptoms, including reflux, dysmotility, and constipation. An otolaryngologist may be needed for airway evaluation and management.[7] Other medical specialties may also be needed for comprehensive management of complex feeding issues. Management of feeding and swallowing difficulties is based on results of interdisciplinary assessment. Oral feedings may need to be limited to 10 to 15 minutes due to physiological fatigue in infants who have difficulties with fatigue due to cardiac defects or hypotonia.[24] The special bottles and nipples discussed in the previous sections may be needed for difficulties noted in creating positive and negative pressure. A more upright position may help reduce nasopharyngeal regurgitation with or without overt palatal cleft. Supplemental feedings via nasogastric tube or gastrostomy tubes may be needed for optimal nutrition and hydration.

## 15.7 Questions

Avery is a female infant born at 40 weeks gestation with unilateral left cleft lip and palate. Despite nursing support and support of the lactation consultant, Avery has had significant difficulty latching and drawing the nipple into her mouth when placed to the breast. When bottles were introduced, she continued to have significant difficulty with taking enough to meet her hydration and caloric needs. Although her mother had regular prenatal care, an ultrasound was not completed during pregnancy; therefore, no prenatal diagnosis was made. The caregivers are anxious and frustrated that their infant girl is having feeding difficulties.

1. What specific feeding difficulties might be expected for an infant with unilateral cleft lip and palate similar to Avery?

A. Drawing the nipple into the mouth
B. Latching onto the nipple
C. Drawing milk from the nipple
D. All of the above

2. Infants with cleft lip and palate have difficulty with feeding due to

A. Reduced ability to create negative pressure (suction) and positive pressure due to anatomical differences
B. Reduced ability to create negative pressure (suction) and positive pressure due to oral motor difficulties
C. Ankyloglossia
D. Difficulty with state regulation

3. Avery's follow-up after discharge from the nursery should include

A. Close monitoring of her intake and growth
B. Parental support
C. Intensive feeding/oral motor therapy
D. A and B
E. A, B, C

Avery and her family were seen in the mother–baby unit of the hospital when she was 6 hours of age. She was seen by the speech-language pathologist for feeding evaluation. A lactation consultant had already spoken with the mother and evaluated a feeding at the breast. Because breastfeeding had been so difficult with the presence of the cleft, bottle feeding had been attempted, and finally syringe feeding was used to prevent hypoglycemia. Avery was alert in her mother's arms. She was rooting, attempting to suck on her fingers, and fussing. Examination revealed left unilateral complete cleft lip and palate. Tongue movement during sucking motions was adequate. Compression was noted with the tongue/jaw against a segment of the upper alveolar ridge and vomer. No negative pressure was observed on a gloved finger or pacifier.

For bottle presentation, Avery was swaddled in a blanket. She was alert and awake. Eager rooting with attempts to latch onto the nipple was observed with touch to her lip. She was held nearly upright. Respirations appeared regular, comfortable, and without obstructive sounds or retractions. Her seal on the nipple was incomplete due to the cleft of her lip and alveolus. Her suck rate was rapid at two sucks per second. Fluid dripped from the nipple but did not appear to be actively expressed. Swallows occurred after every four or five sucks. No coughing, choking, or gagging was noted. Avery appeared to become more upset and frustrated quickly. Caregivers expressed concern about how they could feed their infant as well as disappointment that breastfeeding did not go well.

4. Bottles/nipples with valves compensate for

A. Nasal regurgitation
B. Reduced ability to express milk by allowing the infant to create suction
C. Increased air ingestion
D. Reduced ability to express milk by allowing the infant to use compression

5. Growth concerns are addressed through all of the following except

A. Use of special bottles/nipples
B. Frequent burping
C. Fortification of breastmilk
D. Fortification of formula

6. Positioning for feeding should consider

A. Optimal airway and breathing
B. Reducing nasal regurgitation
C. Parent comfort
D. All of the above

## 15.8 Answers and Explanations

**1. Correct: all of the above (D).**
Due to the anatomical defect, latch, seal, and expression of milk are all difficult, with reduced ability to create negative and positive pressure.

**2. Correct: reduced ability to create negative pressure (suction) and positive pressure due to anatomical differences (A).**
The physical defect associated with cleft prevents an adequate seal for development of negative pressure. Some positive pressure may be created, but it is usually less than that created by infants without clefts. The tongue and jaw typically move appropriately in infants with an isolated cleft lip and palate.

**3. Correct: A and B (D).**
Infants with clefts are at risk for poor growth due to reduced feeding efficiency. Caregivers also need support because feeding needs may change as the infant grows, as well as with other medical concerns related to clefts and craniofacial disorders.

**4. Correct: reduced ability to express milk by allowing the infant to use compression (D).**
The valve seals the bottle side of the nipple, so compression of the nipple results in expression from the cut/hole in the nipple. This compensates for the reduced ability to create negative pressure by using the infant's ability to create compression.

**5. Correct: frequent burping (B).**
Frequent burping may help by reducing spit-ups and improving the infant's comfort. Special bottles and fortification are used to help improve feeding efficiency and growth.

**6. Correct: all of the above (D).**
Infants will feed better if they are supported in a position that allows comfortable breathing through a stable/supported airway. In addition, a more upright position will help reduce nasal regurgitation with the use of gravity. Caregivers need to be as comfortable as the infant for a successful and positive feeding experience.

## Appendix 15.1 Case Presentation Conclusion

Avery's caregivers were educated on the difficulties noted during her feeding attempt and the need for compensations for the difficulties. The options for feeding compensations were presented. The consensus was to first try Dr. Brown's Specialty Feeding System and the Level 1 nipple. Bottle assembly, including the use of the valve, was demonstrated. Avery was held nearly upright, and Dr. Brown's Specialty Feeder was presented. She showed rooting to accept the nipple. Jaw movement resulted in compression of the nipple against the upper right alveolar ridge and the vomer. Her suck rate was initially fast at two sucks per second and quickly slowed to one suck per second. With fluid expression, swallows were audible and occurred after every one or two sucks. Some milk was noted coming from the corner of her mouth as well as from the cleft of her lip/nose. Gulping was noted at times, and the bottle was tipped so no fluid was at the hole in the nipple. When gulping stopped, the bottle/nipple was tipped up to allow fluid to the level of the hole in the nipple, and Avery resumed sucking. Feeding was stopped after 10 minutes, and she had consumed 15 mL. She was supported upright and burped. She was returned to the nearly upright/slightly reclined position, and Dr. Brown's Specialty Feeder was presented again. She rooted again and accepted the nipple. Her suck rate was one suck per second. Swallows occurred after every one or two suck movements. Her suck—swallow—breathe coordination appeared adequate without any signs of incoordination or stress. She fed for another 10 minutes before becoming very drowsy. Feeding was stopped, and she had consumed another 15 mL. She was burped again and fell soundly asleep. The caregiver's questions regarding bottle use, expected weight gain, and follow-up were addressed. Handouts from the Cleft Palate Foundation (http://www.cleftline.org/who-we-are/what-we-do/feeding-your-baby/how-to-order-bottles/) were provided for further information regarding resources available to Avery's family.

## References

[1] Parker SE, Mai CT, Canfield MA, et al; National Birth Defects Prevention Network. Updated National Birth Prevalence estimates for selected birth defects in the United States, 2004-2006. *Birth Defects Res A Clin Mol Teratol* 2010;*88*(12):1008–1016

[2] Winter RM, Baraitser M. The London Dysmorphology Database: A Computerised Database for the Diagnosis of Rare Dysmorphic Syndromes. New York, NY: Oxford University Press Electronic Publishing; 1996

[3] Spranger J, Benirschke K, Hall JG, et al. Errors of morphogenesis: concepts and terms. Recommendations of an international working group. *J Pediatr* 1982;*100*(1):160–165

[4] Evans AK, Rahbar R, Rogers GF, Mulliken JB, Volk MS. Robin sequence: a retrospective review of 115 patients. *Int J Pediatr Otorhinolaryngol* 2006;*70*(6):973–980

[5] Smith MC, Senders CW. Prognosis of airway obstruction and feeding difficulty in the Robin sequence. *Int J Pediatr Otorhinolaryngol* 2006;*70*(2):319–324

[6] Monasterio FO, Molina F, Berlanga F, et al. Swallowing disorders in Pierre Robin sequence: its correction by distraction. *J Craniofac Surg* 2004;*15*(6):934–941

[7] Dailey S. Feeding and swallowing in infants with cleft and craniofacial anomalies. *Perspect Speech Sci Orofac Disord* 2013;*23*(2):62–72

[8] van den Elzen APM, Semmekrot BA, Bongers EM, Huygen PL, Marres HA. Diagnosis and treatment of the Pierre Robin sequence: results of a retrospective clinical study and review of the literature. *Eur J Pediatr* 2001;*160*(1):47–53

[9] Li HY, Lo LJ, Chen KS, Wong KS, Chang KP. Robin sequence: review of treatment modalities for airway obstruction in 110 cases. *Int J Pediatr Otorhinolaryngol* 2002;*65*(1):45–51

[10] Wagener S, Rayatt SS, Tatman AJ, Gornall P, Slator R. Management of infants with Pierre Robin sequence. *Cleft Palate Craniofac J* 2003;*40*(2):180–185

[11] Abadie V, Morisseau-Durand MP, Beyler C, Manach Y, Couly G. Brainstem dysfunction: a possible neuroembryological pathogenesis of isolated Pierre Robin sequence. *Eur J Pediatr* 2002;*161*(5):275–280

[12] Baudon JJ, Renault F, Goutet JM, et al. Motor dysfunction of the upper digestive tract in Pierre Robin sequence as assessed by sucking-swallowing electromyography and esophageal manometry. *J Pediatr* 2002;*140*(6):719–723

[13] Baujat G, Faure C, Zaouche A, Viarme F, Couly G, Abadie V. Oroesophageal motor disorders in Pierre Robin syndrome. *J Pediatr Gastroenterol Nutr* 2001;*32*(3):297–302

[14] Renault F, Baudon JJ, Galliani E, et al. Facial, lingual, and pharyngeal electromyography in infants with Pierre Robin sequence. *Muscle Nerve* 2011;*43*(6):866–871

[15] Renault F, Flores-Guevara R, Soupre V, Vazquez MP, Baudon JJ. Neurophysiological brainstem investigations in isolated Pierre Robin sequence. *Early Hum Dev* 2000;*58*(2):141–152

[16] Habel A, McGinn MJ II, Zackai EH, Unanue N, McDonald-McGinn DM. Syndrome-specific growth charts for 22q11.2 deletion syndrome in Caucasian children. *Am J Med Genet A* 2012;*158A*(11):2665–2671

[17] Cuneo BF. 22q11.2 deletion syndrome: DiGeorge, velocardiofacial, and conotruncal anomaly face syndromes. *Curr Opin Pediatr* 2001;*13*(5):465–472

[18] Goldmuntz E. DiGeorge syndrome: new insights. *Clin Perinatol* 2005;*32*(4):963–978, ix–x

[19] Eicher PS, McDonald-Mcginn DM, Fox CA, Driscoll DA, Emanuel BS, Zackai EH. Dysphagia in children with a 22q11.2 deletion: unusual pattern found on modified barium swallow. *J Pediatr* 2000;*137*(2):158–164

[20] Shprintzen RJ. Velo-cardio-facial syndrome: 30 years of study. *Dev Disabil Res Rev* 2008;*14*(1):3–10

[21] Masarei AG, Sell D, Habel A, Mars M, Sommerlad BC, Wade A. The nature of feeding in infants with unrepaired cleft lip and/or palate compared with healthy noncleft infants. *Cleft Palate Craniofac J* 2007;*44*(3):321–328

[22] Pandya AN, Boorman JG. Failure to thrive in babies with cleft lip and palate. *Br J Plast Surg* 2001;*54*(6):471–475

[23] Arvedson JC, Brodsky L. Pediatric Swallowing and Feeding: Assessment and Management. 2nd ed. Albany, NY: Singular Publishing Group; 2002

[24] Cooper-Brown L, Copeland S, Dailey S, et al. Feeding and swallowing dysfunction in genetic syndromes. *Dev Disabil Res Rev* 2008;*14*(2):147–157

[25] Reid J, Reilly S, Kilpatrick N. Sucking performance of babies with cleft conditions. *Cleft Palate Craniofac J* 2007;*44*(3):312–320

[26] Garcez LW, Giugliani ER. Population-based study on the practice of breastfeeding in children born with cleft lip and palate. *Cleft Palate Craniofac J* 2005;*42*(6):687–693

[27] Glenny AM, Hooper LM, Shaw WC, Reilly S, Kasem S, Reid J. Feeding Interventions for Growth and Development in Infants with Cleft Lip, Cleft Palate, or Cleft Lip and Palate. Cochrane Database of Systematic Reviews. New York, NY: Wiley; 2004

[28] Seth AK, McWilliams BJ. Weight gain in children with cleft palate from birth to two years. *Cleft Palate J* 1988;*25*(2):146–150

[29] Cleft Palate Foundation. Feeding Your Baby. 4th ed. Chapel Hill, NC: Author; 2009

[30] American Cleft Palate-Craniofacial Association. Parameters for Evaluation and Treatment of Patients with Cleft Lip/Palate or Other Craniofacial Anomalies. Chapel Hill, NC:Author; 2009

[31] Cleft Palate Foundation. Introduction to cleft and craniofacial team care. 2015. http://www.cleftline.org/caregivers-individuals/team-care/#intro

[32] Reid J. A review of feeding interventions for infants with cleft palate. *Cleft Palate Craniofac J* 2004;*41*(3):268–278

## Suggested Reading

[1] Cole A, Tomlinson J, Slator R, Reading J. Understanding cleft lip and palate. 3: feeding the baby. *J Fam Health Care* 2009;*19*(5):157–158

[2] Kummer A. Cleft Palate and Craniofacial Anomalies: Effects on Speech and Resonance. Scarborough, ON: Nelson Education; 2013

[3] Miller CK. Feeding issues and interventions in infants and children with clefts and craniofacial syndromes. *Semin Speech Lang* 2011;*32*(2):115–126

[4] Osborn AJ, de Alarcon A, Tabangin ME, Miller CK, Cotton RT, Rutter MJ. Swallowing function after laryngeal cleft repair: more than just fixing the cleft. *Laryngoscope* 2014;*124*(8):1965–1969

[5] Peterson-Falzone SJ, Hardin-Jones MA, Karnell MP. Cleft Palate Speech. St. Louis, MO. Mosby; 2001:266–291

# 16 Congenital Heart Disease

*Jason Nathaniel Johnson*

## Summary

Dysphagia in congenital heart disease can be associated with congenital abnormalities of the aortic arch or a complication of surgery. Congenital anomalies of the aortic arch occur due to an abnormality of the resolution of different paired embryological arches. Aortic arch anomalies and vascular rings can cause compression of the esophagus and trachea, leading to dysphagia and respiratory symptoms. Patients with tight vascular rings will present at an early age with more respiratory symptoms, and patients with loose rings will present later with dysphagia. Esophageal compression is typically seen by barium esophagram or upper gastrointestinal endoscopy. Computed tomography and magnetic resonance angiography allow three-dimensional assessment of the aortic arch anomaly in relationship to the trachea and esophagus. The specific aortic arch anomaly dictates treatment; milder forms can potentially improve with conservative measures, but tighter vascular rings and the presence of a diverticulum require surgical correction.

Dysphagia after congenital heart surgery is common and can occur in up to 50% of patients. Several risk factors have been identified: young age or low weight at surgery, length of intubation, and surgical type and duration. Aspiration of liquids is common, especially in patients with vocal cord dysfunction or paralysis. Evaluation of oral readiness by a speech-language pathologist identifies potential etiologies of dysphagia. Barium swallow can identify patients who aspirate liquids, and laryngoscopy can identify vocal cord abnormalities. Identifying risk factors and evaluation by a multidisciplinary team can successfully treat dysphagia in patients with congenital heart disease requiring surgery.

## Keywords

vascular ring, computed tomography, magnetic resonance angiogram, diverticulum of Kommerell, dysphagia lusoria, congenital heart surgery

### Learning Objectives

- Explain why dysphagia is a common symptom of congenital anomalies of the thoracic arteries and vascular rings
- Identify the diagnostic evaluation and management of the different forms of vascular rings
- Explain why dysphagia is common in congenital heart disease, especially after surgery
- Identify the pre- and postoperative factors that increase the risk of dysphagia following congenital heart surgery

## 16.1 Introduction

Congenital heart disease is the most common type of birth defect. It affects about 1% of all children, or 40,000 births a year, in the United States.[1] Congenital anomalies of the thoracic arteries that surround the trachea and/or esophagus by vascular structures are called **vascular rings** (**Box 16.1**). Dysphagia, inspiratory stridor, wheezing, cough, and recurrent respiratory infections are common symptoms of patients with vascular rings.[2] The presentation of a vascular ring depends on the severity of the compression and the age of the patient, and swallowing difficulties are almost always present. Therefore, recognizing vascular rings and knowing the appropriate diagnostic workup are imperative in understanding dysphagia in congenital heart disease. This chapter describes the many different forms of vascular rings associated with dysphagia and reviews the clinical presentation, diagnostic evaluation, and treatment of vascular rings.

### Box 16.1

**Vascular Ring**
Vascular rings are a malformation of the aorta and/or its surrounding vessels that completely encircle the trachea and esophagus and contribute to breathing, swallowing, and digestive issues.

Most children born with congenital heart disease require at least one surgical procedure in their lifetime, usually in early childhood.[3] Patients that require surgery for congenital heart disease are at an increased risk of dysphagia.[4,5,6] Several factors increase the risk of dysphagia following congenital heart surgery, including preoperative patient status, use of **transesophageal echocardiography**, and length of intubation.[4] Specific congenital heart surgeries increase the risk of dysphagia, specifically patent ductus arteriosus ligation and surgery for left-sided obstructive lesions. A multidisciplinary team can assess dysphagia after congenital heart surgery and recommend treatment. This chapter outlines the congenital anomalies and subsequent surgical repairs associated with dysphagia.

## 16.2 Case Presentation

A 15-year-old girl had a history of chronic dysphagia and wheezing diagnosed with asthma. She was taking multiple asthma medications with no resolution of her symptoms. She had the sensation of food getting stuck, having to vomit to relieve the obstruction several times a week. She denied stridor, chronic respiratory infections, weight loss, or abdominal pain. Her vital signs and physical exam were normal. Her chest X-ray revealed clear lung fields with a right aortic arch (**Fig. 16.1**). Recall that the aortic arch

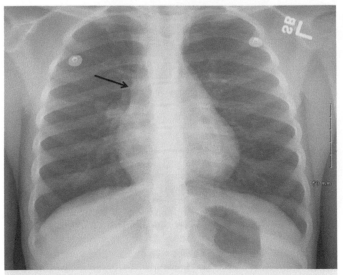

Fig. 16.1 Chest roentgenogram. The anteroposterior chest X-ray shows clear lung fields and normal heart size. The black arrow points to the aortic knob from a right aortic arch.

## Box 16.2

### Diverticulum of Kommerell

A diverticulum of Kommerell refers to the aneurysmal section of the aortic arch that typically is the origin of an aberrant subclavian artery in an aortic arch abnormality. It was first described by Burckhard F. Kommerell, a German radiologist. The presence of a Kommerell diverticulum always indicates a vascular ring because the aneurysmal segment indicates a contralateral ligamentum arteriosum. The typical presentation is a right aortic arch with an aberrant retroesophageal left subclavian artery from a diverticulum of Kommerell where the diverticulum gives rise to a left ligamentum arteriosum that completes the vascular ring (**Fig. 16.6**). Dysphagia and respiratory symptoms are common presentations of patients with this aortic arch abnormality because the vascular ring and diverticulum compress the esophagus and trachea.

## 16.3 Epidemiology

Congenital anomalies of the aortic arch are relatively common, and minor forms can occur in up to 10% of the population. The most common aortic arch anomaly is a left aortic arch with an aberrant retroesophageal right subclavian artery, occurring in 0.5 to 1.5% of the general population.[7] Aortic arch abnormalities are commonly associated with other forms of congenital heart disease, such as tetralogy of Fallot (34%) (**Box 16.3**) and complete transposition of the great arteries (16%) (**Box 16.4**).[7] However, vascular rings are uncommon anomalies and make up less than 1% of all congenital heart disease. Vascular rings can occur with

should be on the left side of the body (**Fig. 16.2**). A transthoracic echocardiogram showed no other congenital heart disease and confirmed the right aortic arch, but the branching pattern could not be confirmed. Chest magnetic resonance angiography (MRA) revealed a right aortic arch with an aberrant retroesophageal left subclavian artery from a **diverticulum of Kommerell** (**Box 16.2; Fig. 16.3**). These findings were consistent with a vascular ring.

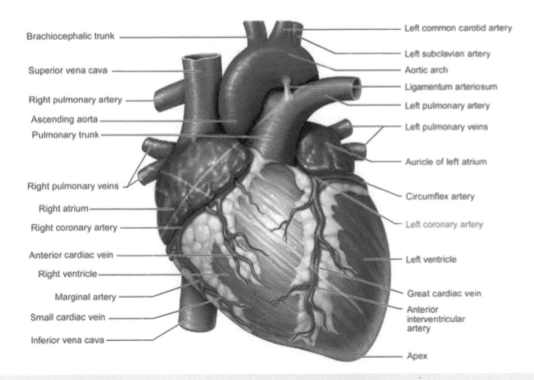

Fig. 16.2 Normal anatomy of the heart.

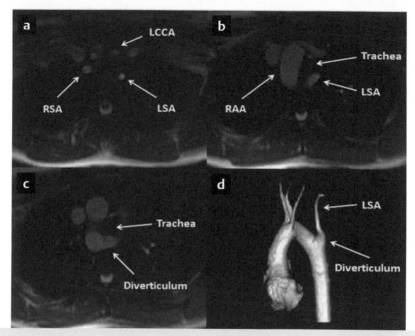

**Fig. 16.3** Right aortic arch with an aberrant retroesophageal left subclavian artery from a diverticulum of Kommerell. **(a–c)** Chest magnetic resonance angiogram axial bright blood slices through the thorax superior to inferior showing a right aortic arch (RAA) with an aberrant retroesophageal left subclavian artery (LSA) arising from a diverticulum of Kommerell. There is a left-sided ligamentum arteriosum that connects the diverticulum to the main pulmonary artery to surround the trachea and esophagus. **(d)** The three-dimensional reconstruction demonstrates the left subclavian artery arising from the diverticulum of Kommerell, which is much larger in caliber than the left subclavian artery and indicates where the ligamentum connects to the aortic arch. (Image courtesy of William E. Boon RT (R), LeBonheur Children's Hospital, Memphis, Tennessee.)

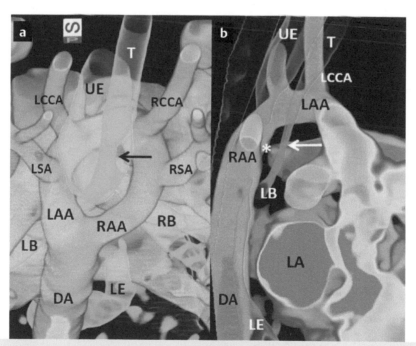

**Fig. 16.4** Double aortic arch. **(a)** Posterior view of a three-dimensional (3D) computed tomographic (CT) scan with contrast showing a double aortic arch with equal size left aortic arch (LAA) and right aortic arch (RAA). The right common carotid artery (RCCA) and right subclavian artery (RSA) arise from the right arch, and the left common carotid artery (LCCA) and left subclavian artery (LSA) arise from the LAA. The left and right arches encircle the trachea (T) and esophagus before rejoining the descending aorta (DA) to complete the vascular ring. The trachea is narrowed, as seen by the caliber change in the area of the vascular ring (black arrow). The upper esophagus (UE) is dilated due to compression from the tight vascular ring with normal caliber of the lower esophagus (LE). **(b)** Sagittal view of the same 3D CT scan with contrast of a double aortic arch. The anterior compression of the trachea by the vascular ring is well seen (white arrow). The complete compression (white asterisk) of the middle esophagus is seen as the esophagus courses inferiorly through the vascular ring and the lower esophagus courses posterior to the left atrium (LA). LB, left bronchus; RB, right bronchus. (Image courtesy of Jason N. Johnson, MD MHS, LeBonheur Children's Hospital, Memphis, Tennessee.)

many different configurations of the aortic arch, and the many different types are listed in **Table 16.1**. The most common type of vascular ring is the double aortic arch (**Fig. 16.4**) followed by the right aortic arch with aberrant retroesophageal left subclavian artery from a diverticulum of Kommerell (**Fig. 16.3**). The true incidence of some vascular rings is difficult to determine because the patients can be asymptomatic and have no associated intracardiac disease.

**Table 16.1** The different congenital aortic arch abnormalities creating a vascular ring

| Aortic arch branching | Vascular ring |
| --- | --- |
| Double aortic arch | • Both aortic arches similar size<br>• Hypoplasia of one aortic arch (usually left)<br>• Atresia of one aortic arch (usually left) |
| Right aortic arch | • Aberrant retroesophageal left subclavian artery from a diverticulum of Kommerell<br>• Left descending aorta and left ligamentum arteriosum<br>• Aberrant retroesophageal innominate artery and left ligamentum arteriosum |
| Left aortic arch | • Aberrant retroesophageal right subclavian artery from a diverticulum of Kommerell<br>• Right descending aorta and right ligamentum arteriosum |
| Cervical aortic arch | • Aberrant retroesophageal subclavian artery from a diverticulum of Kommerell<br>• Contralateral descending aorta and ligamentum arteriosum |

## Box 16.3

**Tetralogy of Fallot**

Tetralogy of Fallot is a congenital heart condition that involves four co-occurring abnormalities: a large ventricular septal defect (VSD), pulmonary stenosis, right ventricular hypertrophy, and an overriding aorta. It is a rare condition and occurs in ~ 5 out of every 10,000 infants, affecting boys and girls equally. A VSD is a hole in the septum of the heart between the ventricles that allows oxygen-rich blood (housed in the left ventricle) to mix with oxygen-poor blood (housed in the right ventricle). Pulmonary stenosis is a narrowing of the pulmonary valve and the subsequent passageway from the right ventricle to the pulmonary artery, which normally carries oxygen-poor blood from the heart to the lungs. Right ventricular hypertrophy involves excessive thickening of the muscle of the right ventricle because of excessive work required to move blood through the narrowed pulmonary valve. An overriding aorta is an aorta that is located between the left and right ventricles, instead of the aorta being attached to the left ventricle, which allows only oxygen-rich blood to flow through the aorta to the body in a typical heart. With an overriding aorta, oxygen-poor blood from the right ventricle flows to the aorta instead of into the pulmonary artery. Together the four abnormalities of tetralogy of Fallot mean that insufficient volumes of blood can reach the lungs for oxygenation, and oxygen-poor blood flows to the body. Cyanosis is a common symptom in tetralogy of Fallot.

## Box 16.4

**Transposition of the Great Arteries**

Transposition of the great arteries is a congenital heart defect that describes a condition in which the two main arteries leaving the heart (aorta and pulmonary arteries) are transposed (reversed). This reversal has implications for the way that blood is circulated around the body, and it results in a shortage of oxygen-rich blood in the body.

The incidence of swallowing dysfunction after congenital heart disease ranges from 18 to 48%, depending on the type of heart disease and required surgery.[4,5,6] In patients following a stage I palliation (Norwood operation) for **hypoplastic left heart syndrome** (HLHS), dysphagia was present in 48% of patients with aspiration present in 24% of patents.[5] In pediatric patients requiring surgery with intraoperative transesophageal echocardiogram assessment, 18% of patients had dysphagia.[4] Finally, in a review of 146 infants who underwent any open-heart surgery, 24% had dysphagia, with 64% of those with dysphagia demonstrating aspiration by videofluoroscopic swallow study.[6] All of these studies represent single-center data, and the true incidence or prevalence of dysphagia after congenital heart surgery is unknown.

## 16.4 Etiology

Aortic arch anomalies encompass many different categories from abnormalities in branching and position to supernumerary or interrupted arches. A vascular ring is an aortic arch anomaly where the trachea and esophagus are completely surrounded by vascular structures that may or may not be patent. Defining aortic arch position, or sidedness, is important in defining potential vascular rings. *Left* and *right aortic arch* refers to the specific bronchus (left or right) that the aortic arch crosses superiorly. The specific arch anomalies that lead to a vascular ring occur due to an abnormality in the appearance and resolution of any of six specific paired embryological vessels (**Fig. 16.4**). A detailed embryological review of each type of vascular ring is outside the scope of this text but has been previously covered in other texts.[7] A normal aortic arch is a left arch with resolution of the embryonic right sixth arch and right dorsal aorta distal to the right subclavian artery (**Fig. 16.5**). A double aortic arch occurs due to persistence of both the right and left embryonic fourth branchial arches. A right aortic arch with retroesophageal left subclavian artery from a diverticulum of Kommerell results from resolution of the left fourth branchial arch and formation of the diverticulum from the left dorsal aorta in the presence of a persistent left sixth branchial arch (**Fig. 16.6**).

The exact etiology of dysphagia in congenital heart disease is unknown but has been linked to several factors. Infants with congenital heart disease have low scores on the evaluation of readiness for oral feeding, similar to premature infants.[3] Clinical evaluation of infants with congenital heart disease showed that dysphagia is characterized by a lack of coordination of the suck–swallow–breath process from several factors: stasis of food in the oral cavity, anterior leaking, and fatigue.[3] Infants with congenital

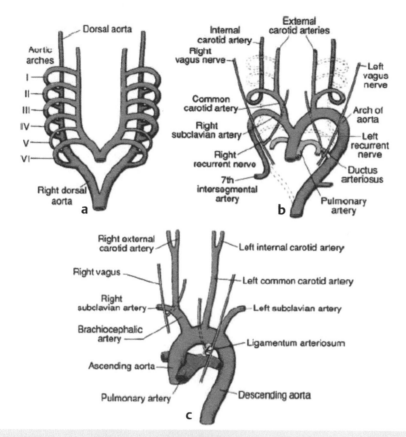

**Fig. 16.5** Typical development of the aortic arch. **(a)** In early development the aortic arches are a bilateral duplicate system with six paired arches (I–VI). **(b)** In later development many of the embryological arches involute, with the left aortic arch becoming prominent. **(c)** After full development there is a left aortic arch with a left-sided ligamentum arteriosum. (Image from Levitt B, Richter JE. Dysphagia lusoria: a comprehensive review. Dis Esophagus 2007;20(6):455–460.[22])

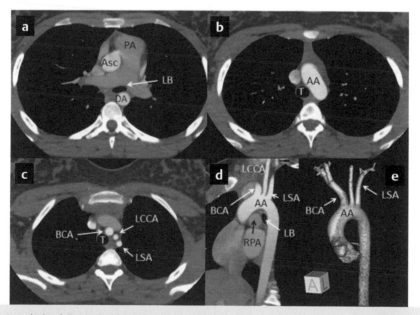

**Fig. 16.6** Normal left aortic arch. **(a–c)** Computed tomography (CT) with contrast, axial slices through the thorax from inferior to superior showing a left aortic arch (AA). The ascending aorta (Asc) starts rightward of the pulmonary artery (PA) and courses leftward of the trachea (T) to course superior to the left bronchus (LB) and the right pulmonary artery (RPA). The normal order of branching from ascending aorta to descending aorta in a left aortic arch is brachiocephalic artery (BCA), left common carotid artery (LCCA), and left subclavian artery (LSA). **(d)** Sagittal CT view of a normal left aortic arch showing the aortic arch coursing superior to the right pulmonary artery and left bronchus. **(e)** Three-dimensional angiogram of the normal left aortic arch. (Image courtesy of Jason N. Johnson, MD MHS, LeBonheur Children's Hospital, Memphis, Tennessee.)

heart disease have long bursts of sucking–swallowing without deep breathing, which forces the infant to perform catch-up breathing while continuing to suck. This leads to the potential for aspiration and limited intake.[6] Significant pharyngoesophageal dysmotility mechanisms exist in infants with congenital heart disease especially among those patients after surgery.[8] The upper esophageal sphincter responses are increased in frequency, whereas the lower esophageal sphincter responses are preserved. Also, infants who have undergone congenital heart surgery have a longer duration of esophageal peristalsis.[8]

Several risk factors have been linked to dysphagia after surgery for congenital heart surgery.[4,5,6] Children less than 3 years of age at the time of surgery, preoperative intubation, lower body weight at operation, intubation for longer than 7 days, longer operation duration, and operations for obstructive left-sided lesions are all clinical predictors of dysphagia after congenital heart surgery.[4,6] The use of transesophageal echocardiography for intraoperative cardiovascular assessment in children weighing less than 12 lb (5.5 kg) is predictive of swallowing difficulties in children requiring surgery for congenital heart disease.[4] Vocal cord dysfunction after congenital heart surgery is associated with dysphagia and aspiration.[9,10,11,12] Different mechanisms for vocal cord dysfunction in congenital heart disease have been previously described: operative injury to the recurrent laryngeal nerve (**Fig. 16.4**), associated congenital laryngotracheal anomalies, prolonged intubation, neurodevelopmental delay, impaired suck–swallow coordination, and injury from a transesophageal echocardiography probe.[12]

## 16.4.1 Pathophysiology

The term **dysphagia lusoria** (**Box 16.5**) (from the Latin, *lusus naturae*, trick or freak of nature) was coined by David Bayford in 1794, after he linked a postmortem case of a left aortic arch with an aberrant retroesophageal right subclavian artery with a history of chronic swallowing difficulty.[13,14] Bayford summarized dysphagia lusoria in his original manuscript as a "distress in swallowing ever so great" with "the obstruction happening in the same place, the very upper part of the thorax."[13,14] Dysphagia secondary to mechanical obstruction is the typical presentation from aortic arch abnormalities.[15] As in the case presented in this chapter, patients commonly describe food being stuck in the mid to upper chest, frequently associated with regurgitation of unchewed food. Symptoms are often more severe for solids than for liquids, and positional changes of the head lead to obstruction.[15]

## Box 16.5

### Dysphagia Lusoria

*Dysphagia lusoria* was originally coined by David Bayford, a British surgeon, in 1794, when he described a postmortem case of a left aortic arch with an aberrant retroesophageal right subclavian artery with a history of chronic dysphagia as a *lusus naturae* (Latin for "trick or freak of nature"). This term has historically been linked to dysphagia in this specific aortic arch abnormality. However, it has slowly evolved to describe swallowing difficulties in patients with any aortic arch abnormality or vascular ring. Dysphagia lusoria occurs as a result of mechanical obstruction, and patients commonly describe food being stuck in the mid to upper chest, frequently associated with regurgitation of food. Symptoms are often more severe for solids than for liquids, and positional changes of the head and neck can lead to obstruction.

Dysphagia lusoria presents as swallowing difficulties arising from a specific aortic arch abnormality that is actually not a true vascular ring. Therefore, the trachea and esophagus are not completely encircled by vascular structures. The exact mechanism of pathophysiology of dysphagia in this disease is not completely understood. Only 20% of patients with this specific abnormality are symptomatic; the incidence of dysphagia lusoria do not equal the incidence of a left aortic arch with aberrant retroesophageal right subclavian artery.[15] The most accepted mechanism for dysphagia lusoria is that the arterial wall of the right subclavian artery becomes more rigid from atherosclerosis with increased age, and symptoms develop from extrinsic compression of the esophagus posteriorly against the trachea anteriorly.[16] This would explain the typical late age of presentation in the mid-40s.[15,17] The other age-related changes that have been associated with dysphagia lusoria are elongation of the aorta and increased esophageal rigidity.[15,17]

*Dysphagia lusoria* is now a term used synonymously with swallowing difficulties arising from aortic arch abnormalities or vascular rings.[18,19,20] Vascular rings typically present with respiratory symptoms in almost all patients (93%) and gastrointestinal symptoms in half of patients.[21] The specific clinical manifestations of a vascular ring are related to the tightness of the ring, specifically the severity of the compression of the trachea and/or esophagus. If the vascular ring is tight, patients typically present early (neonates or infants) with inspiratory stridor. If the vascular ring is loose, patients typically present later (as children or adults) with dysphagia and vague respiratory symptoms like wheezing. In a double aortic arch with both aortic arches widely patent, the ring is tight, and patients present with respiratory symptoms in the first weeks of life. Infants with a tight vascular ring can demonstrate a posture with neck hyperextension and reflex apnea with oral feeds.[7] In a double aortic arch with atresia of the left aortic arch, the ring is loose, and patients present with dysphagia. These patients will have swallowing difficulties and consistently choke on their food, and careful questioning will reveal a vague history of respiratory symptoms as an infant, such as mild stridor, wheezing, or coughing.

Infants with dysphagia after congenital heart surgery have a slightly different presentation than children with vascular rings, and the symptoms can be vague. These patients will have delayed triggering of swallowing, signs of aspiration with choking and coughing with liquid feeds, refusal to feed, disruptive behavior, preference, and lack of feeding competence.[3] Fatigue and cyanosis during feeding are common in children with congenital heart disease both prior to and after surgery.[3]

Feeding difficulties in children with congenital heart disease lead to inadequate nutritional intake resulting in poor growth, especially in postoperative patients. There is a strong association between decreased weight for age and mortality in patients after surgery for congenital heart disease.[8] Specific types of congenital heart disease and surgeries, large patent ductus arteriosus, or systemic-to-pulmonary artery shunts predispose the intestinal mucosa to decreased blood pressure. This increases gut permeability, altering nutrient absorption and placing the patients at risk for necrotizing enterocolitis. Patients who are unable to protect their airway due to vocal cord dysfunction may experience aspiration with oral feeds and are at risk for pneumonia. Signs and symptoms of vocal cord dysfunction are choking with feeds and a weak cry.[3,4,5,6]

## 16.5 Discussion of Diagnosis

The diagnosis of dysphagia from an aortic arch abnormality can be made in a variety of ways. A simple chest roentgenogram can delineate whether the aortic arch is leftward or rightward (Fig. 16.1).[7] Not all rightward aortic arches represent a vascular ring, so a chest roentgenogram cannot confirm the presence of a vascular ring. However, a right aortic arch in the presence of dysphagia warrants further, more detailed, imaging of the aortic arch to determine the arch branching and potential presence of a diverticulum of Kommerell. Barium contrast imaging of the esophagus is an excellent tool to diagnose esophageal compression from a vascular ring or aortic arch anomaly.[17,22,23,24] A barium esophagram shows the characteristic diagonal compression of the esophagus at the level of the third and fourth vertebrae (Fig. 16.7). An upper gastrointestinal endoscopy will show posterior external compression with arterial pulsations of the middle third of the esophagus.[22,25,26] The upper gastrointestinal endoscopy is typically performed to rule out other conditions (e.g., esophagitis) given the symptoms of dysphagia. However, the diagnosis of aortic arch abnormality or vascular ring is made when the pulsatile compression is visualized. Esophageal manometry has not been proven to be an effective way of making the diagnosis of dysphagia from aortic arch abnormalities or predicting which patients may benefit from surgical correction.[17]

A barium esophagram and/or upper gastrointestinal endoscopy can identify symptoms of dysphagia resulting from an aortic arch abnormality; however, a modified barium swallow study/videofluoroscopic swallow study is necessary to diagnose dysphagia and accurately describe the physiology that is resulting in the aberrant symptoms (e.g., aspiration) that might have been detected on the barium esophagram or upper gastrointestinal endoscopy. The specific aortic arch abnormality or vascular ring cannot be made by either a barium esophagram or an upper gastrointestinal endoscopy, and more specific imaging of the aortic arch and its branches is required. The surgical options available to correct an aortic arch abnormality requires further imaging of the aortic arch to determine the exact mechanism of esophageal compression. In neonates or infants a transthoracic echocardiogram (Fig. 16.8) in skilled hands can outline the aortic arch anatomy, but it can be challenging in older patients.[7] Typically, angiography

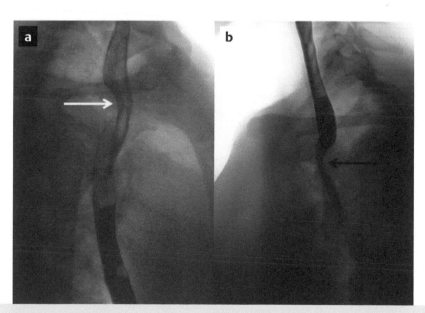

Fig. 16.7 Barium esophagram in an aortic arch abnormality. (a) An anteroposterior view barium esophagram shows lateral indentation of the middle third of the esophagus (white arrow) in a patient with dysphagia from a right aortic arch with an aberrant retroesophageal left subclavian artery. (b) A lateral view barium esophagram shows posterior indentation of the middle third of the esophagus (black arrow) in the same patient with a right aortic arch with a left aortic arch and ligamentum arteriosum completing a vascular ring. (Image courtesy of Jason N. Johnson, MD MHS, LeBonheur Children's Hospital, Memphis Tennessee.)

of the aortic arch is required to completely define aortic arch anatomy with fluoroscopy, computed tomography (CT), or MRA.[2,7,16] Fluoroscopic angiography in the catheterization suite is not commonly performed because other noninvasive options (e.g., CT or MRA), available in most centers, do not require arterial cannulation. Also, it can be difficult to define the exact brachiocephalic branching in anteroposterior fluoroscopic angiography because of projection imaging. CT and MRA allow for three-dimensional imaging to evaluate the entire aortic arch in relationship with the trachea and esophagus, avoiding the pitfalls of projection imaging (**Fig. 16.9**).[7] Both CT and MRA require contrast to evaluate the aortic arch and therefore require a peripheral intravenous line. CT and fluoroscopic angiography use ionizing radiation to acquire images and expose patients to the potential cancer risks of these techniques.[27] MRA does not use radiation in image acquisition, but it typically takes longer than CT. Young patients may require sedation to complete an MRA scan successfully.[2] The decision as to CT versus MRA to diagnose an aortic arch abnormality depends on the clinical situation and is different for each institution and patient.

The diagnosis of the etiology of dysphagia in infants with congenital heart disease typically starts with an evaluation by a speech-language pathologist to determine the infant's readiness for oral feeds.[3] The Preterm Oral Feeding Readiness Assessment scale is used in some centers and assesses the infant's behavior state, oral posture, oral reflexes, and nonnutritive sucking to determine readiness.[3] For a complete discussion of clinical evaluation of swallowing function in infants, please see Chapter 5 in this book. Modified barium swallow studies (MBSSs) and/or fiberoptic endoscopic evaluation of swallowing (FEES) may be performed to diagnose dysphagia in pediatric patients. MBSSs are performed in conjunction with radiology and speech-language pathologists to evaluate swallowing at different liquid consistencies.[5] A modified barium swallow can determine the presence of laryngeal penetration or frank aspiration of liquids at different consistencies. To evaluate for vocal cord dysfunction laryngoscopy is performed by otolaryngologists to assess the appearance of the larynx and vocal cord mobility.[5,9,10,11] FEES may also be performed in conjunction with otolaryngology and speech-language pathologists to document the presence of laryngeal penetration and/or frank aspiration of liquids at different consistencies. For a complete discussion of MBSS and FEES in this book, please consult index.

## 16.6 Management

The management of dysphagia from aortic arch anomalies depends on several factors. The symptoms, age at presentation, and the specific aortic arch anatomy all determine the type of intervention recommended. The presence of symptoms is important to the management of patients with aortic arch abnormalities. Asymptomatic patients with an aortic arch abnormality or vascular ring do not require any intervention, medical or surgical, as long as there is no aneurysm present.[7] In patients with an asymptomatic vascular ring with a coexisting congenital heart disease requiring surgery, the vascular ring should be ligated at the time of the congenital heart surgery. However, patients who experience symptoms related to an aortic arch abnormality or vascular ring require some form of

intervention. Once symptoms of a vascular ring or aortic arch anomaly are present (e.g., dysphagia, stridor, or wheezing), the age at which the symptoms develop dictates the type and timing of the intervention. In patients who present early with tight vascular rings, surgery is required soon after diagnosis to relieve the tracheal compression.[2,7,28] The respiratory symptoms from the tracheal compression typically resolve after surgical repair of the vascular ring. Tracheomalacia from prolonged vascular ring compression could develop if the obstruction is not relieved, and surgical intervention is recommended soon after initial diagnosis.[28]

When patients present at an older age, the symptoms are not as severe. The specific aortic arch anatomy determines the recommended intervention. In patients with an aortic arch abnormality but not a true vascular ring, such as a left aortic arch with an aberrant retroesophageal right subclavian artery, conservative medical management may be of benefit.[17] A majority of patients with a left aortic arch with an aberrant retroesophageal right subclavian artery are asymptomatic and require no intervention. When symptoms are present in this specific aortic arch anatomy, the frequency and severity of the symptoms determine the initial management. In patients with mild and intermittent symptoms, conservative management can be instituted. Typical conservative management involves treatment of coexisting esophageal abnormalities with prokinetic or antireflux drugs.[16] However, if conservative management fails, then surgical treatment is warranted.[16,29,30]

The presence of a diverticulum of Kommerell dictates management regardless of symptoms. Patients with a vascular ring with an associated diverticulum of Kommerell are at risk of spontaneous rupture, dissection, and death.[7,29,30] In one series of 10 patients with a diverticulum of Kommerell, 50% had an associated aortic dissection.[31] Due to this risk several publications advocate for surgical resection of the diverticulum even in asymptomatic patients.[7,29,30,31] Pathological examination of the diverticulum of Kommerell reveals medial degeneration or necrosis commonly found in patients with aortic aneurysms or dissection.[29]

When surgical treatment is warranted, the type of aortic arch abnormality or vascular ring dictates the type of surgical repair. In patients with a vascular ring, surgical division of the ductus arteriosus, ligamentum arteriosum, or hypoplastic aortic arch that completes the vascular ring is the treatment. In most vascular rings the ligamentum is a left-sided structure, and the ligation can occur through a left-sided thoracotomy. However, in rare vascular rings the ductus or ligamentum is right-sided, requiring a right-sided thoracotomy. This further reiterates the importance of knowing the exact aortic arch anatomy prior to surgical correction of a vascular ring. In the presence of a diverticulum of Kommerell several surgeons advocate for division of the ligamentum and resection of the diverticulum with transfer of the left subclavian artery to the left common carotid artery.[7,29] Hybrid and endovascular approaches have been developed in the last 15 years and can be used to surgically treat aortic arch abnormalities.[30,31]

An important management strategy of patients with congenital heart disease is limiting the potential risk factors of dysphagia. Avoiding preoperative intubation, improving weight gain prior to surgery, limiting time on the ventilator, and limiting operation time can decrease the risk of postoperative dysphagia. Identification of the recurrent laryngeal nerve by the cardiovascular surgeon is

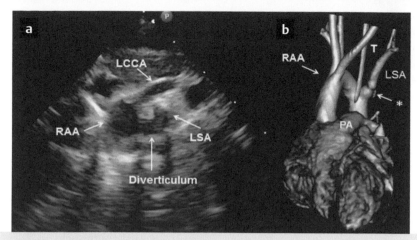

**Fig . 16.8** Transthoracic echocardiogram and chest computed tomography in aortic arch abnormality. **(a)** Suprasternal coronal view of a transthoracic echocardiogram in a patient with a right aortic arch (RAA) with an aberrant retroesophageal left subclavian artery (LSA) from a diverticulum of Kommerell. **(b)** A three-dimensional computed tomographic reconstruction of the same patient showing the large-caliber diverticulum of Kommerell (*) where the left ligamentum arteriosum connects anterior to the pulmonary artery (PA), completing the vascular ring and encircling the trachea (T) and esophagus. LCCA, left common carotid artery. (Image courtesy of Victoria Schroder RDCS, LeBonheur Children's Hospital, Memphis, Tennessee.)

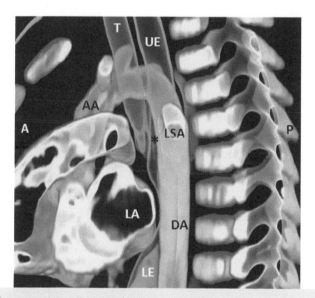

**Fig. 16.9** Three-dimensional computed tomography. Hollow vessel reconstruction of the esophagus and trachea (T) showing the posterior esophageal compression (black asterisk) from the left subclavian artery (LSA) in a patient with a right aortic arch with an aberrant retroesophageal left subclavian artery. A, anterior; AA, ascending aorta; DA, descending aorta; LA, left atrium; LE, lower esophagus; P, posterior; UE, upper esophagus. (Image courtesy of Jason N. Johnson, MD MHS, LeBonheur Children's Hospital, Memphis, Tennessee.)

important so it can be avoided in procedures that require augmentation of the aortic arch or patent ductus arteriosus. The use of mini-multiplane transesophageal echocardiography probes should be considered in neonates weighing less than 12 lb (5.5 kg).[4]

The treatment of dysphagia in infants with congenital heart disease or after congenital heart disease surgery is extensive and requires a multidisciplinary team. Evaluation by a speech-language pathologist is not only diagnostic but therapeutic as well. Identifying abnormalities in the infant's behavior state, oral posture, oral reflexes, or nonnutritive sucking and discussing techniques to optimize oral feeding can be communicated to the caregiver. Working with a nutritionist to identify optimal caloric intake to achieve weight gain in the setting of congestive heart failure is essential. Due to the increased caloric demand it is often necessary to fortify the formula or breastmilk to optimize caloric density and decrease the volume of intake. In infants with frank aspiration many centers limit oral feeds, and nasogastric, naso-duodenal, or gastrointestinal tube feeds would be instituted.[5] In patients with aspiration of only thin liquids, thickened liquids to the consistency where no aspiration occurs will be prescribed. Infants with vocal cord paralysis rarely require a tracheostomy to protect the airway.[10,11] Typically vocal cord dysfunction will spontaneously recover over time, and conservative measures (e.g., oral proton pump inhibitors) are all that is required. The speech-language pathologist caring for patients with congenital heart disease will work with the medical team (parents/caregivers, physicians, nurses, lactation specialists, and nutritionists) to support early oral feeding milestones while ensuring safe and adequate intake of sufficient nutrition to meet the increased caloric demands of this population. Often this will involve allowing modified oral intake via breast or bottle with nonoral supplementation. Thickened liquids are not typically prescribed for this population due to the increased work of sucking required to extract the thickened expressed breastmilk or formula from the nipple. Speech-language pathologists should consider the method of oral intake (breast or bottle) and how to optimize safe oral intake for the infant. For review of specific treatment considerations for supporting oral intake in high-risk neonatal populations, please review Chapter 14 in this book.

# 16.7 Questions

1. Which statement about aortic arch abnormalities is false?

A. The most common vascular ring is the double aortic arch.
B. The most common aortic arch abnormality is the right aortic arch with aberrant retroesophageal left subclavian artery.
C. Aortic arch abnormalities are commonly associated with other forms of congenital heart disease.
D. The aortic arch forms from the appearance and resolution of specific paired embryological vessels.
E. Vascular rings can form from many different variations of appearance and resolution of the paired embryological vessels that form the aortic arch.

2. Which statement regarding dysphagia associated with aortic arch abnormalities is true?

A. The most common symptom associated with vascular rings is dysphagia.
B. When patients with vascular rings present early, as in a neonate or an infant, the most common symptom is dysphagia.
C. Patients with a "loose" vascular ring typically present early, as in a neonate or an infant, with vague respiratory symptoms.
D. Almost all patients with a left aortic arch and aberrant retroesophageal right subclavian artery have gastrointestinal symptoms such as dysphagia.
E. *Dysphagia lusoria* is a term used to define swallowing difficulties originally described in patients with a left aortic arch with an aberrant retroesophageal right subclavian artery.

3. A left aortic arch with an aberrant retroesophageal right subclavian artery is not a vascular ring because the esophagus and trachea are not completely encircled by vascular structures. What is the proposed mechanism of dysphagia in this common aortic arch abnormality?

A. The esophagus loses rigidity with age and becomes more susceptible to the posterior right subclavian artery.

B. There is always an associated diverticulum of Kommerell that leads to esophageal compression.
C. The arterial wall of the right subclavian artery becomes more rigid from atherosclerosis with increased age.
D. The aorta shortens as the patient ages, creating more crowding of the esophagus.
E. Symptoms only present with concomitant bicarotid truncus, a common trunk to both carotid arteries.

4. A 4-day-old boy with hypoplastic left heart syndrome will undergo congenital heart surgery tomorrow. The mother asks what factors would predict feeding difficulties for her son in the future. You tell her that all of the following factors are risk factors for dysphagia in infants after heart surgery except

A. Preoperative intubation
B. Use of transesophageal echocardiography in an infant weighing less than 12 lb (5.5 Kg)
C. Surgery for a left-sided obstructive lesion
D. Long operation time
E. Intubation for fewer than 7 days

5. A 15-year-old girl is being seen by her primary physician for difficulty swallowing once or twice a week for the last several years, with frequent regurgitation of food. A chest X-ray shows a right aortic arch, and a barium esophagram shows posterior compression of the esophagus at the fourth vertebral level, with the report stating "findings consistent with dysphagia lusoria." The patient asks you about the next step in her management, and you tell her:

A. The finding on the barium esophagram confirms a vascular ring. Her symptoms are relatively severe, and treatment by surgical repair is indicated.
B. The finding on the barium esophagram confirms that her symptoms of dysphagia are related to an aortic abnormality. However, further testing will be required to define her specific aortic arch anatomy to plan further management.
C. The finding on the barium esophagram confirms a vascular ring. Her symptoms are not severe, and medical management will be initiated.
D. The finding on the barium esophagram confirms that her symptoms of dysphagia are related to an aortic arch abnormality. Further evaluation with esophageal manometry will determine whether she will respond well to surgery.
E. The finding on the barium esophagram confirms her symptoms of dysphagia are related to an aortic abnormality. Given the presence of a right aortic arch on the chest X-ray, the aortic arch abnormality is likely a right aortic arch with an aberrant retroesophageal left subclavian artery from a diverticulum of Kommerell, and surgery will be scheduled soon.

6. A 42-year-old man has a 5-year history of intermittent dysphagia with difficulty swallowing two or three times a month and occasional regurgitation of food. Upper gastrointestinal endoscopy shows mild esophagitis and a

pulsatile mass in the middle third of the esophagus, and MRA shows a left aortic arch with an aberrant retroesophageal right subclavian artery with no diverticulum of Kommerell. What is the next step in his management?

A. Surgical correction will never be indicated because there is no diverticulum of Kommerell.
B. Surgical correction will never be indicated because a left aortic arch with an aberrant retroesophageal right subclavian artery with no diverticulum of Kommerell is not a vascular ring.
C. Surgical correction is warranted now because a left aortic arch with an aberrant retroesophageal right subclavian artery is a vascular ring.
D. Conservative measures should be tried given his mild esophagitis and intermittent symptoms. If there is no improvement, surgical correction is indicated.
E. Conservative measures will not work because there is esophageal compression.

7. A 3-month-old girl has inspiratory stridor at rest with worsening reflux. She has a chest X-ray that shows a right aortic arch, and a computed tomographic scan shows a double aortic arch with a hypoplastic left arch. A transthoracic echocardiogram shows no other congenital heart disease. What is the next step in management?

A. A trial of conservative management with antireflux medications is indicated prior to surgical repair being scheduled.
B. Surgical division of the hypoplastic left arch is indicated through a left thoracotomy.
C. A barium esophagram is indicated to evaluate for esophageal compression given the presence of a double aortic arch.
D. Surgical division of the right arch is indicated because the normal aortic arch anatomy is a left arch.
E. The early presentation of the patient predicts conservative management will be effective, and surgery can likely be avoided.

8. A 4-year-old girl has an umbilical hernia and is scheduled for surgery. She has a routine chest X-ray with a right aortic arch, and a computed tomographic scan shows a right aortic arch with an aberrant retroesophageal left subclavian artery from a diverticulum of Kommerell consistent with a vascular ring. She has no symptoms of dysphagia, wheezing, or stridor, and a transthoracic echocardiogram shows normal intracardiac anatomy. What is the next step in her management?

A. The umbilical hernia surgery should be canceled.
B. The vascular ring should be surgically repaired at the same time as the umbilical hernia surgery.
C. The umbilical hernia surgery should continue as planned.
D. The vascular ring should be surgically repaired prior to the umbilical hernia surgery.
E. A barium esophagram should be scheduled to evaluate for esophageal compression.

9. A 5-month-old boy with hypoplastic left heart syndrome has already had two heart surgeries and now has dysphagia with difficulty gaining weight consistently. Which of the following is not part of routine treatment for infants with dysphagia following congenital heart surgery?

A. A nutritionist can help increase the caloric density of his formula to promote weight gain.
B. A speech-language pathologist can evaluate his suck–swallow–breath response to oral feeds.
C. If he is found to have left vocal cord paralysis, he will certainly require a tracheostomy.
D. If he is found to have aspiration of liquids, he would be a candidate for gastrointestinal-tube feeds.
E. An otolaryngologist can evaluate his vocal cord function with a laryngoscope.

## 16.8 Answers and Explanations

1. **Correct: the most common aortic arch abnormality is the right aortic arch with aberrant retroesophageal left subclavian artery (B).**

A right aortic arch with aberrant retroesophageal left subclavian artery is an aortic arch abnormality, but it is not the most common. When the left subclavian arises from an associated diverticulum of Kommerell, there is a left-sided ligamentum arteriosum that completes the vascular ring. This aortic arch abnormality represents the second most common form of vascular rings. The most common aortic arch abnormality is a left aortic arch with aberrant retroesophageal right subclavian artery, present in about 1% of the population. The most common vascular ring is the double aortic arch, and several types exist, as described in **Table 16.1**. The typical double aortic arch involves a dominant right aortic arch with a hypoplastic left aortic arch (**A**). Aortic arch abnormalities are more commonly associated in patients with congenital heart disease than in those without. The incidence of aortic arch abnormalities varies depending on the specific congenital lesion. They are common in tetralogy of Fallot (34%) and complete transposition of the great arteries (16%) (**C**). There is a specific, complicated order of appearance and resolution of paired embryological vessels that determine the aortic arch. The normal left aortic arch results from resolution of the right sixth aortic arch and the right dorsal aorta distal to the origin of the seventh intersegmental artery (**D**). There are many different aortic arch abnormalities that result in a vascular ring, and they are listed in **Table 16.1**. The different combinations of appearance and resolution of the paired embryological vessels that form the aortic arch determine the ultimate aortic arch anatomy (**E**).

2. **Correct: *dysphagia lusoria* is a term used to define swallowing difficulties originally described in patients with a left aortic arch with an aberrant retroesophageal right subclavian artery (E).**

*Dysphagia lusoria* was first coined in 1794 by a British surgeon, David Bayford, to describe this specific aortic arch abnormality. The term *dysphagia lusoria* is now used to describe swallowing difficulties associated with any aortic arch abnormality. The most common symptom associated with vascular rings is respiratory (stridor, wheezing, coughing, or recurrent respiratory infections) present in almost all patients (93%). Gastrointestinal symptoms are present in only half of cases of vascular rings (**A**). When a vascular ring presents early in life, the ring is considered "tight," and respiratory symptoms like stridor are the most common presentation (**B**). When vascular rings are "loose," the typical presentation is dysphagia later in life, typically in adulthood. Vague respiratory symptoms like wheezing are common in loose vascular rings (**C**). Very few patients with a left aortic arch and aberrant retroesophageal right subclavian artery have symptoms (20%) (**D**).

3. **Correct: the arterial wall of the right subclavian artery becomes more rigid from atherosclerosis with increased age (C).**

The most accepted mechanism for dysphagia in this specific aortic arch abnormality is that the right subclavian artery becomes more rigid. Symptoms develop from extrinsic compression of the esophagus posteriorly from the rigid right subclavian artery against the trachea, anteriorly. The esophagus actually becomes more rigid with age, and is one of the proposed mechanisms for dysphagia in this anatomy (**A**). A diverticulum of Kommerell is usually not associated with a left aortic arch with an aberrant retroesophageal right subclavian artery. There are only rare case reports where a diverticulum is present with this aortic arch abnormality, and they always represent a true vascular ring (**B**). The elongation of the aorta is one of the proposed mechanisms for dysphagia in this specific aortic arch abnormality (**D**). Concomitant bicarotid truncus is one of the proposed mechanisms for dysphagia in this specific aortic arch abnormality. However, a bicarotid truncus is not present in all cases of dysphagia associated with a left aortic arch with an aberrant retroesophageal right subclavian artery (**E**).

4. **Correct: intubation for fewer than 7 days (E).**

Intubation for fewer than 7 days is *not* a risk factor for dysphagia in children after heart surgery. Patients who require more than 1 week of intubation after heart surgery are at an increased risk of dysphagia. Preoperative intubation is a risk factor for dysphagia in children with heart disease requiring surgery. Every effort is made to avoid preoperative intubation prior to congenital heart surgery (**A**). Use of transesophageal echocardiography in an infant weighing less than 12 lb (5.5 kg) is a risk factor for dysphagia in children with heart disease requiring surgery. Evaluation of complicated heart surgery during the operation is sometimes essential, and the use of transesophageal echocardiography is warranted. There are new mini-multiplane transesophageal echocardiography probes that should be used in infants weighing less than 12 lb (5.5 kg) (**B**). Surgery for a left-sided obstructive lesion is a risk factor for dysphagia in children with heart disease requiring surgery. Specific operations, such as left-sided obstructive lesions (hypoplastic left heart syndrome) or patent ductus arteriosus ligation, put children at risk for postoperative dysphagia (**C**). Long operation time

is a risk factor for dysphagia in children with heart disease requiring surgery. There are many complications of longer operation time, with feeding difficulties representing an important risk. Every effort is made to perform successful surgery in a timely manner (**D**).

5. **Correct: the finding on the barium esophagram confirms that her symptoms of dysphagia are related to an aortic abnormality. However, further testing will be required to define her specific aortic arch anatomy to plan further management (B).**

The barium esophagram finding confirms her symptoms of dysphagia are related to an aortic arch abnormality. However, the specific aortic arch anatomy has not been defined, which is essential prior to surgical repair. Therefore, MRA or CT should be ordered. The barium esophagram cannot confirm the exact type of vascular ring, which also warrants further imaging. The patient's symptoms are relatively severe and will likely require surgical repair (**A, C**). Esophageal manometry cannot determine the specific aortic arch anatomy, nor can it predict her response to surgical repair (**D**). The specific vascular anatomy described in this answer is the most common vascular ring associated with a right aortic arch. However, there are at least three different types of vascular rings associated with a right aortic arch, and further imaging should be performed to aid in the surgical repair (**Table 16.1**) (**E**).

6. **Correct: conservative measures should be tried given his mild esophagitis and intermittent symptoms. If there is no improvement, surgical correction is indicated (D).**

Left aortic arch with an aberrant retroesophageal right subclavian artery is the most common aortic arch abnormality and is frequently asymptomatic. Therefore, his symptoms may improve with conservative management and surgery can be avoided. Surgery may not be indicated in this specific aortic arch anatomy, but it should be considered if conservative measures fail. Dysphagia from aortic arch anomalies can require surgical correction even without the presence of a diverticulum of Kommerell (**A**). Surgical repair may be indicated to repair this anatomy if dysphagia persists after failure of conservative management (**B**). Left aortic arch with an aberrant retroesophageal right subclavian artery is *not* a vascular ring (**C**). A majority of patients with a left aortic arch with an aberrant retroesophageal right subclavian artery are asymptomatic despite some esophageal compression. Conservative measures should be tried as the initial management (**E**).

7. **Correct: surgical division of the hypoplastic left arch is indicated through a left thoracotomy (B).**

This is an early presentation of a tight vascular ring, and surgery is indicated soon. Tracheomalacia can develop if tight vascular rings are not released. The approach through a left thoracotomy is indicated to divide the hypoplastic left arch to relieve the ring. This is a presentation of a tight vascular ring with symptoms. Conservative management is not indicated, and only surgical repair will relieve the symptoms (**A**). A barium esophagram is not indicated because the diagnosis of a vascular ring has been made by the CT scan. The CT scan will also show the esophageal compression, making it an ideal imaging modality in symptomatic patients with concern for a vascular ring (**C**). A majority of patients with a double aortic arch will have a hypoplastic left arch with a majority of the systemic blood flow through the right aortic arch. Therefore, ligating the right aortic arch is not feasible because the left aortic arch is not large enough to handle systemic outflow (**D**). The early presentation of a vascular ring supports a tight ring, and surgery is always indicated. A trial of conservative measures will delay the appropriate treatment: the surgical division of the vascular ring (**E**).

### 8. Correct: the umbilical hernia surgery should continue as planned (C).

She has an asymptomatic vascular ring that does not currently require intervention. She should have her umbilical hernia surgery as planned. Should she develop symptoms, then the vascular ring should be repaired (**D**). There is no reason to cancel the umbilical hernia surgery (**A**). The umbilical hernia surgery is in a different region than the vascular ring surgery and would not be performed at the same time. If she had a congenital heart disease that required surgery, then the vascular ring would be ligated at the same time (**B**). The barium esophagram is not needed in this case. The CT scan shows the anatomy of the vascular ring and the esophageal compression. Therefore, the barium esophagram does not add anything to this case (**E**).

### 9. Correct: if he is found to have left vocal cord paralysis, he will certainly require a tracheostomy (C).

Very rarely do children with dysphagia and vocal cord paralysis require tracheostomy. Increasing the caloric density of formula is a common treatment of dysphagia in children with heart disease requiring surgery. Increasing the caloric density of the formula allows the infants to reach a caloric goal with limited volume (**A**). A speech-language pathologist will identify potential etiologies for dysphagia (**B**). When infants are found to aspirate, oral feeds are no longer safe and other routes of feeding are required. This can be performed by a gastrointestinal or nasogastric tube (**D**). Specific heart surgeries place infants at risk for vocal cord paralysis, so evaluation of vocal cord function is important in postoperative patients with dysphagia (**E**).

## References

[1] Hoffman JI, Kaplan S. The incidence of congenital heart disease. *J Am Coll Cardiol* 2002;*39*(12):1890–1900

[2] Humphrey C, Duncan K, Fletcher S. Decade of experience with vascular rings at a single institution. *Pediatrics* 2006;*117*(5):e903–e908

[3] Pereira KdaR, Firpo C, Gasparin M, et al. Evaluation of swallowing in infants with congenital heart defect. *Int Arch Otorhinolaryngol* 2015;*19*(1):55–60

[4] Kohr LM, Dargan M, Hague A, et al. The incidence of dysphagia in pediatric patients after open heart procedures with transesophageal echocardiography. *Ann Thorac Surg* 2003;*76*(5):1450–1456

[5] Skinner ML, Halstead LA, Rubinstein CS, Atz AM, Andrews D, Bradley SM. Laryngopharyngeal dysfunction after the Norwood procedure. *J Thorac Cardiovasc Surg* 2005;*130*(5):1293–1301

[6] Yi S-H, Kim S-J, Huh J, Jun T-G, Cheon HJ, Kwon J-Y. Dysphagia in infants after open heart procedures. *Am J Phys Med Rehabil* 2013;*92*(6):496–503

[7] Weinberg PM, Natarajan S, Rogers LS. Aortic arch and vascular anomalies. In: Allen HD, Driscoll DJ, Shaddy RE, Feltes TF, eds. Moss and Adams' Heart Disease in Infants, Children, and Adolescents: Including the Fetus and Young Adult. Philadelphia, PA: Lippincott Williams & Wilkins: 2013:780–821

[8] Sachdeva R, Hussain E, Moss MM, et al. Vocal cord dysfunction and feeding difficulties after pediatric cardiovascular surgery. *J Pediatr* 2007;*151*(3):312–315, 315.e1–315.e2

[9] Nichols BG, Jabbour J, Hehir DA, et al. Recovery of vocal fold immobility following isolated patent ductus arteriosus ligation. *Int J Pediatr Otorhinolaryngol* 2014;*78*(8):1316–1319

[10] Pereira KD, Webb BD, Blakely ML, Cox CS Jr, Lally KP. Sequelae of recurrent laryngeal nerve injury after patent ductus arteriosus ligation. *Int J Pediatr Otorhinolaryngol* 2006;*70*(9):1609–1612

[11] Rukholm G, Farrokhyar F, Reid D. Vocal cord paralysis post patent ductus arteriosus ligation surgery: risks and co-morbidities. *Int J Pediatr Otorhinolaryngol* 2012;*76*(11):1637–1641

[12] Truong MT, Messner AH, Kerschner JE, et al. Pediatric vocal fold paralysis after cardiac surgery: rate of recovery and sequelae. *Otolaryngol Head Neck Surg* 2007;*137*(5):780–784

[13] Bayford D. An account of a singular case of obstructed deglutition. *Mem Med Soc London* 1794;*2*:275–286

[14] Asherson N. David Bayford. His syndrome and sign of dysphagia lusoria. *Ann R Coll Surg Engl* 1979;*61*(1):63–67

[15] Morris ME, Benjamin M, Gardner GP, Nichols WK, Faizer R. The use of the Amplatzer plug to treat dysphagia lusoria caused by an aberrant right subclavian artery. *Ann Vasc Surg* 2010;*24*(3):416.e5–416.e8

[16] Feezor RJ, Lee WA. Dysphagia lusoria. *J Vasc Surg* 2007;*46*(3):581

[17] Janssen M, Baggen MGA, Veen HF, et al. Dysphagia lusoria: clinical aspects, manometric findings, diagnosis, and therapy. *Am J Gastroenterol* 2000;*95*(6):1411–1416

[18] McNally PR, Rak KM. Dysphagia lusoria caused by persistent right aortic arch with aberrant left subclavian artery and diverticulum of Kommerell. *Dig Dis Sci* 1992;*37*(1):144–149

[19] Morris CD, Kanter KR, Miller JI Jr. Late-onset dysphagia lusoria. *Ann Thorac Surg* 2001;*71*(2):710–712

[20] Sitzman TJ, Mell MW, Acher CW. Adult-onset dysphagia lusoria from an uncommon vascular ring: a case report and review of the literature. *Vasc Endovascular Surg* 2009;*43*(1):100–102

[21] Grathwohl KW, Afifi AY, Dillard TA, Olson JP, Heric BR. Vascular rings of the thoracic aorta in adults. *Am Surg* 1999;*65*(11):1077–1083

[22] Gnanapandithan K, Rahni DO, Habr F. Intermittent esophageal dysphagia: an intriguing diagnosis. Dysphagia lusoria. *Gastroenterology* 2014;*146*(4):e3–e4

[23] Jalal H, El Idrissi R, Azghari A, et al. Dysphagia lusoria: report of a series of six cases. *Clin Res Hepatol Gastroenterol* 2014;*38*(3):e45–e49

[24] Levitt B, Richter JE. Dysphagia lusoria: a comprehensive review. *Dis Esophagus* 2007;*20*(6):455–460

[25] Breaux J, Gupta N, Smith R, Connolly SE. The third esophageal sphincter: a case of dysphagia lusoria. *ACG Case Rep J* 2014;*2*(1):6–7

[26] Kang MS. Dysphagia lusoria caused by Kommerell's diverticulum of the aberrant left subclavian artery. *Clin Gastroenterol Hepatol* 2014;*12*(6):e47–e48

[27] Johnson JN, Hornik CP, Li JS, et al. Cumulative radiation exposure and cancer risk estimation in children with heart disease. *Circulation* 2014;*130*(2):161–167

[28] Bonnard A, Auber F, Fourcade L, Marchac V, Emond S, Révillon Y. Vascular ring abnormalities: a retrospective study of 62 cases. *J Pediatr Surg* 2003;*38*(4):539–543

[29] Kim KM, Cambria RP, Isselbacher EM, et al. Contemporary surgical approaches and outcomes in adults with Kommerell diverticulum. *Ann Thorac Surg* 2014;*98*(4):1347–1354

[30] van Bogerijen GH, Patel HJ, Eliason JL, et al. Evolution in the management of aberrant subclavian arteries and related Kommerell diverticulum. *Ann Thorac Surg* 2015;*100*(1):47–53

[31] Idrees J, Keshavamurthy S, Subramanian S, Clair DG, Svensson LG, Roselli EE. Hybrid repair of Kommerell diverticulum. *J Thorac Cardiovasc Surg* 2014;*147*(3):973–976

# 17 Oropharyngeal Dysphagia in Children with Cerebral Palsy

*Georgia A. Malandraki and Jaime Bauer Malandraki*

## Summary

Cerebral palsy (CP), a neurodevelopmental disorder caused by nonprogressive lesions of the developing fetal or infant brain, is the most common cause of physical disability in childhood. CP is often accompanied by other disturbances in cognition, sensation, communication, perception, as well as feeding and swallowing. Feeding and swallowing disorders (i.e., dysphagia) are rather common in CP and may manifest as inability to self-feed, oral motor discoordination, abnormal oropharyngeal tone, reduced strength, frequent coughing and choking, and overall poor feeding development, increasing the risk for malnutrition and dehydration. Therefore, optimal dysphagia evaluation and treatment approaches are essential in the management of children with CP. This chapter begins by defining the term *cerebral palsy* and describing the epidemiology and pathophysiology of this multifaceted condition. The main classifications of CP are discussed, as well as how CP affects feeding and swallowing in children. The chapter then explores evidence-based ways to evaluate and treat feeding and swallowing in this population within a multidisciplinary approach. A case study illustrates the important points and the takeaway messages of the text.

## Keywords

cerebral palsy, spasticity, dyskinesias, prematurity, motor learning, neuroplasticty

### Learning Objectives

- Describe cerebral palsy (CP) and its major clinical manifestations, classifications, and pathophysiological features
- Identify the main types of feeding and swallowing disorders observed in children with CP
- Describe feeding and swallowing evaluation and treatment strategies for children with CP and identify the research evidence behind them

## 17.1 Introduction

Cerebral palsy (CP) is a neurodevelopmental disorder that begins early in a child's life and persists throughout the life span. It is known to be the most common cause of physical disability in childhood.[1] The first comprehensive description of the musculoskeletal symptoms seen in CP is attributed to William Little, an English orthopedic surgeon, in 1843,[2] and CP was originally known as Little's disease. Since then, many descriptions and definitions of CP have been proposed. Interestingly, even today there is no fully accepted universal definition for this well-recognized neurodevelopmental condition. In 2006 an executive committee, including an international team of esteemed neurologists, clinicians, and scientists, published a new proposed definition of CP to ensure a more comprehensive inclusion of the many etiological, diagnostic, and activity limitations that are manifestations of the condition. This definition appears to be the most widely accepted to date and is reported herein.

According to this definition, cerebral palsy (CP) is a group of permanent disorders of the development of movement and posture, causing activity limitation, that are attributed to nonprogressive disturbances that occurred in the developing fetal or infant brain. The motor disorders of cerebral palsy are often accompanied by disturbances of sensation, perception, cognition, communication, and behavior, by epilepsy, and by secondary musculoskeletal problems.[3]

## Case Presentation Part 1: Case History

GL is a 2-year, 7-month-old boy with a diagnosis of mixed spastic/athetoid cerebral palsy caused by diffuse cerebral dysplasia of unknown etiology. Pre- and postnatal history were unremarkable; however, GL's mother (who is an occupational therapist) noted delayed gross motor development at approximately 3 months of age. GL has had a history of feeding difficulties and inability to breastfeed, leading to gastrostomy tube dependency for the first 2 months of life. Regarding gross motor development, he now presents with reduced head and trunk control, athetoid limb movements, and inability to sit and walk independently (Gross Motor Function Classification System [GMFCS] level V). His speech/language and cognitive development is delayed. Specifically, GL produces many isolated sounds, but no intelligible words; he appears to comprehend simple one-step commands. Regarding feeding and swallowing, he is currently on thin liquids (using a sippy cup) and semisolids (mashed pureed foods), and is not an independent feeder. Solids have not been introduced. He has no history of respiratory infections, but his parents report frequent coughing and gagging during feeding. He is at the 20th percentile for weight/height for children of his age with CP.

The case of GL clearly illustrates many of the key components of the definition presented in the Introduction. In addition to the severe motor impairments caused by a nonprogressive neurologic condition (dysplasia), GL also exhibits disruptions in sensation, cognition, and communication. Furthermore, in accordance with the World Health Organization (WHO) International Classification of Functioning, Disability and Health (ICF) (which has been taken into consideration in devising the definition),[4,5] GL's motor impairments have caused severe limitations in his daily activities because he is unable to sit, walk, or communicate effectively.

Moreover, it is evident that GL also exhibits a feeding and swallowing disorder (i.e., dysphagia). This is common in many, if not most, children with CP. Specifically, between 30 and 99% of children with CP have been reported to experience feeding and swallowing disorders.[6,7,8,9] Without effective treatment for dysphagia, the risk for malnutrition, failure to thrive, respiratory compromise, or even death greatly increases.[10,11,12] Taking into consideration these large numbers, as well as the potentially devastating complications of swallowing and feeding disorders in the quality of life, health, and growth of a child with CP, the need for accurate identification and effective treatment is crucial.

The present chapter provides an overview of the epidemiology and pathophysiology of CP, followed by the main classifications used to describe the clinical manifestations of the disorder and a description of the main feeding and swallowing symptomatology seen in this population. The discussion then turns to the main steps in the evaluation and treatment of dysphagia in CP as well as the most widely used diagnostic and treatment modalities for this population, along with the evidence behind them.

## 17.2 Epidemiology of Cerebral Palsy with and without Associated Impairments

Epidemiology studies across the world report prevalence estimates of CP between 1.5 and 4 per 1,000 births/cases studied.[13,14,15,16,17] In the United States, a recently published population-based study completed by the Autism and Developmental Disabilities Monitoring Network in four U.S. states (Alabama, Georgia, Missouri, and Wisconsin) revealed a prevalence of 3.1 per 1,000 children.[18] CP has been found to be relatively more common in males than females,[18,19] as well as in black children compared to white and Hispanic children.[18]

Furthermore, CP is frequently seen with one or more associated impairments. The underlying motor disorders seen in CP, especially spasticity, often result in musculoskeletal impairments,

such as contractures, hip luxations, and scoliosis (see **Table 17.1** for key definitions), all of which are seen in 72–75% of children with quadriplegic CP.[20] Intellectual disability is reported in almost half of children with CP[21] and is also more common in severely disabled children.[20] Epilepsy/seizure disorder is seen in 30–40% of this population,[18,21] and this incidence also increases with severity of disability.[20] In addition, 50 to 85% of children with CP present with communication and motor speech disorders,[1,22] whereas visual impairments/cortical blindness are seen in 9.5–15%,[23] and hearing impairment in 4–13%.[23,24] Recently the diagnosis of autism was also found to be significantly higher in children with CP (7%) than in children without CP (1%).[18] These frequent comorbidities often significantly complicate the clinical presentation of the condition and emphasize the importance of comprehensive and multidisciplinary evaluation and management plans for this population.

## 17.3 Pathophysiology and Risk Factors

According to the definition of CP, the prevailing theory is that it is caused by an injury (i.e., permanent static lesion) in the developing central nervous system, which can occur in utero, during delivery, or during the first 1–2 years of life. Thus, depending on the timing of the insult, etiologies/risk factors can be categorized as prenatal, natal, or postnatal.[31]

### 17.3.1 Pathophysiological Features

When examining clinical brain magnetic resonance imaging (MRI) scans of children with CP, abnormalities of brain development are among the most common findings. Specifically, periventricular leukomalacia (PVL) (**Fig. 17.1a**) is the most frequently reported brain abnormality,[32] followed by basal ganglia lesions, cortical/subcortical lesions (**Fig. 17.1b**), brain malformations, and focal infarcts.[32] However, in some children (~ 10%) no significant MRI findings are observed.

**Table 17.1** Key terms relating to motor function in cerebral palsy and brief definitions

| Key motor terms | Definition |
| --- | --- |
| Abnormal muscle tone | The amount of activity in a muscle when we are not moving |
| Hypertonia | "Abnormally increased resistance to externally imposed movement about a joint"[25] |
| Spasticity | A velocity-dependent resistance of muscle to stretch or excessive, inappropriate involuntary muscle activity usually associated with upper-motor-neuron involvement[26] |
| Rigidity | Hypertonia characterized by resistance to movement regardless of the speed or direction of the passive movement. Rigid muscles often feel heavy and like "a lead pipe" when they are moved[25] |
| Hypotonia | Tone lower than normal (muscles that are "loose" or "floppy") |
| Dyskinesias<br>• Dystonia<br><br>• Athetosis<br>• Chorea | Excessive, involuntary movements<br>Involuntary, sustained, or intermittent muscle contractions that cause twisting and repetitive movements, abnormal postures, or both[27]<br>"A slow, continuous, involuntary writhing movement that prevents maintenance of a stable posture"[28]<br>"An ongoing random-appearing sequence of one or more discrete involuntary movements or movement fragments"[28]; may present as a symptom in the shoulders, trunk, and head and neck |
| Contractures | Limitations of the passive range of motion of a joint.[29] Contractures can be the result of changes in muscles, tendons, skin, or bones and cartilages. |
| Scoliosis | Lateral curvature of the spine[30] |

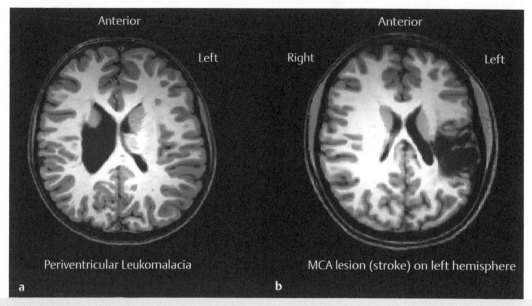

**Fig. 17.1** **(a)** Magnetic resonance imaging (MRI) scan of a 13-year-old boy who was diagnosed with periventricular leukomalacia. **(b)** MRI scan of a 17-year-old girl who had a perinatal middle cerebral artery cerebrovascular accident (stroke). (Images courtesy of the Purdue I-EaT Swallowing Research Lab.)

The type, location, and extent of the brain injury and the resulting motor disability are strongly dependent on the gestational age at which brain development was disrupted. For the first 6 months (24 weeks) of pregnancy, when the nervous system is being developed (e.g., proliferation and migration of cells), genetic abnormalities and viral infections can significantly alter brain development and lead to cortical dysplasia, schizencephaly, polymicrogyria, and other brain malformations.[31] In the subsequent weeks of gestation, when significant neuronal growth is taking place (e.g., growth of axons and dendrites, myelination, and emerging specialization of neural functions) several environmental factors have been associated with CP, such as viral infections, hypoxia/ischemia, and brain injuries.[31] Currently researchers believe that the causes of CP are multifactorial, including the interaction of multiple predisposing/risk factors (**Table 17.2**) that will lead to a deficit in the nervous system and will later manifest as the constellation of symptoms seen in CP.

## Risk Factors

Several *prenatal risk factors* have been associated with the development of CP. Perhaps the most commonly reported such factor is *prematurity*. Specifically, studies have reported that the prevalence of CP ranges between 35 and 43.7 per 1,000 live births in children born at 28–31 weeks gestation, compared to 1.1 to 1.4 per 1,000 births in children born at term.[33] This is likely because preterm birth separates the fetus's brain from its natural environment and can disrupt its normal development.[34] *Low birth weight* and *multiple pregnancies* have also been associated with a significantly increased risk of a CP diagnosis.[35] Multiple pregnancy has been found to increase the CP diagnosis risk by twofold, with in vitro fertilization twins having a fourfold increased risk.[35] This risk is due to the high rate of prematurity and co-twin death in multiple pregnancies.[36] *Viral* or *bacterial infections* (such as toxoplasma, cytomegalovirus, Epstein–Barr virus, rubella, varicella-zoster, etc.)[37,38] and *toxicity* caused by

alcohol or drugs[39] have also been associated with an increased risk for brain malformations leading to a CP diagnosis. In addition, a large number of children with CP are born with *birth defects* or *congenital malformations*, such as hydrocephalus and schizencephaly.[40] This finding, along with the increased risk of CP in multiple pregnancies, has led investigators to start exploring genetic factors as contributors to the development of CP.[41] Several genes possibly associated with the diagnosis of CP have been identified. As genetic science advances it is likely that more cases may be explained genetically, and more complex gene interactions may be discovered.[41]

*Perinatal events* that have been associated with the development of CP include birth asphyxia or trauma (although only in 14.5% of cases)[42] and maternal inflammation/infections (chorioamnionitis or urinary tract infection) that have been found to be associated with neonatal encephalopathy.[43,44] For years birth asphyxia was reported as the main etiological factor for CP occurrence; however, epidemiological studies have revealed a small number of cases (~ 8%)[45] associated with birth asphyxia.

*Postnatal factors* are typically seen in preterm infants for whom brain development has to continue outside of its natural environment[31] and include stress and separation of mother/baby, extrauterine growth retardation, nosocomial infections, enterocolitis, or drugs.[46] These factors can significantly hinder brain development in this early stage of life (see **Table 17.2**).

**Table 17.2** Risk/etiological factors for the development of cerebral palsy

| Prenatal | Perinatal | Postnatal |
|---|---|---|
| Prematurity | Hypoxic asphyxia | Hypoxia |
| Low birth weight | Infections/inflammations | Stress and |
| Multiple pregnancies | | parent/infant |
| Viral and bacterial | | separation |
| infections | | Medications |
| Genetic factors | | Infections |

## 17.4 Cerebral Palsy Classifications/ Symptomatology

Classification of the clinical features of CP frequently involves difficult decisions about the exact boundaries of specific tools or measures used to classify the disorder.[3] Assigning a child with CP to a specific classification category is not always easy and will depend on the specific features used to classify CP, as well as on parameters such as predominant motor involvement, and the purpose of the classification.

### 17.4.1 Motor Disorder Classification

Perhaps the most popular classification of CP is based on the type of movement disorder or abnormal muscle tone that *predominates* in each child. According to this classification, CP is categorized as spastic, dyskinetic, or ataxic.[47] Spastic CP (also known as pyramidal CP) is the most common type (affecting 70–80% of cases)[47] and is typically associated with muscle hypertonia (**Table 17.1**). Spasticity is theorized to be the result of lesions affecting the upper motor neurons and their pathways.[48] Dyskinetic CP is associated with excessive involuntary movements that can manifest as dystonic, athetoid, or choreic movements (**Table 17.1**),[49,50] and is theorized to be associated with involvement of the basal ganglia.[51] Ataxic CP is less common than the aforementioned two types (affecting 5 to 10% of all cases), and is primarily characterized by ataxia (defined as abnormal postural control and incoordination of movements[52]). The main features of ataxic CP include loss of muscle coordination resulting in movements with abnormal force, accuracy, and rate, tremor, and low tone.[50] The dyskinetic and ataxic CP types are considered as subcategories of extrapyramidal CP, which affects the indirect motor pathways. Finally, mixed CP involves a combination of two or more of the previously defined types; this is a term that needs to be further specified when used.[3] Our case, GL, is an example of a child with a diagnosis of mixed CP. It is important to note that most children will actually have more than one type of abnormal muscle tone or movement disorder (e.g., spasticity and dyskinesia), but typically one will predominate. Clinicians are highly encouraged to describe all types of abnormal tone seen in a child in order to help understand the underlying pathophysiology and thereby optimize treatment.[25]

### 17.4.2 Anatomical Distribution Classification

The second most prevalent classification refers to the anatomical distribution of the disorder (i.e., essentially to what body parts have been mostly affected). According to this classification, CP can be subdivided into the following main categories: hemiplegia, diplegia, and quadriplegia. Hemiplegia indicates that both the upper and lower extremity on one side of the body have been affected. Diplegia indicates that the two lower limbs are affected more than the upper limbs, and quadriplegia implies that all four limbs are affected to a similar degree.[53] Although these terms have been prevalent in the literature and in clinical practice, their inability to fully capture all movement symptomatology in CP, including trunk and bulbar involvement, has led investigators to propose the replacement of these terms with the simpler binary classification of *unilateral vs. bilateral motor involvement.*[47] Given, however, the historic and wide use of the traditional anatomical distribution classification (-plegia), this chapter includes both. Importantly, in clinical practice it is essential to individually describe all body regions and how they may be affected in CP,[3] which is the reason why functional classifications for different body functions have now emerged.

### 17.4.3 Classifications Based on Functional Abilities

In recent years the World Health Organization (WHO) International Classification of Functioning, Disability and Health (ICF) has emphasized the importance of evaluating and treating the *functional consequences* of medical conditions.[5] This has led to the development of functional scales that are used to classify the consequences of CP on the function of the upper and lower extremities, communication, and eating.

For the function of the lower extremities and ambulation, the Gross Motor Function Classification System (GMFCS) has been devised and is widely used to group individuals with CP into one of five levels of gross motor function or functional mobility (GMFCS Score I = children can walk without significant limitations; GMFCS Score V = children are transported by wheelchair or by full manual assistance).[54] The GMFCS has descriptors broken down into four age bands (0–2, 2–4, 4–6, 6–12) allowing for use with different age groups.[55] To assess upper extremity function, the Manual Ability Classification System (MACS) has been developed.[56] MACS also categorizes children to one of five levels of manual functional ability (Level I = children handle objects easily and successfully; Level V = children are unable to handle objects).[56]

The Communication Functional Classification System (CFCS) also uses a similar five-level scale to describe the everyday communication performance of individuals with CP and other developmental disabilities (Level I = children are effective receivers and senders of communication; Level V = children are rarely effective receivers and senders of communication).[57] Recently, the Eating and Drinking Ability Classification System (EDACS) for individuals with CP was also published. EDACS is a similar functional scale used to classify the eating and drinking functional abilities of children with CP on five functional levels (Level I = eats and drinks safely and efficiently; Level V = unable to eat or drink safely—tube feeding may be considered to provide nutrition).[58]

These classification systems can be valuable tools when evaluating children with CP because they allow universally accepted terms to be used in describing the functional limitations of the child. In addition, because most are validated and have good interrater reliability, they can be used as outcome variables in clinical trials and cohort treatment studies, and thus can be useful for research.

Given the wide variability of clinical manifestations seen in CP, health care professionals are encouraged to use a combination of these classification systems, as well as descriptive narratives of symptoms not otherwise addressed within these schemes, to ensure a comprehensive diagnosis that addresses the sensorimotor and other characteristics and activity limitations of a child with CP. Such a comprehensive description is essential in ensuring all symptomatology has been documented and taken into account when devising treatment plans.

## 17.5 Feeding and Swallowing Disorders in Cerebral Palsy

### 17.5.1 Neural Control and Adaptations

Now that we have an understanding of the pathophysiology and the clinical manifestations of CP, we can begin to describe the feeding and swallowing symptomatology in this population, with the caveat that symptoms can vary greatly from individual to individual, as well as between stages of the swallow. Overall, there is a well-documented stepwise correlation between higher GMFCS levels and dysphagia severity,[59,60] indicating a clear relationship between gross motor involvement and swallowing difficulties. This is why most research on swallowing in CP has focused on investigating the swallowing and feeding functions in children with moderate or severe motor impairments, such as those with GMFCS levels of III and higher.[6,8,61] Recent evidence, however, supports that dysphagia can be present even in milder forms of CP (GMFCS I–II).[59,62,63,64,65]

In addition, through the years we have observed a wide variability of feeding and swallowing symptoms across GMFCS levels. For example, it is not uncommon to evaluate children with GMFCS level V and observe moderate to severe oral dysphagia but a relatively functional pharyngeal swallow; similarly in an experiment including children with GMFCS level I (hemiplegia) we documented signs of pharyngeal dysphagia (e.g., frequent coughing during meals) in 30% of our sample.[66]

This variability in the severity and specificity of swallowing symptomatology in CP relates in part to the areas of the nervous system affected in each individual with CP, as well as to the remarkable ways the central and peripheral nervous systems have been able to adapt to the early occurring brain lesions. As a field we know a lot more about the specificity of the neural control of healthy swallowing than about the brain adaptations that result in the wide range of normal to profound swallowing symptomatology in this population.

Specifically, we are now well aware that swallowing is not just a reflex but involves the complex coordination of receptors, muscles, nerves, *and the brain* and has both automatic and voluntary control mechanisms.[67,68,69] Thus we have begun to refer to pharyngeal swallowing as a patterned response (i.e., a response triggered at the brainstem but regulated by higher centers in the brain).[69,70] We have further identified that these higher centers have a relative specificity, with cortical centers being more influential in oral components of deglutition, and subcortical centers being more important in more automatic aspects of the swallowing sequence (e.g., laryngeal closure).[71] In other words, pharyngeal involvement is expected more frequently in lesions affecting mostly the subcortical and brainstem swallowing areas, and oral involvement is considered more likely in upper motor neuron lesions.

In addition to the area of the lesion, the type and extent of the lesion and the neuroplastic adaptations developed as a response to the lesion are equally important to understand. Unfortunately, to date these additional factors influencing swallowing/feeding development in CP remain largely understudied. In an effort to begin exploring this topic, our research team recently investigated the volumetry (i.e., brain volume) and resting-state neural activity (i.e., functional communication between brain areas at rest) of swallowing related brain areas in a group of 19 children with unilateral spastic CP.[72,73] We found that children with unilateral CP and clinical signs of dysphagia were more likely to exhibit reduced functional communications (resting-state functional connectivity) between areas of interest of the contralesional hemisphere, although their brain volumes were similar to the children with unilateral CP without signs of dysphagia.[72,73] These findings indicate that even when brain volume is preserved, if functional communications between areas of interest are disrupted, varying degrees of swallowing difficulties may be observed. These preliminary findings provide the first evidence of swallowing-related neural adaptations that have occurred in the brains of children with CP and unilateral brain lesions. The continuation of this line of research is crucial because it will enable us to understand better how the brain adapts for swallowing function, and it has the potential to lead to the development of new or better neurorehabilitative treatment targets for dysphagia in this population.

### 17.5.2 Feeding and Swallowing Symptomatology by Stage

Although focal brain lesions may affect specific swallowing components or stages, in most cases of CP the brain lesions have affected multiple brain areas and pathways, and it is not uncommon for children to exhibit difficulties in one or more of the swallowing stages, including the preoral, oral, pharyngeal, and esophageal stages.[61,62,74,75] The most common symptoms associated with each stage are detailed here and are briefly summarized in **Table 17.3**.

#### Preoral Stage and Symptomatology

The preoral stage, a relatively new term in the literature, involves anticipatory events, such as motivation and readiness for eating, posture and positioning, and food acceptance in the mouth, and involves many of the actions more commonly associated with the term *feeding*.[76,77] Difficulties associated with this stage relate to both abnormal gross motor development and reduced or abnormal development of oropharyngeal sensorimotor control. Frequently in children with CP, poor head and trunk control and abnormal muscle tone in the arms result in suboptimal positioning for oral feeding,[78] difficulty orienting to the food,[79] and partial or complete inability to self-feed.[6] In addition, tactile hypersensitivity in the orofacial area may also cause difficulties with oral reception and acceptance.[74] Drooling, or sialorrhea, is known to occur in 10–58% of children with CP[80,81] and is typically the result of either impaired oral sensorimotor function or infrequent saliva swallowing. Drooling can make it difficult for a child to adequately accept food in the oral cavity and may affect the subsequent oral and pharyngeal stages of deglutition as well.[75] In addition, excessive drooling can increase the risk for perioral infections and the buildup of bacteria that can be potentially aspirated. These difficulties in the preoral stage can be further complicated by cognitive and perceptual challenges that frequently accompany CP.[1]

## Oral Stage and Symptomatology

In the oral stage, foods and liquids are accepted, contained, processed, and then transported to the posterior part of the mouth. Oral stage difficulties are reported in up to 93.8% of pre-school children with CP[62] and have been extensively described, mainly because, clinically, they are easily observable. Typical symptoms that may affect the oral stage in children with CP include reduced labial seal,[82] reduced bolus control,[60] difficulty with oral reception,[82] difficulty drinking from a cup or straw,[62,63,64,65,66,67,68,69,70,71,72,73,74,75,76,77,78,79,80,81,82,83] tongue thrust, oral hypersensitivity, and hypersensitive reflexes (e.g., the gag reflex and the tonic bite reflex),[74] and immature or abnormal biting and chewing.[62,84,85] These symptoms may result in difficulties with oral reception and containment, tongue propulsion, and the efficient transportation of the food from the anterior to the posterior oral cavity.

## Pharyngeal Stage and Symptomatology

The pharyngeal stage involves the highly coordinated transportation of the food from the oropharynx to the esophagus adjacent to a well-protected airway. Perhaps the most frequently documented symptom that involves the pharyngeal stage in children with CP is a delay in the triggering of the pharyngeal response,[86] leading to an increased risk for aspiration and respiratory compromise.[87,88,89,90,91] Diffuse pharyngeal weakness or dysmotility is also often reported and is associated with increased instances of residue in the pharynx and a subsequent increase of the risk for aspiration after the swallow has been completed.[61,74] Wet voice, multiple swallows, gagging, and coughing during eating are also commonly reported as signs of pharyngeal difficulty.[66,75] At times increased spasticity in the pharynx and the upper esophageal sphincter (UES) may cause reduced UES opening, further reducing pharyngeal clearance. Aspiration is known to occur in up to 70% of children with severe CP.[87,88] When aspiration occurs, it is often silent without a cough or any other overt response and may delineate sensory, as well as motor, neural involvement.[61,91]

## Esophageal Stage and Lower Gastrointestinal System Symptomatology (Briefly)

The final, esophageal stage of swallowing involves the transportation of the foods through the esophagus and into the stomach. Gastroesophageal reflux disease (GERD), reported in approximately 50% of children,[92] is probably the most common esophageal disturbance in CP. Esophageal dysmotility is also frequently reported and may result in esophageal backflow and severe discomfort during and after eating.[93] Conditions of the lower gastrointestinal (GI) system may also negatively impact the motivation and ability of a child with CP to eat adequately by mouth.

Among the many lower GI conditions associated with CP, the most frequent include constipation and dumping syndrome. Constipation in CP relates to musculoskeletal abnormalities, abnormal neurological control of the lower GI system, and prolonged immobility,[94] and is most common in children with severe CP. Dumping syndrome is a constellation of symptoms describing the rapid movement of the food or liquid into the small intestine.[95]

**Table 17.3** Common swallowing symptomatology in children with cerebral palsy

| Feeding/swallowing stage | Common difficulties |
|---|---|
| Preoral stage | • Poor positioning<br>• Poor head control (often hyperextension)<br>• Inability to self-feed or difficulty with self-feeding<br>• Drooling/sialorrhea and decreased frequency of saliva swallows |
| Oral stage | • Tongue thrust<br>• Reduced bolus control and anterior loss of food<br>• Poor labial seal<br>• Oral hypersensitivity<br>• Hypersensitive gag reflex<br>• Drooling/sialorrhea<br>• Tonic bite reflex<br>• Immature biting and chewing |
| Pharyngeal stage | • Delayed pharyngeal response<br>• Pharyngeal dysmotility/incoordination<br>• Residue/multiple swallows<br>• Chronic aspiration (frequently silent)<br>• Reduced upper esophageal sphincter opening |
| Esophageal stage and lower gastrointestinal symptoms | • Gastroesophageal reflux disease<br>• Esophageal dysmotility<br>• Dumping syndrome<br>• Constipation<br>• And more |

This syndrome may lead to discomfort, nausea, retching, diarrhea, and lethargy and may also impact a child's ability to eat adequately.

# 17.6 Assessment of Feeding and Swallowing in Cerebral Palsy

## 17.6.1 Interdisciplinary Approach

Given the highly complex symptomatology and pathophysiology of dysphagia in CP and its potentially devastating consequences, a thorough and holistic assessment of a child's feeding and swallowing function is of utmost importance. In addition to the specific feeding/swallowing deficits that need to be noted and quantified, we must also consider the individual's gross motor development, positioning, neurological development, communication abilities, other medical diagnoses and complications, and medication use, because all of these areas have an impact on feeding, swallowing, and nutritional outcomes.[11,66,74] A comprehensive multidisciplinary assessment is needed to address all of the areas listed. Depending on the institution the team members involved may vary, but likely collaborators would include neurologists, pulmonologists, developmental pediatricians, gastroenterologists, psychologists, orthopedic surgeons, otorhinolaryngologists, dieticians, physical therapists, occupational therapists, speech-language pathologists, and, most importantly, the *individual with CP* and the *family*. The patient and the family are vital team members whose importance on the team cannot be overlooked; they can provide important insights into the day-to-day feeding and swallowing challenges of the individual with CP as well as the at-home feasibility of various adaptations or proposed treatment approaches (feeding strategies, positioning, etc.).

## 17.6.2 Assessment Aims

Strudwick describes a rather inclusive list of aims for the assessment of feeding and swallowing in children with neurodevelopmental disorders.[96] Of those aims, we consider two as primary and the remaining ones secondary. The *primary aims* of the assessment are to evaluate swallow safety and adequacy of nutritional intake and to identify potential risk factors for respiratory compromise and reduced growth. Secondary, though not less important, aims include increasing the individual's eating and drinking potential; reducing anxiety and stress around the eating process; helping the individual and family make informed decisions on feeding options when oral feeding is not adequate; developing management and rehabilitation/habilitation plans; and educating the family or caregivers about feeding and swallowing and the difficulties that are specific to their family member with CP.[96] Through these primary and secondary aims, the outline of a comprehensive evaluation can be seen—a swallowing evaluation of the "whole patient." It is important to note that a feeding and swallowing evaluation cannot be complete without a comprehensive nutritional assessment. The combination of these assessments will adequately capture all aspects of health, growth, and development of a child with CP. This chapter focuses on strategies relating specifically to evaluating feeding and swallowing function; however, the importance of the nutritional assessment (conducted by a dietitian) should not be overlooked.

## 17.6.3 Feeding and Swallowing Assessment Types

Dysphagia diagnosis in CP requires a combination of clinical and instrumental assessments to fully evaluate the feeding and swallowing processes and determine the areas of dysfunction and treatment targets.

### Clinical Assessment of Dysphagia

In the clinical assessment of dysphagia the clinician makes an initial determination of the dysphagia diagnosis and the potential causes and decides whether or not further instrumental evaluations or referrals are necessary to fully describe the parameters of the swallowing and feeding disorder.[66] As such, the clinical assessment typically includes the case history, the oropharyngeal sensorimotor evaluation of swallowing, and a clinical functional eating assessment (i.e., a clinical observation during swallowing of saliva, foods, and liquids).

### Case History

For children with CP a case history should include detailed questions pertaining to family, medical (especially neurologic), nutritional, and developmental history as well as feeding/swallowing and communication milestones.[74] Questions about gross motor skills and seating/positioning (or referrals to physical and occupational therapists for assessing these skills)[96] are also essential in order to inform decisions that may impact how the clinical swallowing evaluation will be performed, as well as for future treatment planning.

### Oropharyngeal Sensorimotor Evaluation of Swallowing

The oropharyngeal sensorimotor evaluation of swallowing is, in essence, a detailed cranial nerve examination and includes examination of oral, pharyngeal, facial, and thoracic anatomy; examination of motor and sensory innervation (cranial nerves) of the oropharynx; and examination of oral and pharyngeal reflexes.[66] There are six pairs of cranial nerves that are involved in feeding and swallowing.[69] This examination elicits responses (spontaneously, via verbal command, or upon imitation) from these nerves to gain insight into the integrity of the peripheral nervous system and the amount of involvement by the central nervous system. During this assessment, the clinician also assesses the adequacy of body postural control and alignment, breath support, and swallow–breathing coordination.[66] A comprehensive oropharyngeal sensorimotor evaluation in individuals with CP should also include an examination of infant reflexes.[74,96] The presence of primitive reflexes beyond the expected time of disappearance can provide valuable insight into the presence of a neurodevelopmental delay or disorder.

### Clinical Functional Eating Assessment

The clinical functional eating assessment consists of trial swallows of various foods and liquids and is typically completed after the oropharyngeal sensorimotor evaluation so that the clinician can make note of what skills were observed or not observed and then assess how they carry over to actual feeding and swallowing function. The difficulty with clinical functional assessments is that there is no standardization between clinicians or institutions, either in the protocol for feeding trials or in the interpretation of the data. To address this discrepancy, a number of groups have sought to standardize pediatric clinical feeding/swallowing assessments. These assessments can reduce clinician bias and thus can be valuable in standardizing a rather subjective clinical procedure.[66] That said, they are not free of psychometric limitations.[79,97]

A critical review published by Benfer and colleagues on standardized assessments of feeding and swallowing for children with CP identified three standardized clinical functional feeding/swallowing assessments as having the highest clinical utility and relatively good psychometric properties[97]: the Dysphagia Disorder Survey (DDS),[79] the Schedule for Oral Motor Assessment (SOMA),[98] and the Pre-Speech Assessment Scale (PSAS).[99] Major features of each assessment and a qualitative summary of their psychometric properties are presented in **Table 17.4**.

**Table 17.4** Summary of three standardized clinical feeding and swallowing assessments for children with cerebral palsy

| Assessment tool | Target population | Purpose: evaluative[a] or discriminative[b] | Reliability | Sensitivity/ specificity | Validity | Training required? |
|---|---|---|---|---|---|---|
| Dysphagia Disorders Survey (DDS)[79] | Children and adults with developmental disabilities | Evaluative[97] | Intrarater: good Interrater: moderate to good[63,79,100] | Sensitivity: high Specificity: low to moderate[63,79,97] | Strong content convergent, and discriminative validity[79,97] | Yes, training and certification required |
| Schedule for Oral Motor Assessment (SOMA)[98] | NOFT and CP 10–42 months[97] | Discriminative[97] | Intrarater: high Interrater: high[97] | Sensitivity: low to moderate Specificity: high[63,97] | Strong content, limited convergent, limited discriminative[97] | Yes, training and certification required |
| Pre-Speech Assessment Scale (PSAS)[99] | CP and neurologic impairments 3–13 years[97] | Evaluative[97] | Intrarater: moderate Interrater: moderate[63,97] | Sensitivity: high Specificity: moderate[63,97] | Moderate content, no studies for convergent or discriminative[97] | No, self-study only |

*Abbreviations:* CP, cerebral palsy; NOFT, nonorganic failure to thrive.

[a]*Evaluative assessment:* designed to identify deviations in specific oral-sensorimotor skills.

[b]*Discriminative assessment:* designed to differentiate infants/children with oropharyngeal dysphagia from those with typical oral-sensorimotor skills.

## Instrumental Assessments

Clinical assessments provide useful information regarding feeding and swallowing behaviors, but they are limited to what can be observed clinically and thus cannot provide adequate information regarding the pharyngeal and esophageal stages of deglutition.[66] When the oropharyngeal dysphagia has not been fully characterized by the clinical assessment, and treatment decisions cannot be reached, instrumental evaluation procedures are essential.

According to Arvedson,[74] four criteria can be used to determine the need for instrumental assessments for a child with CP: (1) risk of aspiration (as assessed via the case history or during the clinical assessment), (2) prior history of aspiration pneumonia, (3) suspicion of a pharyngeal or laryngeal problem, and (4) a wet/gurgling voice quality. To these criteria we would add the following: significant concern for failure to thrive (weight gain and growth), history of recurrent respiratory infections, other clinical signs of aspiration (e.g., frequent throat clearing, coughing, or gagging), and the child's ability to tolerate the procedure so that the appropriate information can be obtained.

Several instrumental assessments are available; however, the two most widely accepted instrumental evaluation procedures in pediatric dysphagia are videofluoroscopy (videfluoroscopic swallowing study [VFSS]) and fiberoptic endoscopy (fiberoptic endoscopic evaluation of swallowing [FEES]). VFSS is a dynamic real-time radiologic assessment that is considered the gold standard for evaluating swallowing biomechanics and airway safety.[66] It is frequently used in the assessment of children with CP. The main advantage of this procedure is that all stages of the swallow can be viewed and evaluated in terms of timing, biomechanics, and bolus flow and clearance, delineating the occurrence of pathological findings (e.g., aspiration and penetration), as well as the possible physiological reasons for these findings.[101] The main limitations of VFSS include radiation exposure, short duration of the examination, use of barium, and the non-child-friendly examination environment.[66] FEES is conducted using a flexible nasopharyngoscope inserted through the nose and into the oropharynx to allow viewing of pharyngeal and laryngeal anatomy, and selective pharyngeal swallowing events.[102] FEES has several advantages over VFSS: it is radiation-free, it can be completed for longer periods of time, and it uses real food (not barium).[102] However, it is minimally invasive and thus may be challenging for patients with severe motor disorders and dyskinesias (as is the case for some children with CP). In addition, during the pharyngeal stage of swallowing a complete whiteout occurs that obstructs the view of the oropharyngeal areas, thus limiting the information provided. The oral and esophageal stages are also not visible when using FEES. Overall, both instrumental tools can be valuable to a clinician evaluating the swallowing function of a child with CP. The decision for which may be preferred will depend on the child's current eating/feeding status, respiratory health, movement disorder profile and symptomatology, and the clinical questions that have arisen from the preceding clinical noninstrumental assessment.

It is worth noting that a few less invasive instrumental procedures have also been used for the evaluation of swallowing in children with dysphagia; however, evidence for their use and their clinical utility has been limited. These include the use of surface electromyography, ultrasonography, and cervical auscultation. Surface electromyography provides information on the electrical activity of groups of muscles during a task and thus can provide input on the peripheral neurophysiology of chewing and swallowing; however, its use in CP has been limited to research endeavors.[103,104] Similarly, ultrasonography has mostly been used in the evaluation of fetal and infant sucking[105,106] and in providing feedback for oral and articulatory events.[107] Cervical auscultation uses a stethoscope that is placed laterally by the thyroid notch and allows the clinician to listen to the sounds of swallowing and breathing before, during, and after the swallow.[96] Despite the ease of use and the economic nature of this tool, its use in evaluating pharyngeal aspects of swallowing physiology has been questioned.[108] A recent randomized controlled trial examined the use of cervical auscultation as an adjunctive tool to the clinical swallowing assessment in improving the reliability of predicting aspiration in children.[109] Results revealed that the use of cervical auscultation as an adjunct to the clinical assessment improved the sensitivity of predicting aspiration by ~ 20% compared to conducting only a clinical assessment, but that cervical auscultation alone was not sensitive enough to predict aspiration.[109]

## Parent Report Measures

Recently it has been increasingly recognized that patient and parent report measures can provide insightful information on a patient's nutritional and feeding capabilities and function. Although parents may not have the same technical expertise as clinicians, they are experts on their own children, and their input is vital to a comprehensive assessment. A few parent report measures have emerged. Although no such measures are specifically designed for children with CP, a number of them can be used with this population (**Table 17.5**).

**Table 17.5** Parent-report measures on feeding/swallowing

| Parent-report assessment | Target population | Aim of the assessment |
|---|---|---|
| Pediatric Assessment Scale for Severe Feeding Problems (PASSFP)[110] | Tube-fed children with various underlying medical conditions | Assesses development of oral feeding skills in tube-fed children |
| Feeding/Swallowing Impact Survey (FS-IS)[111] | Children with medically based feeding/swallowing disorders | Measures the impact of feeding/swallowing issues on caregivers |
| Drooling Impact Scale (DIS)[112] | Children with developmental disabilities | Measures outcome of saliva-control interventions based on impact of drooling on child, parents/caregivers |

## Case Presentation Part 2: Swallowing Assessment

As reported earlier, GL is a 2-year, 7-month-old boy diagnosed with severe mixed spastic/athetoid cerebral palsy (GMFCS V), who is unable to independently walk and sit and presents with reduced head and trunk control and athetoid limb movements. Although his speech-language development is severely delayed, he is able to understand simple commands. Regarding feeding and swallowing, he is currently on thin liquids (using a sippy cup) and semisolids (mashed pureed foods), and is not an independent feeder. Solids have not been introduced. He has no history of respiratory infections, but his parents report frequent coughing and gagging during feeding. He is at the 20th percentile for weight and height for children of his age with CP.

The logical next step is to consider how we would assess his feeding and swallowing skills. Consider the questions posed at the end of the chapter to apply the knowledge gained from this section.

## 17.7 Management of Feeding and Swallowing in Cerebral Palsy

The prevailing wisdom for years had been that the feeding and swallowing disorders commonly associated with CP are chronic and relatively unresponsive to therapeutic intervention. As such, feeding and swallowing have not been given much attention in this population, with roughly two-thirds of parents reporting that their child has never had a swallowing or dietary assessment.[113] Thankfully, times are changing; neuroscience and developmental research are advancing, and we are beginning to discover that what we once thought to be chronically damaged and unchanging brains are perhaps more active and adaptive than we ever imagined.[73,100,114,115]

With that in mind, the main feeding/swallowing management goal for the child with CP is to optimize the health and quality of life of the child and the family. Health and safety are once more prioritized with primary aims to minimize or eliminate aspiration,

choking, and respiratory infections and to optimize nutrition and hydration. Secondarily, clinicians should also aim to advance the eating and drinking skills of the child by improving swallowing skills and taking advantage of developmental neuroplasticity to maximize motor learning.[66] It is important to emphasize once more that, as in dysphagia evaluation, these management goals require a team approach to be comprehensively addressed. To achieve these aims, a combination of compensatory and habilitative/rehabilitative strategies can be considered that have varying degrees of research evidence supporting them.

### 17.7.1 Compensatory Strategies

Compensatory strategies are interventions that compensate for a swallowing symptom, do not address the underlying physiology, and have only temporary effects.[116] In addition, compensatory interventions may be also used in children and adults during practice of new or challenging eating tasks in order to improve eating skills.[66,117] The most common compensatory strategies that have been used for children with CP and dysphagia include seating and positioning recommendations, dietary modifications, environmental and feeding adaptations, adaptive oral and feeding equipment, and tube feeding. These strategies and the evidence available are discussed next.

### Seating and Positioning

Appropriate seating and positioning are essential in the development of eating for all children and even more so for children with CP.[118,119] Several positioning strategies, such as stabilization of the head, neck, and trunk, and neck flexion have been proposed to improve eating skills in these children.[78] Evidence in this area is scarce and stems mostly from small-scale cohort studies or case series designs. Specifically, in a study of five children with quadriplegic CP, a 30-degree reclined position with supported neck flexion was found to reduce the incidence of aspiration in all five subjects.[118] Also, a study of 14 children with CP who underwent videofluoroscopy showed that a semireclined position was more beneficial for children with oral-stage difficulties, whereas an upright (erect position) was more helpful for children with disorders of the pharyngeal stage.[120] Finally, another small-scale study included 15 children with CP and feeding difficulties who were fitted with a special thoracic–lumbar–sacral orthosis with a flexible frame for a period of months to years. The parents of these children were asked to complete a questionnaire regarding several feeding/swallowing behaviors at baseline and at the end of the application of this orthotic device (variable for each subject). According to the parents' reports 14/15 children showed some improvements in eating skills, 13 children improved in their ability to accept different textures, and 11 children improved in speed of eating.[121] Despite the positive results reported by this study, several methodological limitations, including the use of a parent-report measure instead of direct evaluation measures, limit the conclusions we can make regarding the use of this specific device on feeding outcomes.

The aforementioned studies, albeit representing a lower level of research evidence, highlight that postural adaptations may have an impact on feeding and swallowing behavior for children with CP. It is of note that a functional sitting position has been found to reduce abnormal movements and increase hand and arm coordination in children with CP[122,123] and has been recommended during feeding as well. This position includes seating in a forward-tipped seat, having a backrest that allows good support of the pelvis and the upper and lower body, forearm support on an anterior surface, and feet stability on supporting surfaces.[122]

## Dietary Modifications

Modifications of food and liquid viscosities (e.g., thickening liquids or pureeing solids), tastes, temperature, and texture are also used in pediatric dysphagia as compensatory strategies for functional deficiencies and as interventions for improving sensorimotor tolerances and developmental skills.[66] In children these modifications are typically completed using food additives (more often) or commercial thickeners.[124]

Evidence for the impact of dietary modifications on the swallowing safety and swallowing behaviors of children with CP is also limited. Specifically, in a study of 67 children with CP and 64 healthy controls, where investigators observed (via video recordings) the behaviors of these children while they ate a mashed (pureed) and a soft, boiled potato (mechanical soft), the children with CP and severe dysphagia exhibited significantly longer eating durations and more signs of aspiration (e.g., coughing) when consuming the soft, boiled potato compared to the mashed food,[124] suggesting that mashed foods may be safer for these individuals. In another study the respiratory–swallow patterns of eight young individuals with quadriplegia and 13 healthy controls were examined via pneumotachographic and acoustic methods while they consumed different viscosities of liquids and pudding.[125] The results showed that the CP group more often exhibited an unsafe postswallow breathing pattern (i.e., inspiration) after a thin liquid swallow compared to the control group,[125] but this was not evident with consumption of thicker liquids or pudding. The authors suggested that thicker liquids might elicit safer respiratory–swallow coordination in individuals with CP[125]; however, they emphasize that their findings are rather preliminary.

As can be seen when reviewing these two studies, the limited sample size and significant limitations in the instrumental procedures used to evaluate swallowing behaviors also limit the

scientific or clinical conclusions that can be made, emphasing the need for additional and more rigorous research in this area. Nevertheless, dietary modifications are a frequent compensatory strategy used for individuals with CP, and with the lack of high levels of research evidence, clinicians are cautioned to critically use their clinical judgment and to consider a variety of factors before determining the need for such interventions. Specifically, we encourage clinicians to consider such alterations in the context of a multidisciplinary team (in close collaboration with the dietician and the physician) and after carefully examining factors such as preoral and oral preparation tolerances, oropharyngeal skills, and competencies of the children, including their ability to protect their airway during swallowing, esophageal motility issues, as well as demands for nutrition and hydration.

## Environmental and Feeding Adaptations

Several environmental and feeding adaptations have been clinically reported to be useful in facilitating functional eating and swallowing in children and adults with neurogenic dysphagia. Common environmental adaptations include monitoring and assisting the feeding process, encouraging/allowing independence, moderating acoustic and visual complexity of the environment (e.g., turning off the TV), maintaining familiarity, establishing optimum eating time, and moderating stressful environments.[126] Common feeding adaptations include altering bite/sip size, rate of presentations, encouraging the use of multiple swallows, and alternating solids with liquids. To our knowledge no systematic research has been conducted as yet on the effects of these adaptations in the feeding and swallowing performance of children with CP.

## Adaptive Oral and Feeding Equipment

The use of oral appliances and specialized feeding equipment has also been examined in children with CP. Perhaps the best known oral appliance that has been used for children with CP is the Innsbruck Sensorimotor Activator and Regulator (ISMAR).[127] The ISMAR appliance is an intraoral device that promotes sensorimotor stimulation and practice. Two clinical trials have been conducted using ISMAR; one compared the use of the device for 6 versus 12 months in 20 children with CP,[128] and the other compared the use of ISMAR for 12 months versus the use of standard rehabilitation therapy for 6 months followed by 6 months of ISMAR use also in 20 children with CP.[129] Both studies reported that use of the device (especially for 12 months) resulted in improvements in oral-motor skills, jaw stabilization, and oral-motor control that, according to the authors, further improved generalized postural control during sitting.[129] A few case series have also reported positive oral-motor outcomes post-ISMAR use in CP.[127,130] However, an older observational cohort study of 71 children with CP using a similar oral appliance did not support significant improvements in oral-motor functions.[131]

In addition to oral appliances, specialized feeding devices and equipment to support swallowing may include specialized spoons, cups, and straws, as well as electric feeders that may be used to enhance oral acceptance of the food and to regulate/standardize bolus size and rate of presentation. The research on the effects of such devices and equipment on feeding and swallowing in CP is similarly limited. A small-scale cohort study on the use of electric feeders versus feeding by a caregiver for children with severe CP and dysphagia has shown the use of electric feeders to be beneficial for maintenance of weight but result in reductions in eating efficiency.[132]

## Tube Feeding

Arvedson states that "total oral feeding is not a realistic goal for all children with CP but the aim should be to introduce some feeding that is physiologically possible and fits in with the social situation of the child and their family."[74] In cases where total oral feeding is not an option (i.e., in children with CP who have profound dysphagia), tube feeding in the form of gastrostomy or jejunostomy tubes is an alternative.[6,133] Most of the evidence on the effects of tube feeding also stems from observational cohort studies with several methodological limitations. From such studies we know that weight gain is a frequent positive outcome of tube feedings in malnourished children with severe CP.[133,134] Similarly, reduction in chest infections for children with CP who were fed via tube versus oral feeding has also been reported.[11,135] Outcomes on quality of life and health-related outcomes, however, for both children and their families, have been mixed.[11,136,137,138] As with many of the prior interventions discussed, no randomized controlled trials have been conducted to date on the impact of tube feeding versus oral feeding for children with CP,[139] and the limited evidence available showcases potentially positive effects on some outcomes but is inconclusive on others. Given the medical complexities and health care and personal costs associated with tube feeding, the need for a well-designed, large-scale, randomized controlled trial on this topic is urgent.

In cases where tube feeding is the treatment of choice, there are some special considerations that need to be made for dysphagia treatment. Specifically, the determination of tube feedings and the process of transitioning from tube to oral feedings will be a determination made by the team, including the dietitian, speech-language practitioner, and developmental pediatrician.[140] In addition, things to consider include tube feeding schedule and type, inclusion of the child in family and classroom meals, and the possibility of providing at least therapeutic tastes and pleasure feedings if full oral feeding is not safe.[140,141]

## 17.7.2 Habilitative Management of Dysphagia in Cerebral Palsy

Habilitative strategies include interventions that aim at improving or helping the child to acquire the underlying neuromuscular and neurophysiological elements and skills needed to functionally swallow. Similar to the compensatory strategies, the evidence for the use of habilitative interventions for this population is limited. Hereafter we discuss the main habilitative interventions that have been used for the treatment of feeding and swallowing disorders in children with CP and the evidence behind them.

## Oral Sensorimotor Treatments

Oral sensorimotor treatments include a wide variety of sensory stimulation and oral motor strategies used to either inhibit or excite neuromuscular functions. According to Clark[142] these treatments can be typically divided into active exercises, passive exercises, and sensory application techniques. Active exercises include exercises targeting strength, stretching, and range of motion of muscles; passive exercises include massage, vibration, stimulation, brushing, stroking, and tapping or passive range of motion; finally, sensory application techniques include the use of heat, cold, electrical stimulation, or other agents to muscle tissue.[142] These techniques are widely used in the dysphagia management of children with CP. A relatively recent systematic review on the role of these treatments in pediatric dysphagia management presented a careful critical review of 16 studies using a variety of oral sensorimotor treatments to treat dysphagia in children (with CP and other diagnoses).[143] This comprehensive review revealed that most of these studies have several methodological challenges, small or (at best) moderate effect sizes (many are case series or case studies), and often conflicting results. The authors conclude that at this time there is insufficient evidence to support the effects of these oral sensorimotor interventions on the management of pediatric dysphagia and that more research is needed.[143]

## Neuromuscular Electrical Stimulation

In the past 10 to 15 years the use of neuromuscular electrical stimulation (NMES) as a treatment modality for dysphagia has become rather popular. NMES of the submental and/or suprahyoid muscles includes low-current stimulation of nerves through surface electrodes, which leads to sensory responses or muscle contractions in the neck area. Research on the effects of NMES on swallowing and feeding performance of children has been limited. In a retrospective analysis of VFSS studies of 93 children with dysphagia (of varying etiologies) of whom half underwent an NMES treatment protocol and half underwent traditional oral sensorimotor treatment and dietary modifications, results revealed that both groups benefited equally from their respective treatments.[144] Despite these limited and largely neutral findings, NMES remains a popular modality that several clinicians use with children and adults. Current research is conducted to help us better understand the optimal situations, diagnoses, and patient groups that this modality may be beneficial for and to obtain more information on the habilitative potential of this modality for CP may emerge in the near future.

## Motor Learning Strategies and Neuroplasticity Principles

In recent years, skill training using motor learning strategies[145] and principles of experience-dependent brain plasticity[146] has been introduced in dysphagia practice and research.[117,147,148,149,150] Indeed, in children with CP, skill training may be a better treatment target because strength may be adequate (or even increased, such as in hypertonia), but skill, coordination, and accuracy are often reduced or abnormal. Sheppard has reported that skill acquisition for oropharyngeal swallowing is more effective when principles of motor learning (e.g., systematic motor learning using blocked vs. random practice, internal and external feedback, specificity of learning, maximizing opportunities for practice, etc.) are consistently applied.[149,151] It has also been theorized that the application of principles of experience-dependent brain plasticity (e.g., the "use it or lose it" principle; the principle of specificity, intensity, and repetition matters; the principle of salience, etc.)[146] in rehabilitation may improve neurogenic patients' rehabilitation potential. The combination of applying motor learning strategies and neuroplasticity principles (some are essentially underlying each other) can maximize the effects of practice for acquiring or improving specific motor skills and competencies and encourage the maintenance of performance.[146,149,152]

In swallowing, a recent effort to systematically apply an intensive and systematic motor learning approach while using neuroplasticity principles was shown to significantly improve functional swallowing outcomes in a case series study of adult patients with neurogenic dysphagia.[117] Other protocols using a motor learning hierarchy for adult dysphagia have also started to emerge.[148,150] Although specific protocols using this approach for dysphagia management in CP have not yet been developed, the clinical use of such an approach has the ability to influence motor learning outcomes and swallowing skills. However, in children with CP specifically, caution should be exercised when training advancement of eating skills, as the risks for nutritional, growth, and respiratory compromise may be high.[74]

## Case Presentation Part 3: Management

GL underwent a comprehensive swallowing assessment, including an oropharyngeal sensorimotor evaluation and a VFSS study. Feeding was conducted with the mother feeding the child on her lap (as done at home) with a slight extension of the head posteriorly. Utensils used during all feeding attempts included the utensils used at home (sippy cup, a nuk spoon), and an open cup. The assessment included thin liquids, nectar-thick liquids, and semisolid (pudding) consistencies. Results of the clinical assessment revealed, in short: reduced head and trunk postural control requiring maximum help from mother, generalized hypotonic orofacial muscles, open mouth at rest, no primitive reflexes present (other than gag), and reduced range of motion of tongue. In addition, videofluoroscopically we observed reduced labial seal and reduced oral control resulting in frequent anterior loss of food (all consistencies), tongue thrust, no masticatory skills, emerging cup drinking skills with an open cup, mildly delayed pharyngeal swallow with thin liquids, mild vallecular residue with thicker liquids and semisolids, adequate hyolaryngeal complex displacement, and no penetration or aspiration at any time during the study.

Given this information and what you know about GL from the aforementioned descriptions, consider the questions posed at the end of the chapter to apply the knowledge gained from this section.

## 17.8 Conclusion

Feeding and swallowing disorders are very common in children with CP and may manifest as sensorimotor difficulties in any of the stages of deglutition. Optimal evaluation and treatment of feeding and swallowing disorders necessitate the coordinated efforts of a multidisciplinary team to maximize these children's potential for adequate growth and development. Interventions for oropharyngeal dysphagia include several compensatory and habilitative strategies that, unfortunately, at this time have limited research evidence. Although more research is urgently needed, compensatory strategies should be used as stepping-stones on the road to achieving oropharyngeal swallowing skills acquisition and improvement. Although CP was once thought to be a static condition with reduced habilitation potential, we now know that the brain of children with CP is a lot more plastic than previously thought, and we owe it to these children to explore new methods for dysphagia habilitation and give them the chance for improved quality of life. To further increase therapeutic and learning outcomes, applying treatment strategies using an approach driven by motor learning and neuroplasticity appears to be a promising clinical and research endeavor and warrants future investigation in this population.

## 17.9 Questions

1. Based on the information provided in the chapter text, and given you had the expertise and training to conduct a standardized functional clinical assessment of swallowing in order to *describe/define oral-sensorimotor functions in this child*, which one of the following assessments would be the most appropriate?

   A. Schedule for Oral Motor Assessment (SOMA)
   B. Dysphagia Disorders Survey (DDS)
   C. Pre-Speech Assessment Scale (PSAS)
   D. None of the above; there are no standardized assessments for the functional clinical assessment of swallowing for children with CP.

2. Based on the information provided in the chapter text, would you proceed to complete an instrumental assessment for this child? Choose the best response.

   A. Yes, I would proceed to complete a FEES.
   B. No, since the child has no history of pneumonia, I would base my recommendations on the clinical evaluation alone.
   C. Yes, I would proceed to complete a VFSS.
   D. Yes, I would proceed with ultrasound to minimize radiation exposure and to increase safety given the patient's potential for unpredictable movements.

3. Of the following *compensatory* strategies, which one may be most appropriate (and evidence based) to address GL's oropharyngeal challenges?

   A. Thickening liquids
   B. Improving positioning using the Myhr and von Wendt (1991) positioning suggestions during feeding

C.   Tube feeding as an alternative to oral feeding (given his low percentile)

D.   Use of a sippy cup (only) for drinking

4.   If you decided to enroll GL in a habilitative swallowing program using a motor learning approach, which *one* of the following functional swallowing skills would you choose to improve or help him acquire *first* based on his current skills level? Choose the best response.

A.   Cup drinking skills

B.   Chewing

C.   Labial closure

D.   Reducing tongue protrusion/tongue thrust

# 17.10 Answers and Explanations

### 1. Correct: Dysphagia Disorders Survey (DDS) (B).

The DDS is an evaluative assessment designed to identify specific deviations in oral-sensorimotor function. (**A**) is incorrect because the SOMA is a discriminative assessment tool, meaning it is designed to identify children with dysphagia versus those without it and is not aimed at describing specific deviations. (**C**) is incorrect because the PSAS is designed for use with children aged 3–13 years; GL is less than 3 years old. (**D**) is incorrect because some (few) standardized functional clinical assessments of swallowing for children with CP exist.

### 2. Correct: yes, I would proceed to complete a VFSS (C).

The child is presenting with clinical signs of pharyngeal dysphagia and aspiration (gagging, frequent coughing) and is at a low percentile for weight/height for children of his age with CP; thus he warrants a comprehensive instrumental swallowing assessment. VFSS will provide information on biomechanical and physiological aspects of all swallowing stages and will help guide the treatment decisions in a comprehensive manner. (**A**) is incorrect because this child presents with reduced head and trunk control and athetoid limb movements; thus the use of FEES could increase the risk of harm from unpredictable movements. (**B**) is incorrect because not having a diagnosis of pneumonia does not mean that the child does not have dysphagia, which if present may increase the likelihood of respiratory infections in the future. The child is noted to cough and gag during meals and is at a low percentile for weight/height for children of his age with CP; thus an instrumental assessment is warranted. (**D**) is incorrect because ultrasound is not yet a reliable or comprehensive means with which to evaluate oropharyngeal dysphagia.

### 3. Correct: improving positioning using the Myhr and von Wendt (1991) positioning suggestions during feeding (B).

The child is presenting with trunk and head stability difficulties that may be contributing to his difficulty feeding and swallowing. Improving positioning will stabilize the child's body and likely improve his feeding behaviors. (**A**) is incorrect because this child did not present with penetration or aspiration of thin liquids. He presented with mild pharyngeal delay, but despite the poor positioning during the study he did not penetrate or aspirate. Thus there is no videofluoroscopic evidence that we would need to modify his liquid intake. (**C**) is incorrect because this child has a relatively safe pharyngeal swallow and can safely consume liquids and semisolids by mouth. Although his weight/height percentile is relatively low, other strategies (e.g., improving positioning and adding supplements to the diet) and management options should be considered first before tube feeding is considered. (**D**) is incorrect because GL has emerging drinking skills from an open cup; thus use of an open cup needs to be at least introduced and reinforced, although the use of a sippy cup for regular hydration purposes may need to be continued until cup drinking skills fully develop.

### 4. Correct: cup drinking skills (A).

GL already presents with emerging skills in drinking from an open cup; thus improving these skills would be the logical next step. (**B**) is incorrect because he does not have any masticatory skills at this time; before chewing skills can be developed and practiced several precursory strategies may be needed (e.g., tongue lateralization, oral stimulation techniques, and oral clearance skills). (**C**) is incorrect because labial closure issues are likely as a result of his hypotonia; given this neurological feature training labial closure using a motor learning hierarchy could be challenging and would take more time. (**D**) is incorrect because tongue thrust is also a neurologic sign, which cannot be easily manipulated using a motor learning hierarchy outside of the context of eating food.

## References

[1]   Bax M, Goldstein M, Rosenbaum P, et al; Executive Committee for the Definition of Cerebral Palsy. Proposed definition and classification of cerebral palsy, April 2005. *Dev Med Child Neurol* 2005;47(8):571–576

[2]   Morris C. Definition and classification of cerebral palsy: a historical perspective. *Dev Med Child Neurol Suppl* 2007;109:3–7

[3]   Rosenbaum P, Paneth N, Leviton A, et al. A report: the definition and classification of cerebral palsy April 2006. *Dev Med Child Neurol Suppl* 2007;109:8–14

[4]   World Health Organization (WHO). International Classification of Functioning, Disability and Health: ICF. Geneva: World Health Organization; 2001

[5]   World Health Organization (WHO). International Classification of Functioning, Disability, and Health: Children & Youth Version: ICF-CY. Geneva: World Health Organization; 2007

[6]   Calis EA, Veugelers R, Sheppard JJ, Tibboel D, Evenhuis HM, Penning C. Dysphagia in children with severe generalized cerebral palsy and intellectual disability. *Dev Med Child Neurol* 2008;50(8):625–630 doi: 10.1111/j.1469-8749.2008.03047.x

[7]   Parkes J, Hill N, Platt MJ, Donnelly C. Oromotor dysfunction and communication impairments in children with cerebral palsy: a register study. *Dev Med Child Neurol* 2010;52(12):1113–1119 doi: 10.1111/j.1469-8749.2010.03765.x

[8]   Reilly S, Skuse D, Poblete X. Prevalence of feeding problems and oral motor dysfunction in children with cerebral palsy: a community survey. *J Pediatr* 1996;129(6):877–882 doi: 10.1016/S0022-3476(96)70032-X

[9]   Wilson EM, Hustad KC. Early feeding abilities in children with cerebral palsy: A parental report study. *J Med Speech-Lang Pathol* 2009;MARCH(608):a57357

[10] Lefton-Greif MA, McGrath-Morrow SA. Deglutition and respiration: development, coordination, and practical implications. *Semin Speech Lang* 2007;28(3):166–179 doi: 10.1055/s-2007-984723

[11] Fung EB, Samson-Fang L, Stallings VA, et al. Feeding dysfunction is associated with poor growth and health status in children with cerebral palsy. *J Am Diet Assoc* 2002;102(3):361–373

[12] Stevenson RD, Hayes RP, Cater LV, Blackman JA. Clinical correlates of linear growth in children with cerebral palsy. *Dev Med Child Neurol* 1994;36(2):135–142

[13] Arneson CL, Durkin MS, Benedict RE, et al. Prevalence of cerebral palsy: Autism and Developmental Disabilities Monitoring Network, three sites, United States, 2004. *Disabil Health J* 2009;2(1):45–48 doi: 10.1016/j.dhjo.2008.08.001

[14] Paneth N, Hong T, Korzeniewski S. The descriptive epidemiology of cerebral palsy. *Clin Perinatol* 2006;33(2):251–267 doi: 10.1016/j.clp.2006.03.011

[15] Winter S, Autry A, Boyle C, Yeargin-Allsopp M. Trends in the prevalence of cerebral palsy in a population-based study. *Pediatrics* 2002;110(6):1220–1225 doi: 10.1542/peds.110.6.1220

[16] Colver AF, Gibson M, Hey EN, Jarvis SN, Mackie PC, Richmond S; The North of England Collaborative Cerebral Palsy Survey. Increasing rates of cerebral palsy across the severity spectrum in north-east England 1964-1993. *Arch Dis Child Fetal Neonatal Ed* 2000;83(1):F7–F12 doi: 10.1136/fn.83.1.F7

[17] Liu JM, Li S, Lin Q, Li Z. Prevalence of cerebral palsy in China. *Int J Epidemiol* 1999;28(5):949–954 doi: 10.1093/ije/28.5.949

[18] Christensen D, Van Naarden Braun K, Doernberg NS, et al. Prevalence of cerebral palsy, co-occurring autism spectrum disorders, and motor functioning - Autism and Developmental Disabilities Monitoring Network, USA, 2008. *Dev Med Child Neurol* 2014;56(1):59–65 doi: 10.1111/dmcn.12268

[19] Odding E, Roebroeck ME, Stam HJ. The epidemiology of cerebral palsy: incidence, impairments and risk factors. *Disabil Rehabil* 2006;28(4):183–191 doi: 10.1080/09638280500158422

[20] Edebol-Tysk K. Epidemiology of spastic tetraplegic cerebral palsy in Sweden. I. Impairments and disabilities. *Neuropediatrics* 1989;20(1):41–45 doi: 0.1055/s-2008-1071263

[21] Hou M, Sun DR, Shan RB, et al. [Comorbidities in patients with cerebral palsy and their relationship with neurologic subtypes and Gross Motor Function Classification System levels]. *Zhonghua Er Ke Za Zhi* 2010;48(5):351–354

[22] Hustad KC, Allison K, McFadd E, Riehle K. Speech and language development in 2-year-old children with cerebral palsy. *Dev Neurorehabil* 2014;17(3):167–175 doi: 10.3109/17518423.2012.747009

[23] Shevell MI, Dagenais L, Hall N; REPACQ Consortium. Comorbidities in cerebral palsy and their relationship to neurologic subtype and GMFCS level. *Neurology* 2009;72(24):2090–2096 doi: 10.1212/WNL.0b013e3181aa537b

[24] Reid SM, Modak MB, Berkowitz RG, Reddihough DS. A population-based study and systematic review of hearing loss in children with cerebral palsy. *Dev Med Child Neurol* 2011;53(11):1038–1045 doi: 10.1111/j.1469-8749.2011.04069.x

[25] Sanger TD, Delgado MR, Gaebler-Spira D, Hallett M, Mink JW; Task Force on Childhood Motor Disorders. Classification and definition of disorders causing hypertonia in childhood. *Pediatrics* 2003;111(1):e89–e97

[26] Goldstein EM. Spasticity management: an overview. *J Child Neurol* 2001;16(1):16–23

[27] Fahn S. Concept and classification of dystonia. *Adv Neurol* 1988;50:1–8

[28] Sanger TD, Chen D, Fehlings DL, et al. Definition and classification of hyperkinetic movements in childhood. *Mov Disord* 2010;25(11):1538–1549 doi: 10.1002/mds.23088

[29] Campbell M, Dudek N, Trudel G. Joint contractures. In: Frontera WR, Silver JK, Rizzo Jr. TD, eds. Essentials of Physical Medicine and Rehabilitation. 3rd ed. Philadelphia, PA: Saunders; 2014

[30] Weiss H-R, Negrini S, Manuel R, et al. Indications for conservative management of scoliosis (SOSORT guidelines). In: Grivas TB, ed. The Conservative Scoliosis Treatment. Amsterdam, Netherlands: IOS Press; 2008:164–172

[31] Marret S, Vanhulle C, Laquerriere A. Pathophysiology of cerebral palsy. *Handb Clin Neurol* 2013;111:169–176

[32] Bax M, Tydeman C, Flodmark O. Clinical and MRI correlates of cerebral palsy: the European Cerebral Palsy Study. *JAMA* 2006;296(13):1602–1608

[33] CDC. gov. Data & statistics for cerebral palsy. Updated May 2, 2016. Accessed June 10, 2016. http://www.cdc.gov/ncbddd/cp/data.html

[34] Livinec F, Ancel P-Y, Marret S, et al; Epipage Group. Prenatal risk factors for cerebral palsy in very preterm singletons and twins. *Obstet Gynecol* 2005;105(6):1341–1347

[35] Davies MJ, Moore VM, Willson KJ, et al. Reproductive technologies and the risk of birth defects. *N Engl J Med* 2012;366(19):1803–1813

[36] Scher AI, Petterson B, Blair E, et al. The risk of mortality or cerebral palsy in twins: a collaborative population-based study. *Pediatr Res* 2002;52(5):671–681

[37] McMichael G, MacLennan A, Gibson C, et al. Cytomegalovirus and Epstein–Barr virus may be associated with some cases of cerebral palsy. 2012. http://dx.doi org/103109/147670582012666587

[38] O'Callaghan ME, MacLennan AH, Gibson CS, et al; Australian Collaborative Cerebral Palsy Research Group. Epidemiologic associations with cerebral palsy. *Obstet Gynecol* 2011;118(3):576–582

[39] Guerri C. Neuroanatomical and neurophysiological mechanisms involved in central nervous system dysfunctions induced by prenatal alcohol exposure. *Alcohol Clin Exp Res* 1998;22(2):304–312

[40] Garne E, Dolk H, Krägeloh-Mann I, Holst Ravn S, Cans C; SCPE Collaborative Group. Cerebral palsy and congenital malformations. *Eur J Paediatr Neurol* 2008;12(2):82–88

[41] MacLennan AH, Thompson SC, Gecz J. Cerebral palsy: causes, pathways, and the role of genetic variants. *Am J Obstet Gynecol* 2015;213(6):779–788 doi: 10.1016/j.ajog.2015.05.034

[42] Graham EM, Ruis KA, Hartman AL, Northington FJ, Fox HE. A systematic review of the role of intrapartum hypoxia-ischemia in the causation of neonatal encephalopathy. *Am J Obstet Gynecol* 2008;199(6):587–595 doi: 10.1016/j.ajog.2008.06.094

[43] Wu YW, Escobar GJ, Grether JK, Croen LA, Greene JD, Newman TB. Chorioamnionitis and cerebral palsy in term and near-term infants. *JAMA* 2003;290(20):2677–2684 doi: 10.1001/jama.290.20.2677

[44] Grether JK, Nelson KB. Maternal infection and cerebral palsy in infants of normal birth weight. *JAMA* 1997;278(3):207–211

[45] Blair E, Stanley FJ. Intrapartum asphyxia: a rare cause of cerebral palsy. *J Pediatr* 1988;112(4):515–519

[46] Glass HC, Bonifacio SL, Chau V, et al. Recurrent postnatal infections are associated with progressive white matter injury in premature infants. *Pediatrics* 2008;122(2):299–305 doi: 10.1542/peds.2007-2184

[47] Cans C; Surveillance of Cerebral Palsy in Europe. Surveillance of cerebral palsy in Europe: a collaboration of cerebral palsy surveys and registers. Surveillance of Cerebral Palsy in Europe (SCPE). *Dev Med Child Neurol* 2000;42(12):816–824 doi: 10.1111/j.1469-8749.2000.tb00695.x

[48] Mandigo CE, Anderson RCE. Management of childhood spasticity: a neurosurgical perspective. *Pediatr Ann* 2006;35(5):354–362

[49] Balf CL, Ingram TT. Problems in the classification of cerebral palsy in childhood. *BMJ* 1955;2(4932):163–166

[50] Christine C, Dolk H, Platt MJ, Colver A, Prasauskiene A, Krägeloh-Mann I; SCPE Collaborative Group. Recommendations from the SCPE collaborative group for defining and classifying cerebral palsy. *Dev Med Child Neurol Suppl* 2007;109:35–38

[51] Bax MCO, Flodmark O, Tydeman C. Definition and classification of cerebral palsy. From syndrome toward disease. *Dev Med Child Neurol Suppl* 2007;109:39–41

[52] De Souza LH. Multiple Sclerosis: Approaches to Management. London, UK: Chapman & Hall; 1990

[53] Gorter JW, Rosenbaum PL, Hanna SE, et al. Limb distribution, motor impairment, and functional classification of cerebral palsy. *Dev Med Child Neurol* 2004;46(7):461–467

[54] Palisano R, Rosenbaum P, Walter S, Russell D, Wood E, Galuppi B. Development and reliability of a system to classify gross motor function in children with cerebral palsy. *Dev Med Child Neurol* 1997;39(4):214–223

[55] Wood E, Rosenbaum P. The gross motor function classification system for cerebral palsy: a study of reliability and stability over time. *Dev Med Child Neurol* 2000;42(5):292–296

[56] Eliasson A-C, Krumlinde-Sundholm L, Rösblad B, et al. The Manual Ability Classification System (MACS) for children with cerebral palsy: scale development and evidence of validity and reliability. *Dev Med Child Neurol* 2006;48(7):549–554 doi: 10.1017/S0012162206001162

[57] Hidecker MJC, Paneth N, Rosenbaum PL, et al. Developing and validating the Communication Function Classification System for individuals with cerebral palsy. *Dev Med Child Neurol* 2011;53(8):704–710 doi: 10.1111/j.1469-8749.2011.03996.x

[58] Sellers D, Mandy A, Pennington L, Hankins M, Morris C. Development and reliability of a system to classify the eating and drinking ability of people with cerebral palsy. *Dev Med Child Neurol* 2014;56(3):245–251 doi: 10.1111/dmcn.12352

[59] Benfer KA, Weir KA, Bell KL, Ware RS, Davies PSW, Boyd RN. Oropharyngeal dysphagia and gross motor skills in children with cerebral palsy. *Pediatrics* 2013;131(5):e1553–e1562 doi: 10.1542/peds.2012-3093

[60] Kim J-S, Han Z-A, Song DH, Oh H-M, Chung ME. Characteristics of dysphagia in children with cerebral palsy, related to gross motor function. *Am J Phys Med Rehabil* 2013;92(10):912–919 doi: 10.1097/PHM.0b013e318296dd99

[61] Rogers B, Arvedson J, Buck G, Smart P, Msall M. Characteristics of dysphagia in children with cerebral palsy. *Dysphagia* 1994;9(1):69–73

[62] Benfer KA, Weir KA, Bell KL, Ware RS, Davies PSW, Boyd RN. Oropharyngeal dysphagia in preschool children with cerebral palsy: oral phase impairments. *Res Dev Disabil* 2014;35(12):3469–3481 doi: 10.1016/j.ridd.2014.08.029

[63] Benfer KA, Weir KA, Bell KL, Ware RS, Davies PSW, Boyd RN. Validity and repro-ducibility of measures of oropharyngeal dysphagia in preschool children with cerebral palsy. Dev Med Child Neurol 2015;57(4):358–365 doi: 10.1111 dmcn.12616

[64] Lopes PAC, Amancio OMS, Araújo RFC, Vitalle MS, Braga JA. Food pattern and nu-tritional status of children with cerebral palsy. Rev Paul Pediatr 2013;31(3):344–349

[65] Malandraki GA, Friel K, Mishra A, Kantarcigil C, Gordon A, Sheppard JJ. Swallow-ing disorders in pediatric hemiplegia: frequency, types and associations with neurological findings. Poster presented at: Annual Dysphagia Research Meeting. Chicago, IL

[66] Sheppard JJ, Malandraki GA. Pediatric dysphagia. In: Swallowing—Physiology, Disorders, Diagnosis and Therapy. New Delhi: Springer India; 2015:161–188

[67] Miller AJ. The search for the central swallowing pathway: the quest for clarity. Dysphagia 1993;8(3):185–194

[68] Martin RE, Sessle BJ. The role of the cerebral cortex in swallowing. Dysphagia 1993;8(3):195–202

[69] Malandraki GA, Johnson S, Robbins J. Functional MRI of swallowing: from neurophysiology to neuroplasticity. Head Neck 2011;33(Suppl 1):S14–S20 doi: 10.1002/hed.21903

[70] Kahrilas PJ, Dodds WJ, Dent J, Logemann JA, Shaker R. Upper esophageal sphinc-ter function during deglutition. Gastroenterology 1988;95(1):52–62

[71] Malandraki GA, Sutton BP, Perlman AL, Karampinos DC, Conway C. Neural activation of swallowing and swallowing-related tasks in healthy young adults: an attempt to separate the components of deglutition. Hum Brain Mapp 2009;30(10):3209–3226 doi: 10.1002/hbm.20743

[72] Malandraki GA, Cameron E, Friel K, Dyke JP, Sheppard JJ, Gordon A. Children with unilateral spastic cerebral palsy and dysphagia present with maladaptive morphometry in cortical areas associated with swallowing. Paper presented at Annual Dysphagia Research Society Meeting. Tucson, AZ

[73] Malandraki GA, Abbas K, Friel K, Dreyer N, Sheppard JJ, Gordon A. Functional neuroplastic adaptations of the swallowing network in children with unilateral spastic cerebral palsy and dysphagia: A resting-state fMRI study. Paper presented at: Annual Dysphagia Research Society Meeting. Tucson, AZ

[74] Arvedson JC. Feeding children with cerebral palsy and swallowing difficulties. Eur J Clin Nutr 2013;67(Suppl 2):S9–S12 doi: 10.1038/ejcn.2013.224

[75] Benfer KA, Weir KA, Bell KL, Ware RS, Davies PSW, Boyd RN. Clinical signs suggestive of pharyngeal dysphagia in preschool children with cerebral palsy. Res Dev Disabil 2015;38:192–201 doi: 10.1016/j.ridd.2014.12.021

[76] Delaney AL, Arvedson JC. Development of swallowing and feeding: prenatal through first year of life. Dev Disabil Res Rev 2008;14(2):105–117 doi: 10.1002 ddrr.16

[77] Matsuo K, Palmer JB. Coordination of Mastication, Swallowing and Breathing. Jpn Dent Sci Rev 2009;45(1):31–40 doi: 10.1016/j.jdsr.2009.03.004

[78] Redstone F, West JF. The importance of postural control for feeding. Pediatr Nurs 2004;30(2):97–100

[79] Sheppard JJ, Hochman R, Baer C. The dysphagia disorder survey: validation of an assessment for swallowing and feeding function in developmental disability. Res Dev Disabil 2014;35(5):929–942 doi: 10.1016/j.ridd.2014.02.017

[80] Tahmassebi JF, Curzon MEJ. The cause of drooling in children with cerebral palsy—hypersalivation or swallowing defect? Int J Paediatr Dent 2003;13(2):106–111

[81] Van De Heyning PH, Marquet JF, Creten WL. Drooling in children with cerebral palsy. Acta Otorhinolaryngol Belg 1980;34(6):691–705

[82] Reilly S, Skuse D. Characteristics and management of feeding problems of young children with cerebral palsy. Dev Med Child Neurol 1992;34(5):379–388

[83] Ortega AdeO, Ciamponi AL, Mendes FM, Santos MTBR. Assessment scale of the oral motor performance of children and adolescents with neurological damages. J Oral Rehabil 2009;36(9):653–659 doi: 10.1111/j.1365-2842.2009.01979.x

[84] Gisel EG, Alphonce E, Ramsay M. Assessment of ingestive and oral praxis skills: children with cerebral palsy vs. controls. Dysphagia 2000;15(4):236–244 doi: 10.1007/s004550000033

[85] Schwartz S, Gisel EG, Clarke D, Haberfellner H. Association of occlusion with eat-ing efficiency in children with cerebral palsy and moderate eating impairment. J Dent Child (Chic) 2003;70(1):33–39

[86] Wright RER, Wright FR, Carson CA. Videofluoroscopic assessment in chil-dren with severe cerebral palsy presenting with dysphagia. Pediatr Radiol 1996;26(10):720–722 doi: 10.1007/BF01383388

[87] Griggs CA, Jones PM, Lee RE. Videofluoroscopic investigation of feeding disorders of children with multiple handicap. Dev Med Child Neurol 1989;31(3):303–308

[88] Mirrett PL, Riski JE, Glascott J, Johnson V. Videofluoroscopic assessment of dys-phagia in children with severe spastic cerebral palsy. Dysphagia 1994;9(3):174–179 doi: 10.1007/BF00341262

[89] Gerek M, Çiyiltepe M. Dysphagia management of pediatric patients with cerebral palsy. Br J Dev Disabil. 2005;51(100):57–72

[90] Morton R, Minford J, Ellis R, Pinnington L. Aspiration with dysphagia: the interaction between oropharyngeal and respiratory impairments. Dysphagia 2002;17(3):192–196 doi: 10.1007/s00455-002-0051-x

[91] Weir KA, McMahon S, Taylor S, Chang AB. Oropharyngeal aspiration and silent aspiration in children. Chest 2011;140(3):589–597 doi: 10.1378/chest.10-1618

[92] Spiroglou K, Xinias I, Karatzas N, Karatza E, Arsos G, Panteliadis C. Gastric emp-tying in children with cerebral palsy and gastroesophageal reflux. Pediatr Neurol 2004;31(3):177–182 doi: 10.1016/j.pediatrneurol.2004.02.007

[93] Staiano A, Cucchiara S, Del Giudice E, Andreotti MR, Minella R. Disorders of oesophageal motility in children with psychomotor retardation and gastro-oesophageal reflux. Eur J Pediatr 1991;150(9):638–641 doi: 10.1007/ BF02072624

[94] Staiano A, Del Giudice E. Colonic transit and anorectal manometry in children with severe brain damage. Pediatrics 1994;94(2 Pt 1):169–173

[95] Sullivan PB. Gastrointestinal disorders: assessment and management. In: Sullivan PB, ed. Feeding and Nutrition in Children with Neurodevelopmental Disability. London, UK: Mac Keith Press; 2009:106–117

[96] Strudwick S. Oral motor impairment and swallowing dysfunction: assessment and management. In: Sullivan PB, ed. Feeding and Nutrition in Children with Neurodevelopmental Disability. London, UK: Mac Keith Press; 2009:35–56

[97] Benfer KA, Weir KA, Boyd RN. Clinimetrics of measures of oropharyngeal dysphagia for preschool children with cerebral palsy and neurodevelopmental disabilities: a systematic review. Dev Med Child Neurol 2012;54(9):784–795 doi: 10.1111/j.1469-8749.2012.04302.x

[98] Skuse D, Stevenson J, Reilly S, Mathisen B. Schedule for oral-motor assessment (SOMA): methods of validation. Dysphagia 1995;10(3):192–202

[99] Morris SE. Pre-Speech Assessment Scale: A Rating Scale for the Measurement of Pre-Speech Behaviors from Birth through Two Years. Rev. ed. Washington, DC: ERIC; 1982

[100] Kantarcigil C, Sheppard JJ, Gordon AM, Friel KM, Malandraki GA. A telehealth approach to conducting clinical swallowing evaluations in children with cerebral palsy. Res Dev Disabil 2016;55:207–217 doi: 10.1016/j.ridd.2016.04.008

[101] Logemann JA. Evaluation and Treatment of Swallowing Disorders. 2nd ed. Austin, TX: Pro-Ed; 1997

[102] Langmore SE. Evaluation of oropharyngeal dysphagia: which diagnostic tool is superior? Curr Opin Otolaryngol Head Neck Surg 2003;11(6):485–489

[103] Ozdemirkiran T, Secil Y, Tarlaci S, Ertekin C. An EMG screening method (dysphagia limit) for evaluation of neurogenic dysphagia in childhood above 5 years old. Int J Pediatr Otorhinolaryngol 2007;71(3):403–407 doi: 10.1016/j ijporl.2006.11.006

[104] Santos MTBR, Manzano FS, Chamlian TR, Masiero D, Jardim JR. Effect of spastic cerebral palsy on jaw-closing muscles during clenching. Spec Care Dentist 2010;30(4):163–167

[105] Miller JL, Sonies BC, Macedonia C. Emergence of oropharyngeal, laryngeal and swallowing activity in the developing fetal upper aerodigestive tract: an ultrasound evaluation. Early Hum Dev 2003;71(1):61–87 doi: 10.1016/S0378-3782(02)00110-X

[106] Miller JL, Kang SM. Preliminary ultrasound observation of lingual movement patterns during nutritive versus non-nutritive sucking in a premature infant. Dysphagia 2007;22(2):150–160 doi: 10.1007/s00455-006-9058-z

[107] Cleland J, Scobbie JM, Wrench AA. Using ultrasound visual biofeedback to treat persistent primary speech sound disorders. Clin Linguist Phon 2015;29(8-10):575–597 doi: 10.3109/02699206.2015.1016188

[108] Lagarde MLJ, Kamalski DMA, van den Engel-Hoek L. The reliability and validity of cervical auscultation in the diagnosis of dysphagia: a systematic review. Clin Rehabil 2016;30(2):199–207 doi: 10.1177/0269215515576779

[109] Frakking TT, Chang AB, O'Grady KF, David M, Walker-Smith K, Weir KA. The use of cervical auscultation to predict oropharyngeal aspiration in children: a randomized controlled trial. Dysphagia 2016;31(6):738–748 doi: 10.1007 s00455-016-9727-5

[110] Crist W, Dobbelsteyn C, Brousseau AM, Napier-Phillips A. Pediatric assessment scale for severe feeding problems: validity and reliability of a new scale for tube-fed children. Nutr Clin Pract 2004;19(4):403–408

[111] Lefton-Greif MA, Okelo SO, Wright JM, Collaco JM, McGrath-Morrow SA, Eakin MN. Impact of children's feeding/swallowing problems: validation of a new

caregiver instrument. *Dysphagia* 2014;29(6):671–677 doi: 10.1007/s00455-014-9560-7

[112] Reid SM, Johnson HM, Reddihough DS. The Drooling Impact Scale: a measure of the impact of drooling in children with developmental disabilities. *Dev Med Child Neurol* 2010;52(2):e23–e28 doi: 10.1111/j.1469-8749.2009.03519.x

[113] Sullivan PB, Lambert B, Rose M, Ford-Adams M, Johnson A, Griffiths P. Prevalence and severity of feeding and nutritional problems in children with neurological impairment: Oxford Feeding Study. *Dev Med Child Neurol* 2000;42(10):674–680

[114] Staudt M, Niemann G, Lotze M, Erb M, Kraegeloh-Mann I, Grodd W. Sensorimotor reorganization in prenatally acquired hemiparesis. *Neuroimage* 2000;11(5):S135

[115] Staudt M, Braun C, Gerloff C, Erb M, Grodd W, Krägeloh-Mann I. Developing somatosensory projections bypass periventricular brain lesions. *Neurology* 2006;67(3):522–525 doi: 10.1212/01.wnl.0000227937.49151.fd

[116] Miller CK, Willging JP. Compensatory strategies and techniques. In: Shaker R, Easterling C, Belafsky PC, Postma GN, eds. Manual of Diagnostic and Therapeutic Techniques for Disorders of Deglutition. New York, NY: Springer; 2013:349–388

[117] Malandraki GA, Rajappa A, Kantarcigil C, Wagner E, Ivey C, Youse K. The intensive dysphagia rehabilitation approach applied to patients with neurogenic dysphagia: a case series design study. *Arch Phys Med Rehabil* 2016;97(4):567–574 doi: 10.1016/j.apmr.2015.11.019

[118] Larnert G, Ekberg O. Positioning improves the oral and pharyngeal swallowing function in children with cerebral palsy. *Acta Paediatr* 1995;84(6):689–692 doi: 10.1111/j.1651-2227.1995.tb13730.x

[119] Snider L, Majnemer A, Darsaklis V. Feeding interventions for children with cerebral palsy: a review of the evidence. *Phys Occup Ther Pediatr* 2011;31(1):58–77 doi: 10.3109/01942638.2010.523397

[120] Morton RE, Bonas R, Fourie B, Minford J. Videofluoroscopy in the assessment of feeding disorders of children with neurological problems. *Dev Med Child Neurol* 1993;35(5):388–395

[121] Vekerdy Z. Management of seating posture of children with cerebral palsy by using thoracic-lumbar-sacral orthosis with non-rigid SIDO frame. *Disabil Rehabil* 2007;29(18):1434–1441 doi: 10.1080/09638280601055691

[122] Myhr U, von Wendt L. Improvement of functional sitting position for children with cerebral palsy. *Dev Med Child Neurol* 1991;33(3):246–256

[123] Myhr U, von Wendt L, Norrlin S, Radell U. Five-year follow-up of functional sitting position in children with cerebral palsy. *Dev Med Child Neurol* 1995;37(7):587–596

[124] Croft RD. What consistency of food is best for children with cerebral palsy who cannot chew? *Arch Dis Child* 1992;67(3):269–271

[125] Rempel G, Moussavi Z. The effect of viscosity on the breath-swallow pattern of young people with cerebral palsy. *Dysphagia* 2005;20(2):108–112 doi: 10.1007/s00455-005-0006-0

[126] Malandraki GA, Robbins J. Dysphagia. In: Aminoff MJ, Boller F, Swaab DF, eds. Neural Rehabilitation: Handbook of Clinical Neurology. Atlanta, GA: Elsevier; 2013:255–271

[127] Gisel EG, Schwartz S, Haberfellner H. The Innsbruck Sensorimotor Activator and Regulator (ISMAR): construction of an intraoral appliance to facilitate ingestive functions. *ASDC J Dent Child* 1999;66(3):180–187, 154

[128] Haberfellner H, Schwartz S, Gisel EG. Feeding skills and growth after one year of intraoral appliance therapy in moderately dysphagic children with cerebral palsy. *Dysphagia* 2001;16(2):83–96 doi: 10.1007/PL00021293

[129] Gisel EG, Schwartz S, Petryk A, Clarke D, Haberfellner H. "Whole body" mobility after one year of intraoral appliance therapy in children with cerebral palsy and moderate eating impairment. *Dysphagia* 2000;15(4):226–235 doi: 10.1007/s004550000032

[130] Haberfellner H, Rossiwall B. Appliances for treatment of oral sensorimotor disorders. *Am J Phys Med* 1977;56(5):241–248

[131] Fischer-Brandies H, Avalle C, Limbrock GJ. Therapy of orofacial dysfunctions in cerebral palsy according to Castillo-Morales: first results of a new treatment concept. *Eur J Orthod* 1987;9(2):139–143

[132] Pinnington L, Hegarty J. Effects of consistent food presentation on efficiency of eating and nutritive value of food consumed by children with severe neurological impairment. *Dysphagia* 1999;14(1):17–26 doi: 10.1007/PL00009580

[133] Sullivan PB, Juszczak E, Bachlet AME, et al. Gastrostomy tube feeding in children with cerebral palsy: a prospective, longitudinal study. *Dev Med Child Neurol* 2005;47(2):77–85

[134] Arrowsmith F, Allen J, Gaskin K, Somerville H, Clarke S, O'Loughlin E. The effect of gastrostomy tube feeding on body protein and bone mineralization in children with quadriplegic cerebral palsy. *Dev Med Child Neurol* 2010;52(11):1043–1047 doi: 10.1111/j.1469-8749.2010.03702.x

[135] Sullivan PB, Morrice JS, Vernon-Roberts A, Grant H, Eltumi M, Thomas AG. Does gastrostomy tube feeding in children with cerebral palsy increase the risk of respiratory morbidity? *Arch Dis Child* 2006;91(6):478–482 doi: 10.1136/adc.2005.084442

[136] Thorne SE, Radford MJ, McCormick J. The multiple meanings of long-term gastrostomy in children with severe disability. *J Pediatr Nurs* 1997;12(2):89–99

[137] Strauss DJ, Shavelle RM, Anderson TW. Life expectancy of children with cerebral palsy. *Pediatr Neurol* 1998;18(2):143–149 doi: 10.1016/S0887-8994(97)00172-0

[138] Smith SW, Camfield C, Camfield P. Living with cerebral palsy and tube feeding: A population-based follow-up study. *J Pediatr* 1999;135(3):307–310 doi: 10.1016/S0022-3476(99)70125-3

[139] Gantasala S, Sullivan PB, Thomas AG. Gastrostomy feeding versus oral feeding alone for children with cerebral palsy. *Cochrane Database Syst Rev* 2013;(7):CD003943 doi: 10.1002/14651858.CD003943.pub3

[140] McKirdy LS, Sheppard JJ, Osborne ML, Payne P. Transition from tube to oral feeding in the school setting. *Lang Speech Hear Serv Sch* 2008;39(2):249–260 doi: 10.1044/0161-1461(2008/024)

[141] Rempel G. The importance of good nutrition in children with cerebral palsy. *Phys Med Rehabil Clin N Am* 2015;26(1):39–56 doi: 10.1016/j.pmr.2014.09.001

[142] Clark HM. Neuromuscular treatments for speech and swallowing: a tutorial. *Am J Speech Lang Pathol* 2003;12(4):400–415 doi: 10.1044/1058-0360(2003/086)

[143] Arvedson J, Clark H, Lazarus C, Schooling T, Frymark T. The effects of oral-motor exercises on swallowing in children: an evidence-based systematic review. *Dev Med Child Neurol* 2010;52(11):1000–1013 doi: 10.1111/j.1469-8749.2010.03707.x

[144] Christiaanse ME, Mabe B, Russell G, Simeone TL, Fortunato J, Rubin B. Neuromuscular electrical stimulation is no more effective than usual care for the treatment of primary dysphagia in children. *Pediatr Pulmonol* 2011;46(6):559–565 doi: 10.1002/ppul.21400

[145] Schmidt RA, Lee TD. Motor Learning and Performance: From Principles to Application. 5th ed. Champaign, IL: Human Kinetics; 2014

[146] Kleim JA, Jones TA. Principles of experience-dependent neural plasticity: implications for rehabilitation after brain damage. *J Speech Lang Hear Res* 2008;51(1):S225–S239 doi: 10.1044/1092-4388(2008/018)

[147] Crary MA, Carnaby GD, LaGorio LA, Carvajal PJ. Functional and physiological outcomes from an exercise-based dysphagia therapy: a pilot investigation of the McNeill Dysphagia Therapy Program. *Arch Phys Med Rehabil* 2012;93(7):1173–1178 doi: 10.1016/j.apmr.2011.11.008

[148] Martin-Harris B, McFarland D, Hill EG, et al. Respiratory-swallow training in patients with head and neck cancer. *Arch Phys Med Rehabil* 2015;96(5):885–893 doi: 10.1016/j.apmr.2014.11.022

[149] Sheppard JJ. Using motor learning approaches for treating swallowing and feeding disorders: a review. *Lang Speech Hear Serv Sch* 2008;39(2):227–236 doi: 10.1044/0161-1461(2008/022)

[150] Athukorala RP, Jones RD, Sella O, Huckabee M-L. Skill training for swallowing rehabilitation in patients with Parkinson's disease. *Arch Phys Med Rehabil* 2014;95(7):1374–1382 doi: 10.1016/j.apmr.2014.03.001

[151] Maas E, Robin DA, Austermann Hula SN, Freedman SE, Wulf G, Ballard KJ, Schmidt RA. Principles of motor learning in treatment of motor speech disorders. *Am J Speech Lang Pathol*, 2008;17(3):277-98. doi: 10.1044/1058-0360(2008/025)

[152] Sheppard JJ. Motor learning approaches for improving negative eating-related behaviors and swallowing and feeding skills in children. In: Handbook of Behavior, Food and Nutrition. New York, NY: Springer; 2011:3271–3284. doi: 10.1007/978-0-387-92271-3_204

## Suggested Reading

[1] Arvedson J, Clark H, Lazarus C, Schooling T, Frymark T. The effects of oral-motor exercises on swallowing in children: an evidence-based systematic review. *Dev Med Child Neurol* 2010;52(11):1000–1013

[2] Sheppard JJ. Using motor learning approaches for treating swallowing and feeding disorders: a review. *Lang Speech Hear Serv Sch* 2008;39(2):227–236

[3] Sullivan PB, ed. Feeding and Nutrition in Children with Neurodevelopmental Disability. London, UK: Mac Keith Press; 2009

# 18 Behaviorally Based Feeding Problems

*Kay A. Toomey and Erin Sundseth Ross*

## Summary

Behavioral feeding disorders are typically feeding problems that do not appear to have a direct medical etiology. However, the research indicates 80–98% of children with feeding difficulties have both physical and behavioral components that interfere with their eating. Treatment approaches vary in large part by the theoretical approach that is used as the foundation for the feeding program. This chapter reframes a "behavioral feeding disorder" as a learned avoidance behavior, typically resulting from aversive experiences due to medical conditions or skill deficits. These aversive experiences do not need to be ongoing; they can be historical. Seven areas of functioning are identified as underlying appropriate feeding skill development. Maladaptive behaviors during mealtimes are reinterpreted as learned avoidance behaviors secondary to the child's lack of abilities. The learning theories of classical and operant conditioning, which provide the basis for all therapy programs, are described as they apply to feeding. Positive (apply) and negative (remove) behavioral therapies, as well as reinforcement (increase) or punishment (decrease) techniques are also discussed and applied to feeding therapy approaches. Although these treatment approaches work, specific programs may be more appropriate for specific children. Advantages and disadvantages of the various approaches are described to assist the therapist in determining which approach is best for a specific child.

## Keywords

disorders, developmental, eating, nutrition, learned avoidance, behaviors, sensory, oral-motor

### Learning Objectives
- List the seven areas of function involved in the process of eating
- Describe the classical conditioning principles leading to associative learning and how this impacts feeding
- Define the operant conditioning principles of positive and negative reinforcement and punishment as they apply to feeding
- Discuss the pros and cons of the main operant conditioning procedures for changing feeding behavior: positive and negative reinforcement
- Delineate the differences between the classical conditioning strategies of systematic desensitization and flooding in feeding therapy

## 18.1 Introduction

The term *behavioral feeding disorder* is used to describe children who do not have a known medical etiology for their feeding struggles. In the past, this disorder was referred to as nonorganic failure to thrive. However, the terminology *failure to thrive* has fallen out of favor in support of a more comprehensive approach to thinking about children with feeding disorders. One reason is that there are children who are growing or thriving from a weight standpoint, but who do not eat enough appropriate types of foods (i.e., they are food restricted). Likewise, there are children who do not eat any food at all by mouth and receive their nutrition through tube feedings (i.e., nonoral). Although these children may be thriving from a weight standpoint, they are not thriving from the perspective of being able to sit and have a meal with their family. On the other hand, there are children who have difficulties gaining weight but who may be thriving in other areas of development (e.g., social skills, cognition, academics, emotional control). The term *failure to thrive* is often seen as punitive and judgmental by the caregivers of these children, which has also contributed to its demise. In 2001, Crist and Napier-Phillips presented a new way of conceptualizing the field as "a biopsychosocial model in which physiological, behavioral, and social factors are all viewed as contributing to the development of feeding difficulties."[1]

The etiology of a feeding disorder is complicated and most often multifactorial, including medical, developmental/skill, environmental, nutritional, and learning components. In addition to addressing skill deficits, feeding treatment programs have adopted the principles of learning theory and behavior modification strategies to successfully increase caloric intake and expand the food repertoire of these children. Both classical and operant conditioning principles are employed to improve mealtime behaviors and consumption. The key to therapeutic success is to understand these principles and to match the needs of the child to the best treatment approach to achieve the goals set for therapy.

Whereas a child may not be growing appropriately because of an organ system/medical (organic) disorder, many other children are either not growing or not eating age-appropriate foods because of developmental issues. It is more often that these developmental problems are the etiology of the food refusal. Prevalence of a combined medical/physical/behavioral etiology in children seen for food refusal ranges from 78 to 97.5%.[2,3,4] When the task of eating the food is too difficult, or the skills needed are lacking, children may develop behaviors to avoid eating. "Children with minor organic disorders may fail to thrive, not because of any direct effect upon metabolism, but because the child is thereby very difficult to feed."[5] Alternatively, children who have medical reasons that interfere with eating often learn to stop eating because eating is painful or makes them feel uncomfortable (e.g., GERD). This in turn creates a high level of stress for the caregivers because they often lack the knowledge and ability to help their child who doesn't want to eat. Even after the medical issues are resolved, the learned avoidance behaviors often remain. In some cases, these children still avoid eating because they have yet to learn that feeding is no longer painful or difficult. However, in other cases, the medical issues may have directly interfered with the child reaching the developmental milestones necessary for learning to eat a wide variety of age-appropriate foods. "Feeding problems often result from multi factorial causes and the classification of disorders based on an organic versus nonorganic dichotomy fails to provide a system that fully represents the often complex interactions between medical problems, family systems, and behavioral difficulties associated with feeding disorders."[6] This chapter addresses these children who either (1) have learned that eating is too difficult/painful and now need to undo this learning, or (2) have delayed development of skills that support the transitions from liquids to textured food diets, and consequently use maladaptive behaviors to avoid eating.

## 18.2 Case Presentation

Jonathan was born at 27 weeks gestation and was intubated in the delivery room. He demonstrated difficulty with suck–swallow–breathe coordination from the start of nipple feedings and was never able to establish breastfeeding. Jonathan had a cranial ultrasound that was normal, but he was diagnosed with gastroesophageal reflux while he was in the neonatal intensive care unit (NICU). Jonathan struggled to eat sufficient volumes of expressed breastmilk by his due date; thus he was discharged with a **nasogastric (NG)** tube. At the time of discharge, Jonathan was meeting only 20% of his nutritional needs with a bottle. Oral stimulation was initiated after discharge to increase his acceptance of the bottle, but Jonathan became increasingly resistant and eventually rejected any attempts to offer tastes, smells, or even the pacifier. At 2 months adjusted age, Jonathan was referred to a feeding therapist to help with his feeding refusal. At 3 months Jonathan underwent surgery to place a **percutaneous endoscopic gastrostomy (PEG) tube**. He was seen regularly by a feeding therapist for 16 months but was still 100% tube dependent after all this treatment. He was no longer considered medically fragile, was off oxygen, and had demonstrated normal swallowing skills. Although he had been diagnosed with **gastroesophageal reflux disease (GERD)**, Jonathan was no longer being treated medically because he did not show any signs of GERD and was no longer vomiting on a regular basis. Jonathan's refusal to eat was considered behaviorally based because he would not put food into his mouth despite having demonstrated the ability to swallow safely. At 18 months corrected age, Jonathan was referred to a multidisciplinary feeding clinic to address his behavioral feeding problem and to establish a plan for transitioning off his gastrostomy tube.

## 18.3 Prevalence

Pediatric feeding disorders are a spectrum of disorders that may include limited volume, poor growth, or limited variety in the diet. Many children with significant medical comorbidities require supplemental tube feedings to achieve adequate nutrition and growth. In a study of U.S. pediatric admissions during 1997–2009, gastrostomy tubes (G-tubes) (either surgically placed or PEG) were placed in 173/100,000 children < 1 year of age in 2009.[7] In this same study, G-tubes accounted for 18.5 procedures/100,000 children in 2009. However, many parents of toddlers and young children report that their child is picky and simply lacks variety in his or her diet. In a longitudinal study of over 4,000 children, the prevalence of picky eating varied according to age, with 26.5% of 18-month-old children reported to be picky, rising to 27.6% by age 3 years, and dropping to 13.2% in this cohort at age 6 years.[8] However, 4% of children in this same study were considered picky at all three age ranges; 55% of children were never described as picky by their parents. In children with known developmental challenges, the prevalence of picky eating is even higher. Two-thirds of parents of children with autism spectrum disorders (ASDs) complain of poor variety and difficult mealtime behaviors.[9] Within a group of 349 children referred for feeding assessments, 93% of the children diagnosed with ASD had a restricted range of foods; 45% of children with trisomy 21 rejected foods based on texture.[2] Many children seen later in feeding clinics fail to successfully negotiate the multiple transitions in food (liquid, puree, meltable, table foods; soft mechanicals) that typically occur across the first year.[10] Poor variety may be due to difficulty with the mechanics of eating, to overresponsivity to textures or tastes, or to preferences established for other reasons. Children without a current, or in some cases obvious, medical condition may be thought of as having a behavioral feeding disorder. Children who can talk, or appear to be developing typically, may yet have subtle skill deficits that influence their eating. For instance, eating requires lateral movement of the tongue and/or jaw; talking requires only vertical movement of both. In a study of 47 children who were diagnosed with "nonorganic failure to thrive," over one-third had an oral-motor deficit that had not been diagnosed.[11] Both for children who require tube feedings and for those with a restricted diet, the key to understanding treatment options begins with a thorough assessment of the underlying cause for the feeding disorder.

## 18.4 Model for Feeding Assessment

A model that considers the whole child (including the family system) is required to best understand the complexity of feeding disorders. There are seven areas of functioning that need to be assessed and addressed each time a child presents with a feeding difficulty:

1. Organ systems/medical diagnoses
2. Motor/muscle systems (including oral-motor skills)
3. Sensory systems
4. Learning (what they have learned in the past, learning style, learning capacity)
5. Developmental/cognitive stage
6. Nutritional status
7. Environment.

Not only do children need to be functional in each of these seven areas; they need to be able to integrate between and across these seven areas. Therefore, when a child isn't eating, it is most helpful to conceptualize the child's feeding challenge as an indication that something is not going well from a physical or developmental standpoint, the "tip of the iceberg" (**Fig. 18.1**). Only after physical/skill deficits have been addressed can behaviors that the child uses to escape eating be fully addressed.

For many children, because their skills in isolation appear to be within normal limits, their feeding refusal may be considered behaviorally based. However, if the child is lacking skills and abilities, focusing solely on changing the child's behaviors during mealtimes will be ineffective. How the problem is conceptualized influences the decision-making process for treatment. According to Dunn-Klein, "If we believe the child has an emotional or behavioral problem, we will try to control and 'fix' the child. If we believe the child is having a stress response because they cannot manage the task, we will teach the skills in a manner that respects the child's readiness for the task"[12] (M. Dunn-Klein, pers. comm., 2010). This chapter focuses on treatment models and therefore will not describe the areas in detail; however, the following is a brief description of the seven areas of functioning.

## 18.5 Organ Systems/Medical Diagnoses

In a brief online search, over 204 medical diagnoses were identified that listed "poor feeding" as a clinical sign.[12] GERD, neurologic, cardiac, pulmonary, and food allergies/intolerances top the list of most common medical issues seen in 349 infants and young children referred to an interdisciplinary feeding team, with 69% of children with GERD demonstrating food refusal.[2] In a study of 40 children with G-tubes, half had congenital anomalies and one-quarter had GERD as their only known medical issue; the remaining 25% had lung or other medical issues.[13] Children with GERD typically have significant food refusal across food textures, even after their GERD has been medically managed, and may reach a point of needing supplemental tube feedings.[4]

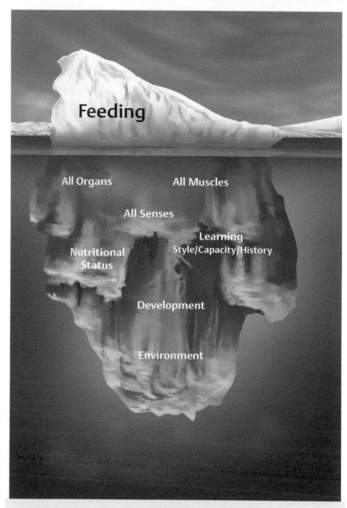

**Fig. 18.1** Model for assessment of feeding disorders.

## 18.6 Motor/Muscle Systems

The muscle systems (gross and fine motor, oral-motor, and internal muscles, such as the gastrointestinal tract) develop over time and support the transition from a totally liquid to a textured table-food diet. Muscle tone and strength develop, providing a framework for more sophisticated movements. Low muscle tone has been identified in over half of children previously diagnosed as nonorganic failure to thrive.[14] Between 5 and 7 months of age, children develop postural stability, which is necessary for sitting.[15] This stability, combined with improved head control, provides stability for more fine motor function of the hands and mouth.[15] Gross motor milestones precede the acquisition of oral motor milestones, beginning as early as 5 months of age.[15] For instance, the skills of grasping and bringing the hands to midline emerge prior to midline movements of the tongue during chewing.[15] Postural control also underlies stability in the jaw, necessary for both drinking from a cup and eating. There is a backward shift of the body, head, and neck during chewing and drinking from cups in 12-month-old infants.[16]

Increased dietary variety and texture diversity are observed between 6 and 12 months of age. The tongue begins to move independently from the jaw. The ability to properly manage these changes in texture of foods requires that children move foods laterally to the jaws with their tongue, as well as grind the foods between the jaws and teeth using either munching or rotary chewing patterns. Chewing becomes more efficient over the 6- to 48-month age range.[17,18,19,20] Children who are inefficient at moving and chewing textured foods often struggle with learning to eat meat, fruits with skins, and a variety of hard raw vegetables. These children may gravitate toward unhealthy snack food, which is typically easy to eat from an oral-motor standpoint. Many commercially prepared snack foods melt in the mouth (e.g., cheese puffs) or are easily chewed (e.g., fries). Children who transition to textured foods prior to developing the oral skills for chewing may be at risk for nutritional deficits.[21,22] They may also be at increased risk for choking and aspiration due to poor oral-phase preparatory skills.

## 18.7 Sensory Systems

Eating is a multisensory task. It involves not only the sight, smell, taste, and texture of food but also the sound of the food when it is chewed in the mouth. Textured food challenges the sensory system on an ongoing basis. Not only are there a myriad of different foods, each with their own sensory inputs, but these sensory inputs change as the food is masticated. For instance, when a saltine cracker is eaten, the shape of the food changes both outside (the piece remaining after a bite) and inside the mouth. The bite begins as one, or a few, pieces of food that must be tracked by the tongue, but progressively becomes multiple pieces as the teeth break the bite apart. The pieces then are collected and become a bolus. This is both a tactile and a mechanical task. Additionally, the smell/taste changes from a somewhat salty flavor to a blander, starchy flavor, and the texture changes from rather sharp pieces into a soft mash.

There is a constant interaction between the sensory and the motor systems that controls the food and supports safe swallowing. Eating also creates internal sensations during swallowing and digestion (shifts in balance during chewing and swallowing, movement of the esophagus and stretching in the stomach, and movement of food through the intestines). Many children seen in feeding clinics have sensory processing disorders. Their atypical sensory ability likely impedes their tolerance for the ever-changing sensory inputs found in textured foods. In two studies, between 68% ($n$ = 65) and 100% ($n$ = 16) of children referred for feeding difficulties scored in the atypical range on sensory profiles.[23,24]

## 18.8 Learning

Children are engaged in learning every time they are involved in any activity, whether they are simply sitting, playing imaginatively, climbing, reading, writing, or eating. Young children eat 5 to 11 times per day, according to a World Health Organization study.[25] Given the high correlation between medical diagnoses and feeding difficulties, a child could have multiple negative experiences while eating each week and hundreds of aversive conditioning events across a month. These negative experiences teach a child with a medical problem that eating is something to be avoided (e.g., it is painful, or it interferes with breathing). Children who have poor sensory or oral-motor skills learn that eating may make them shudder or gag and is an action that should be avoided. This learning may remain well after the medical issue has been resolved or the skill has been learned. What and how a child learns, as well as the child's capacity to learn, should be considered when determining the best treatment approach.

## 18.9 Developmental/ Cognitive Stage

Eating is the most challenging thing children do because it requires an integration of multiple motor, oral-motor, medical, sensory, cognitive, and interactive skills.[26] In a review of 38 studies of children ($n$ = 218) seen for "food refusal," 34 studies reported on developmental skill. Seventy-eight percent of children were diagnosed with some level of developmental delay.[4] Because children's developmental status influences skill development, it is to be expected that their ability to eat is limited by their highest developmental skill level. And yet, many caregivers as well as some therapists offer children foods that are above their capability to eat due to their developmental delays.

The way children think and interact with others and their world also influences their acceptance of novel foods.[26] Developmental and cognitive stages need to be considered when developing an intervention program to improve a child's eating. For instance, role modeling eating the target food may improve intake for some children, while talking about a food may improve acceptance for older children.[27,28]

## 18.10 Nutritional Status

Specific nutritional deficits influence a child's eating abilities, and they go beyond just a lack of calorie intake. Many children meet their total caloric needs and therefore are growing adequately, but they have a limited variety in their diet. In the Feeding Infants and Toddlers study, half of parents of infants 19–24 months of age felt their child was a very picky eater.[29] In two studies of preschoolers ranging from 2 to 6 years of age, 30% of parents felt their child was a picky eater.[30,31] Picky eating may become a chronic problem. In a longitudinal study of 120 children 2 to 11 years of age, parents reported a duration of more than 2 years in 40% of children identified as being a picky eater.[32] For those children who are consistently described as picky, eventually their diet may suffer and their growth may be affected.[33] A severely restricted diet can lead to vitamin and mineral deficiencies, which in turn can influence endurance, energy, and attention. For example, zinc has been implicated in the role of hunger, and iron deficits negatively impact endurance, energy, and attention. While specialized liquid/puree diets may meet the nutritional needs of the child, they do not provide the variety that is inherent in a typical textured diet. The quality of the diet is a major concern for many caregivers, especially caregivers of children on the autism spectrum, or children born preterm.[34,35,36]

Another significant area of nutrition that must be considered includes the roles of food intolerance or sensitivity, and allergy. Although these are considered medical factors as well, restrictions in the diet may affect the quality of the diet.[37] Caregivers may also restrict the diet based on a fear of or concern about a food intolerance.[38] This is an extensive area, and it is not the focus of this chapter. For a complete discussion of this expansive topic, the reader is referred to Brostoff and Gamlin.[39]

## 18.11 Environment

The environment has historically been viewed as a major cause of feeding disorders. It is beyond the scope of this chapter to discuss the underpinnings of this in any detail. However, although the environment (and caregiver behaviors) are often supporting maladaptive behaviors, this is only one part in the etiology of feeding disorders.[40] In fact, theories now posit that the child's feeding difficulties are at the root of the changes that are observed in parent–child interactions at mealtimes.[41] Nutrition research has often categorized caregiver behaviors as parenting "styles," and recent research shows that parents use different parenting behaviors with different children within their own home. They often become more permissive (allowing the child to eat whatever and whenever he or she wants) or authoritarian (directing the child to eat specific amounts and types of foods) when their child has been diagnosed as underweight.[42]

## 18.12 Case Presentation Part 2

Although Jonathan was physically able to eat small volumes by 18 months of age (he could swallow and he was no longer on oxygen), there were many areas of development still influencing his ability to eat. The organ systems/medical diagnoses are but one of the seven areas that must be coordinated for Jonathan to learn to eat a wide variety of age-appropriate foods in sufficient quantities to maintain appropriate growth. A full assessment of his current medical issues, as well as his developmental skills and skill deficits, is needed to understand all the component parts that are interfering with Jonathan's ability to learn about eating.

### 18.12.1 Case Assessment

Jonathan's multidisciplinary team evaluation now shows the following:

- Jonathan's overall developmental skill level is 8 months of age. He is scooting on his bottom rather than crawling, he is vocalizing a few vowels and bilabial sounds (m, b) but rarely babbles.
- Given his lack of experience with oral feedings, even though Jonathan does not show overresponses or obvious tactile issues to sensory input on his hands, he may have sensory overresponses to foods or liquids in his mouth. This needs to be further assessed because he refuses to put most things in his mouth (objects or foods).
- Jonathan occasionally takes a small amount of puree from a spoon and liquid from a sippy cup, but this is a rare occurrence.
- His learned avoidance behaviors need to be understood in the context of his history, especially given that Jonathan continues to vomit once or twice a day. He typically vomits first thing in the morning and when he gets upset. His physician feels Jonathan vomits as a behavioral reaction. Jonathan refuses to put foods and most toys and objects in his mouth, and his refusal to do so appears to be the natural consequence of learning that food makes him uncomfortable (an overgeneralized, learned, avoidant response).
- Jonathan's mother is very involved, and would like to transition him off his tube feedings and onto any type of oral feeding. However, Jonathan's ability to transition off his G- tube needs to be determined based on his developmental age and nutritional status.

Since he was 2 months of age, Jonathan has been attending weekly physical and occupational therapy, as well as speech therapy, to work on gross, fine, and oral-motor skills as well as communication. He has also been in feeding therapy since that time, as already noted.

## 18.13 Behavioral Therapy Strategies for Children with Feeding Disorders

One of the challenges in any discussion of behavioral approaches to feeding therapy is that therapists use behavior modification

daily. Every feeding program is a behavioral feeding program. Therefore, when discussing behavioral approaches to treating children who don't eat, it is important to begin by understanding what it means to use a behavioral approach to treat any type of childhood problem. Using a behavioral approach to treatment requires that the therapist use behavior modification strategies to change targeted behaviors. The American Psychological Association defines behavior modification as "the systematic use of principles of learning to increase the frequency of desired behaviors and decrease the frequency of problem behaviors."[43]

Behavior modification includes the direct use of both classical and operant conditioning and may include the principles of social learning theory. Therefore, any feeding therapy program that uses the principles of operant and/or classical conditioning and/or social learning theory is using a behavioral approach to feeding. However, most feeding approaches that are labeled as behavioral feeding programs actively use and primarily discuss only operant conditioning strategies. Even if a program is primarily using operant conditioning, there is always classical conditioning involving the environmental cues present during the operant strategies. These cues become part of a conditioning cue complex (more on this in the following section). This classical conditioning must be addressed for the child to learn to eat foods across a wide variety of settings (home, school, clinics, hospitals, etc.).

The terminology used needs to be accurate and specific. It is too broad of a classification, as well as an incorrect use of the definition of *behavior modification* to refer to programs that use or discuss predominantly operant conditioning as behavioral, and exclude those that rely more on classical conditioning. Therefore, to correctly and accurately discuss behavioral feeding therapy programs one must delineate the strategies used on both the operant and the classical conditioning dimensions as well as on the focus (goal) of that program.

Two primary sets of strategies are used in every behavioral program treating children who have feeding problems: (1) the use of systematic desensitization or flooding (i.e., techniques from classical conditioning), and (2) the use of positive and/or negative reinforcement and/or punishment (i.e., strategies from operant conditioning). Although all feeding programs ultimately have the goal of helping children learn to eat a wide variety of foods with good skills in appropriate volumes, different feeding approaches will use various ways to achieve this goal. One feeding approach may focus on a short-term goal of working on skill development first and then gradually achieving adequate volumes of food. Another feeding approach will focus in the short-term on increasing the volume the child will eat of any food, to increase caloric intake. These programs may then work on teaching the child to eat age-appropriate table foods as the long-term goal. Each approach will address skill development in varying degrees to reach its goals. The principles of each of these types of approaches follows, along with a discussion of which type of program falls into which category of learning. The advantages and disadvantages of the various behavioral approaches are then discussed.

## 18.14 Classical Conditioning

**Classical conditioning** is otherwise known as learning through association. Much of classical conditioning is also what is referred to as body-based learning. This is because learning in classical conditioning begins with a naturally occurring stimulus that causes an organism to have a natural physiological response. In classical conditioning, the naturally occurring stimulus is an object, thing, or activity in the world that is called an **unconditioned stimulus (UCS)**. The naturally occurring physiological body response to the natural stimulus is called the **unconditioned response (UCR)**. For example, if you give a dog food powder, the dog will salivate (Ivan Pavlov's classic experiment). If another, ideally neutral, stimulus (e.g., a bell) is paired with the UCS (i.e., the food powder), the person or animal will have the natural body response (i.e., salivation) to the UCS. Over many trials of the UCS (food) being paired with the other stimulus (bell), connections are made in the brain (i.e., learning) such that when the previously neutral stimulus is presented by itself, the dog now salivates in response to just hearing the bell. The bell has become a **conditioned stimulus (CS)** that leads to a **conditioned response (CR)** (i.e., salivation). The CR of salivation is a smaller body reaction, which is now occurring with the presentation of the previously neutral stimulus. The bell is then a CS because the dog would not typically salivate in response to it. The animal has learned to associate the UCS of food powder with a CS, the bell (**Fig. 18.2**).

How does classical conditioning impact feeding? There are certain naturally occurring stimuli in the world that directly influence whether a child will or will not eat. When human beings are ill or nauseated, neurochemical changes in the gut send signals to the brain to turn off the appetite. Nausea paired with the presentation of food, over time, will create a conditioned response of appetite suppression when the food is presented (**Fig. 18.3**). If a child is fed from a bottle and then has GERD every time, that child may withdraw from the bottle because the bottle has become associated with the pain of the reflux. The bottle becomes a CS. Similarly, if a child is fed a food that creates an aversive sensory response to the feel or flavor of that food, the child will then attempt to escape from that food.

Very often adults forget that the body's natural reaction is to escape or withdraw from painful or uncomfortable stimuli. This is because adults insert a cognitive process in the learning sequence where they tell themselves, "I can do this because it is good for me." However, children do not do things just because it is good for them until around the age of 5 years, when they are shifting cognitively from prelogical thinking to logical thinking. For children, if it hurts, you cry. If it makes you mad, you throw it on the floor or you scream. If something is hard work, young children either run away or cheat. One way to cheat during feeding is to eat only the easiest possible foods. Another way to cheat is to fuss at your caregivers until they make your food easier to eat. For children with sensory challenges, eating the same food prepared the same way allows them to have a more predictable experience that provides less of a sensory challenge. Most prepackaged food is created to be as similar as possible every time; quality control ensures a similar sensory experience for the consumer. Homemade food, on the other hand, varies due to the food and its preparation. The consistency in the sensory properties of prepackaged foods, compared to homemade food, may be more easily recognized and accepted by children with sensory processing difficulties.

The other way that classical conditioning impacts feeding is through the associative learning between eating and the conditioning cues in the eating environment. No one learns to do any behavior in isolation. There are always cues in our environment that become classically conditioned to the foods during our meals and snacks. Just because a child learns to eat one food at school does not necessarily guarantee that the child will also eat that same exact food in the home environment. Depending on how microscopically the child learns or how visually hypersensitive the child is, every visual cue in the environment may become part of the conditioning cue complex. For example (**Fig. 18.4**), to the child who notices every cue in the environment, a chicken nugget offered at school may be a small, round, brown, warm, breaded,

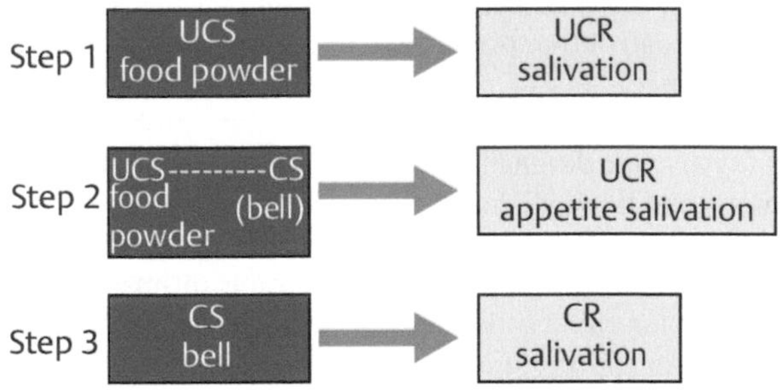

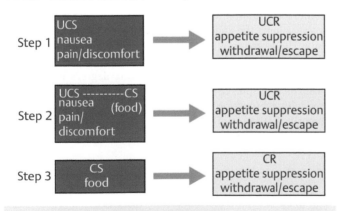

Fig. 18.2 Classical conditioning.

Fig. 18.3 Classical conditioning applied to food.

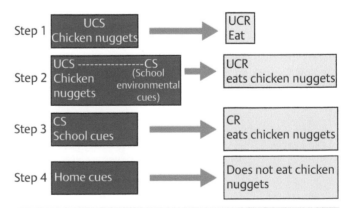

Fig. 18.4 Classical conditioning applied to food.

prechewed piece of meat that comes on a white plastic plate on a red plastic tray, on top of a gray table while the child sits on a bench in a large, noisy room with tiles on the floor. The food is not just the chicken nugget—the food is the chicken nugget in the context of the other visual cues. If the caregiver takes that same chicken nugget from school and brings it into the kitchen at home, the child may not eat that chicken nugget. Why? Because now this food has been placed on a nice pottery plate on a cloth placemat on top of a table while the child is sitting on a regular chair in a small, quiet room that has carpeting on the floor. Too many of this child's conditioning cues have been changed, and the child no longer recognizes or eat that food. Children on the autism spectrum may not be able to separate the important detail (the chicken nugget) from the rest of the conditioning cues.

## 18.15 Operant Conditioning

**Operant conditioning** is also known as learning through consequences. Social learning theory posits that people also learn by watching others receive consequences for their actions.[44] B. F. Skinner is the theorist who presented the principles of operant conditioning. He used two words, *positive* and *negative*, in his theory to describe these principles. Unfortunately, most people attach a judgment value to these words by thinking *positive* means good, and *negative* means bad. In operant conditioning there is no judgment value assigned to learning. Operant conditioning does not label behaviors as good or bad. Behaviors are either adaptive or maladaptive for that child in that situation or within that set of conditioning cues. Consequences are not good or bad either.

Consequences are either desirable or undesirable to that child in that situation. In operant conditioning, *positive* means to apply a stimulus. *Negative* means to remove a stimulus. Reinforcement causes a behavior to increase, and punishment causes a behavior to decrease. There is no judgment value involved.

Operant conditioning states that if a behavior (adaptive or maladaptive) is followed by a desirable consequence, that behavior will increase. In operant conditioning, a behavior (maladaptive or adaptive) that is followed by an undesirable consequence will lead to a decrease in that behavior (**Fig. 18.5**).

Operant conditioning plays a large role in children's eating and in feeding environments. Operant conditioning is a strong influence on how children learn to eat after 5–6 months of age. It is also how maladaptive behaviors (e.g., learned avoidance) around eating are accidentally maintained. Operant conditioning is also how adaptive feeding behaviors can be accidentally eliminated. If a child is eating and the caregiver praises the child, the child will eat more (**Fig. 18.6**). But what if the child has auditory hypersensitivity resulting in a physiological overreaction to very loud noises, and the caregiver cheers loudly when the child takes a bite of food (**Fig. 18.7**)?

In the first scenario, the caregiver's praise is a desirable consequence and the adaptive eating behavior increases, or has been reinforced (reinforcement = behaviors increase). In the second scenario, the loud cheering is an undesirable consequence for the child with auditory overreactivity, and the adaptive eating behavior has now been punished (punishment = behaviors decrease). Some children with sensory difficulties are unintentionally being punished during eating because they can't handle the stimulation occurring at the meal or with the food.

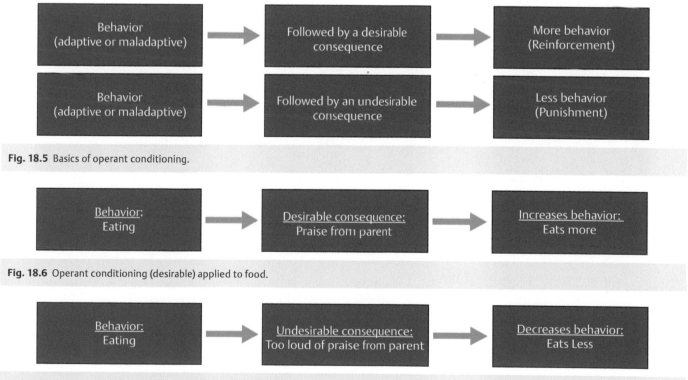

**Fig. 18.5** Basics of operant conditioning.

**Fig. 18.6** Operant conditioning (desirable) applied to food.

**Fig. 18.7** Operant conditioning (undesirable) applied to food.

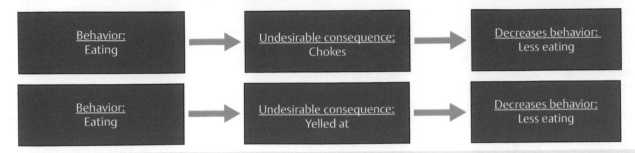

**Fig. 18.8** Operant conditioning (undesirable) applied to food.

Another situation that frequently happens during feedings is that the child is eating and has an uncomfortable experience, such as accidentally choking, aspirating, biting their tongue, or being yelled at by a caregiver (e.g., "Just eat it without whining"). These aversive experiences will cause the child to learn *not* to eat (**Fig. 18.8**). In addition to this type of aversive operant conditioning occurring and causing a child to eat less, there is also classical conditioning occurring, which further interferes with the child's

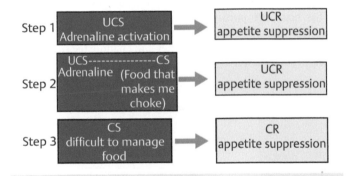

**Fig. 18.9** Classical conditioning added to operant conditioning.

eating. When children are upset, their adrenaline system is activated, the result of which is appetite suppression (**Fig. 18.9**).

Much of what adults interpret as a child engaging in bad behaviors during meals actually consists of learned avoidance behaviors because the child has had an aversive experience occur with that food, causing a loss of appetite. It is important to understand that when a child is asked to do a task (eating) that he or she doesn't have the skills to do correctly (e.g., oral-motor problems or sensory overreactions), it can lead to aversive experiences. Children who repeatedly bite their tongue because of oral-motor incoordination, or who gag because they can't tolerate the texture of the food, are going to learn to avoid that food in the future because of conditioning experiences. Children who have skill deficits, whether those deficits are postural, oral-motor, or sensorimotor in origin, have repeated aversive conditioning experiences in which they are learning to *not* eat (**Fig. 18.10**). Even if their skills improve, they may continue to avoid eating because of the learning that has occurred.

Unfortunately, caregivers can then accidentally reinforce these avoidance/refusal behaviors because caregivers are so concerned about getting children to eat that they give them a preferred food, or try to coax them to eat, or play games to distract them from the

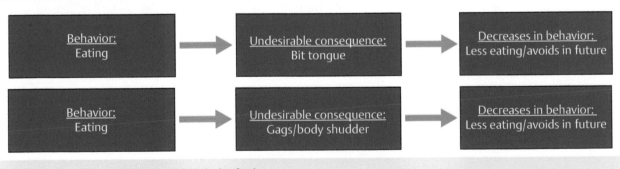

**Fig. 18.10** Operant conditioning (undesirable) applied to food.

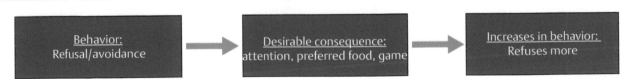

**Fig. 18.11** Operant conditioning (desirable) applied to food.

experience. These caregiver reactions are desirable consequences for the maladaptive behavior of refusing to eat (**Fig. 18.11**).

When the concepts of positive and negative reinforcement and punishment are combined, caregivers and professionals can sometimes become confused when discussing the role of operant conditioning in feeding. It is easy to understand **positive reinforcement** of adaptive behaviors and **positive punishment** of maladaptive behaviors. Positive reinforcement would be to apply a desirable consequence, which increases the eating behavior. Positive punishment would be applying an undesirable consequence to decrease the food refusal/learned avoidance behaviors. Understanding **negative reinforcement** and **negative punishment** is a bit more challenging (**Fig. 18.12**).

Negative punishment occurs when a behavior causes the removal of a desirable stimulus, leading to the child doing less of that behavior. For example, a caregiver might remove a child's preferred food if the child spits it at someone (**Fig. 18.13**).

Negative reinforcement occurs when engaging in a behavior causes the removal of an undesirable stimulus that is occurring. For example, a caregiver may keep a child belted into a high chair until the child consumes a preset volume of food that the caregiver determines is necessary for the child to eat. By eating that preset volume of food (even if the child doesn't want to eat that much or any at all), the child can escape being restrained in the chair. Typically, negative reinforcement is referred to as escape conditioning (**Fig. 18.14**).

## 18.16 Behavioral Feeding Problems

Many of the bad behaviors that children engage in at mealtimes are learned avoidance behaviors resulting from classical and operant conditioning, created by an interplay of physiological reactions, skill deficits, and repeated experiences. If a child throws a food that makes her shudder because she cannot tolerate the touch input to her hand, she is reacting to the sensory input that is aversive. Having the food remain on the floor reinforces the throwing behavior (operant conditioning). In addition, the child's physiological reaction to wet sensations becomes associated with food, and now she avoids certain textures of foods (classical conditioning) (**Fig. 18.15**).

What then constitutes a behavior being a real problem, or not, and from whose perspective? Babies who refuse to eat because they have silent GERD (e.g., nonregurgitory) may be diagnosed with a behavioral feeding disorder because they are not eating enough calories. Whereas the professional believes eating is the adaptive behavior in this situation, it is a maladaptive behavior from the child's perspective, because necessary eating causes more GERD. This is why a thorough evaluation is necessary. Food refusal is often a result of current, or past, learned avoidance reactions (**Fig. 18.16**).

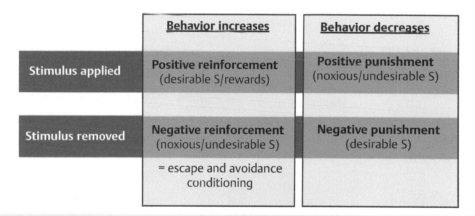

|  | **Behavior increases** | **Behavior decreases** |
|---|---|---|
| **Stimulus applied** | Positive reinforcement (desirable S/rewards) | Positive punishment (noxious/undesirable S) |
| **Stimulus removed** | Negative reinforcement (noxious/undesirable S) = escape and avoidance conditioning | Negative punishment (desirable S) |

**Fig. 18.12** Operant conditioning.

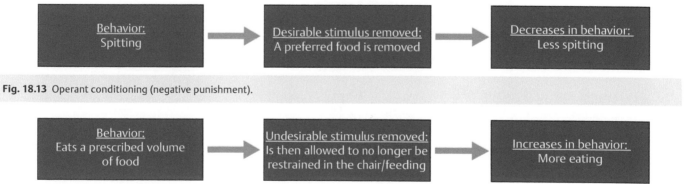

Behavior: Spitting → Desirable stimulus removed: A preferred food is removed → Decreases in behavior: Less spitting

**Fig. 18.13** Operant conditioning (negative punishment).

Behavior: Eats a prescribed volume of food → Undesirable stimulus removed: Is then allowed to no longer be restrained in the chair/feeding → Increases in behavior: More eating

**Fig. 18.14** Operant conditioning (negative reinforcement).

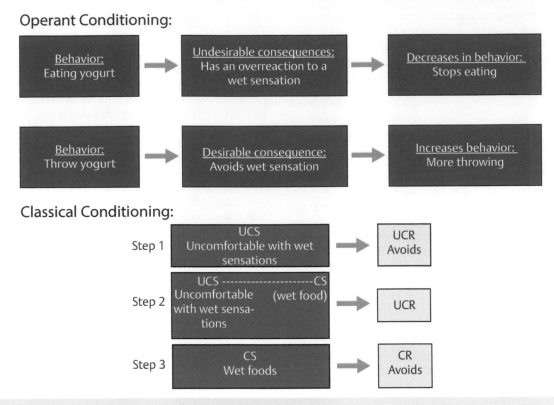

**Fig. 18.15** Operant conditioning and classical conditioning applied to food.

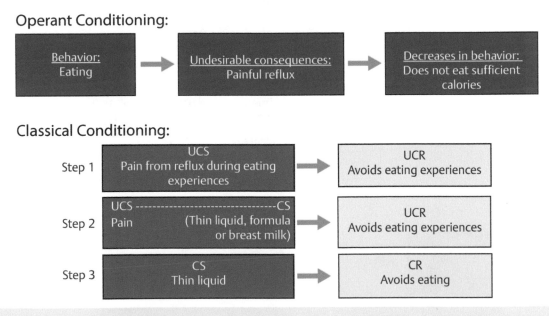

**Fig. 18.16** Operant conditioning and classical conditioning applied to food.

A behavior is classified as a problem behavior when that behavior (1) interferes with the child's ability to learn new skills; (2) interferes with the child exhibiting skills he has already learned; and/or (3) is harmful or disruptive to self and/or others. Drinking in the scenario just described could be considered a problem behavior because it is harmful to the self. The avoidance of drinking could also be classified as a problem behavior because this avoidance causes the child to fail to gain weight. Eating is the appropriate response to hunger. When a child is not eating, the professional should ask why, and a thorough evaluation should be conducted to understand the etiology.

## 18.17 Behavioral Feeding Therapy Programs

As discussed earlier in this chapter, there are two primary dimensions along which the techniques used to teach children to eat are delineated: (1) systematic desensitization and flooding, which are the strategies primarily using classical conditioning; and (2) positive and negative reinforcement, which are primarily operant conditioning strategies. These different sets of strategies often have quite different short-term feeding goals: (1) skill development versus (2) increased consumption of volume of food (**Table 18.1**).

Programs that use systematic desensitization are based primarily in the classical conditioning theoretical perspective that children don't eat because of the associative aversive conditioning that occurs when children are in pain or discomfort during the process of eating. Very often, this pain or discomfort is a result of these children being given foods that they do not have the sensory tolerance for or the oral-motor skills required to eat them (i.e., developmental problems). The pain or discomfort could also be present secondary to some type of medical problem or nutritional deficit as discussed earlier (**Fig. 18.17**).

To learn to eat using systematic desensitization, a child would need to start at the lowest possible component skill level and acquire that skill without physical discomfort or distress. Positive reinforcement is applied when the child achieves that skill level, either (1) naturally because of the success of mastering that skill level or via social reinforcers (e.g., being smiled at, praised, imitated), or (2) via an object reinforcer (e.g., toy, sticker) for completing that skill step. The child then moves on to learning the next skill step in the sequence of necessary actions required for eating (i.e., a hierarchy of steps to eating). An example of a hierarchy of steps to eating that would be used in the Sequential-Oral-Sensory (SOS) Approach[45] (copyright Toomey, 1990–2015) would start with the skill of eating beginning with looking at a food, then interacting with the food in some manner. Smelling, touching, tasting, and finally eating are higher steps in this approach. Systematic desensitization builds on a successive skill acquisition approach to teaching children to eat.

Any program that requires a child to swallow a bite of food (which would be the highest skill) to receive a reinforcer (e.g.,

access to an iPad or tablet, money, or a TV show) is using both flooding and positive reinforcement. Any program that employs a strategy in which a child must stay in the chair until a prescribed amount of food is consumed is also using flooding, paired with negative reinforcement. This is learning through negative reinforcement because this technique teaches the child to eat the prescribed amount of food to avoid/escape the undesirable experience of being made to stay in the chair and/or being force-fed.

## 18.18 Focus of Feeding Therapy Programs

Both types of approaches (flooding; systematic desensitization), and both types of reinforcement programs (positive; negative) can be used to teach most children to eat sufficient volumes of food to meet their nutritional goals and, if needed, to transition off nutritional supplements and feeding tubes. However, the goals of these different types of approaches and programs frequently occur in a different order. Systematic desensitization programs typically focus on teaching skill development in the short term, with a goal of transitioning to an age-appropriate diet and off any supplements or tube feedings as the long-term goal. In flooding and negative reinforcement programs, frequently the treatment plan focuses initially on increasing the volume of foods (fluids and purees) that a child eats in the short term. If the child is being tube fed, a typical initial goal would be to transition the child off the tube feedings and onto a liquid and pureed diet. After the child learns to consume the prescribed amount of purees and liquids, the treatment focus then may shift to teaching the additional skills needed to transition the child to an age-appropriate diet (i.e., fluids, purees, meltable table foods, soft cubes, soft mechanicals, hard mechanicals). The focus is frequently on increasing volume of foods that the child has the skill to eat first, and then teaching the skills needed to eat more challenging foods.

Both approaches reach the same long-term end goal of the child eating adequate volumes of an age-appropriate diet, but they do so in very different manners. It is therefore important to consider the differing short-term goals when one is comparing the two basic types of feeding programs. Outcomes should be similar

**Table 18.1** Approaches to feeding therapy

| Classical conditioning strategy | Operant conditioning strategy | Primary feeding goal |
|---|---|---|
| Systematic desensitization | Positive reinforcement<br>1. Program uses natural reinforcers (e.g., praise, smile, play, enjoyment of food sensation)<br>2. Program uses object reinforcers (e.g., iPad, toy, sticker, favorite food) | Skill development |
| Flooding | Negative reinforcement<br>1. Paired with object reinforcement<br>2. Paired with access to caregiver | Volume consumed |
| Flooding | Positive reinforcement using object reinforcers | Volume consumed |

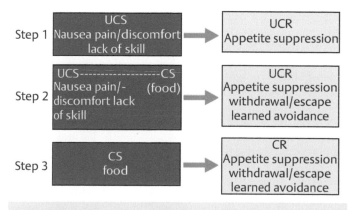

**Fig. 18.17** Classical conditioning applied to food.

for any comparative research study between the two types of approaches. It would not be expected that a child using systematic desensitization with positive reinforcement would necessarily be eating a lot of foods in the short term. It would be expected that the child be demonstrating progress in advancing up a series of steps to eating. Systematic desensitization programs often focus on skill development as the primary goal and do not necessarily focus on immediate increased volume as the primary goal. One benefit of using such a program is the ability of the team to continue exploring medical/skill issues that might be subtle, while beginning the process of teaching a child to enjoy eating.

When a child is being weaned from tube feedings, the two approaches might do things in different orders, while eventually reaching the same goal. Systematic desensitization programs might begin with slow skill development and use the PEG feedings to ensure adequate nutrition. Once skill has been achieved the child would be weaned onto an age-appropriate diet. Flooding programs might focus on increasing calories from liquids and purees, weaning off the tube feedings onto liquids and purees. Once the child is taking adequate nutrition from these simpler-texture sources, therapy would shift focus to transitioning onto a more age-appropriate diet. Caregivers and professionals should take this difference into account when choosing the right approach for a specific child.

Most intervention programs use a combination of strategies to achieve increased volume while increasing skill. In a review of outcomes for 38 behavioral feeding programs, 97% used positive reinforcement strategies with food/drink reinforcers and/or object/game/activity reinforcers.[4] In this same review, escape prevention strategies were used in 60% of the studies. In a second review of 13 psychological intervention studies of food refusal, 82% used behavioral treatment, 54% used nutrition manipulation (e.g., cutting tube feedings), 73% included caregiver training, and 46% included oral-motor therapy strategies.[46]

When volume is the initial goal (typically flooding programs), research studies report 40–90% of children wean off their tube feedings within the specified time of the study, with a range of time to transition between 1 month and 2 years of treatment. The range was highly influenced by the number of oral calories that the child was eating before the treatment was initiated. The studies used both negative and positive reinforcement techniques, with up to 33% relapse reported 4 months after discharge.[4,13,46,47] Medically complex infants and young children are the most likely population to fail out of these programs.[47,48] This is probably due to the ongoing medical issues as well as the significant skill deficits seen in younger children.

When increased food repertoire is the primary goal (reflective of skill development—typically the primary goal of systematic desensitization programs), fewer studies are available. Many published studies lack information on food variety. Boyd[49] evaluated the growth of food repertoires in children treated using the SOS Approach to Feeding. This program uses a very structured, systematic desensitization approach with natural, positive reinforcement to teach children the skills to eat a wide variety of age-appropriate foods. In this program, the necessary sensory and oral-motor skills for eating the age-appropriate diet are taught first, and then the focus shifts to increased volume of foods/fluid consumed, followed by weaning off any tube or supplement dependency if possible. Using the SOS Approach to Feeding, half of

children seen for feeding disorders ($n = 37$) increased the number of foods represented on a 3-day diet history by 41% across a 12-week period.[49] For children who were 100% tube-dependent ($n = 3$), this approach took between 60 and 72 weekly sessions to transition off a G-tube. However, on average, the children with G-tubes had demonstrated the ability to eat 102 different foods across the course of treatment and were regularly eating at least 10 different proteins, starches, fruits, and/or vegetables at the time they transitioned fully off their G-tube (100% oral feeding). In an unpublished study of 30 children using this systematic desensitization approach, those children who could eat some type of food/fluid by mouth at the start of therapy took approximately 1 year to transition off their tube and onto an age-appropriate diet. Those children who started therapy who were 100% G-tube dependent (0% oral intake), took an average of 2 years to transition off the G-tube onto an age-appropriate diet. None of these children had to have their G-tube replaced later (up to 1 year informal update).

All behavioral feeding approaches have advantages and disadvantages. Families and therapists need to recognize these and make informed decisions regarding the best approach(s) to achieve the desired goals (**Table 18.2**).

## 18.19 Case Presentation Part 3

In returning to Jonathan, there are several questions that should be asked when one is determining what treatment approach might be used to achieve the caregivers' goal of tube weaning. First, what progress can be expected in terms of transitioning to an age-appropriate diet? To look to the answer for this question, one must recall that Jonathan is currently 18 months of age, corrected. He has received developmental services, including feeding, for 16 months, and his highest functioning is at a developmental age of 8 months. Therefore, developmentally, his age-appropriate sources of nutrition would be liquids and purees, with an expectation of beginning to explore meltable foods. At 18 months of age, Jonathan is occasionally consuming both liquids and purees, although in very small volumes. He reportedly takes a few sips of fluid, twice a day, and will take a few small bites of baby foods from a spoon as well. Jonathan is unable to chew meltable foods because he lacks the ability to move his tongue off midline to place foods along his molars. From this perspective, his current food source would be appropriate for a negative reinforcement program approach focused on increasing volume.

The second question to ask is "What are the chances Jonathan will succeed with a tube weaning now?" Jonathan's parents believe he is not eating enough food because he is not hungry secondary to the tube feedings. They feel if the tube feedings were decreased, Jonathan would eat more. However, given his skill deficits Jonathan may not be able to increase his intake even if he is hungry. Also, even if he increases his oral intake, he may not be able to increase sufficiently to equal the amount cut from his tube feedings, and his growth may suffer as a result.

A third question asks how much fluid and puree Jonathan would need to consume orally to transition fully off his G-tube. For typical 16- to 18-month-old children, 60% of their calories would normally be consumed in table foods and 40% in fluids.[50] Children in Jonathan's chronological age range usually have transitioned all or most of the way off baby food purees and onto textured table

**Table 18.2** Advantages and disadvantages of feeding therapy approaches

| Positive reinforcement + systematic desensitization | | Negative reinforcement + flooding | |
| Advantage | Disadvantage | Advantage | Disadvantage |
|---|---|---|---|
| Creates lasting behavior change as child learns to eat because of the skills acquired | Takes time to learn new skills fully | Quickly teaches swallowing of liquids/purees | Learns to eat to escape the punishment of being force-fed and/or made to stay in chair |
| Is similar to how typically developing children learn to eat | May not necessarily lead to increased volume of foods consumed initially | Increases caloric intake by mouth in a short time frame, resulting in decreased volume through tube feedings | Child may relapse and lose gains in volume achieved |
| Builds intrinsic motivation | Child may learn to eat only for the reward when object reinforcers are used | | Creates external motivation |
| Is enjoyable for child and adults | | | May be aversive, which creates high adrenaline and leads to appetite disruption |
| Involves active participation | | | Cannot use with textured table foods, so all children are placed on puree and fluid diets |

food diets, which are more calorie-dense. They are also generally drinking regular milk versus a nutritional supplement. However, despite Jonathan being the physical size of a 16- to 18-month-old child, his developmental age is only 8 months. This can create a challenge in deciding what foods and fluids to use for transitioning Jonathan off his PEG feedings. Of course, the question of how to transition Jonathan off his PEG feedings (and onto what foods and fluids) is best left to his medical team and his dietitian. However, close collaboration with Jonathan's occupational therapist and speech pathologist, who are both working on his skill deficits, will be necessary.

## 18.19.1 For This Case, What Would Be a Best Approach?

Given his developmental feeding age, Jonathan could possibly begin weaning off his 100% tube dependency by orally increasing the volume he takes from a cup and from purees. Jonathan is currently taking formula; the expected primary nutritional source for children who are 8 months of age. Jonathan could be a candidate for a systematic desensitization/positive reinforcement approach to transitioning off his G-tube, as well as a flooding/negative reinforcement approach.

However, it is important to recall that Jonathan had very aversive reactions to oral stimulation when he was a baby, which caused him to stop eating by mouth at 2 months of age. Jonathan would therefore likely do poorly in an approach that was based on flooding. Additionally, given his unresolved medical issues (he continues to vomit, although he has not been diagnosed with GERD at this time), he is at high risk to fail in his G-tube transitioning if a flooding approach is taken. Children who are the least successful with flooding include those born prematurely, those with developmental delays, those with difficulty chewing and/or moving foods around in the mouth, and those with GERD or lung disease.[47,48] Jonathan meets all of these criteria (prior oxygen use and GERD diagnosis, as well as his premature birth and skill deficits).

In Jonathan's case, the therapist and family decided to begin a slow weaning process. He was referred once more to a gastroenterologist to work toward optimal comfort given his unresolved vomiting. At that time, Jonathan was diagnosed with a food intolerance and was placed on a specialized formula that improved his vomiting frequency. A systematic desensitization program was developed to overcome Jonathan's learned avoidance behaviors, using repeated pairing of food with play. Given his developmental delays, as well as his slow progress despite intensive therapy interventions, it is probably unrealistic to believe Jonathan will transition to a textured table-food diet soon. It would be much easier for Jonathan to meet the calorie requirements he needs to transition off his G-tube if he could eat textured table foods versus just purees. However, it may be possible for Jonathan to slowly learn to consume enough volume of liquids and purees to transition off his G-tube while he builds the skills for eating more textured foods. He will need to remain in his developmental therapies to work toward advancing his global developmental skills first. As he progresses in those therapies, Jonathan can hopefully gain the feeding skills needed to make the transition to a more advanced diet.

## 18.20 Questions

1. Positive reinforcement is a behavioral principle used to change behavior and is used in many feeding programs. The definition of positive reinforcement is

A. Being nice to a child when he does what you want

B. Applying a consequence that is desirable to that child, with the intent of increasing a desired behavior

C. Giving candy to a child every time she takes a bite of a new food

D. Using a sticker chart in a classroom to improve children's behavior

E. Keeping a child in a chair until he takes a bite of food—and then letting him down to play

**2.** Behavioral techniques are used in many feeding programs. When using a behavioral technique, it is important to:

A. Use a consistent, single approach to all children within the same program

B. Make sure there is no skill deficit that needs to be addressed

C. Pick the correct technique, or set of techniques, to meet the stated goals

D. Use trained therapists exclusively; caregivers are not important because, once the behaviors are changed, the behaviors will remain

E. Keep the child in the hospital until she can eat everything orally

**3.** Feeding problems are often multifactorial. A child may demonstrate skills that appear within normal limits in play but struggle in eating because:

A. The coordination of multiple systems is more complex than any use of single skills.

B. Children like to get attention for not eating.

C. The child is not hungry enough.

D. Sensory skills are limited to just tasting and the texture of the food, and are the most important skill for eating.

E. Children who are not growing are not truly thriving.

**4.** Operant conditioning focused behavioral feeding programs are very successful. The population of children who demonstrate the least success in these programs are:

A. Children who are older than 4 years of age

B. Children with mental health problems

C. Children who are very picky

D. Children with sensory issues

E. Children with medical complications or who were born prematurely

**5.** Different behavioral feeding programs all may work for certain populations. The key issues when determining which program is best for a child include which of the following?

A. The amount of food the child currently eats

B. The priority of the family—volume or variety

C. The severity of the temper tantrums during mealtimes

D. The amount of money the insurance will pay for a program

E. The age of the child

# 18.21 Answers and Explanations

**1. Correct: applying a consequence that is desirable to that child, with the intent of increasing a desired behavior (B).**
*Positive* means apply, *reinforcement* means to increase desired behavior. But the key to reinforcement is that it must be specific to that child. (**A, C, D**) are incorrect because they do not consider the child's specific desirable consequences. (**E**) is incorrect because it is an example of a negative reinforcement approach.

**2. Correct: pick the correct technique, or set of techniques, to meet the stated goals (C).**
Most behavioral programs use a variety of techniques, and specific children react best to specific approaches. (**A**) is not correct because different children require different approaches, and most programs use a variety of approaches. (**B**) is not correct because skill deficits can be addressed using behavioral approaches. (**D**) is incorrect because many studies show a regression in volume at home. (**E**) is incorrect because behavioral programs can be done in the hospital and at home.

**3. Correct: the coordination of multiple systems is more complex than any use of single skills (A).**
There are seven different areas that must coordinate for eating to be successful. (**B, C, D, E**) are incorrect because they do not consider the synaction across the seven areas of function.

**4. Correct: children with medical complications or who were born prematurely (E).**
(**A, B, C, D**) are incorrect for they have not been shown to be risk factors for failing from a behavioral feeding program.

**5. Correct: the priority of the family—volume or variety (B).**
Behavioral programs approach this disorder with an initial focus on increasing volume to decrease reliance on tube feedings, or with an initial focus on decreasing distress during mealtimes and teaching the skill of eating a wide variety of age-appropriate foods. (**A, C, D, E**) may be considerations, and they may inform the therapy team about the length of time therapy may take, but they are not the key differences seen between different therapy approaches.

## References

[1] Crist W, Napier-Phillips A. Mealtime behaviors of young children: a comparison of normative and clinical data. *J Dev Behav Pediatr* 2001;22(5):279–286

[2] Field D, Garland M, Williams K. Correlates of specific childhood feeding problems. *J Paediatr Child Health* 2003;39(4):299–304

[3] Sharp WG, Jaquess DL, Morton JF, Herzinger CV. Pediatric feeding disorders: a quantitative synthesis of treatment outcomes. *Clin Child Fam Psychol Rev* 2010;13(4):348–365 doi: 10.1007/s10567-010-0079-7

[4] Williams KE, Field DG, Seiverling L. Food refusal in children: a review of the literature. *Res Dev Disabil* 2010;31(3):625–633

[5] Skuse D. Identification and management of problem eaters. *Arch Dis Child* 1993;69(5):604–608

[6] Bryant-Waugh R, Markham L, Kreipe RE, Walsh BT. Feeding and eating disorders in childhood. *Int J Eat Disord* 2010;43(2):98–111 doi: 10.1002/eat.20795

[7] Fox D, Campagna EJ, Friedlander J, Partrick DA, Rees DI, Kempe A. National trends and outcomes of pediatric gastrostomy tube placement. *J Pediatr Gastroenterol Nutr* 2014;59(5):582–588 doi: 10.1097/MPG.0000000000000468

[8] Cardona Cano S, Tiemeier H, Van Hoeken D, et al. Trajectories of picky eating during childhood: a general population study. *Int J Eat Disord* 2015;48(6):570–579 doi: 10.1002/eat.22384

[9] Williams PG, Dalrymple N, Neal J. Eating habits of children with autism. *Pediatr Nurs* 2000;26(3):259–264

[10] Levine A, Bachar L, Tsangen Z, et al. Screening criteria for diagnosis of infantile feeding disorders as a cause of poor feeding or food refusal. *J Pediatr Gastroenterol Nutr* 2011;52(5):563–568 doi: 10.1097/MPG.0b013e3181ff72d2

[11] Reilly SM, Skuse DH, Wolke D, Stevenson J. Oral-motor dysfunction in children who fail to thrive: organic or non-organic? *Dev Med Child Neurol* 1999;41(2):115–122

[12] Anak K. My Picky Eaters. 2009. http://mypickyeaters.wordpress.com/2009/08/24/picky-eaters-poor-feeding (Accessed August 12, 2012)

[13] Cornwell SL, Kelly K, Austin L. Pediatric feeding disorders: effectiveness of multidisciplinary inpatient treatment of gastrostomy-tube dependent children. *Child Health Care* 2010;39:214–231

[14] Wilensky DS, Ginsberg G, Altman M, Tulchinsky TH, Ben Yishay F, Auerbach J. A community based study of failure to thrive in Israel. *Arch Dis Child* 1996;75(2):145–148

[15] Telles MS, Macedo CS. Relationship between the motor development of the body and the acquisition of oral skills [in Portuguese]. *Pro Fono* 2008;20(2):117–122

[16] Stolovitz P, Gisel EG. Circumoral movements in response to three different food textures in children 6 months to 2 years of age. *Dysphagia* 1991;6(1):17–25

[17] Gisel EG. Chewing cycles in 2- to 8-year-old normal children: a developmental profile. *Am J Occup Ther* 1988;42(1):40–46

[18] Gisel EG. Effect of food texture on the development of chewing of children between six months and two years of age. *Dev Med Child Neurol* 1991;33(1):69–79

[19] Green JR, Moore CA, Ruark JL, Rodda PR, Morvée WT, VanWitzenburg MJ. Development of chewing in children from 12 to 48 months: longitudinal study of EMG patterns. *J Neurophysiol* 1997;77(5):2704–2716

[20] Tamura F, Chigira A, Ishii H, Nishikata H, Mukai Y. Assessment of the development of hand and mouth coordination when taking food into the oral cavity. *Int J Orofacial Myology* 2000;26:33–43

[21] Briefel RR, Reidy K, Karwe V, Jankowski L, Hendricks K. Toddlers' transition to table foods: Impact on nutrient intakes and food patterns. *J Am Diet Assoc* 2004;104(1, Suppl 1):s38–s44

[22] Enneman A, Hernández L, Campos R, Vossenaar M, Solomons NW. Dietary characteristics of complementary foods offered to Guatemalan infants vary between urban and rural settings. *Nutr Res* 2009;29(7):470–479

[23] Davis AM, Bruce AS, Khasawneh R, Schulz T, Fox C, Dunn W. Sensory processing issues in young children presenting to an outpatient feeding clinic. *J Pediatr Gastroenterol Nutr* 2013;56(2):156–160 doi: 10.1097/MPG.0b013e3182736e19

[24] Yi SH, Joung YS, Choe YH, Kim EH, Kwon JY. Sensory processing difficulties in toddlers with nonorganic failure-to-thrive and feeding problems. *J Pediatr Gastroenterol Nutr* 2015;60(6):819–824 doi: 10.1097/MPG.0000000000000707

[25] WHO Multicentre Growth Reference Study Group. Complementary feeding in the WHO Multicentre Growth Reference Study. *Acta Paediatr Suppl* 2006;450:27–37

[26] Ross E. Eating development in young children: understanding the complex interplay of developmental domains. In: Saavedra J, Dattilo A, eds. Early Nutrition and Long-Term Health: Mechanisms, Consequences, and Opportunities. London, UK: Elsevier; 2006:230–264

[27] Blissett J, Bennett C, Donohoe J, Rogers S, Higgs S. Predicting successful introduction of novel fruit to preschool children. *J Acad Nutr Diet* 2012;112(12):1959–1967

[28] Houston-Price C, Butler L, Shiba P. Visual exposure impacts on toddlers' willingness to taste fruits and vegetables. *Appetite* 2009;53(3):450–453

[29] Carruth BR, Ziegler PJ, Gordon A, Barr SI. Prevalence of picky eaters among infants and toddlers and their caregivers' decisions about offering a new food. *J Am Diet Assoc* 2004;104(1, Suppl 1):s57–s64

[30] Dubois L, Farmer A, Girard M, Peterson K, Tatone-Tokuda F. Problem eating behaviors related to social factors and body weight in preschool children: a longitudinal study. *Int J Behav Nutr Phys Act* 2007;4:9

[31] Lewinsohn PM, Holm-Denoma JM, Gau JM, et al. Problematic eating and feeding behaviors of 36-month-old children. *Int J Eat Disord* 2005;38(3):208–219 doi: 10.1002/eat.20175

[32] Mascola AJ, Bryson SW, Agras WS. Picky eating during childhood: a longitudinal study to age 11 years. *Eat Behav* 2010;11(4):253–257 doi: 10.1016/j.eatbeh.2010.05.006

[33] Dubois L, Farmer AP, Girard M, Peterson K. Preschool children's eating behaviours are related to dietary adequacy and body weight. *Eur J Clin Nutr* 2007;61(7):846–855

[34] Bandini LG, Anderson SE, Curtin C, et al. Food selectivity in children with autism spectrum disorders and typically developing children. *J Pediatr* 2010;157(2):259–264

[35] Emond A, Emmett P, Steer C, Golding J. Feeding symptoms, dietary patterns, and growth in young children with autism spectrum disorders. *Pediatrics* 2010;126(2):e337–e342

[36] Ross ES, Browne JV. Feeding outcomes in preterm infants after discharge from the neonatal intensive care unit (NICU): a systematic review. *Newborn Infant Nurs Rev* 2013;13(2):87–93

[37] Christie L, Hine RJ, Parker JG, Burks W. Food allergies in children affect nutrient intake and growth. *J Am Diet Assoc* 2002;102(11):1648–1651

[38] McHenry M, Watson W. Impact of primary food allergies on the introduction of other foods amongst Canadian children and their siblings. *Allergy Asthma Clin Immunol* 2014;10(1):26 doi: 10.1186/1710-1492-10-26

[39] Brostoff J, Gamlin L. Food Allergies and Food Intolerance: The Complete Guide to Their Identification and Treatment. Rochester, VT: Inner Traditions/Bear & Co; 2000

[40] Wright C, Birks E. Risk factors for failure to thrive: a population-based survey. *Child Care Health Dev* 2000;26(1):5–16

[41] Gueron-Sela N, Atzaba-Poria N, Meiri G, Yerushalmi B. Maternal worries about child underweight mediate and moderate the relationship between child feeding disorders and mother-child feeding interactions. *J Pediatr Psychol* 2011;36(7):827–836 doi: 10.1093/jpepsy/jsr001

[42] Farrow CV, Galloway AT, Fraser K. Sibling eating behaviours and differential child feeding practices reported by parents. *Appetite* 2009;52(2):307–312 doi: 10.1016/j.appet.2008.10.009

[43] Gerrig RJ, Zimbardo PG. Psychology and Life. 16th ed. Boston, MA: Allyn and Bacon; 2002

[44] Bandura A, Walters RH. Social Learning Theory. New York, NY: General Learning Press; 1977

[45] Toomey KA, Ross ES. SOS Approach to Feeding. Perspectives on swallowing and swallowing disorders. *Dysphagia* 2011;20(3):82–87

[46] Lukens CT, Silverman AH. Systematic review of psychological interventions for pediatric feeding problems. *J Pediatr Psychol* 2014;39(8):903–917 doi: 10.1093/jpepsy/jsu040

[47] Foy T, Czyewski D, Phillips S, Ligon S, Baldwin J, Klish W. Treatment of severe feeding refusal in infants and toddlers. *Infants Young Child* 1997;9(3):26–35

[48] Benoit D, Coolbear J. Post-traumatic feeding disorders in infancy: behaviors predicting treatment outcome. *Infant Ment Health J* 1998;19:409–421

[49] Boyd K. The Effectiveness of the Sequential Oral Sensory Approach Group Feeding Program. Colorado Springs: Colorado School of Professional Psychology; 2007

[50] Fox MK, Reidy K, Karwe V, Ziegler P. Average portions of foods commonly eaten by infants and toddlers in the United States. *J Am Diet Assoc* 2006;106(1, Suppl 1):S66–S76

## Suggested Reading

[1] Edelman GM. Neural Darwinism: The Theory of Neuronal Group Selection. New York, NY: Basic Books; 1987

[2] Pavlov IP, Anrep GV. Conditioned Reflexes: An Investigation of the Physiological Activity of the Cerebral Cortex. Oxford, UK: Oxford University Press; 1927

[3] Skinner BF. About Behaviorism. New York, NY: Knopf; 1974

[4] VanDahm K, Ed. Pediatric Feeding Disorders: Evaluation and Treatment. Framingham, MA: Therapro, Inc.; 2013

# 19 Neurodegenerative Disease

*Lauren Tabor Gray and Emily K. Plowman*

## Summary

The three neurodegenerative diseases discussed in this chapter represent populations at high risk for the development of dysphagia. A multidisciplinary approach is likely to facilitate the best management and care for these specialized patient populations, whose rehabilitation potential is unique. It is imperative that clinicians be knowledgeable on the disease pathophysiology, expected trajectories, and available evidence-based treatment options. Further, proactive patient and caregiver education is of paramount importance for the prevention of pulmonary sequelae, malnutrition, and dehydration.

## Keywords

deglutition, dysphagia, dysarthria, neurodegenerative disease, management, evaluation

### Learning Objectives

- Understand the pathophysiology of three prevalent neurodegenerative diseases:
  - Amyotrophic lateral sclerosis (ALS)
  - Parkinson's disease (PD)
  - Multiple sclerosis (MS)
- Define prominent swallowing impairments observed in ALS, PD, and MS and describe the underlying neuropathophysiological framework that gives rise to these impairments
- Describe evidence-based treatment and management strategies for dysphagia in patients with neurodegenerative disease

## 19.1 Introduction

This chapter discusses dysphagia in neurodegenerative disease, with a focus on amyotrophic lateral sclerosis (ALS), Parkinson's disease (PD), and multiple sclerosis (MS). **Table 19.1** provides an overview of each of the diseases discussed. Detailed information is provided regarding the underlying neuropathophysiology and the associated swallowing impairment profiles. The chapter then summarizes current evidence-based treatment strategies and provides recommendations for the care of these individuals.

Typically, neurodegenerative diseases affect the central and peripheral neural components of deglutition, including the cortex, basal ganglia, brainstem, cranial nerves, corticobulbar tracts, and, peripherally, the muscles of bulbar function. The extent to which the neural control and function are impaired depends on the specific disease type, the associated progression rates, and the availability of evidence-based treatment options. Understanding the basic neuroanatomical and pathological framework of each of these diseases and how they relate to swallowing function will facilitate the best possible management and prognosis of dysphagia in these special patient populations. Neurodegenerative diseases necessitate careful monitoring, frequent reevaluation, and early and proactive patient and caregiver education. Treatment trajectories are unique in neurodegenerative patient populations, with a typical focus on the *maintenance* of function rather than improvement or gains. Management of dysphagia in these populations is complex and multidisciplinary, and it involves many variables that change at varying rates (dependent on disease type) over time. Therefore, the health care provider, patient, and caregivers must understand the nature and typical course of the disease and associated risks of dysphagia to facilitate learning and to maximize functional outcomes.[1] Case studies will be presented

**Table 19.1** Summary of the underlying pathophysiology, disease onset, symptoms, and prognosis for three prominent neurodegenerative diseases

|  | Pathophysiology | Typical onset | Hallmark symptoms | Prognosis |
|---|---|---|---|---|
| Amyotrophic lateral sclerosis | Both UMN and LMN degeneration in the cortex, brainstem, spinal cord, corticospinal tracts, corticobulbar tracts, NMJ, muscles | 65 years[1]<br>M/F ratio: 1.5:1[1] | • Spasticity<br>• Flaccidity<br>• Fasciculations<br>• Weakness<br>• Fatigue | Terminal, leading cause of death is respiratory insufficiency<br>Rapidly progressing with typical survival 2–5 years (depending on onset type) |
| Parkinson's disease | Loss of dopaminergic neurons in the substantia nigra and basal ganglia | 62 years[2]<br>M/F ratio: 1.49:1[3] | • Bradykinesia<br>• Tremor<br>• Cogwheel rigidity<br>• Postural instability | Mortality attributed to complications of the disease, such as falling and aspiration pneumonia (leading cause of death), not the disease itself<br>Life expectancy 5–10 years less than general population depending on age of diagnosis[6] |
| Multiple sclerosis | Demyelination of nerve fibers in the central nervous system, brain, and spinal cord | 20–40 years[5]<br>M/F ratio: 1:2.3[5] | • Weakness<br>• Spasticity<br>• Sensory impairment | Life expectancy 10 years less than general population; highly variable dependent upon type |

*Abbreviations:* LMN, lower motor neuron; NMJ, neuromuscular junction; UMN, upper motor neuron.
*Sources:* Mehta, 2014,[1] Factor & Weiner, 2008[2]; Wirdefeldt et al, 2011,[3] Oosterveld et al, 2014,[4] Miller & Britton, 2011.[5]

throughout the chapter to provide illustrative examples of key concepts and to facilitate learning of the material.

## 19.2 Amyotrophic Lateral Sclerosis

### 19.2.1 Case Presentation: Patient History

BH is a 64-year-old woman who has worked in administration for the past 17 years. Her responsibilities at work include speaking on the telephone, typing, and writing throughout the day. Over the past year, she has noticed changes in the quality of her voice characterized by increased hoarseness, imprecise articulation, strain, and reduced volume. BH has also noted intermittent difficulty swallowing characterized by coughing with thin liquids and difficulty swallowing her medications, and she complains of foods (tough solids, such as meats and breads) sticking in her throat. Due to these complaints, BH is having great difficulty fulfilling her responsibilities as an administrator at work. BH is becoming increasingly concerned as she perceives increased generalized weakness and fatigue; therefore, she schedules an appointment with her primary care physician.

### 19.2.2 Overview of Amyotrophic Lateral Sclerosis

Amyotrophic lateral sclerosis (ALS), or Lou Gehrig's disease, is a rapidly progressing degenerative disease that involves gradual destruction of both upper and lower motor neurons. *Amyotrophic* is derived from the Greek language elements *a* ("no"), *myo* ("muscle"), and *trophic* ("nourishment")—literally, no muscle nourishment. *Lateral* denotes the areas in the spinal cord where nerve cells are affected, but in this disease the damage includes both the upper (cortex, brainstem) and lower (corticobulbar/spinal tracts, neuromuscular junction, myofibers) motor neurons in the brain and spinal cord. *Sclerosis* (hardening) occurs as the motor neuron cells degenerate. ALS is the most commonly occurring of the motor neuron diseases, a classification of disorders in which motor neurons that control muscle movement, tone, and contraction gradually deteriorate with unknown etiology. Other motor neuron diseases include progressive bulbar palsy, primary progressive muscle atrophy, primary lateral sclerosis, and Kennedy's disease (spinal muscular atrophy). Some of these other motor neuron diseases may eventually advance to ALS, which is the most aggressive form of motor neuron disease.[2]

A diagnosis of ALS is made using the El-Escorial World Federation of Neurology criterion[3] and requires confirmation of the involvement of both upper motor neurons (UMNs) and lower motor neurons (LMNs) with progressive spread of signs to other regions of the body on clinical examination, electromyographic testing, and/or neuropathological examination.[3] The prevalence of ALS is 3.9 per 100,000 individuals in the United States and is more common in men than in women (M:F ratio, 1.5:1), with typical disease onset occurring between 55 and 65 years of age.[4] Average survival rates vary between 2 and 5 years and are largely dependent on disease onset type.[5] Diagnosis is usually considered sporadic (of unknown etiology); however, 10% of cases are familial with autosomal dominant, recessive, or X-linked transmission.[6]

Generalized weakness is the primary symptom and is observed in impairments due to both UMN and LMN involvement. Cognitive abilities typically remain intact during onset and progression, although recent studies highlight the development of impairments in executive functioning that overlap with symptoms of frontotemporal dementia (FTD) in 30–50% of individuals with ALS.[7] FTD involves degeneration of spindle fibers in the frontal and temporal lobes, leading to impairments in language and behavior as well as symptoms associated with dementia, such as personality changes, mental rigidity, and impaired regulation of personal conduct.[8]

Onset of ALS is typically classified by the involvement of spinal or bulbar (cranial) nerves, and involvement of upper and/or lower motor neurons. Involvement of spinal nerves results in reduced upper- and lower-extremity function. Bulbar nerve involvement leads to impairments in the muscles involved in speech and swallowing. Onset is usually dominated by either spinal or bulbar presentation; however, as the disease progresses, both spinal and bulbar symptoms are eventually observed. Limb motor involvement is the most prevalent site of disease onset, occurring in 70% of cases, whereas bulbar disease onset is reported in 30% of ALS cases.[5]

The neurologic underpinnings of ALS involve both the central and the peripheral nervous system. The central nervous system comprises the cerebral cortex, brainstem, and cervical and lumbar spinal cord and is affected by loss of pyramidal neurons that make up the descending pathway of the corticospinal motor tract, which controls voluntary muscle movement. Disease within the central nervous system leads to changes in neuromuscular status affecting inhibitory and stimulatory actions of the muscles. Therefore, hypertonicity (inhibitory impairment) and hypotonicity (stimulatory impairment) are observed as the disease progresses.

The peripheral nervous system includes the cranial nerves and myoneural junction, as well as nerves to muscles and sensory organs. Degeneration of neurons leads to impaired function of cranial nerves V, VII, IX, X, and XII, leading to common symptoms of dysphagia and dysarthria.[9] Oculomotor function is generally well preserved because cranial nerves III, IV, and VI are spared.

Spasticity caused by UMN degeneration leads to muscle stiffness, muscle slowness, hyperreflexia (overactive reflexes, such as the gag reflex), and hypertonicity (muscles with increased tone).[9] LMN degeneration leads to muscle atrophy or weakening that functionally relates to decreased strength, decreased force, fasciculations (involuntary muscle twitches and contractions), and flaccidity (reduction or loss of voluntary muscle movement).[10] Both the UMN and LMN degeneration lead to increasing difficulties and a typical constellation of speech and swallowing signs in individuals with ALS; **Fig. 19.1** provides an overview. Further, UMN and LMN degeneration contributes to respiratory symptoms and breathing complications due to muscle weakness and stiffness of the diaphragm, which can further impair airway defense mechanisms during deglutition (such as cough).

### 19.2.3 Case Presentation: BH Diagnosis

BH underwent a general physical evaluation with her primary care physician following her 1-year history of progressively worsening dysarthria, dysphagia, and generalized weakness.

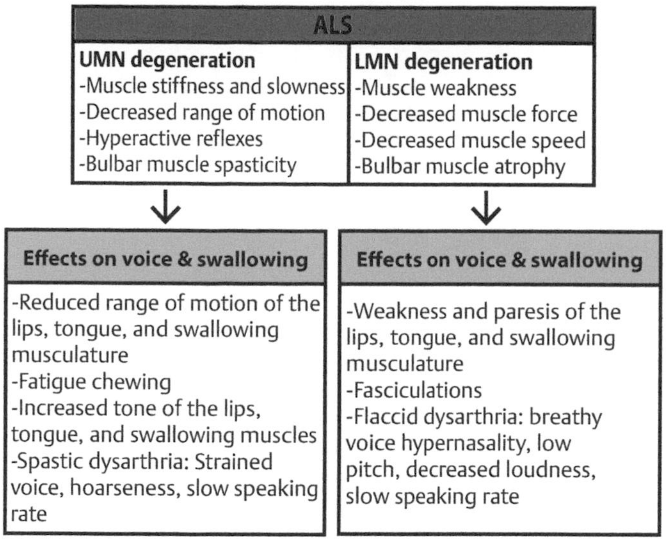

| ALS | |
|---|---|
| **UMN degeneration** | **LMN degeneration** |
| -Muscle stiffness and slowness | -Muscle weakness |
| -Decreased range of motion | -Decreased muscle force |
| -Hyperactive reflexes | -Decreased muscle speed |
| -Bulbar muscle spasticity | -Bulbar muscle atrophy |

| **Effects on voice & swallowing** | **Effects on voice & swallowing** |
|---|---|
| -Reduced range of motion of the lips, tongue, and swallowing musculature | -Weakness and paresis of the lips, tongue, and swallowing musculature |
| -Fatigue chewing | -Fasciculations |
| -Increased tone of the lips, tongue, and swallowing muscles | -Flaccid dysarthria: breathy voice hypernasality, low pitch, decreased loudness, slow speaking rate |
| -Spastic dysarthria: Strained voice, hoarseness, slow speaking rate | |

**Fig. 19.1** Underlying neuropathology with associated voice and swallowing symptoms (or symptomology) in amyotrophic lateral sclerosis.

Upon report of her concerns, her primary care physician recommended evaluation by a neurologist and speech-language pathologist (SLP). BH arrived at her neurology appointment and expressed her concerns. The neurologist reported BH's current signs:

Patient BH is a 64-year-old woman referred from her primary care physician for progressively worsening complaints of generalized weakness, difficulty swallowing, and changes in speech and voice quality. She presents with the following:

1. Mixed flaccid-spastic dysarthria characterized by slow rate, hypernasality, imprecise consonant production, breathiness, strain, and reduced volume
2. Dysphagia characterized by prolonged mastication, intermittent coughing with thin liquids, difficulty swallowing medications, and sensation of food sticking in her throat
3. Pseudobulbar affect characterized by emotional lability and uncontrolled laughing and crying
4. Difficulty with upper extremity fine motor movements, including gripping utensils and cutting foods during mealtime. She reports unintentional weight loss of 30 lb over the past 4 months

BH's rapidly progressing symptoms remained undiagnosed despite a multitude of testing that included imaging studies (i.e., magnetic resonance imaging [MRI] of the brain, computed tomographic [CT] scan of the cervical spine), blood tests, review of family history, as well as pharmacological trials for suspected myasthenia gravis and Lyme disease. Following referral to a secondary neurologist, a diagnosis of ALS was confirmed following electromyographic testing. BH's neurologist explained that ALS is a progressive neurologic disease with no cure and very few pharmacological, surgical, or behavioral treatment options. He recommended she start Rilutek, the only medication approved by the U.S. Food Drug Administration to prolong survivorship in ALS (by approximately 2–3 months), as well as attending the university's multidisciplinary ALS clinic, where she will see[7] various health care specialists to assist in the management of her symptoms.

## 19.2.4 Dysphagia and Malnutrition in Amyotrophic Lateral Sclerosis

Given the progressive and terminal nature of this disease, ALS treatments typically focus on proactive symptom management, patient and caregiver education, compensations, and environmental support within a multidisciplinary setting. Although respiratory insufficiency represents the primary cause of death in persons with ALS (PALS), dysphagia-related complications resulting in malnutrition and aspiration pneumonia account for approximately one quarter of disease morbidity,[11] and a reported 85% of PALS will experience dysphagia at some point during the disease process, regardless of onset type.[12,13] Swallowing impairment typically occurs during later stages of disease progression; however, bulbar-onset patients will experience dysphagic symptoms much earlier in the disease. It is important to note that the presence of dysphagia increases the risk of malnutrition due to reduced intake, fatigue during mealtimes, and chronic aspiration,[11,14,15,16] which in turn increases the risk of death in this patient population.[11,17] PALS are particularly susceptible to malnutrition due to two confounding factors. First, they are in a hypermetabolic state and therefore function with a higher resting metabolic rate.[11,18] Second, they typically take in fewer calories because of difficulties with self-feeding due to limb involvement, fatigue in feeding, and dysphagia or because of decreased appetite.[11,16] This clinical scenario is referred to as the perfect storm for the development of malnutrition, decreased functional reserve, and further muscle wasting.[14] A sevenfold increase in mortality is present in PALS who are malnourished,[11,17] underscoring the importance of adequate nutrition in this patient population. Research also indicates that difficulty swallowing by mouth creates a significant burden, longer mealtimes, and reduced enjoyment of eating, all of which can contribute to food aversion behaviors and further weight loss.[19,20] To maintain weight and prevent malnutrition, dehydration, and respiratory complications, alternative methods of feeding may need to be introduced early in this specific patient population. Placement of a percutaneous endoscopic gastrostomy (PEG) tube is typically well tolerated and recommended by the American Academy of Neurology in ALS.[14] PEG placement has been shown to increase survival by 104 days in a recent retrospective study of 2,172 PALS in the United States[21] and by 120 days in a similar retrospective review of 150 Italian PALS.[22] The prevention of malnutrition is of paramount importance in PALS, and health care professionals need to proactively educate patients of the associated nutritional risks and the importance of nutritional intake, particularly in those patients whose body mass index is average or low at the time of diagnosis.

Swallowing difficulty may occur throughout any stage of deglutition in PALS (**Table 19.2**). The most common impairments experienced in ALS are primarily due to muscle weakness, slowness, and stiffness. The hallmark UMN and LMN degeneration in ALS contributes to muscle weakness in the oropharyngeal musculature and weakness and stiffness of the upper airway and diaphragm

**Table 19.2** Typical swallowing impairments in individuals with amyotrophic lateral sclerosis

| Oral preparatory/oral stage | Pharyngeal stage | Esophageal stage |
|---|---|---|
| • Difficulty managing saliva<br>• Fatigue with mastication<br>• Labial leakage<br>• Premature spillage<br>• Drooling<br>• Reduced anterior-posterior movement of bolus<br>• Oral residue/pocketing | • Vallecular/piriform sinus residue<br>• Nasal regurgitation<br>• Inadequate laryngeal vestibule closure<br>• Penetration/aspiration<br>• Shortness of breath and fatigue during mealtime<br>• Reduced cough strength and effectiveness | • Regurgitation or retropulsion of food/liquid into the pharynx and oral cavity<br>• Pharyngeal residue in the throat/base of neck |

*Sources:* Chen & Garrett, 2005[13]; Britton & Miller, 2011[5]; Greenwood, 1999.[16]

muscles that can further contribute to impaired airway defense mechanisms during swallowing. Due to these impairments, PALS may not be able to generate adequate subglottic air pressure to produce a productive and effective cough. During the oral stage of swallowing, patients may report a sensation of a "heavy tongue" that makes it difficult to manipulate the bolus within the oral cavity, masticate, and move the bolus posteriorly when initiating the swallow. Due to weakness of the orbicularis oris and muscles of the tongue, food or liquid may uncontrollably spill anteriorly or posteriorly during the swallow. Impairments in the pharyngeal stage of the swallow may include diffuse pharyngeal residue with solids and liquids, resulting in increased coughing during the meal, or nasal regurgitation due to incomplete velopharyngeal closure due to muscle weakness. Regurgitation of food or liquid during or after the meal may be an indication of cricopharyngeal or esophageal-related impairment.

## 19.2.5 Evaluation and Management of Dysphagia in Amyotrophic Lateral Sclerosis

Management of dysphagia in PALS is best approached with an interdisciplinary team with particular coordination between the SLP, dietitian, respiratory therapist, and neurologist. Due to the rapid progression of symptoms and the high risk of aspiration, it is recommended that swallowing impairment and cough function be routinely monitored in PALS. Research completed in our laboratory indicates that aspiration occurs in approximately 30% of PALS (confirmed via videofluoroscopic evaluation) attending a specialized ALS multidisciplinary clinic.[23] Of the PALS who aspirated, 58% did so without a cough response, whereas 42% demonstrated an ineffective cough response that did not clear aspirant material.[23] Therefore, in this convenience sample of ALS patients, none were able to effectively defend the airway when aspiration occurred.[23] Given the noted high prevalence of silent aspiration in this patient population, the modified barium swallow study (MBSS, the gold standard) is recommended for evaluating and managing dysphagia (**Fig. 19.2**).

Current swallowing management recommendations for PALS include dietary modifications, postural changes, compensations, and PEG placement.[10] Dietary modifications include the addition of thickeners to liquids and downgrading diets to softer, more manageable textures, depending on the patients presenting symptoms. Avoidance of particulate foods is also recommended because these can represent a choking hazard for PALS. Although the impact of postural adjustments or maneuvers has not been extensively studied, Solazzo and colleagues noted that a throat clear, chin tuck, head turn, and head tilt were effective at reducing penetration and/or aspiration in 79% of PALS.[24] Other compensations that may benefit PALS include the effortful swallow, use of a liquid wash or a "dry" swallow (double swallow). **Table 19.3** summarizes commonly prescribed compensations and postural adjustments to aid specific swallow signs in PALS.

The implementation of a PEG tube is highly recommended in PALS and represents one of only a few treatments noted to significantly increase survival in PALS.[21,22] As previously mentioned in this chapter, prophylactic PEG placement is often recommended to avoid malnutrition and ensure adequate nutritional intake prior to significant respiratory compromise. The American Academy of Neurology Practice parameter currently indicates that PEG placement occur before forced vital capacity drops below 50% of predicted or greater than 10% of baseline body weight is lost.[7,16]

Although an instrumental evaluation of swallowing function is highly recommended in PALS, patients are typically seen by SLPs in multidisciplinary clinics where the clinician typically has a short time frame to *screen* for swallowing function and aspiration risk. We have recently studied the discriminant ability of voluntary cough and patient self-report screening tests to predict aspiration status in PALS. The Eating Assessment Tool-10 (EAT-10)[25] is a validated, easy-to-administer, 10-item patient self-report tool of swallowing impairment. We gave this survey to 70 PALS and noted that ALS patients scoring ≥ 8 on the EAT-10 were *three times* more likely to aspirate (determined on videofluoroscopy), and this cutoff value had 88% sensitivity, 56.7% specificity, and 95.5% negative predictive value.[10] We also investigated the utility of voluntary cough testing in PALS and noted that cough volume acceleration was three times lower in PALS with unsafe swallowing compared to those with adequate airway protection (Plowman, *Chest*, submitted). Additional commonly used tools to track progression of dysphagia over time and aid in identifying possible swallowing impairment include the Swallowing-Related Quality of Life (SWAL-QOL) survey,[26] the Yale Swallow Protocol,[27] and the Dysphagia Outcome and Severity Scale.[28]

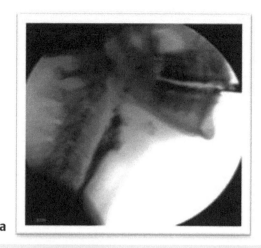 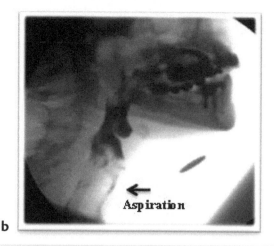

a          b

**Fig. 19.2** Modified barium swallow study images of two individuals with amyotrophic lateral sclerosis (ALS) illustrating the varying degree of swallowing function in this patient population. **(a)** The patient has spinal-onset ALS and demonstrates functional swallowing abilities with good airway protection during swallowing. **(b)** The patient has bulbar-onset ALS and demonstrates deep tracheal aspiration during the swallow with subsequent residue of materials in the vallecula and piriform sinuses due to decreased base of tongue and pharyngeal constrictor movement. A circular calibration ring has been placed on the patient's neck.

**Table 19.3** General recommendations for management of dysphagia in individuals with amyotrophic lateral sclerosis

| Swallowing impairment | Pharyngeal stage |
|---|---|
| Longer mealtime duration | • Take smaller, more frequent meals throughout the day<br>• Add high-calorie snacks |
| Difficulty chewing | • Moisten foods with gravies and/or sauces<br>• Smaller bite size<br>• Downgrade to softer consistency |
| Weight loss | • Include high-calorie, high-fat foods in diet<br>• Include smoothies and shakes with full cream milk and the addition of peanut butter, chocolate, or other calorically dense items<br>• Supplement nutrition with Boost or Ensure drinks, Resource Benecalorie<br>• Supplement with percutaneous endoscopic gastrostomy tube feedings<br>• Take appetite-stimulant aids |
| Fatigue<br>Shortness of breath | • Take smaller, more frequent meals throughout the day<br>• Drink high-calorie smoothies to reduce effort required for oral intake<br>• Minimize exertion during meals (i.e., side conversations, distractions)<br>• Utilize respiratory aids prior to and after meals |

*Sources:* Britton & Miller, 2011[5]; Yorkston, Miller & Strand, 2004.[2]

## 19.2.6 Case Presentation: BH Management and Recommendations

### Clinical Assessment

BH attended her first multidisciplinary ALS clinic at her local university and was seen by a team of health care professionals that included a neurologist, an SLP, a dietitian, an occupational therapist, a physical therapist, a social worker, and a respiratory therapist. Each specialist made recommendations and helped to educate BH on safety, expectations, prophylactic treatment options, and disease management. During the SLP evaluation, BH completed the validated EAT-10 and obtained a score of 14,

indicating the presence of a self-reported swallowing impairment. Our recent research findings would indicate that this patient has a three times higher likelihood of aspirating given this score. On oral-motor examination she demonstrated significant lingual and labial weakness and a hyperactive gag reflex, and she failed the 3-ounce water screen (cough elicited). Given these symptoms, the SLP requested a referral from the patient's neurologist to perform an MBSS to determine the specific physiological impairments and degree of airway safety to optimize treatment recommendations and management strategies. Results of the MBSS indicated the following swallowing impairments: prolonged mastication and lingual weakness resulting in oral residue on the base of the tongue, and oral pocketing and reduced pharyngeal contraction resulting in piriform sinus residue with solid consistency trials. Aspiration occurred during the swallow with consecutive sips of thin liquids, but did not occur on any of five trials using a single cup sip of thin liquid. Pharyngeal residue of solid bolus trials (graham cracker coated with barium paste) cleared completely with a single sip of thin liquid. The 13 mm barium tablet was unable to pass from the anterior to the posterior tongue despite multiple liquid washes. **Fig. 19.3** depicts two images from BH's MBSS exam.

## Treatment Recommendations

Due to patient-reported symptoms and clinical and instrumental evaluation results, the SLP recommended that BH downgrade to a mechanical soft-consistency diet, with compensations including small, single bites/sips, and alternating liquids and solids during meals. The SLP also recommended that BH take smaller meals more frequently throughout the day, and utilize supplemental nutrition, such as Boost and Ensure, as needed. The clinician reviewed the instrumental swallowing evaluation video with the patient to demonstrate how consistent implementation of the recommended compensations would ensure safe swallowing. Patient education included red flags of aspiration and deterioration in swallow function, importance of adherence to diet modifications and compensations, and strategies to maintain nutrition and keep her weight stable.

# 19.3 Parkinson's Disease

## 19.3.1 Case Presentation: CD Patient History

CD is a 66-year-old man with primary complaints of unilateral hand tremor and difficulties with gait. Symptoms began 4 years ago and have progressively worsened over time; however, CD has not previously seen a physician regarding these symptoms. CD is otherwise healthy and reports no changes in memory or cognition. Upon review of his history, CD was a college psychology professor and recently retired, though reportedly not due to impairments related to the current symptoms. CD's wife accompanied him to the evaluation and reported she has noticed frequent coughing during mealtimes. She also noted changes in vocal quality that she describes as being harder to understand (particularly when background noise is present) and "softer." CD presented to his neurologist following referral from his primary care physician.

PD was first described by James Parkinson in 1817 as a neurologic disease that caused the "propensity to bend the trunk forward and to pass from a walking to a running pace: the senses and intellects being uninjured."[29] Although the etiology of PD is unknown, there exist genetic and molecular epidemiological theories on the contribution of environmental and genetic risk factors.[30] PD is the second most common neurodegenerative disease following Alzheimer's disease, and lifetime risk of developing PD increases with age.[30] PD is associated with Parkinson plus syndromes or atypical Parkinsonism, which subdivide into multiple system atrophy, progressive supranuclear palsy, dementia with Lewy bodies, drug-induced Parkinsonism, corticobasal degeneration, and vascular Parkinsonism. Parkinsonism and Parkinson plus syndromes generally present much like PD but are typically resistant to traditional pharmacological treatment and progress more rapidly than idiopathic PD.[2] Idiopathic PD is most common, and symptoms typically respond more positively to medical and pharmacological management. Onset of PD is relatively slow progressing and characterized by gradual death of dopamine-generating cells in the substantia nigra and presence of Lewy bodies in the brain.[31] The substantia nigra in the brainstem plays an integral role in movement and coordination. PD is classified as a movement disorder due to the associated motor symptoms affecting gait, movement, and coordination due to death of dopamine neurons within the substantia nigra pars compacta of the basal ganglia.[31] Dopaminergic neurons play an important role in volitional movements, motor planning, sequencing, cognition, mood,

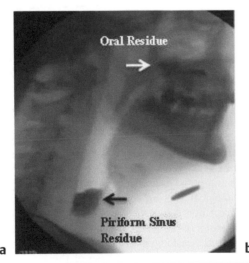 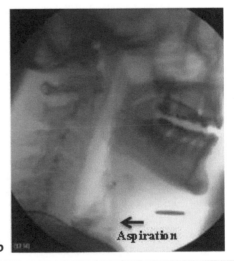

**Fig. 19.3** Still frames of the modified barium swallow study performed on case study BH demonstrating **(a)** significant residue in the piriform sinus and moderate residue in the oral cavity following a solid bolus trial (barium-coated cracker) and **(b)** aspiration on a thin-liquid trial. A calibration tool is placed on the patient's chin.

addiction, and stress. Dopamine depletion leads to accumulation of cytoplasmic inclusion bodies composed of α–synuclein (Lewy bodies).[31] As a result, the aforementioned symptoms, including hypokinetic (reduced and slow) movements are observed in PD due to underactivation (inhibition) of the thalamus and cortical motor areas, including the primary motor cortex, supplementary motor area, and premotor cortex. In addition to dopamine degeneration, neurochemicals, including noradrenalin, serotonin, and acetylcholine, are also thought to be affected in PD.[31] There is currently no cure for PD,[32] and therapies consist of treating symptoms and preserving function and quality of life.

## 19.3.2 Diagnoses and Prevalence of Parkinson's Disease

Much as in ALS, a diagnosis of PD requires extensive clinical and instrumental assessment because a single lab test cannot definitively diagnose the disease. As much as 80% of dopaminergic neurons may degenerate before clinical symptoms appear,[31] and the overall progression of PD varies among patients. A diagnosis of PD is made from observation of clinical symptoms, diagnostic imaging (e.g., a dopamine transporter or positron emission topography scan), and documentation of symptoms on the Movement Disorder Society United Parkinson's Disease Rating Scale (MDS-UPDRS).[29] The MDS-UPDRS is a validated comprehensive scale used to document disease severity and progression over time.

PD is more prevalent in older adults with an increase from 1 to 4% between the ages of 60 to 80 years, and lifetime risk indicates PD will affect approximately 1 in every 100 people.[33] Approximately 85–90% of PD diagnoses are sporadic in nature (no genetic link), whereas the disease is inherited in the remaining cases.[34] PD is not considered a fatal disease, although mortality rates in persons with the disease are 35 to 65% higher due to complications associated with PD that include deep vein thrombosis, pulmonary embolism, pneumonia, and falls.[35] Aspiration pneumonia is the primary cause of mortality in patients with PD.[33,35] Early signs of PD may be general and nonspecific to neurodegenerative disease, such as generalized fatigue or weakness, muscle cramping, and gait disturbance. Hallmark clinical symptoms of PD include asymmetric resting tremor, rigidity, and bradykinesia.[36] Postural instability affecting gait is also considered a prominent presenting symptom. Mild cognitive decline is noted in approximately 25% of newly diagnosed PD cases,[37] whereas dementia occurs in 80% of PD cases at some point during the disease process[38] and is more common as age at diagnosis increases.[39] Cognitive domains of memory, executive function, and visuospatial skills are commonly impaired. Additionally, masked facial expressions, dysarthria, dysphagia, and insomnia are more common later in the disease process.[36]

## 19.3.3 Dysphagia and Related Complications in Parkinson's Disease

The prevalence of dysphagia in persons with PD varies widely from an estimated 40 to 95%, depending on disease severity, patient awareness of difficulties with swallowing, and presence of dementia.[36] Research also indicates that 100% of individuals with PD eventually develop dysphagia at some point during the disease process.[2,36] It is generally recognized that dysphagia is more common and severe as the disease progresses to more severe stages.[40] In some individuals, speech and swallowing impairment may also be the presenting symptom of the disease.[41,42] For this reason, baseline evaluation and consistent monitoring of swallow function are recommended throughout the disease process. Despite signs of swallowing difficulties, weight loss, dehydration, and malnutrition, individuals with PD may be unaware of their swallowing deficits due to the slow progression of the disease and online compensations and dietary modifications they subconsciously employ. Further, persons with PD are reported to have poor self-awareness of swallowing difficulties and are noted to underreport their swallowing impairments.[43] Sequelae from dysphagia in PD are serious, and aspiration pneumonia constitutes the leading cause of death in this patient population.[35] In addition to the medical consequences of dysphagia, significant reductions in quality of life and mental well-being have been associated with the presence of swallowing impairment in PD.[40,44] Specifically, individuals with PD reported reduced enjoyment in eating out due to drooling, slow feeding rate, and fear of choking, as well as reduced ability to engage in social settings and participation in vocational and leisure activities.[40,44]

Movement dysfunction is a hallmark feature of PD and functionally results in weakened and slowed movement of the swallowing muscles (**Table 19.4**). Swallowing difficulties can occur during any stage of swallowing. Oral stage movement dysfunction may include lingual tremor, lingual pumping, impaired mastication, and mandible rigidity.[45] In turn, oral-stage swallowing impairments may be characterized by poor bolus control, increased oral transit time, oral pocketing, and premature spillage into the vallecula. Delayed swallow initiation and prolonged mastication may be affected, attributing to premature spillage and increased oral transit time.[46,47] Reduced pharyngeal contraction, hyolaryngeal elevation, and incomplete laryngeal vestibule closure during the pharyngeal stage result in pharyngeal residue, laryngeal penetration, and tracheal aspiration.[47] Impairment can also occur at the level of the upper esophageal sphincter (UES)

**Table 19.4** Typical swallowing impairments in Parkinson's disease

| Movement dysfunction | Resulting swallowing impairment |
|---|---|
| • Lingual tremor<br>• Lingual pumping<br>• Impairment mastication<br>• Mandible rigidity | • Poor bolus control<br>• Increased oral transit time<br>• Oral pocketing<br>• Premature spillage to the pharynx |
| • Reduced pharyngeal contraction<br>• Decreased hyolaryngeal elevation<br>• Impaired laryngeal vestibule closure | • Diffuse pharyngeal residue<br>• Laryngeal penetration<br>• Tracheal aspiration |
| • Decreased upper esophageal sphincter opening<br>• Esophageal dysmotility | • Piriform sinus residue<br>• Retropulsion into the pharynx |

*Sources:* Groher & Crary, 2010[48]; Rosenbek & Jones, 2009[40]; Sung et al, 2010.[42]

and during the esophageal stage of swallowing.[48] The UES may be reduced in opening, contributing to increased piriform sinus residue. Esophageal dysmotility and poor bolus clearance or bolus redirection may also occur.[42]

In addition to the impairments found in the oropharyngeal and esophageal stages of swallowing, pulmonary and respiratory muscle function impairment are commonly observed in individuals with PD.[49] The swallowing and respiratory systems are required to work integrally together in order to protect the airway during the swallow and produce an effective and timely cough in the event of penetration or aspiration. In individuals with PD, impairments in respiratory function can be detrimental to cough function, swallowing, and speech production.[50] As in other neurological patient populations, the co-occurrence of dystussia and dysphagia has been noted in PD patients whose voluntary cough[51,52,53] and urge to cough[54] have been shown to differ between safe and unsafe PD swallowers. Considering the high incidence of pulmonary complications, aspiration pneumonia, and poor self-awareness of swallowing impairments, consistent monitoring and evaluation of cough and swallowing function are vital for preservation of function and preventing pulmonary sequelae.

## 19.3.4 Evaluation and Dysphagia Management in Parkinson's Disease

Although PD typically progresses at a relatively slow rate, patient and caregiver education, dietary modifications, and mealtime compensations may be necessary early during the disease course to maintain adequate nutrition and avoid unintentional weight loss. Modifications may be as simple as taking smaller meals throughout the day to avoid fatigue during meals, or adding supplemental nutrition such as Boost, Ensure, or homemade smoothies.

Intervention strategies are either compensatory or rehabilitative in nature. Compensatory strategies involve the implementation of postural adjustments, swallow maneuvers, and dietary modifications. These strategies are recommended in order to create short-term adjustments in swallow function, but they do not alter swallow physiology or extend beyond the treatment period. Rehabilitative interventions are implemented to target and improve physiological impairments observed during the instrumental evaluation of the swallow mechanism and produce enduring changes that extend beyond the treatment period (**Table 19.5**).[48]

Commonly recommended compensatory strategies include the use of postural adjustments and swallowing maneuvers, such as a chin tuck, effortful swallow, and supersupraglottic swallow.[47,55,56,57] Implementation of compensatory strategies depends on the observed impairment and pathophysiology of the swallow, and the patient's ability to consistently utilize the recommended strategies. The benefits of the intervention (i.e., eliminating aspiration, reducing pharyngeal residue) have been shown to vary across individuals with neurogenic dysphagia; therefore, several compensations may need to be tried in order to identify appropriate strategies.[47,57] Further, limitations in cognition, movement, and range of motion may interfere with proper use of strategies and need to be taken into careful consideration. Other environmental modifications may include the use of adaptive feeding equipment,

**Table 19.5** Parkinson's disease: interventions and expected outcomes

| Intervention | Outcome |
|---|---|
| **Compensatory** | |
| Effortful swallow | Increased base of tongue retraction[1] Reduced pharyngeal residue[1,3] |
| Chin tuck | Improved airway protection[2,3] Reduced penetration/aspiration[2,3] |
| **Rehabilitative** | |
| Expiratory muscle strength training (EMST) | Improved airway protection[4] Improved cough function[5] Improved quality of life[6] |
| Video-assisted swallowing therapy (VAST) | Reduced pharyngeal residue[7,8] Reduced swallowing impairment[7,8] |
| Biofeedback in Swallowing Skill Training (BiSSkiT) | Improved timing/durational measures (i.e., time per swallow, preswallow timing)[9] Improved quality of life[9] |

*Sources:* Logemann, 1998[1]; Groher & Crary, 2010[2]; Ramig et al, 2011[3]; Troche et al, 2010[4]; Pitts et al, 2009[5]; Sapienza et al, 2014[6]; van Hooren et al, 2014,[7] Manor et al, 2013,[8] Huckabee et al, 2014[9]

such as a weighted utensil, to reduce the impact of hand tremors to assist with feeding during mealtimes.

Research has been conducted on the impact of two rehabilitative strategies in PD, namely expiratory muscle strength training (EMST) and the Lee Silverman Voice Treatment (LSVT). EMST involves forcefully exhaling into a small portable handheld device with a pressure-loaded spring valve set to a specific resistance level.[58] The patient exhales quickly and forcefully to break the seal of the spring valve, which constitutes a completed repetition. A preliminary investigation in EMST and PD conducted by Silverman and colleagues[49] first identified the potential benefit of respiratory strength training on maximum expiratory pressure and functionally related tasks, such as cough, swallowing, and speech. Pitts and colleagues[50] investigated the impact of EMST on voluntary cough airflow and airway protection during swallowing in PD and reported increased cough volume acceleration and improved airway protection (reduced Penetration-Aspiration Scale scores) during swallowing.[50] Results of a randomized sham control trial performed in 60 PD patients concluded that EMST improved airway protection, cough function, and patient-reported quality of life.[59] Additionally, hyolaryngeal elevation and excursion were increased following the 4-week training period of EMST.[59] Although the LSVT program was originally developed to target voice impairments in PD, a cross-systems effect on swallowing function has been reported, with noted improvements in oral and pharyngeal transit times as well as reduced pharyngeal residue in individuals with PD.[60] Both EMST and LSVT incorporate many key principles of plasticity that include repetition, load, transference, and the "use it or lose it" concept.[61]

Biofeedback is a therapy tool documented to facilitate learning novel motor tasks or relearning motor tasks following injury.[1,48] As an adjunct to therapy, biofeedback techniques involve utilizing additional modalities to demonstrate, teach, monitor, and, in turn, enhance function and performance.[1] Visual biofeedback using surface electromyography of submental muscle activation and the Biofeedback in Swallowing Skill Training (BiSSkiT) program have been shown to improve kinematic and temporal swallowing measures and patient-reported swallow-related quality of life.[62] Video-assisted swallowing therapy (VAST) utilizes visual cueing to improve motor and coordination skills in swallowing through guided observation of the patient's swallow via fiberoptic endoscopic evaluation of swallowing (FEES), in conjunction with consistent implementation of compensatory strategies and swallowing exercises.[63] In a randomized controlled trial of 42 PD patients, those who completed the VAST program had significantly less pharyngeal residue on FEES examination and improved patient-reported swallowing quality of life as measured by the SWAL-QOL survey.[63,64] Biofeedback is likely especially useful for individuals with PD who are known to have sensory awareness issues of their bulbar deficits by raising their proprioceptive awareness.

Medical management of PD includes dopamine replacement therapy with levodopa and deep brain stimulation (DBS). DBS involves surgically implanting a small device that delivers high-frequency electrical stimulation to targeted parts of the brain. Although pharmacological and surgical interventions have been efficacious for limb motor functions, improvements in speech and swallowing in PD have typically been less responsive and reliable for these interventions.[65,66,67] When comparing PD patients with DBS on versus off, Ciucci et al observed significant improvements in pharyngeal transit time and pharyngeal clearance with solid consistency trials with DBS on; however, no improvements were observed for oral-stage impairments or maximum hyoid displacement.[68] Unfortunately, bulbar functions are typically more resistant to medical management, and DBS seems to have relatively little positive effect on speech and swallow physiology.[66,69] It is generally recommended that dysphagia treatment in PD consist of behavioral modifications and rehabilitative exercise programs.[46]

Timing of meals with medications for an individual patient is recommended because motor function impairments, including dyskinesia, tremor, and bradykinesia, affecting feeding and mealtime duration have been shown to improve.[70,71] For some patients this may occur on or soon after taking PD medications.

## 19.3.5 Case Presentation: CD Management and Recommendations

Following his appointment with the neurologist, CD commenced a regimen of levodopa and was recommended to complete a baseline voice and swallowing evaluation, including videostroboscopy and an MBSS. Although he was initially resistant because he did not believe it was necessary, CD's wife and avid supporter convinced him to complete the evaluation. Results of the voice evaluation, including videostroboscopy, revealed incomplete adduction of the true vocal folds characterized by a small, spindle-shaped gap. Functionally, this finding contributes to CD's reduced volume and difficulty projecting during speaking. Results of the MBSS revealed prolonged mastication, lingual pumping, oral residue on the base of the tongue, vallecular residue with solid consistencies, and deep penetration with consecutive cup sips of thin liquids (throat clear elicited). Deep penetration was eliminated with single sips of thin liquid. Vallecular residue was reduced with modified bite size and liquid wash. Results of the evaluations indicated mild hypokinetic dysarthria characterized by reduced volume and slow speaking rate, and mild–moderate oropharyngeal dysphagia characterized by the aforementioned impairments in speech and swallow function (**Fig. 19.4**). Recommendations included intensive voice treatment using the LSVT approach, in addition to education on consistent implementation of safe swallowing strategies, including single sips of thin liquid and small, single bites of food with alternating liquids and solids throughout the meal. Patient and caregiver education included explanation of normal swallow function using visual feedback from the MBSS, red flags of aspiration, and deterioration in swallow function, as well as importance of adherence to prandial compensations. The LSVT approach was reviewed and discussed in terms of intensity and commitment required for success in the program. CD and his wife agreed to the recommendations given as a result of the evaluation, and CD is slated to commence therapy with the SLP.

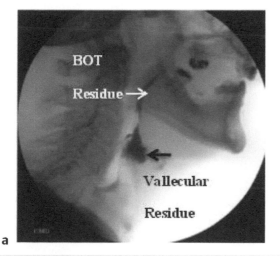
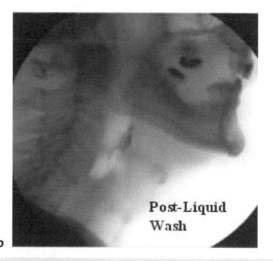

**Fig. 19.4** Parkinson's disease case study CD: modified barium swallow study (MBSS). **(a)** MBSS image demonstrating residue on the base of the tongue (BOT) and in the vallecula after swallowing a solid bolus trial (graham cracker coated with barium). **(b)** MBSS image demonstrating cleared residue following use of the recommended compensations (liquid wash, alternating liquids/solids, modified bolus size).

# 19.4 Multiple Sclerosis

MS is an inflammatory disease of the central nervous system that causes gradual degeneration of the myelin sheath. Myelin is a white matter insulating covering found along most neuronal axons in the brain and spinal cord that enables them to propagate signals at rapid speeds.[72] Therefore, demyelination of neurons within the central nervous system causes slowed signal transduction and eventually leads to neuronal death.[73] Although MS is the most common and well-known demyelinating disease,[72] additional demyelinating diseases include Guillain–Barré syndrome and Charcot–Marie–Tooth disease. Unlike the previous two neurodegenerative diseases discussed in this chapter, MS symptoms typically present suddenly. Common MS symptoms include sudden-onset paresthesias, or tingling of the limbs, motor weakness, visual disturbances, incoordination, dizziness, and fatigue.[74] Impairments may also be observed in cognition and autonomic, sensory, and motor systems. Common sensory symptoms include Uhthoff's phenomenon, or exacerbation in symptoms following exposure to heat (e.g., after a hot bath, during a hot day, or following exercise). Pain is often reported due to neuralgia, spasms, inflammation, and joint stiffness.[72] Motor system involvement can lead to spasticity, weakness, dysarthria, and dysphagia.[75] Further, the scattered nature of lesions within the brain can result in variable presenting symptoms among individuals with MS. Due to the broad range of impairments and severity levels, prognosis for MS can be difficult to determine and is based on MS type and success in treatment of individual symptoms.[76] Additionally, treatment of one symptom may adversely affect a co-occurring symptom. For example, pharmacological treatment for spasticity has side effects, such as drowsiness, weakness, and incoordination, that may exacerbate fatigue and weakness.[72]

There are four clinical case presentations (i.e., onset types) of MS that are summarized in **Table 19.6**. Remitting-relapsing MS (RRMS) accounts for 85–90% of individuals and typically has the best prognosis, characterized by continually mild symptoms, positive response to drug therapy, and slow progression. Primary-progressive MS (PPMS) accounts for approximately 10% of MS cases and progresses more rapidly and with more severe symptoms.[72,73,76] Onset of PPMS is associated with the poorest outcomes and the least effective treatment options.[77] In 90% of RRMS cases, the disease progresses to a secondary-progressive disease course (SPMS) within 25 years.[76] Progressive-relapsing (PRMS) is rare, accounting for only 5% of individuals diagnosed with MS.[73,76] PRMS is characterized by progressive neurologic decline with acute periods of exacerbation that may or may not be followed by recovery (**Table 19.6**).[76] The progressive decline and relapse-remitting characteristics of MS eventually lead to permanent neurological damage and disability, which varies based on disease onset type and impact of treatment.

## 19.4.1 Diagnosis and Prevalence

MS is the most common neurologic disability in young adults in the United States affecting more than 400,000 people.[76] MS onset typically occurs between the ages of 20 and 40 and is rare after 60 years of age.[72] The disease is more common in females (F:M ratio of 2.3:1).[72] Similar to the other diseases presented in this chapter, there is currently no cure for MS, with intervention generally focused on treatment of individual symptoms of the disease. Of the known prognostic indicators, increased age and male sex are associated with poorer outcomes.[78] Although etiology of this disease is unknown, there are theories on the contribution of environmental factors, compromised immune system, and genetic markers that contribute to the development of MS.[73] Mortality occurs approximately 7–10 years prior to average life expectancy for the general population when matched by age and gender.[72,74,77] In an epidemiological study, cause of death in individuals with MS was attributed to infections, cardiovascular disease, and pulmonary problems.[79] Of the mortality attributed to pulmonary problems, 58.7% were due to aspiration.[79]

A diagnosis of MS typically requires thorough evaluation, instrumental testing, and imaging. In addition to the case history and physical exam, MRI is the standard diagnostic tool because it can determine the presence of focal lesions and diffuse degeneration within the white matter of the brain and spinal cord.[74,80] MRI can be repeated throughout the disease course to monitor progression, the impact of treatment, and/or the relapsing-remitting nature of MS. Disease onset type is not typically distinguishable using MRI alone.[80] Cerebrospinal fluid analysis and visual evoked potential testing are also used to aid in a definitive diagnosis. In

**Table 19.6** Characteristics and prevalence of multiple sclerosis described by onset type

| Multiple sclerosis onset type | Characteristics | Prevalence |
|---|---|---|
| Remitting-relapsing (RRMS) | • Continually mild symptoms<br>• Response to anti-inflammatory therapy<br>• Slow progression | 85–90% (with eventual progression to SPMS)<br>10–15% benign |
| Primary-progressive (PPMS) | • Rapid progression<br>• More severe symptomology<br>• No exacerbation/remission | 10% |
| Progressive-relapsing (PRMS) | • Slow progression<br>• Periods of exacerbation without remission | 5% |
| Secondary-progressive (SPMS) | • Following 10–25 years of RRMS<br>• Progressive decline<br>• Periods of exacerbation/remission | 85–90% (progresses from RRMS to SPMS) |

*Sources:* Chen & Garrett, 2005[13]; Britton & Miller, 2011[5]; Greenwood, 1999.[16]

some cases, a thorough physical exam and clinical evaluation can garner necessary information for a reliable diagnosis. However, the revised McDonald diagnostic criterion describes the archetypal clinical presentation and additional data for diagnosing MS and includes imaging evaluations.[80] Disease progression in MS is most commonly monitored using the standardized Expanded Disability Status Scale (EDSS), which classifies disease severity on a scale from 0 (normal neurological examination) to 10 (death due to MS).[81] Each subcategory on the scale broadly considers impairment level for the following functional systems: pyramidal, cerebellar, brainstem, sensory, bowel and bladder, visual, cerebral/mental, and other.

## 19.4.2 Pathophysiology

The neurological pathology characteristic of MS includes numerous small lesions or plaques distributed throughout the space that comprises the central nervous system, which therefore serve as a hallmark diagnostic feature of the disease.[73] A combination of the presence of small lesions, gradual demyelination, and progressive axonal loss contributes to the neurological impairment and disability in MS. Lesions can vary in size and location, resulting in varying patient presentations of the disease.[82] However, much like the deterioration of dopaminergic neurons in individuals with PD, impairments may not be clinically apparent until significant and chronic demyelination has occurred.[73] Depending on the characteristics of the onset type, there are several possible mechanisms that describe axonal degeneration, including elevated levels of the neurotransmitter glutamate, resulting in glutamate-mediated excitotoxicity, and increased vulnerability to degeneration due to an imbalance of energy demand and supply within the axon.[73] The precise way in which each of these mechanisms evolves partially depends on the disease onset type. In the remission period of a remitting-relapsing onset type, the demyelinated axons regain their ability to conduct action potentials at reduced speeds. As edema and inflammation resolve, the axons remyelinate and function is restored. The transition from RRMS to SPMS is believed to occur once the compensatory mechanism (remyelination of axons) is depleted and the axons are no longer able to recover.[73] This leads to chronic and irreversible damage to the neurons and eventual neuronal death.

## 19.4.3 Dysphagia in Multiple Sclerosis

Prevalence reports of dysphagia in MS vary between 36 and 81%.[72,75] Complications resulting from swallowing impairment, such as pulmonary sequelae, may arise if symptoms of dysphagia are not closely monitored as the disease progresses. Involvement of the corticobulbar tract, cerebellum, and brainstem in MS contributes to symptoms of dysphagia, with swallowing impairments more common and severe in MS individuals who have more widespread neurological involvement.[32] Just as the presenting symptoms of MS vary, swallowing impairments may vary depending on the site and involvement of lesions.[47] Cerebellar and brainstem lesions may affect timing and sequencing within the oral and pharyngeal stages of swallowing and have been identified in individuals with MS with varying severity levels.[32]

Swallowing impairments can occur during the oral, pharyngeal, and esophageal phases in individuals with MS. In a study of 525 individuals with varying types of MS, patient-reported symptoms of dysphagia included prandial coughing (26%), choking (19%), anxiety related to swallowing (19%), and patient-reported changes in swallow function (11%).[83] DePauw and colleagues characterized specific swallowing impairments associated with MS severity status as determined by the EDSS. These authors noted that individuals with mild MS (EDSS ≤ 7.5) demonstrated difficulties with bolus formation, swallow initiation, and mild vallecular stasis following instrumental evaluation.[84] Individuals classified as having severe MS (EDSS ≥ 8) demonstrated impairments with bolus formation, swallowing initiation, diffuse pharyngeal residue, multiple swallows per bolus, and penetration and aspiration.[85] Therefore, dysphagia symptoms were more severe and occurred more often in individuals with more advanced MS.[77] Hypertonicity of the cricopharyngeal muscle in the upper esophageal sphincter (UES) has also been observed as a prevalent impairment in MS.[8,32,86]

## Evaluation and Management of Dysphagia in Multiple Sclerosis

It is generally recommended that the evaluation of dysphagia in MS include an instrumental evaluation of swallowing in order to identify the specific pathophysiology of dysphagia and implement appropriate interventions.[85] In addition to the presence of dysphagia, oral intake may be affected by restricted mobility, fatigue, tremor, cognitive impairment, and depression associated with MS. Therefore, a multidisciplinary approach including an SLP, a dietitian, and a neurologist is ideal for developing a treatment plan.[87] Due to the varying signs of dysphagia in MS, research in treatment of dysphagia in MS is relatively limited.[72] Developing a treatment plan is dependent on the impairments observed during the clinical and instrumental swallowing evaluations.[72] Appropriate compensatory and rehabilitative strategies should focus on the impaired physiology, as well as the ability of the individual to implement strategies effectively (**Fig. 19.5**).

Chiara et al investigated the impact of EMST on expiratory pressure-generating capability, pulmonary function, and maximal voluntary cough in individuals with MS. Results indicated improved voluntary cough volume and improved expiratory pressure-generating capability across the entire cohort.[88] The effect of neuromuscular electrostimulation (NMES) on dysphagia in individuals with MS has been investigated in a pilot study of 17 individuals with MS.[89] In this study, patients with MS underwent a 3-week treatment of twice weekly NMES with completion of 12 saliva, 24 water, and 24 yogurt bolus trials during each 20-minute treatment period. Reported outcomes included reduced pooling of saliva in the piriform sinus and improved Penetration-Aspiration Scale scores in 9 of 17 (53%) patients. Interpretation of these findings is limited, however, due to the lack of a control group to determine the impact of active swallowing exercises without simultaneous NMES. Further research is needed to determine the potential benefit of both of these treatment modalities in MS.

The use of botulinum neurotoxin type A (BoNT/A) is a medical intervention for individuals with MS. BoNT/A has been used in individuals with MS with severe oropharyngeal dysphagia and hypertonicity of the UES following evaluation under videofluoroscopy. Injection of BoNT/A into the cricopharyngeal muscle of

24 individuals with MS and hypertonicity of the UES resulted in improved swallowing outcome measures, including decreased Penetration-Aspiration Scale scores and reduced pharyngeal residue.[86]

In cases of severe oropharyngeal dysphagia in individuals with MS, the risk of aspiration pneumonia, respiratory complications, malnutrition, dehydration, and weight loss must be considered. Alternative forms of feeding, including the placement of a PEG tube, may be necessary to supplement or replace oral intake. The development of malnutrition in MS further exacerbates immune insufficiency and respiratory muscle weakness, in turn worsening symptoms of fatigue, weakness, and muscle spasms.[87] This further supports the need for multidisciplinary intervention in this patient population.

# 19.5 Questions

## 19.5.1 Amyotrophic Lateral Sclerosis (ALS) Pathophysiology

**1.** ALS involves the degeneration of:

A. Upper motor neurons
B. Lower motor neurons
C. Both upper and lower motor neurons
D. Basal ganglia
E. Primary motor cortex

**2.** ALS with bulbar involvement will lead to:

A. Deterioration in the function of the lower extremity musculature
B. Cognitive impairments
C. Deterioration in the muscles involved in speech and swallowing
D. Difficulty with fine motor movements
E. Sensory impairment

**3.** In the absence of lower motor neuron involvement, you will likely not observe:

A. Spasticity
B. Hypertonicity
C. Fasciculations
D. Slowed muscle movement
E. Hyperactive reflexes

## 19.5.2 Management of Dysphagia in ALS

**4.** To avoid the risk of malnutrition in ALS it is important to:

A. Monitor body weight and appetite levels
B. Consistently reevaluate swallow function and use of swallow strategies
C. Consider alternative feeding methods, such as percutaneous endoscopic gastrostomy (PEG) tube placement
D. Educate the patient on importance of nutrition
E. All of the above

**5.** To manage symptoms of dysphagia, useful compensations may include:

A. Avoiding high-calorie supplements and additives to avoid weight gain
B. Taking smaller, more frequent meals with high-calorie snacks between meals
C. Taking larger bite sizes to get the meal finished quickly and avoid fatigue
D. Choosing food items that require thorough mastication to engage the muscles
E. Eating one large meal per day to ensure adequate caloric intake

**6.** The Eating Assessment Tool-10 is a good adjunct to the clinical swallowing evaluation in individuals with ALS because:

A. It is a quick, easy to administer patient survey.
B. It predicts aspiration with 95% accuracy.
C. It demonstrated that ALS patients scoring ≥ 8 were three times more likely to aspirate.
D. It accurately identifies silent aspirators.
E. A and C only.

**7.** True or False: In individuals with ALS, silent aspiration is rare and typically does not occur in this patient population.

## 19.5.3 CD: Diagnosis

Patient CD arrived at his neurological evaluation and completed a series of clinical tests. Although CD's primary concerns are regarding changes in gait and his hand tremor, his wife also expresses concerns regarding changes in CD's vocal quality and choking episodes. The neurologist completed the evaluation and recorded her findings, including a potential diagnosis of Parkinson's disease and comorbidities in the following report:

Patient CD is a 66-year-old man who reports gradually worsening symptoms of hand tremor and impaired gait. CD was accompanied by his wife, who reported additional changes she recognized over the past year, including coughing during meals and changes in vocal quality. On examination, patient CD demonstrated clinical signs of dysphagia and dysarthria characterized by

**1.** Mild hypokinetic dysarthria: changes in voice and speech characterized by hypophonia, breathiness, and reduced prosody.

2. Dysphagia characterized by increased prandial coughing and choking as observed by the patient's wife and confirmed during the 3-ounce water swallow screen today, requiring further examination by instrumental evaluation and speech-language pathology referral.

3. Motor symptoms: asymmetric resting tremor in the left hand, shuffling gait, postural instability.

4. Cognition within normal limits: no impairments in memory, cognition, or language.

## 19.5.4 Overview of PD

8. The hallmark features of Parkinson's disease include:

A. Resting tremor
B. Rigidity
C. Bradykinesia
D. Postural instability
E. All of the above

9. Which of the following is considered the primary cause of mortality in individuals with PD is considered?

A. Falls
B. Aspiration pneumonia
C. Dementia
D. Deep vein thrombosis
E. Stroke

10. Parkinson's disease is classified as a movement disorder due to the associated motor symptoms affecting gait, movement, and coordination as a result of:

A. Underactivation of neurons within the thalamus and cortical motor areas
B. Lower motor neuron involvement
C. Death of dopamine neurons within the substantia nigra pars compacta of the basal ganglia
D. Serotonin depletion resulting in overactivation in the primary and sensorimotor cortex
E. A and C

## 19.5.5 Management of Dysphagia in PD

11. Common oral-stage impairments in individuals with PD include:

A. Lingual pumping
B. Incomplete laryngeal vestibule closure
C. Prolonged mastication
D. Impaired UES relaxation
E. A and C

12. Results of use of expiratory muscle strength training (EMST) in individuals with PD indicated positive effects on:

A. Improved cough function and airway protection
B. Reduced pharyngeal residue
C. Improved labial seal and reduced labial leakage
D. Improved base of tongue retraction
E. Improved velopharyngeal closure

13. True or False: Patient and caregiver education, including use of safe swallow strategies, biofeedback, and signs of deterioration in swallow function, is not important in this patient population.

14. Which of the following principles of plasticity do the Lee Silverman Voice Treatment (LSVT) and EMST incorporate for the management of dysphagia?

A. Specificity
B. Repetition
C. Use it or lose it
D. Interference
E. B and C

## 19.5.6 Multiple Sclerosis

15. Multiple sclerosis is considered:

A. A progressive disease of the peripheral nervous system
B. Curable if diagnosed within the first 10 years post onset
C. Primarily attributed to genetic mutation
D. Caused by traumatic brain injury
E. A progressive disease of the central nervous system

16. The most common onset type of multiple sclerosis is:

A. Primary-progressive multiple sclerosis (PPMS)
B. Remitting-relapsing multiple sclerosis (RRMS)
C. Progressive-relapsing multiple sclerosis (PRMS)
D. Continuous multiple sclerosis
E. Benign multiple sclerosis

17. True or False: The clinical presentation (i.e., initial signs and symptoms) of MS is very similar from patient to patient.

## 19.5.7 Management of Dysphagia in MS

18. Evaluation and treatment of dysphagia in MS should focus on:

A. Patient-reported swallowing impairment
B. Case history and clinical evaluation
C. Results of instrumental evaluation of swallowing
D. Results of evaluations by professionals from other disciplines (e.G., Neurology, dietitian)
E. All of the above

**19.** True or False: Dysphagia treatment in individuals with MS should be tailored to the specific impairments observed during the clinical and instrumental swallowing evaluation in order to treat each patient's deficits appropriately.

**20.** In individuals with MS diagnosed with dysphagia, the use of botulinum neurotoxin type A has been shown to treat

A. Reduced base of tongue retraction
B. Mandibular spasticity
C. Hypertonicity of the ues
D. Reduced pharyngeal contraction
E. None of the above

# 19.6 Answers and Explanations

**1. Correct: both upper and lower motor neurons (C).**
A diagnosis of ALS requires the involvement of *both* upper and lower motor neurons to meet El-Escorial World Federation of Neurology criterion. Impairments due to insult to the basal ganglia and primary motor cortex are not included in the diagnostic criterion for ALS.

**2. Correct: deterioration in the muscles involved in speech and swallowing (C).**
Bulbar nerve involvement leads to impairments in the muscles involved in speech and swallowing. Upper and lower extremity function is affected with progression of spinal nerve involvement.

**3. Correct: fasciculations (C).**
*Upper motor neuron* involvement causes spasticity resulting in muscle slowness, stiffness, and hyperreflexia. Fasciculations occur due to *lower motor neuron* involvement, which also causes muscle atrophy resulting in flaccidity and reduced muscle speed and force.

**4. Correct: all of the above (E).**
Management of dysphagia in ALS requires an interdisciplinary approach (e.g., SLP, dietitian, and neurologist), addressing swallow safety, nutrition maintenance, patient education, and alternative feeding methods, in order to avoid the consequences of aspiration and malnutrition.

**5. Correct: take smaller, more frequent meals with high-calorie snacks between meals (B).**
Taking smaller, more frequent meals and high-calorie snacks throughout the day aids in avoiding fatigue during meals and ensuring adequate caloric intake. Weight gain is not a concern in this patient population, and larger bite size is contraindicated due to the commonly observed impairments in mastication and lingual strength and movement.

**6. Correct: A and C only (E).**
The EAT-10 is useful in clinical swallowing evaluation, but has not been shown to predict aspiration with 95% accuracy or identify silent aspiration. To identify silent aspiration, an instrumental swallowing evaluation, such as a modified barium swallow study or fiberoptic endoscopic evaluation of swallowing, is necessary.

**7. Correct: False.**
In this particular patient population, silent aspiration may occur. Recent findings indicate that aspiration occurs in approximately 30% of ALS patients (confirmed via videofluoroscopic evaluation) attending a specialized ALS multidisciplinary clinic. Of the persons with ALS who aspirated, 58% did so without a cough response, whereas 42% demonstrated an ineffective cough response that did not clear aspirant material.[23]

**8. Correct: all of the above (E).**
All of the above are considered hallmark symptoms of PD. Additional early signs of PD may include fatigue, generalized weakness, and gait disturbance.

**9. Correct: aspiration pneumonia (B).**
Aspiration pneumonia is considered the primary cause of mortality in individuals with PD. Additional leading causes of death include pulmonary embolism and falls.

**10. Correct: A and C (E).**
Both underactivation of neurons and death of dopamine neurons contribute to the impairment movements observed in PD, including but not limited to gait disturbance, bradykinesia, dyskinesia, impaired coordination, and postural instability.

**11. Correct: A and C (E).**
Both lingual pumping and prolonged mastication are hallmark oral-stage impairments in PD. Although incomplete laryngeal vestibule closure and impaired UES relaxation may be observed in PD, they do not occur during the oral stage of swallowing.

**12. Correct: improved cough function and airway protection (A).**
Results of a randomized controlled trial investigating EMST in individuals with PD, conducted by Troche and colleagues, found improvements in cough function and airway protection. Specific temporal and kinematic measures (tongue base retraction, residue ratings) of swallowing were not considered during this particular study.

**13. Correct: False.**
Biofeedback and caregiver education is particularly useful and important in this patient population given the concomitant cognitive impairments and poor self-awareness of impairments.

**14. Correct: B and C (E).**
Repetition refers to repeated practice of a novel task in order to cause lasting neural changes and avoid or reduce detraining in the absence of practice. The use it or lose it principle speaks to the degradation of neural circuits within a system when not trained over a period of time. Both the repetition and use it or lose it principles of plasticity are incorporated in LSVT and EMST regimens.

### 15. Correct: a progressive disease of the central nervous system (E).

MS is a progressive disease of the central nervous system and, unfortunately, is not curable regardless of when it is diagnosed. Although theories exist as to the etiology of MS, including environmental factors, compromised immunity, and genetic markers, it is not definitely due to genetics and is not caused by traumatic brain injury.

### 16. Correct: remitting-relapsing multiple sclerosis (RRMS) (B).

RRMS accounts for 85–90% of MS cases, the majority of which progress to secondary-progressive MS (SPMS) within 25 years. PPMS and PRMS are less common at 10% and 5% prevalence, respectively.

### 17. Correct: False.

MS symptoms vary tremendously from individual to individual, making treatment difficult. Intervention is symptom specific and tailored to each patient's specific symptoms.

### 18. Correct: all of the above (E).

Intervention for dysphagia should be centered on a multidisciplinary approach and include all aspects, including both clinical and instrumental swallowing evaluations, with frequent monitoring and reevaluation as symptoms continually evolve.

### 19. Correct: True.

As in any population, dysphagia treatment should be focused on the impairment visualized during clinical and instrumental swallowing evaluations, as well as results of other professionals on the multidisciplinary care team.

### 20. Correct: hypertonicity of the UES (C).

The use of botulinum neurotoxin type A has been shown to improve hypertonicity of the UES when injected into the cricopharyngeal muscle of 24 individuals with MS. This resulted in reduced pharyngeal residue and decreased Penetration-Aspiration Scale scores.[86]

## References

[1] Huckabee ML, Pelletier CA. Management of Adult Neurogenic Dysphagia. Dysphagia Series. San Diego, CA: Singular: 1999

[2] Yorkston KM, Miller RM, Strand EA. Management of Speech and Swallowing in Degenerative Diseases. Tucson, AZ: Communication Skill Builders; 1995

[3] Brooks BR, Miller RG, Swash M, Munsat TL; World Federation of Neurology Research Group on Motor Neuron Diseases. El Escorial revisited: revised criteria for the diagnosis of amyotrophic lateral sclerosis. Amyotroph Lateral Scler Other Motor Neuron Disord 2000;1(5):293–299

[4] Mehta P, Antao V, Kaye W, et al; Division of Toxicology and Human Health Sciences, Agency for Toxic Substances and Disease Registry, Atlanta, Georgia; Centers for Disease Control and Prevention (CDC). Prevalence of amyotrophic lateral sclerosis - United States, 2010-2011. MMWR Suppl 2014;63(7):1–14

[5] Wijesekera LC, Leigh PN. Amyotrophic lateral sclerosis. Orphanet J Rare Dis 2009;4:3

[6] Blumenfeld H. Neuroanatomy through Clinical Cases. Sunderland, MA: Sinauer; 2002

[7] Lomen-Hoerth C, Anderson T, Miller B. The overlap of amyotrophic lateral sclerosis and frontotemporal dementia. Neurology 2002;59(7):1077–1079

[8] Papps B, Abrahams S, Wicks P, Leigh PN, Goldstein LH. Changes in memory for emotional material in amyotrophic lateral sclerosis (ALS). Neuropsychologia 2005;43(8):1107–1114

[9] Kühnlein P, Gdynia HJ, Sperfeld AD, et al. Diagnosis and treatment of bulbar symptoms in amyotrophic lateral sclerosis. Nat Clin Pract Neurol 2008;4(7):366–374

[10] Plowman EK. Is there a role for exercise in the management of bulbar dysfunction in amyotrophic lateral sclerosis? J Speech Lang Hear Res 2015;58(4):1151–1166

[11] Desport JC, Preux PM, Truong CT, Courat L, Vallat JM, Couratier P. Nutritional assessment and survival in ALS patients. Amyotroph Lateral Scler Other Motor Neuron Disord 2000;1(2):91–96

[12] Carpenter RJ III, McDonald TJ, Howard FM Jr. The otolaryngologic presentation of amyotrophic lateral sclerosis. Otolaryngology 1978;86(3 Pt 1):ORL479–ORL484

[13] Chen A, Garrett CG. Otolaryngologic presentations of amyotrophic lateral sclerosis. Otolaryngol Head Neck Surg 2005;132(3):500–504

[14] Plowman EK. Nutrition and Feeding Tube Placement for People with ALS: Best Practice in Clinical Decision Making. Dysphagia Cafe; 2014. https://dysphagiacafe.com/2014/10/23/nutrition-and-feeding-tube-placement-for-people-with-als-best-practice-in-clinical-decision-making/

[15] Ngo ST, Steyn FJ, McCombe PA. Body mass index and dietary intervention: implications for prognosis of amyotrophic lateral sclerosis. J Neurol Sci 2014;340(1-2):5–12

[16] Greenwood DI. Nutrition management of amyotrophic lateral sclerosis. Nutr Clin Pract 2013;28(3):392–399

[17] Goyal NA, Mozaffar T. Respiratory and nutritional support in amyotrophic lateral sclerosis. Curr Treat Options Neurol 2014;16(2):270

[18] Braun MM, Osecheck M, Joyce NC. Nutrition assessment and management in amyotrophic lateral sclerosis. Phys Med Rehabil Clin N Am 2012;23(4):751–771

[19] Paris G, Martinaud O, Petit A, et al. Oropharyngeal dysphagia in amyotrophic lateral sclerosis alters quality of life. J Oral Rehabil 2013;40(3):199–204

[20] Tabor L. Defining Swallowing-Related Quality of Life in Individuals with Amyotrophic Lateral Sclerosis. Kimberly, WI: Dysphagia Research Society; 2015

[21] Plowman EK. Pecutaneous Gastronomy Tube Placement Increases Survival in Amyotrophic Lateral Sclerosis. Kimberly, WI: Dysphagia Research Society; 2015

[22] Spataro R, Ficano L, Piccoli F, La Bella V. Percutaneous endoscopic gastrostomy in amyotrophic lateral sclerosis: effect on survival. J Neurol Sci 2011;304(1-2):44–48

[23] Gaziano J. Prevalence, Timing and Source of Aspiration in Individuals with ALS. Kimberly, WI: Dysphagia Research Society; 2015

[24] Solazzo A, Del Vecchio L, Reginelli A, et al. Search for compensation postures with videofluoromanometric investigation in dysphagic patients affected by amyotrophic lateral sclerosis. Radiol Med (Torino) 2011;116(7):1083–1094

[25] Belafsky PC, Mouadeb DA, Rees CJ, et al. Validity and reliability of the Eating Assessment Tool (EAT-10). Ann Otol Rhinol Laryngol 2008;117(12):919–924

[26] McHorney CA, Bricker DE, Kramer AE, et al. The SWAL-QOL outcomes tool for oropharyngeal dysphagia in adults: I. Conceptual foundation and item development. Dysphagia 2000;15(3):115–121

[27] Leder SB, Suiter DM. The Yale Swallow Protocol: An Evidence-Based Approach to Decision Making. New York, NY: Springer; 2014

[28] O'Neil KH, Purdy M, Falk J, Gallo L. The Dysphagia Outcome and Severity Scale. Dysphagia 1999;14(3):139–145

[29] Goetz CG. The history of Parkinson's disease: early clinical descriptions and neurological therapies. Cold Spring Harb Perspect Med 2011;1(1):a008862

[30] Wirdefeldt K, et al. Epidemiology and Etiology of Parkinson's Disease: A Review of the Evidence. New York, NY: Springer; 2011

[31] Factor SA, Weiner WJ. Parkinson's Disease: Diagnosis and Clinical Management. 2nd ed. New York, NY: Demos; 2008

[32] Poorjavad M, Derakhshandeh F, Etemadifar M, Soleymani B, Minagar A, Maghzi AH. Oropharyngeal dysphagia in multiple sclerosis. Mult Scler 2010;16(3):362–365

[33] Levine CB, Fahrbach KR, Siderowf AD, Estok RP, Ludensky VM, Ross SD. Diagnosis and treatment of Parkinson's disease: a systematic review of the literature. Evid Rep Technol Assess (Summ) 2003; (57):1–4

[34] Verstraeten A, Theuns J, Van Broeckhoven C. Progress in unraveling the genetic etiology of Parkinson disease in a genomic era. Trends Genet 2015;31(3):140–149

[35] Hely MA, Morris JG, Traficante R, Reid WG, O'Sullivan DJ, Williamson PM. The Sydney multicentre study of Parkinson's disease: progression and mortality at 10 years. J Neurol Neurosurg Psychiatry 1999;67(3):300–307

[36] Rosenbek J, Jones H. Dysphagia in Movement Disorders. Vol 1. San Diego, CA: Plural Publishing; 2008

[37] Aarsland D, Brønnick K, Larsen JP, Tysnes OB, Alves G; Norwegian ParkWest Study Group. Cognitive impairment in incident, untreated Parkinson disease: the Norwegian ParkWest study. Neurology 2009;72(13):1121–1126

[38] Rongve A, Aarsland D. Dementia with Lewy Bodies and Parkinson's Disease Dementia. Oxford, UK: Oxford University Press; 2013

[39] Lin C-H, Wu R-M. Biomarkers of cognitive decline in Parkinson's disease. *Parkinsonism Relat Disord* 2015;*21*(5):431–443

[40] Rosenbek JC, Jones HN. Dysphagia in Movement Disorders. Clinical Dysphagia Series. San Diego, CA: Plural Publishing; 2009:265

[41] Robbins JA, Logemann JA, Kirshner HS. Swallowing and speech production in Parkinson's disease. *Ann Neurol* 1986;*19*(3):283–287

[42] Sung HY, Kim JS, Lee KS, et al. The prevalence and patterns of pharyngoesophageal dysmotility in patients with early stage Parkinson's disease. *Mov Disord* 2010;*25*(14):2361–2368

[43] Hammer MJ, Murphy CA, Abrams TM. Airway somatosensory deficits and dysphagia in Parkinson's disease. *J Parkinsons Dis* 2013;*3*(1):39–44

[44] Plowman-Prine EK, Sapienza CM, Okun MS, et al. The relationship between quality of life and swallowing in Parkinson's disease. *Mov Disord* 2009;*24*(9):1352–1358

[45] Leopold NA, Kagel MC. Pharyngo-esophageal dysphagia in Parkinson's disease. *Dysphagia* 1997;*12*(1):11–20

[46] Ciucci MR, Grant LM, Rajamanickam ES, et al. Early identification and treatment of communication and swallowing deficits in Parkinson disease. *Semin Speech Lang* 2013;*34*(3):185–202

[47] Logemann JA. Evaluation and Treatment of Swallowing Disorders. Austin, TX: Pro-Ed; 1998:406

[48] Groher M, Crary M. Dysphagia: Clinical Management in Adults and Children. Vol 1. Maryland Heights, MO: Mosby Elsevier; 2010:336

[49] Silverman EP, Sapienza CM, Saleem A, et al. Tutorial on maximum inspiratory and expiratory mouth pressures in individuals with idiopathic Parkinson disease (IPD) and the preliminary results of an expiratory muscle strength training program. *NeuroRehabilitation* 2006;*21*(1):71–79

[50] Pitts T, Bolser D, Rosenbek J, Troche M, Okun MS, Sapienza C. Impact of expiratory muscle strength training on voluntary cough and swallow function in Parkinson disease. *Chest* 2009;*135*(5):1301–1308

[51] Pitts T, Troche M, Mann G, Rosenbek J, Okun MS, Sapienza C. Using voluntary cough to detect penetration and aspiration during oropharyngeal swallowing in patients with Parkinson disease. *Chest* 2010;*138*(6):1426–1431

[52] Wheeler Hegland K, Troche MS, Brandimore AE, Davenport PW, Okun MS. Comparison of voluntary and reflex cough effectiveness in Parkinson's disease. *Parkinsonism Relat Disord* 2014;*20*(11):1226–1230

[53] Hegland KW, Okun MS, Troche MS. Sequential voluntary cough and aspiration or aspiration risk in Parkinson's disease. *Lung* 2014;*192*(4):601–608

[54] Troche MS, et al. Decreased Cough Sensitivity and Aspiration in Parkinson Disease. Northbrook, IL: American College of Chest Physicians; 2014:1294

[55] Ramig LO, Theodoros DG. Communication and Swallowing in Parkinson Disease. San Diego, CA: Plural Publishing; 2011

[56] Luchesi KF, Kitamura S, Mourão LF. Dysphagia progression and swallowing management in Parkinson's disease: an observational study. *Rev Bras Otorrinolaringol (Engl Ed)* 2015;*81*(1):24–30

[57] Ashford J, McCabe D, Wheeler-Hegland K, et al. Evidence-based systematic review: Oropharyngeal dysphagia behavioral treatments. Part III—impact of dysphagia treatments on populations with neurological disorders. *J Rehabil Res Dev* 2009;*46*(2):195–204

[58] Chiara T, Martin D, Sapienza C. Expiratory muscle strength training: speech production outcomes in patients with multiple sclerosis. *Neurorehabil Neural Repair* 2007;*21*(3):239–249

[59] Troche MS, Okun MS, Rosenbek JC, et al. Aspiration and swallowing in Parkinson disease and rehabilitation with EMST: a randomized trial. *Neurology* 2010;*75*(21):1912–1919

[60] El Sharkawi A, Ramig L, Logemann JA, et al. Swallowing and voice effects of Lee Silverman Voice Treatment (LSVT): a pilot study. *J Neurol Neurosurg Psychiatry* 2002;*72*(1):31–36

[61] Kleim JA, Jones TA. Principles of experience-dependent neural plasticity: implications for rehabilitation after brain damage. *J Speech Lang Hear Res* 2008;*51*(1):S225–S239

[62] Athukorala RP, Jones RD, Sella O, Huckabee ML. Skill training for swallowing rehabilitation in patients with Parkinson's disease. *Arch Phys Med Rehabil* 2014;*95*(7):1374–1382

[63] Manor Y, Mootanah R, Freud D, Giladi N, Cohen JT. Video-assisted swallowing therapy for patients with Parkinson's disease. *Parkinsonism Relat Disord* 2013;*19*(2):207–211

[64] van Hooren MRA, Baijens LW, Voskuilen S, Oosterloo M, Kremer B. Treatment effects for dysphagia in Parkinson's disease: a systematic review. *Parkinsonism Relat Disord* 2014;*20*(8):800–807

[65] Plowman-Prine EK, Okun MS, Sapienza CM, et al. Perceptual characteristics of Parkinsonian speech: a comparison of the pharmacological effects of levodopa across speech and non-speech motor systems. *NeuroRehabilitation* 2009;*24*(2):131–144

[66] D'Alatri L, Paludetti G, Contarino MF, Galla S, Marchese MR, Bentivoglio AR. Effects of bilateral subthalamic nucleus stimulation and medication on parkinsonian speech impairment. *J Voice* 2008;*22*(3):365–372

[67] De Letter M, Santens P, Estercam I, et al. Levodopa-induced modifications of prosody and comprehensibility in advanced Parkinson's disease as perceived by professional listeners. *Clin Linguist Phon* 2007;*21*(10):783–791

[68] Ciucci MR, Barkmeier-Kraemer JM, Sherman SJ. Subthalamic nucleus deep brain stimulation improves deglutition in Parkinson's disease. *Mov Disord* 2008;*23*(5):676–683

[69] Lengerer S, Kipping J, Rommel N, et al. Deep-brain-stimulation does not impair deglutition in Parkinson's disease. *Parkinsonism Relat Disord* 2012;*18*(7):847–853

[70] Rodriguez-Oroz MC, Obeso JA, Lang AE, et al. Bilateral deep brain stimulation in Parkinson's disease: a multicentre study with 4 years follow-up. *Brain* 2005;*128*(Pt 10):2240–2249

[71] Troche MS, Brandimore AE, Foote KD, Okun MS. Swallowing and deep brain stimulation in Parkinson's disease: a systematic review. *Parkinsonism Relat Disord* 2013;*19*(9):783–788

[72] Miller RM, Britton D. Dysphagia in Neuromuscular Diseases. Clinical Dysphagia Series. San Diego: Plural Publishing; 2011

[73] Dutta R, Trapp BD. Mechanisms of neuronal dysfunction and degeneration in multiple sclerosis. *Prog Neurobiol* 2011;*93*(1):1–12

[74] Milo R, Miller A. Revised diagnostic criteria of multiple sclerosis. *Autoimmun Rev* 2014;*13*(4-5):518–524

[75] Guan X-L, Wang H, Huang HS, Meng L. Prevalence of dysphagia in multiple sclerosis: a systematic review and meta-analysis. *Neurol Sci* 2015;*36*(5):671–681

[76] Peterson JW, Trapp BD. Neuropathobiology of multiple sclerosis. *Neurol Clin* 2005;*23*(1):107–129, vi–vii

[77] Koch M, Zhao Y, Yee I, et al; UBC MS Clinic Neurologists. Disease onset in familial and sporadic primary progressive multiple sclerosis. *Mult Scler* 2010;*16*(6):694–700

[78] Koch M, Kingwell E, Rieckmann P, Tremlett H; UBC MS Clinic Neurologists. The natural history of secondary progressive multiple sclerosis. *J Neurol Neurosurg Psychiatry* 2010;*81*(9):1039–1043

[79] Goodin DS, Corwin M, Kaufman D, et al. Causes of death among commercially insured multiple sclerosis patients in the United States. *PLoS One* 2014;*9*(8):e105207

[80] Polman CH, Reingold SC, Banwell B, et al. Diagnostic criteria for multiple sclerosis: 2010 revisions to the McDonald criteria. *Ann Neurol* 2011;*69*(2):292–302

[81] Kurtzke JF. Rating neurologic impairment in multiple sclerosis: an expanded disability status scale (EDSS). *Neurology* 1983;*33*(11):1444–1452

[82] Lublin FD, DeAngelis TM. Multiple sclerosis as a model neurologic disease. *Mt Sinai J Med* 2011;*78*(2):159–160

[83] Abraham S, et al. Neurologic impairment and disability status in outpatients with multiple sclerosis reporting dysphagia symptomatology. *Neurorehabil Neural Repair* 1997;*11*(1):7

[84] Blonder LX, Heilman KM, Ketterson T, et al. Affective facial and lexical expression in aprosodic versus aphasic stroke patients. *J Int Neuropsychol Soc* 2005;*11*(6):677–685

[85] De Pauw A, Dejaeger E, D'hooghe B, Carton H. Dysphagia in multiple sclerosis. *Clin Neurol Neurosurg* 2002;*104*(4):345–351

[86] Restivo DA, Marchese-Ragona R, Patti F, et al. Botulinum toxin improves dysphagia associated with multiple sclerosis. *Eur J Neurol* 2011;*18*(3):486–490

[87] Habek M, Hojsak I, Brinar VV. Nutrition in multiple sclerosis. *Clin Neurol Neurosurg* 2010;*112*(7):616–620

[88] Chiara T, Martin AD, Davenport PW, Bolser DC. Expiratory muscle strength training in persons with multiple sclerosis having mild to moderate disability: effect on maximal expiratory pressure, pulmonary function, and maximal voluntary cough. *Arch Phys Med Rehabil* 2006;*87*(4):468–473

[89] Bogaardt H, van Dam D, Wever NM, Bruggeman CE, Koops J, Fokkens WJ. Use of neuromuscular electrostimulation in the treatment of dysphagia in patients with multiple sclerosis. *Ann Otol Rhinol Laryngol* 2009;*118*(4):241–246

# 20 Dysphagia Following Stroke

*Giselle Carnaby*

## Summary

Dysphagia after stroke is a common and underrecognized problem associated with significant and negative health outcomes. Speech-language pathologists have a critical role to play in the early identification and management of this issue. To enhance this goal, clinicians need to remain updated on specific stroke-related data and, in particular, the application of early intensive interventions to focus motor recovery and eliminate aberrant movements that may prevent effective rehabilitation.

## Keywords

stroke, dysphagia, screening, intervention, compensation, rehabilitation

### Learning Objectives
- Describe common characteristics of dysphagia resulting from stroke
- Identify health issues resulting from swallowing deficits following a stroke
- Describe intervention strategies for swallowing rehabilitation following a stroke and how they may change over time
- Describe novel intervention methods for dysphagia following stroke

## 20.1 Introduction

Dysphagia is a common occurrence following a stroke. It affects almost half of all stroke patients and is associated with negative outcomes, such as respiratory complications, aspiration pneumonia, dehydration, reduced quality of life, and even death. Patients with dysphagia following a stroke are one of the most common groups with whom a speech-language pathologist (SLP) will work. The SLP plays a key role in the screening, assessment, treatment, and management of dysphagia in the stroke survivor. Consequently, it is critical that the practicing clinician understand the factors associated with dysphagia after stroke and its management. This chapter outlines the impact and characteristics of stroke and dysphagia and common complications. It addresses critical information associated with the identification of swallowing problems in stroke patients and reviews state-of-the-art knowledge in dysphagia treatment options available to the SLP working with a stroke patient.

One of the most common diseases affecting the elderly population is cerebrovascular disease. Cerebrovascular disease may manifest gradually as vascular dementia, or abruptly as a stroke. Stroke is defined as a focal or global loss of cerebral function or neurological impairment of sudden onset, lasting more than 24 hours (or leading to death), and of presumed vascular etiology.[1,2] When the brain is damaged from a stroke, it disrupts the flow of information between and to different structures. Information arriving and leaving the brain via the sensory and motor tracts becomes disturbed. Consequently, activities, such as swallowing, that are broadly represented within the brain (i.e., controlled by multiple brain structures in the cortical, subcortical, and brainstem regions) often become affected.

Disturbed swallowing (or dysphagia) following a stroke is also significant and strongly affects outcome. Dysphagia poststroke is associated with aspiration that leads to pneumonia, prolonged hospital stay, increasing cost to the community, and increasing morbidity and mortality.[3,4] For this reason, efforts have focused on early identification and treatment of dysphagia poststroke.

## 20.2 Stroke Incidence/Prevalence

Stroke is the second most common cause of death and one of the most common causes of preventable long-term disability in developed countries.[5,6] In the United States alone, the annual incidence of stroke is estimated at to be greater than 795,000 individuals per year, or one every 40 seconds.[7] Of note, stroke is more often disabling than fatal, and it is a major public health problem resulting in increased health care expenditure and loss of productivity. It is also a disease of aging, the incidence increasing exponentially with increasing age, thus placing a considerable burden on the community. Further, African Americans have almost twice the risk for a first-ever stroke than Caucasians and are more likely to die from the stroke.[8] Death following stroke is often due to nonneurological causes, such as cardiovascular disease and pneumonia. Of the approximately 700,000 Americans who suffer a stroke each year, more than 20% will die within the first year, and nearly 35% of deaths that happen after the acute stroke are associated with the development of pneumonia.[9] In fact, studies of the natural history of stroke have identified a 20% incidence of death from aspiration pneumonia in the first year following a stroke, and 10 to 15% with each successive year.[10] At 12 months following a stroke, about 70% of persons will be dead or disabled.[11,12]

## 20.3 Prevalence of Dysphagia Following Stroke

Dysphagia following stroke is common and often acknowledged as a serious complication that is underappreciated.[13,14] Incidence of dysphagia following stroke has been reported to be between 25 and 60% of patients.[13,14,15] In addition, between 22 and 42% of stroke patients are thought to have aspiration as a result of oropharyngeal dysphagia.[4,16,17,18,19] Although the reported prevalence of dysphagia is variably reported within the literature (22–60%), it has been estimated at its lowest using cursory screening techniques (37–45%), higher using clinical testing (51–55%), and highest using instrumental testing (64–78%).[20] These conflicting pictures suggest that estimates are the result of the wide range of methodology used to identify dysphagia and estimate its prevalence. Similarly, samples evaluated in the research have been restricted to selected groups[13,15] from referred populations only,[21,22] or generated with limited controls over potentially confounding factors, such as time post onset of stroke.[23] Truly prospective investigations of dysphagia incidence in unselected stroke groups are scarce. Moreover, researchers have directed their efforts into other aspects of stroke research. Consequently, our knowledge of the incidence, characteristics (clinical and radiological), survivorship trajectory, prognosis, and optimal treatment for dysphagia following acute stroke remains incomplete.[24]

## 20.4 Mechanisms of Dysphagia Following Stroke

There are two main types of stroke: ischemic and hemorrhagic. Ischemic stroke occurs when an artery that supplies blood to the brain becomes blocked. A hemorrhagic stroke occurs when a blood vessel in the brain ruptures or leaks blood into the surrounding brain tissue. An ischemic etiology is the most frequent cause of stroke (87%), followed by intracerebral hemorrhage and then subarachnoid hemorrhage. Poststroke dysphagia is thought to be due to damage to cortical and subcortical structures involved in the stroke. Research suggests that the type of stroke does not influence dysphagia; however, stroke severity is thought to predict dysphagia.[25] Specifically, a lower level of consciousness is considered most predictive of dysphagia.[26] When considering dysphagia from stroke, the extent of the brain damage and the functional consequences of the damage influence symptoms. In clinical practice these issues are important in helping identify the severity of the swallowing deficits and the likely prognosis for its recovery.

## 20.5 Swallowing Pattern by Lesion Site

Lesions from a stroke, either cortical or subcortical, can produce many and varied combinations of swallow symptoms. Damage to the various areas of the brain can result in dysphagic profiles that range from a lack of intent to swallow to poorly coordinated but functioning swallowing patterns. Conversely, it is difficult to determine the most likely neurological localization from symptoms and signs affecting such a highly coordinated process as swallowing. Many authors have suggested that lesion site does not consistently predict dysphagia.[27,28] The relationship of specific or diagnostic swallowing deficits to the various clinical stroke types remains controversial.

Several studies have attempted to identify a predominant site for dysphagia following a stroke. Traditionally it has been suggested that lesions must occur bilaterally in the cerebral cortex or in the brainstem to produce dysphagia. However, work has also associated dysphagia with unilateral lesions.[17,29,30,31] Daniels, in a retrospective review of 16 unilateral stroke patients referred for

videofluoroscopy, identified patients with significant dysphagia as having lesions that were more anterior than posterior, and cortical rather than purely subcortical. Further, in a follow-up prospective study of 54 consecutive stroke cases, the same authors found that the insular cortex was a common lesion site for patients with dysphagia.[32]

Likewise, data have been published that implicate damage to the primary sensory cortex in dysphagia. The primary sensory areas are believed to have extensive interconnections to the motor cortex of the brain. These sensory interconnections are thought to control or limit voluntary movement.[13] Patients with damage to these areas may demonstrate difficulty in processing and responding to a sensory stimulus. For example, a patient with dysphagia may not recognize when a bolus of food or fluid is in his mouth and may hold it there until cued to swallow.

In contrast, recent metadata from Flower et al suggest that specific neuroanatomical influences may increase the likelihood of dysphagia.[26] For example, the incidence of dysphagia according to stroke region was reported as 43% in the pons, 40% in the medial medulla, and 57% in the lateral medulla. Within these regions, pontine (relative risk 3.7, 95% confidence interval 1.5–7.7), medial medullary (relative risk 6.9, 95% confidence interval 3.4–10.9), and lateral medullary lesions (relative risk 9.6, 95% confidence interval 5.9–12.8) predicted an increased risk of dysphagia.[26] Similarly, unilateral cortical stroke of the nondominant side has been associated with dysphagia in 40%, bilateral lesions of the cortex in 56%, and brainstem lesions in 67% of patients.[33] Similarly, recent diffusion-weighted magnetic resonance imaging studies have reported that lesions to the left periventricular white matter may be more disruptive to swallowing behavior.[32] Similarly, it has been shown that, as the magnitude of damage to the brain increases, so does the likelihood of dysphagia.

In examining whether both hemispheres are necessary for normal deglutition, Hamdy et al demonstrated that the pharyngeal musculature is bilaterally but asymmetrically represented in the cerebral cortex and identified the presence of interhemispheric asymmetry of swallowing motor function.[33,34] In their study using transcranial magnetoelectric stimulation, almost half of the nondysphagic stroke patients demonstrated absent pharyngeal responses from the affected hemisphere. In contrast, the dysphagic patients did show responses to stimulation of the affected hemisphere. The authors concluded that bilateral cortical innervation is not essential for normal swallowing and hypothesized that damage to the "dominant" swallowing hemisphere may underlie the development of dysphagia in stroke patients.

To better understand the mechanisms of dysphagia following stroke, Hamdy et al mapped brain changes in swallowing during stroke recovery in a sample ($n = 28$) of stroke survivors. Nondysphagic stroke survivors were found to have greater pharyngeal cortical representation in the contralesional hemisphere compared to those with dysphagia poststroke.[35] Transcranial magnetoelectric stimulation data reviewed at 1 and 3 months poststroke revealed significantly greater pharyngeal representation in the unaffected hemisphere for those who had recovered from their dysphagia.[35] Several studies have now confirmed this finding, suggesting that reorganization in the nonimpaired hemisphere via cortical neuroplasticity may be the mechanism for dysphagia recovery.[36,37,38]

Some generalizations can be drawn from the studies investigating lesion localization and dysphagia following stroke reviewed so far. Clinically there are some common "truths" that correspond to the evidence brought by the various location studies:

- A variety of lesion locations can produce dysphagia.
- Bilateral strokes and damage to brainstem structures will demonstrate the most severe dysphagia.
- Many patients with unilateral cortical strokes will recover from dysphagia rapidly.
- Patients with damage to the premotor areas are likely to display difficulty with the initiation of the swallowing event or motor coordination of the event.
- Patients with damage to the sensory regions display issues associated with bolus retention and/or clearance.
- The presence of a prior stroke is highly associated with dysphagia.

Dysphagia is clearly a common and significant problem. Variable patterns of impairment are noted, and the site and size/severity of a lesion may determine the characteristics of the swallowing impairment. Lastly, changes within the unimpaired brain, from "cortical plasticity," may be the mechanism that helps dysphagic stroke patients recover their swallowing.

## 20.6 Clinical Characteristics of Poststroke Dysphagia

A variety of swallowing deficits have been described following stroke. Clinically, signs and symptoms of dysphagia often overlap. The overwhelming pattern of swallowing following a stroke is characterized by slowness, delay, and inefficiency in managing food and fluids. However, hemispheric lesions (i.e., cortical and/or subcortical) can produce an array of deficits, such as slowed or reduced oral initiation of swallowing, delayed pharyngeal initiation of the swallow, incoordination of the swallow sequence, increased oral and pharyngeal transit times, reduced pharyngeal clearing or contraction, penetration or aspiration of materials into the airway, and pharyngoesophageal dysfunction (**Box 20.1**).

### Box 20.1

**Common Swallowing Deficits in Patients Following a Stroke**
- Incoordination of oral movements
- Delayed initiation of the swallow
- Increased oral and pharyngeal transit times
- Reduced pharyngeal clearance resulting in multiple swallow attempts
- Penetration or aspiration of the bolus
- Impaired pharyngoesophageal function

During evaluation of an acute stroke patient, the signs or symptoms of dysphagia may not be immediately evident. Following a stroke, a patient may initially demonstrate weakness and reduced alertness or difficulty with attention. In addition, it

is not uncommon for patients to demonstrate reduced stamina along with language comprehension or language production difficulties, such as aphasia or dyspraxia. Factors such as these often impede early, meaningful evaluation of the swallowing function. In response to this, many clinicians will delay a comprehensive swallowing evaluation and spend the intervening time collecting history and status information to better understand the possible deficit associated with the stroke. In this case, patients may be "wait listed" for later in-depth evaluation.

A variety of clinical signs are significantly associated with dysphagia following stroke (**Box 20.2**). These include tongue weakness, palatal weakness, abnormal respiration pattern, weakened cough, dysphonia, wet voice, and dysarthria.[39] Often these signs relate specifically to one or more cranial nerves and their functioning. In fact, the core portion of any clinical swallowing examination is the physical exam. This process evaluates the structure and functioning of the oral, pharyngeal, and laryngeal structures involved in swallowing. Movement of these structures provides critical information on the involvement of the cranial nerves associated with deglutition. **Table 20.1** provides a list of the cranial nerves frequently impaired in stroke and the characteristics associated with the impairment. One recent addition to the evaluation of swallowing signs in the acute stroke patient is the inclusion of respiratory function. Acute stroke patients can demonstrate abnormal respiratory patterns, including weak/inadequate cough response, and episodes of oxygen desaturation associated with changes in respiratory patterning.[40,41,42] Respiratory weakness or alterations in respiratory pattern can place a stroke patient at increased risk for incomplete clearance of materials from the pharynx or airway following a swallow. Given the increased risk of aspiration in stroke patients and subsequent pneumonia, it is important to evaluate respiratory function as part of any clinical examination.

While there are a number of common clinical signs associated with dysphagia following stroke, clinicians' opinions differ on the relative importance of each sign. McCullough et al evaluated clinicians' perceptions of the most frequently used and valued components within a clinical bedside examination for dysphagia.[43] Overall, clinicians working with dysphagia identified 16 separate oromotor and vocal components (in addition to a test

**Table 20.1** Cranial nerves implicated in dysphagia in patients following a stroke

| CN V | Reduced jaw mobility<br>Reduced strength to open/close<br>Difficulty chewing/biting down |
|---|---|
| CN VII | Incomplete ability to purse/retract lips<br>Absent or asymmetrical smile<br>Unable to raise eyebrows<br>Unable to keep lips sealed against resistance |
| CN IX | Absent or minimized gag reflex<br>Palate moves asymmetrically or reduced movement on "ah" |
| CN X | Reduced cough strength<br>Reduced cough quality<br>Impaired voice or difficulty with sustained phonation/speech |
| CN XII | Reduced tongue movement<br>Reduced tongue strength—protrusion/lateralization<br>Difficulty pushing tongue against resistance<br>Tongue atrophy |

swallow) as important indicators of dysphagia. Of those signs rated highly, only seven had research evidence supporting them. Moreover, few of these signs were commonly used as indicators for referral for further instrumental evaluation (e.g., dysarthria, dysphonia, history of pneumonia, no swallow produced, wet voice, reactive cough postswallow).[43,44] Conversely, Mann et al statistically identified a set of important clinical indicators for both dysphagia and aspiration from a large sample of stroke patients. This study reported that the strongest independent predictors of dysphagia (confirmed by videofluoroscopic evaluation) were age > 70 years, male sex, disabling stroke, palatal weakness or asymmetry, incomplete oral clearance, and impaired pharyngeal response (cough/gurgle). The identified clinical predictors of aspiration in stroke patients were delayed oral transit and incomplete oral clearance.[45] Clearly there is a lack of consensus on the most important clinical indicators for predicting dysphagia and or aspiration from dysphagia in stroke patients.[46,47]

## Box 20.2

**Common Signs of Dysphagia in Patients Following a Stroke**
- Tongue weakness
- Palatal weakness/asymmetry
- Abnormal voice/dysphonia
- Wet cough
- Dysarthria
- Dyspraxia
- Weak cough/altered respiratory pattern
- Poor secretion/saliva management
- Poor oral clearance
- Slow swallow initiation

## Prognosis

The prospect of recovery from stroke or its prognosis may be very different from the dysphagia associated with the stroke event.

## 20.6.1 Stroke

The severity of stroke on neurological exam is probably the most important factor affecting short- and long-term outcome. Approximately 25% of patients worsen during the first 24 hours following stroke. Three out of four will survive the acute event, and the vast majority of these survivors will require ongoing health care services.[5] As a general rule, large strokes with severe initial clinical deficits have poorer outcomes compared with smaller strokes. Half of the patients with disabling ischemic stroke will recover within 18 months, and recovery is greatest within the first 6 months.[48] The significant predictors of recovery include the severity of the stroke and no history of peripheral artery disease or diabetes.[49]

## Dysphagia after Stroke

It is well recognized that some patients with dysphagia following stroke can experience a relatively benign clinical course, whereas others suffer repeated negative events.[13,14,50] Dysphagia is reported to resolve quickly in around 90% of patients over the first weeks following stroke.[13,14,20,51] Although many stroke patients will recover swallowing early, between 11 and 50% have been reported to continue to have dysphagia at 6 months.[19,51] A recent analysis of Medicare files revealed that stroke patients who have severe dysphagia are twice as likely to die within a year of stroke (66% vs. 36% of nondysphagic stroke patients), are almost six times as likely to be readmitted to a hospital for aspiration pneumonia (17% vs. 3%), and are more than three times as likely to be readmitted for infections (13% vs. 4%).[51] Consequently, dysphagia and its complications act together to increase the length of hospital stay and are associated with poorer functional ability, institutionalization, increased mortality, and an increased health care cost.[52,53] In fact, more recent studies have suggested that after a stroke the injured swallowing system adapts or compensates for the impairment rather than recovers to prestroke status.[35] Given this association, it is important for health care professionals working with stroke patients to be aware of the range of negative outcomes associated with unresolved dysphagia (**Box 20.3**).

## Box 20.3

**Clinical Impact of Dysphagia Following Stroke**
- Dehydration
- Pneumonia
- Aspiration
- Increased length of hospital stay
- Institutionalization
- Depression
- Poorer functional outcome
- Increased cost for patient and community

## Functional Outcome

Dysphagia is strongly related to a longer hospital stay and poorer functional outcome in patients following stroke.[54,55,57] Patients with dysphagia often display lower levels of cognitive functioning on admission and score lower on functional abilities tests at discharge.[58] Moreover, dysphagia following acute stroke has been reported by several authors to be an independent predictor of mortality following stroke.[4,52,54,59] For example, Barer, in an analysis of the mortality of dysphagic patients, allowing for level of consciousness, showed that even alert stroke patients with dysphagia had an increased chance of dying (33% deceased by 6 months) compared to other alert stroke patients.[14]

## Nutritional Status

The prevalence of nutritional decline following stroke has also been variously reported as between 6 and 62%.[60] Reductions in nutritional status following stroke are important because of the negative impact it can have on functional recovery and mortality. Results from a large multicenter trial of feeding after stroke found poor nutritional status was associated with increased odds of death and disability at 6 months after stroke.[60]

Evidence linking dysphagia poststroke to nutritional decline is less clear.[52,61,62,63,64] Over 11 studies have reported a link between dysphagia and malnutrition. Smithard et al, in a prospective cohort study of 121 stroke patients, reported significant worsening of nutritional indices in patients with dysphagia and postulated that nutritional deficiency resulted in a lowered immune response to infection, initiating a spiral of decline, leading to further swallowing difficulties.[52] Conversely, other researchers have found no relationship between dysphagia and nutritional decline.[65,66] These studies suggest that the gradual deterioration in nutritional status of stroke patients over time may be a function of stroke severity and age rather than swallowing ability. Unfortunately, many prestroke variables and the use of different nutritional tests that are sensitive to rapid changes were not used in all studies. Therefore, debate continues on whether swallowing impairment causes reduced nutritional status following stroke.

## Dehydration

Dehydration is common (30–40%) in patients hospitalized with a stroke.[67,68] Dehydration can be detected by biomarkers in the blood (i.e., urea to creatine or blood urea nitrogen ratio). Patients who are dehydrated often have more severe strokes and worse outcomes. However, it is not clear whether dysphagia during the acute stage of stroke causes significant dehydration. Some studies have reported a tendency for dehydration to occur in patients with swallowing problems.[13,14,66,69] Those studies have demonstrated changes in the blood markers for dehydration from admission to 1 week after stroke in dysphagic patients as compared to nondysphagic patients. However, it is not clear whether this is because patients are not receiving enough fluids or because they do not eat and drink the modified foods or fluids as prescribed. Conversely, in other studies of acute stroke patients using the same dehydration measures, investigators have found no evidence for this claim.[52]

## Infection

Infection following a stroke is also common. The most common sites for infection are the lungs and the urinary tract.[6] Pneumonia accounts for 30% of deaths up to 30 days after stroke, making it the leading cause of death in the postacute phase of stroke.[6] Most pneumonia is the result of a bacterial infection secondary to entry of foreign material into the airways. This usually occurs in those who are weak and immobile. Pneumonia is a significant problem because it is related to increased hospital readmission and increased rates of disability and death following stroke.[25,71]

Chest infection and lower respiratory tract infection associated with swallowing impairment have been reported in between 40 and 70% of dysphagic stroke patients.[13,52,72,73] A recent meta-analysis reviewing the incidence of dysphagia and aspiration-related pneumonia indicated patients with dysphagia were three times more likely to develop pneumonia, and those with confirmed aspiration were 11 times more likely to develop pneumonia.[20]

Dysphagia with aspiration of food resulting in adverse outcome is therefore a significant issue that can affect a stroke patient's quality of life.

## Aspiration in Poststroke Dysphagia

Aspiration has been implicated as a leading cause of mortality in stroke.[184] However, aspiration of oral materials as a source of pneumonia following stroke has been conflictingly reported to contribute to morbidity.[74,75,76,77,78] Aspiration events have been reported in between 42 and 72% of patients following stroke, and aspiration is suggested to resolve rapidly in most cases.[3,20,23,27,57,74,75,76,77,78,79]

The relationship of aspiration associated with dysphagia to both morbidity and mortality is less clear. Aspiration in itself is a common occurrence. About half of normal adults and approximately 70% of patients with depressed consciousness will aspirate oral contents into their lungs during sleep with little detrimental effect.[80] The condition known as aspiration pneumonia is ascribed to the entry of pharyngeal contents with infectious material into the lower airway. When this happens, one of four general syndromes may develop: rapid clearance, chemical pneumonitis, bacterial pneumonia, or laryngeal obstruction. What is more commonly meant by aspiration pneumonia is pneumonia due to normally nonpathogenic agents that cause infection. This may be influenced by several factors working alone or in combination, including the pH of the aspirate, the amount aspirated, the time over which aspiration takes place, and the state of the host's immune defenses.

Many stroke patients are elderly. Elderly patients may suffer poor nutritional status and thus poor immune response.[81] They may also present with associated gastric disorders that predispose them to reflux of gastric contents into the pharynx and, potentially, aspiration pneumonia. A diagnosis of aspiration pneumonia is therefore often difficult to make. In addition, many studies have failed to identify the specific criteria upon which such a diagnosis was made.[82] In most cases this diagnosis is made by convenience. Studies have shown that, in many cases, without the use of sensitive testing for aspiration of oral contents into the lung, a diagnosis of "aspiration pneumonia" is rendered by a speech-language pathologist. Consequently, misleading use of terms, lack of clear definition for the condition, and limited availability of sensitive tests for aspiration pneumonia all contribute to the problem in diagnosis. The role of aspiration as an important symptom in dysphagia that predisposes a patient to the development of pneumonia, therefore, remains unclear. Nevertheless, recent meta-analyses have provided pooled results suggesting that dysphagia and aspiration are both associated with an increase in the odds of developing pneumonia.[79] Consequently, the practicing health care professional is urged to be cautious in the overuse of this term when assessing a stroke patient with dysphagia.

## Hospitalization and Institutionalization

It has been reported that swallowing dysfunction following stroke is associated with an increased length of hospital stay and the likelihood of being discharged to institutionalized care.[14,18,56] In a study by Kalra et al, the presence of dysphagia at 2 weeks poststroke was found to be predictive of admission to a nursing home.[83] Similarly, Smithard et al reported an association between dysphagia and an increased rate of institutionalization. This author suggested that dysphagia is a marker of more severe stroke and poorer long-term outcome, resulting in the need for nursing home care.[52,54]

## Long-Term Outcome of Dysphagia in Stroke Patients

Full recovery from a stroke may take months or years. Many people who have had a stroke never fully recover. Clinically it is important to understand the factors that may predict ongoing dysphagia in the stroke patient. In many patients with dysphagia following stroke, the risk of poorer outcome is highest within the first year following the stroke.[53] After 1 year, the risk diminishes, and the severity of the stroke remains the most important factor.

One issue at the core of the published evidence debate on recovery is the definition of swallowing recovery. Authors have variously defined swallowing recovery as no difficulty with a water challenge task; percent of patients returning to a "normal diet"; improvement in ability to eat different consistencies of food over a specified time period; absence of aspiration while swallowing; and swallowing without the use of compensatory strategies or medical support. In order for clinicians to make better predictions of outcome for patients and their families, a common definition of *recovered* is needed. More research that follows stroke patients with dysphagia for many years is needed in order to clarify this.

## 20.6.2 Impact of Dysphagia

Dysphagia predisposes patients to life-threatening events, such as pneumonia. It also leads to a reduction in quality of life through enforced changes in a patient's diet. Patients may not be able to consume their normal diet, may be restricted to certain consistencies of food, or might not even be able to eat or drink. The resulting limitation in the ability to ingest safe, adequate amounts of food and liquid also places the patient with an acute stroke at risk for complications and an array of negative outcomes.[4,59]

### Psychosocial Impact

Not every patient will recover his or her swallowing ability.[4,54,84] Restrictions in eating due to dysphagia are sometimes significant. When eating is no longer pleasurable and/or social, the inability to eat normally can dramatically affect patient morale and quality of life. For patients who remain dysphagic the likelihood of poorer health outcome and nursing home or assisted placement is high.[54] Moreover, patients with persistent dysphagia commonly suffer from depression that may hamper their recovery or rehabilitation. Depression following a stroke affects around 18% of stroke survivors, and depression may stay with a stroke patient for over 1 year.[85] Symptoms such as losing interest in everyday activities, not being able to enjoy the activities once enjoyed, finding it difficult to concentrate or make decisions, losing self-esteem or confidence, and becoming isolated from society are common signs of depression. Similarly, levels of depression and perceived burden are high in caregivers. Caregivers play a significant role in the longer-term management of dysphagic

stroke patients. However, the caregivers of dysphagic stroke patients are often isolated within the community, with limited support from families and friends. Recent studies have identified that high burden and lower caregiver quality of life are related to increased disability (e.g., dysphagia) following stroke.[86,87]

### Costs of Stroke

The cost of stroke care is staggering. A systematic review estimated the long-term (15 years) costs of a severe stroke at $159,004 and for a minor stroke $58,582. Furthermore, short-term costs (up to 6 months) were driven primarily (73%) by length of stay.[88]

Dysphagia contributes significantly to increased length of stay following stroke. The burden of illness associated with dysphagia following stroke ranges from 287,000 to 573,000 individuals per year in the United States.[88,89,90] Furthermore, dysphagia has been shown to add significantly to the estimated lifetime costs (between $12,031 and $73,542) for stroke survivors.[89,90] Consequently, it is important to identify treatments that offer the most clinical benefit and improved long-term outcome. These are important in directing appropriate health care resources to the problem of dysphagia following stroke.

## 20.6.3 Dysphagia Screening in Stroke

One way to reduce the burden of dysphagia following stroke is by early identification and intervention for swallowing problems. Swallow screening methods are techniques proposed to do this. Successful swallow screening programs have been associated with lower rates of pneumonia in stroke patients.[9] Swallow screening methods consist of some form of brief bedside examination for signs or symptoms of dysphagia. The aim of the swallow screen is to identify those persons who need a formal evaluation for swallowing, from those who can take food, fluids, and medication safely by mouth. Unfortunately, these techniques are not really screening methods because they do not fit with the definition of screening (i.e., "a brief procedure performed to identify or detect disease in apparently well (asymptomatic) individuals"). This is because dysphagic stroke patients have already been admitted to a health facility or have been identified as having a health problem prior to screening. They therefore do not fit the definition for being screened.[91]

Nonetheless, many acute care hospitals and stroke centers have standards in which it is expected that screening for dysphagia will be performed and documented on all stroke patients before food, fluids, or medication are given by mouth (e.g., Joint Commission on the Accreditation of Health Care Organizations, 2009).[92] Suggested screening approaches include, but are not limited to (1) water swallow tests, such as the Burke water swallow test[93] or the 3-ounce water swallow test[93,94,95,96,97]; (2) swallowing screening protocols, including brief assessments of oral-motor and sensory function as well as water swallow tests, the Toronto Bedside Swallowing Screening Test,[98] or the Simple Standardized Bedside Swallowing Assessment[99,100]; or (3) clinical (bedside) swallow sign examinations performed by nurse screeners or physicians.[101,102,103]

Evidence supporting these approaches comes from studies of acute stroke showing that early detection of dysphagia reduces the risk of aspiration pneumonia.[9,20,101,102,103,104,105] To date there is a plethora of clinical screening tools published for detecting dysphagia and aspiration risk with various levels of accuracy.[106,107] However, due to a failure to agree on a single acceptable method, there remains no accepted standard for dysphagia screening in the United States.

## Dysphagia Assessment Following Stroke

Several forms of dysphagia evaluation are available to estimate the function and severity of impairment to the swallowing system following a stroke. These techniques range from a group of noninvasive clinical tasks (e.g., clinical bedside assessment) to comprehensive instrumental procedures (e.g., videofluoroscopy or endoscopy of swallowing).[91]

## Noninstrumental Assessment of Swallowing in Stroke

A variety of forms of noninstrumental "clinical" approaches have been used to evaluate the function of the swallowing system. These predominantly include clinical bedside evaluations. Most evaluations include some form of physical examination and a "trial swallow" of one or more materials. The clinical bedside assessment is often considered the front-line tool for the assessment of swallowing function in stroke patients.[91] It aims to help define the potential causes of the dysphagia and direct a hypothesis of the nature and level of the breakdown in the swallow system. Few formalized clinical instruments with adequate reliability and validity have been published.[91] Most clinical instruments used to measure swallow disability after stroke emphasize or are limited to checking the presence or absence of a constellation of physical symptoms. They may not capture other important issues, such as diminished quality of response or modification of behaviors. Further, many of the tools have been institution-specific, non-validated rating scales that have not demonstrated strength of measurement. In such cases, patients may continue to improve, but the scales used to measure swallowing improvement may not be sensitive enough to detect small but important changes in function. One assessment tool that was specifically developed for stroke patients is the Mann Assessment of Swallowing Ability.[108] This 24-item clinical evaluation was designed to direct the bedside evaluation of swallowing components. Performance is measured using 5- to 10-point ordinal scales for each component. It also provides scores for each skill and a total score (maximum score, 200). Both dysphagia and aspiration are evaluated, and a score is compiled for each. It has been used in numerous studies and treatment trials of stroke.[101,108,109,111]

Despite the method used, clinical assessments of swallowing function have been reported to be less sensitive than instrumental methods in the identification of dysphagia following stroke.[112,113] Nonetheless, these clinical evaluations hold an advantage in that they are cheap, accessible, and time efficient. They provide valuable information to help direct immediate intervention and are often used to direct future, more invasive evaluations.

## Instrumental Assessment of Swallowing in Stroke

Over the last decade, a range of instrumental assessment methods has evolved to measure the nature of dysphagia following stroke.

The most popular of these techniques has been the videofluoroscopic assessment of swallowing. Instrumental assessments are thought to provide a more complete evaluation of the swallowing performance because they provide observable output (e.g., X-ray images, real-time video, or line tracings).[114] Several studies have reported that these observable or dynamic images can help the clinician localize problems and better detect the potential for treatment. The major advantage is believed to be the ability to visualize critical information within the pharyngeal phase of the swallow that is not directly observable from clinical methods. In fact, several studies have found that clinical evaluations can miss about 40% of important information regarding the degree of aspiration and may therefore underestimate the risk for disability in stroke patients.[115] Conversely, videofluoroscopic assessments have been criticized for being unrepresentative of the true swallowing ability and environment and too costly, while exposing patients to additional radiation.[116,117] Nonetheless, many facilities now provide access to a form of instrumental assessment of swallowing as common practice.

Recently, investigators have also validated a scoring and instruction technique for videofluoroscopy to help train accuracy in its interpretation. The Modified Barium Swallow (MBS) impairment scale has now become widely available for the health care professional wishing to learn to evaluate video fluoroscopic swallowing studies.[118] For further in-depth reading on clinical and instrumental swallowing assessments the reader is directed to the listed texts at the end of this chapter.[107-118]

## 20.6.4 Dysphagia Rehabilitation Following Stroke

The primary goals of treatment for swallowing disorders following stroke are to facilitate natural recovery, improve swallowing function, optimize nutrition, and minimize the risk of aspiration and other complications (**Box 20.4**).

### Box 20.4

**Primary Goals of Dysphagia Rehabilitation Following Stroke**
- Prevent aspiration-related complications
- Maintain and promote swallow function
- Meet nutritional and hydration needs

Current treatment for dysphagia involves two distinct approaches: (1) the management of dysphagic complications, including the prevention of aspiration in the form of alternate feeding, modification of food and fluid textures to promote safe swallowing, compensatory maneuvers, and positional changes; and (2) the rehabilitation of damaged or ineffective swallowing actions, which involves the use of oromuscular exercises or techniques to promote movement of the structures involved in swallowing. These may be used independently but are mostly used together. Management also depends on whether the focus is on risk of aspiration or the dysphagic level of impairment, and most treatments are highly individualized (**Box 20.5**).

## Box 20.5

### Best Practice for Managing Dysphagia Following Stroke

- Maintain nothing by mouth until swallow function is determined.
- Assess nutrition/hydration status.
- Perform regular oral care to limit buildup of bacteria.
- Provide feeding assistance with compensations/adjustments for feeding (as prescribed).
- Screen for swallow status and readiness for feeding.
- Educate the family and patient.
- Perform swallow assessment for those who "fail" the screen.
- Evaluate regularly to measure improvement.

As the patient's condition improves, more active intervention for dysphagia is often introduced. At this point the patient's medical condition has stabilized, and the patient is considered to be an active participant in treatment and motivated to improve his swallowing performance. Participation in direct and intense rehabilitation programs has been shown to improve swallowing outcome following stroke. In fact, direct and intense intervention has demonstrated benefits in reduced pneumonia rates, increased variety of diet level, and improved nutrition.[119,120] The choice of treatment technique depends largely on the specific patient characteristics. However, data suggest that more frequent and more intense intervention provides a benefit, even in patients with chronic dysphagia.[119,120,121,122,123,124] Further, recent advances in treatment modalities have expanded the range of rehabilitation techniques available to include surface electromyographic biofeedback, neuromuscular electrical stimulation (NMES), neurostimulation, and muscle conditioning/motor learning integration techniques. All are designed to ensure the easiest, safest, and most effective method of swallowing. The following sections address dysphagia treatment options available to the practicing clinician.

## Nonoral (Enteral) Feeding

Nonoral, or enteral, feeding is recommended when a stroke patient presents with severe dysphagia or cannot meet nutritional needs orally. Food can be taken through a nasogastric tube, which goes from the nose to the stomach or small intestine. More serious or longer-term feeding problems may require a gastrostomy tube, which is surgically placed directly into the stomach. It is often placed within 3–4 days following an initial swallow evaluation. If the dysphagia is severe or likely to be persistent, a percutaneous endoscopic gastrostomy tube (PEG) or jejunostomy tube may be placed. Nasogastric tubes have been found to be less effective and result in greater side effects for those patients requiring longer-term alternate feeding, whereas PEG feeding is associated with fewer failures and less decline in nutritional state poststroke.[120,127,128,129]

Nonoral feeding strategies in stroke patients can also add significantly to health care costs and do not necessarily reduce or eliminate dysphagia-related complications.[127,128,129,130] PEG or alternate feeding is used in approximately 12% of stroke rehabilitation cases.[131] Approximately one-third of feeding tubes are discontinued before patients are discharged from rehabilitation,

and many are reported discontinued by 1 year.[131] Patients with stroke lesions that are bilateral or located in the brainstem areas are less likely to return to oral feeding.

Not all patients will require tube feeding for lengthy periods. Consequently, it is important for those working with stroke patients with dysphagia to understand methods for transitioning off tube feeding and back to oral feeding when ready. A first prerequisite is that the patient is able to manage safe oral intake on a regular basis. Not only should the intake of oral materials be safe; it must also be efficient. Without the required speed of intake, a patient will abandon oral feeding attempts and risk additional nutritional or hydration problems. The patient should also be able to consume adequate amounts of food and fluids to maintain nutritional requirements before transitioning from alternate feeding methods. The patient should be alert and able to maintain attention long enough to complete a meal. Lastly the transition from alternate feeding to oral intake should be staged. Because transition can be cognitively and physically challenging for some patients, specific patient-related variables and swallowing assessment information should be used to make decisions on when to transition off tube feeding. Swallow performance and safety do not always predict whether a patient can consume the required amounts and types of foods to stay healthy once a tube is removed. Careful documentation of all types of intake and coordination with nutritional specialists are critical to ensure a successful transition.[132]

## Diet Modification

One of the most common strategies applied to treat stroke patients with dysphagia is diet modification, or changes in the thickness, volume, temperature, or acidity of foods and fluids to be consumed by the patient.[133,134,135,136,137] In a national survey, it was reported that thickening strategies were used with 80% of all patients in skilled nursing facilities.[137] Although bolus modification via the adaptation of the texture is often the mainstay of a dysphagia treatment protocol, this strategy does not directly change the impaired swallow physiology nor promote recovery of damaged swallowing in stroke patients. The application of diet modification is based on the premise that thickening fluids can slow the bolus and improve bolus flow, leading to a reduction in penetration and aspiration.[133] It is believed that, by slowing the movement of the food or fluid, patients have a better opportunity to swallow with less risk of airway compromise. However, the quality and extent of modification of food and fluids are inconsistent and very subjective. For example, the exact thickness of fluids depends on the type of fluid, the temperature, the individual making the drink, and the type of thickener used, resulting in wide variability within and between patients.[134]

Moreover, the use of thickeners and thickening recipes and definitions of the varying levels of thickening between institutions is not consistent. Similarly, the materials used in assessment of the patient do not match those used in the management of the patient, and this has resulted in an inaccurate application of this "pseudoscientific" practice. Current evidence supporting the use of thickening as a strategy is also conflicting. Some authors suggest benefit is minimal, and over 50% of patients do not adhere to thickened diets when they are prescribed.[137] Additionally, there is little evidence to support decisions as to which patient should receive which diet level and which types of materials are safe or unsafe.[138] Despite the limited data supporting the application of diet modification as a strategy to improve dysphagia, this practice remains widespread. In an attempt to resolve some of the problems associated with diet modification and its definitions, a group of dysphagia experts have initiated the National Dysphagia Diet, in which levels have been determined by exact measures to help define what is meant by thin, nectar-thick, and honey-thick fluids.[139] The utility and broad application of these national recommendations by practicing clinicians is as yet unclear.

## Alternate Use of Food and Fluid Modification

Thickening or altering the characteristics of foods or fluids provided to the stroke patient may also offer a method to alter the physiology of swallowing. Studies have consistently demonstrated the specific timing effects of altering bolus characteristics on the swallow mechanism.[140,141,142] For example, thickening fluids can slow down the transit of a bolus, promote increased lingual–palatal and pharyngeal pressure, and extend the upper esophageal opening.[140,141,142,143,144] Moreover, swallow physiology has been shown to accommodate various changes in bolus characteristics during feeding. Recent work also suggests that these immediate physiological alterations brought about by bolus changes may be different for dysphagic versus nondysphagic patients. Further research is required to expand our understanding of these effects beyond simple timing changes.

## Compensatory Treatments or Maneuvers

Traditionally, a number of activities have been proposed to "correct" the swallowing of patients with stroke. The overarching goal of many of these techniques has been to manage a patient's oral intake and reduce airway compromise in the stroke patient. Collectively, these strategies have been termed compensatory behaviors because they are focused on an "in the moment" change in the physiology of the swallow. They are short-term adjustments and may not improve the physiology of the swallow long term or promote swallow recovery. These strategies or maneuvers include postural changes (e.g., chin tuck, head rotation, side-lying, slowed feeding rate, reduced bolus size, effortful swallow, supraglottic swallow, super-supraglottic swallow,

and the Mendelsohn maneuver).[145,146,147] See **Table 20.2** for a brief description of each maneuver and its effect. Collectively, compensatory actions are considered to help redirect the bolus and change pharyngeal management in the moment. To date, there is limited evidence that they may reduce aspiration or improve outcome in stroke patients. Most studies have evaluated the effect of the maneuvers when performed as single-session intervention under videofluoroscopic review. Few if any long-term studies have been conducted, and, in those performed, the longer-term adherence to these techniques by patients was considered poor.[148] Although there is little evidence to support postural and compensatory techniques, they are widely and variably used, leading to difficulties in establishing standards of care in dysphagia. For a more in-depth definition of each maneuver and its intended effect, the reader is referred to the second entry in the suggested reading section at the end of this chapter.[2]

## Active Rehabilitation Techniques: Muscle Conditioning Interventions

Active rehabilitation procedures (e.g., therapeutic exercises) aim to improve the underlying swallowing function. These approaches often involve progressive strengthening and coordination of the swallowing muscles. The concept of muscle strengthening as a means of improving functional outcome poststroke is not new. Studies of stroke patients who strengthen limb muscles have shown repeated positive functional benefits in treadmill walking and stair climbing. Consequently, the application of strengthening and conditioning of swallowing muscles is an extension of this already recognized approach. This form of exercise-based dysphagia therapy can include techniques such as lingual strengthening, the Shaker technique, the McNeill Dysphagia Therapy program (MDTP) and adjunctive treatments, including surface electromyographic therapy (sEMG), NMES, and neurostimulation.[50,149,150,151,152,153,154] At the core of these approaches is the focus on strengthening and exercising the unimpaired swallowing structures. By making use of the principles of neuroplasticity and exercise physiology these approaches apply the "use it or lose it" phenomenon through their application. More specifically, when a system is not used or is underused, it may lose

Table 20.2 Compensatory techniques for managing dysphagia following stroke

| Technique | Description | Presumed effect |
|---|---|---|
| Head rotation | Turing the head to the affected side | Redirects the bolus down the stronger side Reduces aspiration and residue |
| Chin up | Elevate the chin | Helps push the bolus to the back of the mouth, opens the oropharynx Improves transport of the bolus |
| Side-lying | Lie with the stronger side down | Slows transit of bolus down the stronger side of the pharynx |
| Supraglottic swallow | Hold your breath, swallow, and then cough out | Increases glottal closure and movement of oropharyngeal complex—reduces aspiration |
| Super-supraglottic swallow | Hold your breath, bear down, swallow, and then cough out | Increases glottal closure and movement of oropharyngeal complex—reduces aspiration |
| Effortful swallow | Swallow hard | Increases lingual force on the bolus to speed transit and reduce residue |
| Mendelsohn maneuver | Swallow and hold the swallow at the top of the movement | Increased and extended hyolaryngeal elevation Reduces residue and aspiration |

its ability to function efficiently. Through exercising the various muscles involved in swallowing, the stroke patient may regain muscular strength and control to improve management of the bolus during swallowing. Because a comprehensive presentation of the exercise principles underlying dysphagia rehabilitation is beyond the scope of this chapter, the reader is directed to **Table 20.3** and the third and fourth entries on the suggested reading list at the end of the chapter. [3,4]

Common rehabilitation techniques, such as oral and lingual exercises, tend to focus on strength and endurance. [154] Data to support lingual strengthening programs are increasing. Robbins et al demonstrated positive gains in tongue strength in healthy elderly individuals after exercise. [154] Preliminary data now suggest that a program of 8 weeks of isometric lingual strengthening can also improve lingual pressures, tongue volume, and airway protection. [155] An extension of this approach, isometric progressive resistance oropharyngeal therapy (I-Pro therapy) has been reported. Using a new device developed by the investigators (the Madison oral strengthening [MOST] device), a single chronic dysphagic stroke patient who had failed traditional therapy was treated with lingual strengthening for a period of 8 weeks, then placed on 5 weeks of no therapy and returned to a less intense I-Pro therapy program for an additional 9 weeks. During the I-Pro therapy the patient completed 10 lingual press exercises (anterior and posterior tongue) three times a day, 3 days a week. Results in this single case study revealed improvement in lingual pressures from the I-Pro intervention, along with the return to an unrestricted oral diet, reduced postswallow pharyngeal residue, and improved upper esophageal sphincter opening. [156] These data suggest lingual strengthening performed intensively can result in an increase in isometric pressure and downstream benefit to the swallowing system. At issue, however, is the efficiency of this exercise program. Exercising only the tongue is an approach aimed at only a single part of the swallow. So, it is not clear how efficiently gains in strength generalize to the more dynamic swallow movement.

The Shaker technique or head lift exercise is another popular rehabilitation approach. This technique is intended to strengthen the pharyngoesophageal segment (PES) by building the muscles that contribute to opening. [149] During swallowing the suprahyoid muscle group contributes to the opening of the PES by raising and pulling the PES. The Shaker technique is believed to exercise those muscles by having the patient lie on her back and complete repetitive head-raising actions. There are isometric and isotonic components to the Shaker exercise. During the isometric component, patients are instructed to complete each head raise and hold it for 1 minute with a 1-minute rest period after each. During the isometric component patients are asked to complete 30 consecutive head lifts. Patients are then instructed to complete this exercise three times a day for 6 weeks. [149] Despite several clinical studies demonstrating the physiological benefit of this technique, patient compliance is not strong. [150] Patients with neck damage, tracheostomy, or cervical spine deficits cannot complete the task. Moreover, its conformity with the principles of exercise is limited. This procedure does not include a method by which the clinician can progressively intensify the exercise to gain additional benefit. More research is needed to demonstrate the longer-term rehabilitative benefit to stroke patients from this technique.

Other approaches report a more explicit focus on motor learning principles and the functional swallowing process. One of these with some evidence of effectiveness is the McNeill Dysphagia Therapy program. [124] The MDTP approach uses the physiological benefit of the effortful swallow approach within its rehabilitation program. However, this approach is much more than a simple effortful swallow technique. MDTP incorporates principles of muscle conditioning and motor learning in its approach to swallow rehabilitation. Patients receive daily therapy sessions that are structured to promote mass practice of swallowing movements. The swallowed materials are systematically advanced as the patient tolerates them, and they are selected to facilitate specific challenges in properties of resistance, speed, and coordination. Clinicians follow rules as to how to advance or regress a patient in the program. Results from a series of studies on this technique have demonstrated its benefit in improving oral intake, swallow coordination, timing, and the effort associated with swallowing. [157,158,159] The program has demonstrated efficacy in treating stroke rehabilitation patients in a recent randomized controlled trial. [159]

## 20.7 Adjunctive Therapies

### 20.7.1 Surface Electromyographic Biofeedback

Many behavioral therapies require a stroke patient to perform different or unusual movements during rehabilitation. These

**Table 20.3** Principles of muscle conditioning through exercise

| Frequency | Number of exercise sessions over a period of time | How often? |
|---|---|---|
| Volume | Total repetitions and sets of exercises performed | How much? |
| Intensity | The amount of resistance used in exercise | How hard to lift, push, or pull? |
| Overload | A stimulus greater than normal—above 40% of your maximum needed to change muscle | Must exercise with a load greater than normal to build up muscle |
| Variety | Exercise more than one set of muscles | The sequence of exercises |
| Recovery | Rest allows muscle to repair and recover | Amount of rest per set/over session? |
| Specificity | Type of training will dictate results, so training must mirror the desired outcome | If you want to swallow—"swallow" |
| Progression | To be effective exercise must progress systematically—become more demanding | Start slow and build up |
| Reversibility | Any gain made with exercise will be reversed when training has stopped | Use it or lose it |

novel movements often challenge motor learning. The application of adjunctive modalities such as sEMG to behavioral therapy can act to enhance the learning of these unusual movements.[152] In addition, these techniques can be helpful in enabling patients to monitor their swallowing performance in real time as a form of biofeedback. sEMG is a noninvasive method of objectively measuring and evaluating swallowing physiology. The procedure entails the application of a two-channel surface electrode patch that is placed on the submental region. The electrical activity of the muscles contracting during swallowing underlying the electrode patch is recorded. The shape and amount of muscle activity is quantified in microvolts ($\mu$V).[152] The accuracy of this technique in swallow identification and agreement across judges has been well established.[122,161,162,163,164] Further, its reliability and characteristics have been well established across both swallowing and nonswallowing tasks.[164]

Studies of sEMG as an adjunct to therapy have demonstrated that this form of biofeedback can reduce the time spent in therapy. Moreover, it has been shown to help develop swallowing skill. Further, studies evaluating the effect of sEMG therapy on recovery from poststroke dysphagia have reported improvements in the amount of swallowing work completed, oral intake levels, and coordination of swallowing.[122,161] Similar outcomes have been reported in both acute and chronic stroke patients with dysphagia. These data provide direction to clinicians wishing to improve the application of behavioral therapy for dysphagia. However, it should be emphasized that biofeedback alone is *not* a therapy. As an adjunct to a strong therapy program this technique can act to enhance good therapy. By itself it does nothing to treat the patient. Therapists must first develop the plan of therapy using all the patient's information, including the patient's history, medical information, and underlying disease, before deciding to apply adjunctive devices.

## 20.7.2 Neurostimulation

Another adjunctive tool is neurostimulation. Several different neurostimulation techniques for swallowing rehabilitation have been proposed, such as pharyngeal electrical stimulation (PES) and NMES. These approaches have been developed to help stimulate cortical neuroplasticity to rehabilitate swallowing. They aim to achieve this by either (1) stimulating the peripheral oropharyngeal sensory system by electrical stimulus or (2) directly stimulating the pharyngeal motor cortex. Again, as with sEMG, these approaches are heavily influenced by the behavioral application to which they are paired.

### Neuromuscular Electrical Stimulation

NMES is a form of rehabilitation that has its origins within the field of physical therapy. It is designed to bypass injured central control to activate neural tissue by creating a contraction in a peripheral muscle in an attempt to return function to a nonfunctioning muscle group. NMES involves passing a low electrical current transcutaneously through electrodes to stimulate a muscle contraction. To be successful, it requires an intact peripheral nerve supply to the muscle being stimulated. NMES is delivered through stimulating electrodes attached to the skin over the muscles of swallowing. NMES is predominantly used as an adjunct modality applied concurrently while the patient swallows or performs swallowing exercises.[153,165]

NMES has been extensively studied and applied successfully on large skeletal muscles in many patient groups, including stroke. Numerous studies have demonstrated that it is effective at enhancing functional activity and promoting motor learning for physical tasks. Similarly, several studies have reported improvement in swallowing following the administration of NMES in stroke patients.[166] The main improvements noted have been improved oral intake, reduced aspiration, and elimination of tube or alternate feeding.[167,168] Other studies have demonstrated conflicting results.[169] Studies of NMES using healthy populations have reported an array of outcomes from no differences in outcomes from the application of NMES[169] to reduced hyolaryngeal elevation,[170] with different effects for different electrode placements[171] and interactions between age and NMES amplitude.[172] In stroke populations, the data are similarly muddy. Although some authors variously report reductions in dysphagia symptoms, such as pharyngeal residue, quicker swallowing times,[167] increased hyolaryngeal improvement,[173] improved swallowing scores,[174] and improved diet level,[175] others note no benefit.[176] The conflict appears to lie in the design of both the studies investigating this approach and the therapy paired with the NMES procedure. An accumulation of different patient groups, different stimulation parameters, different electrode placements, and different behavioral therapies attached to the NMES application limit the conclusions that can be drawn. Recently, a meta-analysis of NMES outcome studies reported that the outcomes with this approach were not different from those reported with traditional therapy.[177] However, this analysis was based on nonstroke populations. Similarly, a more recent randomized trial of NMES in subacute stroke ($n = 53$) identified no benefit of NMES beyond that gained from intensive behavioral therapy. In this study, patients in the intensive behavioral therapy plus sham NMES arm demonstrated greater gains in oral intake, swallowing physiology, and 3-month outcome than did either the active NMES arm or the usual care arm.[159] The application of NMES in this study did not enhance therapeutic outcome. Clearly the impact of NMES on the effectiveness of dysphagia rehabilitation for stroke patients is not uniform. Clinicians will need to continue to evaluate future research to determine the most appropriate use of this treatment modality for their patients.

### Pharyngeal Electrical Stimulation and Other Techniques

The Phagenesis technique (Phagenesis Ltd.) uses a device developed by Hamdy[178] that uses pharyngeal electrical stimulation. This therapy involves applying an electrical signal to the pharynx through electrodes positioned in a catheter inserted nasally. This technique is aimed at improving swallowing function by restoring neurological control. The intensity of the electrical stimulation is determined following the calculation of a suitable sensory threshold tailored to the individual stroke patient. After the optimal stimulation intensity has been determined, an electrical stimulation pulse is delivered. In an initial study of pharyngeal electrical stimulation, this technique was provided (in addition to standard care) once daily for 10 minutes on 3 consecutive days to 28 stroke patients with severe dysphagia at baseline, 2 weeks, and 3 months. This study reported that pharyngeal electrical stimulation might act to speed up swallowing poststroke.[179]

Other lesser known neurostimulation techniques, such as transcranial magnetic stimulation (TMS) and transcranial direct current stimulation (tDCS), are also emerging within the stroke dysphagia treatment literature. TMS is a method that uses magnetic fields to stimulate nerve cells in the brain. During TMS a magnetic coil is placed near the patient's head. It has been used to explore the corticomotor physiology associated with swallowing. TMS-induced motor evoked potentials have been noted to change the excitability of nerves projecting to swallowing muscles.

Alternatively, tDCS uses low-intensity direct currents applied to broad areas of the cortex to modify the electrical potential of cortical neurons. Depending on how it is applied, tDCS can enhance or reduce cortical excitability. In a study by Yang et al, stroke patients with dysphagia were randomized to receive tDCS or sham tDCS to the pharyngeal motor cortex of the affected hemisphere while undergoing traditional swallowing therapy.[180] They were treated daily for 30 minutes over a 10-day period. Results revealed improvement in swallowing scores measured on a nonvalidated swallowing scale at 3 months posttreatment in those patients who received the tCDS. While promising, these treatment approaches are clearly early and emerging.

Overall, there is some evidence that neurostimulation approaches may reduce aspiration and pharyngeal residue and improve swallowing performance in stroke patients. However, recent reviews of dysphagia treatments continue to report limited consistency of evidence for interventions, but some evidence of effectiveness for improved function.[181] Of course, further studies will be necessary to compare the effects of these neurostimulation approaches; the swallow system appears bilaterally innervated and displays different neuroplastic behavior. Application of an inappropriate therapy could potentially lead to negative responses that may interfere with swallowing recovery.

## 20.8 Efficacy of Dysphagia Treatments in Stroke

Although several treatments are available, they are frequently applied rather haphazardly to patients with dysphagia following stroke. It is not clear whether they are effective (or even risky), because few studies have adequately evaluated these techniques. The few studies that have attempted to evaluate the effects of dysphagia treatment on patient outcome have been plagued by variable methodology and hence variable results. Although studies have suggested positive outcomes of treatments for stroke patients,[3,15,18,66,119] the majority have been retrospective studies with small samples or noncomparable groups. This raises the possibility that outcomes may have been confounded by population differences. Therefore, the results may not be truly representative of any treatment effects. It is important that, when evaluating the use and effect of the various rehabilitative treatments for swallowing, clinicians be aware of the lack of rigorous research and the impact of this on interpretation of the available evidence.

## 20.9 Controlled Trials of Swallowing Treatment Poststroke

One of the highest forms of evidence for the efficacy of a treatment type is the randomized controlled trial. To date there have been only a few truly randomized controlled trials of rehabilitative treatment for dysphagia following stroke.[119] For example, an early trial conducted by Depippo et al evaluated dysphagia treatment in the subacute phase after stroke. This study attempted to compare effects of graded levels of intervention by a dysphagia therapist on the occurrence of pneumonia, dehydration, calorie-nitrogen deficit, recurrent upper airway obstruction, and death following stroke. Unfortunately, this study was small ($n = 115$), and there was no control ("no treatment") group.[182] These errors in the application of clinical trials methodology are common within the field of dysphagia. Uncertainty therefore remains about the effectiveness of the interventions measured in this study.

Another larger trial was reported by Carnaby et al, who compared two levels of graded behavioral intervention for swallowing following acute stroke.[119] In this trial, 306 patients with clinically identified dysphagia were randomized to one of three arms: usual care, standardized low-intensity behavioral swallowing intervention (compensatory strategies), or standardized high-intensity intervention (direct swallowing exercises). The primary outcome measure was survival without the need for a modified diet. Although this trial failed to support its primary hypothesis, it did report a significant increase in the proportion of patients who achieved functional swallowing and a significant decrease in the number of patients with dysphagia-related medical complications (e.g., pneumonia) (relative risk, 0.56; confidence interval 0.4–0.8).[119] The value of this trial is the methodological rigor with which it was conducted. The authors ensured a secure randomization system, confirmed their sample size, and specified all primary and secondary outcome measures. Further, all measures were assessed blind to the treatment allocation, and the follow-up of patients was rigorous.[183] This single-center trial by Carnaby and colleagues identified for the first time that behavioral intervention may have a positive impact on dysphagia outcome following stroke, and intensity of therapy may be associated with reduced comorbidity. This study offers a guide to the construction of dysphagia trials. Given such promising results, it is important that similar larger studies be conducted to evaluate the outcome of the other interventions for dysphagia commonly used with stroke patients.

## 20.10 Final Thoughts

Dysphagia after stroke is a common and underrecognized problem associated with significant and negative health outcomes. Speech-language pathologists are often at the forefront of health care services for these patients. Early identification and assessment for stroke-related swallowing deficits have the potential to provide significant benefit to patients and their families. The application of different treatment strategies at differing times in a stroke patient's recovery can help remediate critical factors that may speed rehabilitation and promote positive outcomes. Clinicians are encouraged to stay informed about promising new developments and treatment options in stroke dysphagia rehabilitation.

# 20.11 Questions

1. Dysphagia following stroke is localized in which primary areas?

A. Primary motor cortex structure
B. Brainstem structures only
C. Insula
D. Multiple cortical and subcortical structures
E. Primary sensory cortex

2. Which negative outcome of stroke has not been overtly linked to dysphagia?

A. Aspiration
B. Dehydration
C. Increased length of stay
D. Chest infection
E. Malnutrition

3. Why would early identification of dysphagia in stroke patients contribute to reduced morbidity?

A. It would identify patients most at risk and direct quicker, more appropriate care.
B. It would raise awareness of the need for feeding rehabilitation.
C. It would provide time for nurses to do other things.
D. It would ensure scarce resources were spent on the most at-risk cases.
E. It would identify dysphagic stroke patients for the speech pathologists.

4. How can diet modification promote recovery of dysphagia from stroke?

A. It does not promote recovery from dysphagia.
B. It helps challenge and exercise the swallow mechanism and change swallow physiology.
C. It promotes slower movement of the food and fluid to make patients safe when eating.
D. It encourages patients to clear the food more often.
E. It provides increased sensory stimulation to facilitate swallowing recovery.

5. Neurostimulation (tDCS) for swallowing is used primarily

A. as an adjunct to traditional therapy.
B. to excite stroke patients and encourage them to donate money for research.
C. to promote cortical excitability for swallowing.
D. to evaluate cortical plasticity for swallowing.
E. to help brain researchers map the cortex.

# 20.12 Answers and Explanations

**1. Correct: primary motor cortex structure (A).**
(D) is correct because researchers have identified multiple cortical and subcortical structures in swallowing. The others only identify one of many specific sites involved.

**2. Correct: malnutrition (E).**
(E) is correct because evidence linking malnutrition is lacking. All other choices have demonstrated evidence of direct associations.

**3. Correct: it would identify patients most at risk and direct quicker, more appropriate care (A).**
Early identification has been shown to reduce morbidity by redirecting patients to more appropriate care more quickly. The other choices do not ensure appropriate care is provided more rapidly.

**4. Correct: it helps challenge and exercise the swallow mechanism and change swallow physiology (B).**
Evidence supporting benefit from diet modification is limited; data do show that accommodation to different bolus types can promote physiological change.

**5. Correct: to promote cortical excitability for swallowing (C).**
(C) is correct because neurostimulation is thought to excite the cortical projections to the muscles of swallowing. Although it is primarily an adjunct to traditional therapy, its aim is to promote excitability. The other options may be possible but are not the primary reason for its use.

## References

[1] Hatano S. Experience from a multicenter stroke register. *Bull World Health Organ* 1976;54(5):541–553
[2] World Health Organization. Cerebrovascular Disorders (Offset Publications). Geneva: World Health Organization; 1978
[3] Horner J, Massey EW, Riski JE, Lathrop DL, Chase KN. Aspiration following stroke: clinical correlates and outcome. *Neurology* 1988;38(9):1359–1362
[4] Mann G, Hankey GJ, Cameron D. Swallowing function after stroke: prognosis and prognostic factors at 6 months. *Stroke* 1999;30(4):744–748
[5] American Heart Association. Heart and Stroke Statistical Update. Dallas, TX: American Heart Association; 2002
[6] Adams HP Jr, Adams RJ, Brott T, et al; Stroke Council of the American Stroke Association. Guidelines for the early management of patients with ischemic stroke: A scientific statement from the Stroke Council of the American Stroke Association. *Stroke* 2003;34(4):1056–1083
[7] Mozaffarian D, Benjamin EJ, Go AS, et al; American Heart Association Statistics Committee and Stroke Statistics Subcommittee. Heart disease and stroke statistics—2015 update: a report from the American Heart Association. *Circulation* 2015;131(4):e29–e322
[8] Centers for Disease Control and Preventions. Stroke facts. Cerebrovascular disease or stroke. 2016. http://www.cdc.gov/dhdsp/data_statistics/fact_sheets/fs_stroke.htm. Accessed May 3, 2016
[9] Hinchey JA, Shephard T, Furie K, Smith D, Wang D, Tonn S; Stroke Practice Improvement Network Investigators. Formal dysphagia screening protocols prevent pneumonia. *Stroke* 2005;36(9):1972–1976
[10] Aviv JE, Martin JH, Sacco RL, et al. Supraglottic and pharyngeal sensory abnormalities in stroke patients with dysphagia. *Ann Otol Rhinol Laryngol* 1996;105(2):92–97

[11] Anderson CS, Jamrozik KD, Burvill PW, Chakera TM, Johnson GA, Stewart-Wynne EG. Ascertaining the true incidence of stroke: experience from the Perth Community Stroke Study, 1989-1990. *Med J Aust* 1993;*158*(2):80–84

[12] Anderson CS, Jamrozik KD, Burvill PW, Chakera TM, Johnson GA, Stewart-Wynne EG. Determining the incidence of different subtypes of stroke: results from the Perth Community Stroke Study, 1989-1990. *Med J Aust* 1993;*158*(2):85–89

[13] Gordon C, Hewer RL, Wade DT. Dysphagia in acute stroke. *Br Med J (Clin Res Ed)* 1987;*295*(6595):411–414

[14] Barer DH. The natural history and functional consequences of dysphagia after hemispheric stroke. *J Neurol Neurosurg Psychiatry* 1989;*52*(2):236–241

[15] Horner J, Buoyer FG, Alberts MJ, Helms MJ. Dysphagia following brain-stem stroke. Clinical correlates and outcome. *Arch Neurol* 1991;*48*(11):1170–1173

[16] Splaingard ML, Hutchins B, Sulton LD, Chaudhuri G. Aspiration in rehabilitation patients: videofluoroscopy vs bedside clinical assessment. *Arch Phys Med Rehabil* 1988;*69*(8):637–640

[17] Robbins J, Levine RL, Maser A, Rosenbek JC, Kempster GB. Swallowing after unilateral stroke of the cerebral cortex. *Arch Phys Med Rehabil* 1993;*74*(12):1295–1300

[18] Odderson IR, Keaton JC, McKenna BS. Swallow management in patients on an acute stroke pathway: quality is cost effective. *Arch Phys Med Rehabil* 1995;*76*(12):1130–1133

[19] Mann G, Hankey GJ, Cameron D. Swallowing disorders following acute stroke: prevalence and diagnostic accuracy. *Cerebrovasc Dis* 2000;*10*(5):380–386

[20] Martino R, Foley N, Bhogal S, Diamant N, Speechley M, Teasell R. Dysphagia after stroke: incidence, diagnosis, and pulmonary complications. *Stroke* 2005;*36*(12):2756–2763

[21] Gresham SL. Clinical assessment and management of swallowing difficulties after stroke. *Med J Aust* 1990;*153*(7):397–399

[22] Veis SL, Logemann JA. Swallowing disorders in persons with cerebrovascular accident. *Arch Phys Med Rehabil* 1985;*66*(6):372–375

[23] Horner J, Massey EW, Brazer SR. Aspiration in bilateral stroke patients. *Neurology* 1990;*40*(11):1686–1688

[24] Cohen DL, Roffe C, Beavan J, et al. Post-stroke dysphagia: A review and design considerations for future trials. *Int J Stroke* 2016;*11*(4):399–411

[25] Bravata DM, Daggett VS, Woodward-Hagg H, et al. Comparison of two approaches to screen for dysphagia among acute ischemic stroke patients: nursing admission screening tool versus National Institutes of Health stroke scale. *J Rehabil Res Dev* 2009;*46*(9):1127–1134

[26] Flowers HL, Skoretz SA, Streiner DL, Silver FL, Martino R. MRI-based neuroanatomical predictors of dysphagia after acute ischemic stroke: a systematic review and meta-analysis. *Cerebrovasc Dis* 2011;*32*(1):1–10

[27] Alberts MJ, Horner J, Gray L, Brazer SR. Aspiration after stroke: lesion analysis by brain MRI. *Dysphagia* 1992;*7*(3):170–173

[28] Daniels SK, Schroeder MF, DeGeorge PC, Corey DM, Foundas AL, Rosenbek JC. Defining and measuring dysphagia following stroke. *Am J Speech Lang Pathol* 2009;*18*(1):74–81

[29] Meadows JC. Dysphagia in unilateral cerebral lesions. *J Neurol Neurosurg Psychiatry* 1973;*36*(5):853–860

[30] Robbins J, Levin RL. Swallowing after unilateral stroke of the cerebral cortex: preliminary experience. *Dysphagia* 1988;*3*(1):11–17

[31] Daniels SK, Foundas AL. Lesion localization in acute stroke patients with risk of aspiration. *J Neuroimaging* 1999;*9*(2):91–98

[32] Daniels SK, Foundas AL. The role of the insular cortex in dysphagia. *Dysphagia* 1997;*12*(3):146–156

[33] Hamdy S, Aziz Q, Rothwell JC, et al. The cortical topography of human swallowing musculature in health and disease. *Nat Med* 1996;*2*(11):1217–1224

[34] Hamdy S, Aziz Q, Rothwell JC, et al. Explaining oropharyngeal dysphagia after unilateral hemispheric stroke. *Lancet* 1997;*350*(9079):686–692

[35] Hamdy S, Aziz Q, Rothwell JC, et al. Recovery of swallowing after dysphagic stroke relates to functional reorganization in the intact motor cortex. *Gastroenterology* 1998;*115*(5):1104–1112

[36] Li S, Luo C, Yu B, et al. Functional magnetic resonance imaging study on dysphagia after unilateral hemispheric stroke: a preliminary study. *J Neurol Neurosurg Psychiatry* 2009;*80*(12):1320–1329

[37] Barritt AW, Smithard DG. Role of cerebral cortex plasticity in the recovery of swallowing function following dysphagic stroke. *Dysphagia* 2009;*24*(1):83–90

[38] Teismann IK, Suntrup S, Warnecke T, et al. Cortical swallowing processing in early subacute stroke. *BMC Neurol* 2011;*11*:34

[39] McCullough GH, Rosenbek JC, Wertz RT, McCoy S, Mann G, McCullough K. Utility of clinical swallowing examination measures for detecting aspiration post-stroke. *J Speech Lang Hear Res* 2005;*48*(6):1280–1293

[40] Leslie P, Drinnan MJ, Ford GA, Wilson JA. Swallow respiration patterns in dysphagic patients following acute stroke. *Dysphagia* 2002;*17*(3):202–207

[41] Leslie P, Drinnan MJ, Ford GA, Wilson JA. Resting respiration in dysphagic patients following acute stroke. *Dysphagia* 2002;*17*(3):208–213

[42] Butler SG, Stuart A, Pressman H, Poage G, Roche WJ. Preliminary investigation of swallowing apnea duration and swallow/respiratory phase relationships in individuals with cerebral vascular accident. *Dysphagia* 2007;*22*(3):215–224

[43] McCullough GH, Wertz RT, Rosenbek JC, Dinneen C. Clinicians' preferences and practices in conducting clinical/bedside and videofluoroscopic swallowing examinations in an adult, neurogenic population. *Am J Speech Lang Pathol* 1999;*8*:149–163

[44] McCullough GH, Wertz RT, Rosenbek JC. Sensitivity and specificity of clinical/bedside examination signs for detecting aspiration in adults subsequent to stroke. *J Commun Disord* 2001;*34*(1-2):55–72

[45] Mann G, Hankey GJ. Initial clinical and demographic predictors of swallowing impairment following acute stroke. *Dysphagia* 2001;*16*(3):208–215

[46] Daniels SK, McAdam CP, Brailey K, Foundas AL. Clinical assessment of swallowing and prediction of dysphagia severity. *Am J Speech Lang Pathol* 1997;*6*:17–24

[47] Daniels SK, Anderson JA, Willson PC. Valid items for screening dysphagia risk in patients with stroke: a systematic review. *Stroke* 2012;*43*(3):892–897

[48] Saver JL, Altman H. Relationship between neurologic deficit severity and final functional outcome shifts and strengthens during first hours after onset. *Stroke* 2012;*43*(6):1537–1541

[49] Hankey GJ, Spiesser J, Hakimi Z, Bego G, Carita P, Gabriel S. Rate, degree, and predictors of recovery from disability following ischemic stroke. *Neurology* 2007;*68*(19):1583–1587

[50] González-Fernández M, Ottenstein L, Atanelov L, Christian AB. Dysphagia after stroke: an overview. *Curr Phys Med Rehabil Rep* 2013;*1*(3):187–196

[51] Go AS, Mozaffarian D, Roger VL, et al; American Heart Association Statistics Committee and Stroke Statistics Subcommittee. Heart disease and stroke statistics—2013 update: a report from the American Heart Association. *Circulation* 2013;*127*(1):e6–e245

[52] Smithard DG, O'Neill PA, Parks C, Morris J. Complications and outcome after acute stroke. Does dysphagia matter? *Stroke* 1996;*27*(7):1200–1204

[53] Smithard DG, Smeeton NC, Wolfe CD. Long-term outcome after stroke: does dysphagia matter? *Age Ageing* 2007;*36*(1):90–94

[54] Smithard DG, O'Neill PA, England RE, et al. The natural history of dysphagia following a stroke. *Dysphagia* 1997;*12*(4):188–193

[55] Wade DT, Hewer RL. Motor loss and swallowing difficulty after stroke: frequency, recovery, and prognosis. *Acta Neurol Scand* 1987;*76*(1):50–54

[56] Axelsson K, Asplund K, Norberg A, Eriksson S. Eating problems and nutritional status during hospital stay of patients with severe stroke. *J Am Diet Assoc* 1989;*89*(8):1092–1096

[57] Kidd D, Lawson J, Nesbitt R, MacMahon J. The natural history and clinical consequences of aspiration in acute stroke. *QJM* 1995;*88*(6):409–413

[58] Falsetti P, Acciai C, Palilla R, et al. Oropharyngeal dysphagia after stroke: incidence, diagnosis, and clinical predictors in patients admitted to a neurorehabilitation unit. *J Stroke Cerebrovasc Dis* 2009;*18*(5):329–335

[59] Sharma JC, Fletcher S, Vassallo M, Ross I. What influences outcome of stroke-pyrexia or dysphagia? *Int J Clin Pract* 2001;*55*(1):17–20

[60] FOOD Trial Collaboration. Poor nutritional status on admission predicts poor outcomes after stroke: observational data from the FOOD trial. *Stroke* 2003;*34*(6):1450–1456

[61] Finestone HM, Greene-Finestone LS, Wilson ES, Teasell RW. Malnutrition in stroke patients on the rehabilitation service and at follow-up: prevalence and predictors. *Arch Phys Med Rehabil* 1995;*76*(4):310–316

[62] Martineau J, Bauer JD, Isenring E, Cohen S. Malnutrition determined by the Patient-Generated Subjective Global Assessment is associated with poor outcomes in acute stroke patients. *Clin Nutr* 2005;*24*(6):1073–1077

[63] Poels BJ, Brinkman-Zijlker HG, Dijkstra PU, Postema K. Malnutrition, eating difficulties and feeding dependence in a stroke rehabilitation centre. *Disabil Rehabil* 2006;*28*(10):637–643

[64] Foley NC, Martin RE, Salter KL, Teasell RW. A review of the relationship between dysphagia and malnutrition following stroke. *J Rehabil Med* 2009;*41*(9):707–713

[65] Dávalos A, Ricart W, Gonzalez-Huix F, et al. Effect of malnutrition after acute stroke on clinical outcome. *Stroke* 1996;*27*(6):1028–1032

[66] Crary MA, Carnaby-Mann GD, Miller L, Antonios N, Silliman S. Dysphagia and nutritional status at the time of hospital admission for ischemic stroke. *J Stroke Cerebrovasc Dis* 2006;15(4):164–171

[67] Kelly J, Hunt BJ, Lewis RR, et al. Dehydration and venous thromboembolism after acute stroke. *QJM* 2004;97(5):293–296

[68] Rowat A, Graham C, Dennis M. Dehydration in hospital-admitted stroke patients: detection, frequency, and association. *Stroke* 2012;43(3):857–859

[69] Crary MA, Humphrey JL, Carnaby-Mann G, Sambandam R, Miller L, Silliman S. Dysphagia, nutrition, and hydration in ischemic stroke patients at admission and discharge from acute care. *Dysphagia* 2013;28(1):69–76

[70] Crary MA, Carnaby GD, Shabbir Y, Miller L, Silliman S. Clinical variables associated with hydration status in acute ischemic stroke patients with dysphagia. *Dysphagia* 2016;31(1):60–65

[71] Saposnik G, Hill MD, O'Donnell M, Fang J, Hachinski V, Kapral MK; Registry of the Canadian Stroke Network for the Stroke Outcome Research Canada (SORCan) Working Group. Variables associated with 7-day, 30-day, and 1-year fatality after ischemic stroke. *Stroke* 2008;39(8):2318–2324

[72] Rofes L, Arreola V, Almirall J, et al. Diagnosis and management of oropharyngeal dysphagia and its nutritional and respiratory complications in the elderly. *Gastroenterol Res Pract* 2011;2011:1–13

[73] Kumar S, Selim MH, Caplan LR. Medical complications after stroke. *Lancet Neurol* 2010;9(1):105–118

[74] Holas MA, DePippo KL, Reding MJ. Aspiration and relative risk of medical complications following stroke. *Arch Neurol* 1994;51(10):1051–1053

[75] Johnson ER, McKenzie SW, Sievers A. Aspiration pneumonia in stroke. *Arch Phys Med Rehabil* 1993;74(9):973–976

[76] Teasell RW, Bach D, McRae M. Prevalence and recovery of aspiration poststroke: a retrospective analysis. *Dysphagia* 1994;9(1):35–39

[77] Teasell RW, McRae M, Marchuk Y, Finestone HM. Pneumonia associated with aspiration following stroke. *Arch Phys Med Rehabil* 1996;77(7):707–709

[78] Langmore SE, Terpenning MS, Schork A, et al. Predictors of aspiration pneumonia: how important is dysphagia? *Dysphagia* 1998;13(2):69–81

[79] Teasell R, Foley N, Martino R, Richardson M, Bhogal S, Speechley M. Dysphagia and aspiration following stroke. In: Teasell R, Hussein N, Foley N, eds. Evidence Based Review of Stroke Rehabilitation. 2013. www.ebrsr.com. Accessed March 5, 2016

[80] Huxley EJ, Viroslav J, Gray WR, Pierce AK. Pharyngeal aspiration in normal adults and patients with depressed consciousness. *Am J Med* 1978;64(4):564–568

[81] Unosson M, Ek AC, Bjurulf P, von Schenck H, Larsson J. Feeding dependence and nutritional status after acute stroke. *Stroke* 1994;25(2):366–371

[82] Finucane TE, Bynum JP. Use of tube feeding to prevent aspiration pneumonia. *Lancet* 1996;348(9039):1421–1424

[83] Kalra L, Dale P, Crome P. Improving stroke rehabilitation. A controlled study. *Stroke* 1993;24(10):1462–1467

[84] Broadley S, Croser D, Cottrell J, et al. Predictors of prolonged dysphagia following acute stroke. *J Clin Neurosci* 2003;10:300–305

[85] Paolucci S. Epidemiology and treatment of post-stroke depression. *Neuropsychiatr Dis Treat* 2008;4(1):145–154

[86] McCullagh E, Brigstocke G, Donaldson N, Kalra L. Determinants of caregiving burden and quality of life in caregivers of stroke patients. *Stroke* 2005;36(10):2181–2186

[87] Schulz R, Tompkins CA, Rau MT. A longitudinal study of the psychosocial impact of stroke on primary support persons. *Psychol Aging* 1988;3(2):131–141

[88] Dewey HM, Thrift AG, Mihalopoulos C, et al. Lifetime cost of stroke subtypes in Australia: findings from the North East Melbourne Stroke Incidence Study (NEMESIS). *Stroke* 2003;34(10):2502–2507

[89] Wilson RD. Mortality and cost of pneumonia after stroke for different risk groups. *J Stroke Cerebrovasc Dis* 2012;21(1):61–67

[90] Bonilha HS, Simpson AN, Ellis C, Mauldin P, Martin-Harris B, Simpson K. The one-year attributable cost of post-stroke dysphagia. *Dysphagia* 2014;29(5):545–552

[91] Carnaby-Mann G, Lenius K. The bedside examination in dysphagia. *Phys Med Rehabil Clin N Am* 2008;19(4):747–768, viii

[92] The Joint Commission Standardized Stroke Measure Set. [September 21, 2009]

[93] DePippo KL, Holas MA, Reding MJ. The Burke dysphagia screening test: validation of its use in patients with stroke. *Arch Phys Med Rehabil* 1994;75(12):1284–1286

[94] DePippo KL, Holas MA, Reding MJ. Validation of the 3-oz water swallow test for aspiration following stroke. *Arch Neurol* 1992;49(12):1259–1261

[95] Massey R, Jedlicka D. The Massey Bedside Swallowing Screen. *J Neurosci Nurs* 2002;34(5):252–253, 257–260

[96] Suiter DM, Sloggy J, Leder SB. Validation of the Yale Swallow Protocol: a prospective double-blinded videofluoroscopic study. *Dysphagia* 2014;29(2):199–203

[97] Suiter DM, Leder SB. Clinical utility of the 3-ounce water swallow test. *Dysphagia* 2008;23(3):244–250

[98] Martino R, Silver F, Teasell R, et al. The Toronto Bedside Swallowing Screening Test (TOR-BSST): development and validation of a dysphagia screening tool for patients with stroke. *Stroke* 2009;40(2):555–561

[99] Perry L, Love CP. Screening for dysphagia and aspiration in acute stroke: a systematic review. *Dysphagia* 2001;16(1):7–18

[100] Perry L. Screening swallowing function of patients with acute stroke. Part two: Detailed evaluation of the tool used by nurses. *J Clin Nurs* 2001;10(4):474–481

[101] Titsworth WL, Abram J, Fullerton A, et al. Prospective quality initiative to maximize dysphagia screening reduces hospital-acquired pneumonia prevalence in patients with stroke. *Stroke* 2013;44(11):3154–3160

[102] Edmiaston J, Connor LT, Steger-May K, Ford AL. A simple bedside stroke dysphagia screen, validated against videofluoroscopy, detects dysphagia and aspiration with high sensitivity. *J Stroke Cerebrovasc Dis* 2014;23(4):712–716

[103] Antonios N, Carnaby-Mann G, Crary M, et al. Analysis of a physician tool for evaluating dysphagia on an inpatient stroke unit: the modified Mann Assessment of Swallowing Ability. *J Stroke Cerebrovasc Dis* 2010;19(1):49–57

[104] Doggett DL, Tappe KA, Mitchell MD, Chapell R, Coates V, Turkelson CM. Prevention of pneumonia in elderly stroke patients by systematic diagnosis and treatment of dysphagia: an evidence-based comprehensive analysis of the literature. *Dysphagia* 2001;16(4):279–295

[105] Lakshminarayan K, Tsai AW, Tong X, et al. Utility of dysphagia screening results in predicting poststroke pneumonia. *Stroke* 2010;41(12):2849–2854

[106] Courtney BA, Flier LA. RN dysphagia screening, a stepwise approach. *J Neurosci Nurs* 2009;41(1):28–38

[107] Schepp SK, Tirschwell DL, Miller RM, Longstreth WT Jr. Swallowing screens after acute stroke: a systematic review. *Stroke* 2012;43(3):869–871

[108] Mann G. MASA: The Mann Assessment of Swallowing Ability. Clifton Park, NY: Singular; 2002

[109] Vanderwegen J, Guns C, Van Nuffelen G, et al. The reliability of the MASA dysphagia screening protocol compared to FEES for patients in an acute stroke unit. *Dysphagia* 2006;21(4):327

[110] Bours GJ, Speyer R, Lemmens J, Limburg M, de Wit R. Bedside screening tests vs. videofluoroscopy or fibreoptic endoscopic evaluation of swallowing to detect dysphagia in patients with neurological disorders: systematic review. *J Adv Nurs* 2009;65(3):477–493

[111] Mathers-Schmidt BA, Kurlinski M. Dysphagia evaluation practices: inconsistencies in clinical assessment and instrumental examination decision-making. *Dysphagia* 2003;18(2):114–125

[112] Langmore SE. Evaluation of oropharyngeal dysphagia: which diagnostic tool is superior? *Curr Opin Otolaryngol Head Neck Surg* 2003;11(6):485–489

[113] Martin-Harris B, Jones B. The videofluorographic swallowing study. *Phys Med Rehabil Clin N Am* 2008;19(4):769–785, viii

[114] Logemann J. Evaluation and Treatment of Swallowing Disorders. San Diego, CA: College Hill Press; 1983

[115] Smithard DG, O'Neill PA, Park C, et al; North West Dysphagia Group. Can bedside assessment reliably exclude aspiration following acute stroke? *Age Ageing* 1998;27(2):99–106

[116] Ramsey DJ, Smithard DG, Kalra L. Early assessments of dysphagia and aspiration risk in acute stroke patients. *Stroke* 2003;34(5):1252–1257

[117] Martin-Harris B, Brodsky MB, Michel Y, et al. MBS measurement tool for swallow impairment—MBSImp: establishing a standard. *Dysphagia* 2008;23(4):392–405

[118] Carnaby G, Hankey GJ, Pizzi J. Behavioural intervention for dysphagia in acute stroke: a randomised controlled trial. *Lancet Neurol* 2006;5(1):31–37

[119] Foley N, Teasell R, Salter K, Kruger E, Martino R. Dysphagia treatment post stroke: a systematic review of randomised controlled trials. *Age Ageing* 2008;37(3):258–264

[120] Crary MA. A direct intervention program for chronic neurogenic dysphagia secondary to brainstem stroke. *Dysphagia* 1995;10(1):6–18

[121] Crary MA, Baldwin BO. Surface electromyographic characteristics of swallowing in dysphagia secondary to brainstem stroke. *Dysphagia* 1997;12(4):180–187

[122] McCullough GH, Kamarunas E, Mann GC, Schmidley JW, Robbins JA, Crary MA. Effects of Mendelsohn maneuver on measures of swallowing duration post stroke. *Top Stroke Rehabil* 2012;19(3):234–243

[123] Carnaby-Mann GD, Crary MA. McNeill dysphagia therapy program: a case-control study. *Arch Phys Med Rehabil* 2010;91(5):743–749

[124]Dziewas R, Warnecke T, Hamacher C, et al. Do nasogastric tubes worsen dysphagia in patients with acute stroke? *BMC Neurol* 2008;*8*(1):28

[125]Gomes CA Jr, Lustosa SA, Matos D, Andriolo RB, Waisberg DR, Waisberg J. Percutaneous endoscopic gastrostomy versus nasogastric tube feeding for adults with swallowing disturbances. *Cochrane Database Syst Rev* 2010;*8*(11):CD008096

[126]Bath PM, Bath FJ, Smithard DG. Interventions for dysphagia in acute stroke. *Cochrane Database Syst Rev* 2000;(2):CD000323

[127]Dennis MS, Lewis SC, Warlow C; FOOD Trial Collaboration. Routine oral nutritional supplementation for stroke patients in hospital (FOOD): a multicentre randomised controlled trial. *Lancet* 2005;*365*(9461):755–763

[128]Dennis MS, Lewis SC, Warlow C; FOOD Trial Collaboration. Effect of timing and method of enteral tube feeding for dysphagic stroke patients (FOOD): a multicentre randomised controlled trial. *Lancet* 2005;*365*(9461):764–772

[129]Crary MA, Carnaby Mann GD, Groher ME, Helseth E. Functional benefits of dysphagia therapy using adjunctive sEMG biofeedback. *Dysphagia* 2004;*19*(3):160–164

[130]Singh S, Hamdy S. Dysphagia in stroke patients. *Postgrad Med J* 2006;*82*(968):383–391

[131]Crary M, Groher M. Reinstituting oral feeding in tube fed adult patients with dysphagia. *Nutr Clin Pract* 2011;*26*:242–252

[132]Garcia JM, Chambers E IV, Molander M. Thickened liquids: practice patterns of speech-language pathologists. *Am J Speech Lang Pathol* 2005;*14*(1):4–13

[133]Penman J, Thompson M. A review of the textured diets developed for diet. *J Hum Nutr Diet* 1998;*11*:51–60

[134]Garcia JM, Chambers E IV, Clark M, Helverson J, Matta Z. Quality of care issues for dysphagia: modifications involving oral fluids. *J Clin Nurs* 2010;*19*(11-12):1618–1624

[135]Castellanos VH, Butler E, Gluch L, Burke B. Use of thickened liquids in skilled nursing facilities. *J Am Diet Assoc* 2004;*104*(8):1222–1226

[136]Low J, Wyles C, Wilkinson T, Sainsbury R. The effect of compliance on clinical outcomes for patients with dysphagia on videofluoroscopy. *Dysphagia* 2001;*16*(2):123–127

[137]Robbins J, Gensler G, Hind J, et al. Comparison of 2 interventions for liquid aspiration on pneumonia incidence: a randomized trial. *Ann Intern Med* 2008;*148*(7):509–518

[138]National Dysphagia Diet Task Force, and American Dietetic Association. National Dysphagia Diet: Standardization for Optimal Care. Chicago, IL: American Dietetic Association; 2002

[139]Pouderoux P, Kahrilas PJ. Deglutitive tongue force modulation by volition, volume, and viscosity in humans. *Gastroenterology* 1995;*108*(5):1418–1426

[140]Chi-Fishman G, Sonies BC. Effects of systematic bolus viscosity and volume changes on hyoid movement kinematics. *Dysphagia* 2002;*17*(4):278–287

[141]Dantas RO, Kern MK, Massey BT, et al. Effect of swallowed bolus variables on oral and pharyngeal phases of swallowing. *Am J Physiol* 1990;*258*(5 Pt 1):G675–G681

[142]Dantas RO, Dodds WJ, Massey BT, Kern MK. The effect of high- vs low-density barium preparations on the quantitative features of swallowing. *AJR Am J Roentgenol* 1989;*153*(6):1191–1195

[143]Dantas RO, Dodds WJ. Effect of bolus volume and consistency on swallow-induced submental and infrahyoid electromyographic activity. *Braz J Med Biol Res* 1990;*23*(1):37–44

[144]Ertekin C, Keskin A, Kiylioglu N, et al. The effect of head and neck positions on oropharyngeal swallowing: a clinical and electrophysiologic study. *Arch Phys Med Rehabil* 2001;*82*(9):1255–1260

[145]Forster A, Samaras N, Gold G, Samaras D. Oropharyngeal dysphagia in older adults: A review. *Eur Geriatr Med* 2011;*2*(6):356–362

[146]Speyer R. Behavioural treatment of oropharyngeal dysphagia: bolus modification and management, sensory and motor behavioural techniques, postural adjustments, and swallow manoeuvres. In: Ekberg O, ed. Dysphagia: Diagnosis and Treatment. Berlin, Germany: Springer; 2011:477–491

[147]Easterling C, Grande B, Kern M, Sears K, Shaker R. Attaining and maintaining isometric and isokinetic goals of the Shaker exercise. *Dysphagia* 2005;*20*(2):133–138

[148]Antunes EB, Lunet N. Effects of the head lift exercise on the swallow function: a systematic review. *Gerodontology* 2012;*29*(4):247–257

[149]Shaker R, Kern M, Bardan E, et al. Augmentation of deglutitive upper esophageal sphincter opening in the elderly by exercise. *Am J Physiol* 1997;*272*(6 Pt 1):G1518–G1522

[150]Crary M, Groher M. Basic concepts of surface electromyographic biofeedback in the treatment of dysphagia. A tutorial. *Am J Speech Lang Pathol* 2000;*9*(2):116–125

[151]Langdon C, Blacker D. Dysphagia in stroke: a new solution. *Stroke Res Treat.* 2010;*2010*:1–6

[152]Robbins J, Gangnon RE, Theis SM, Kays SA, Hewitt AL, Hind JA. The effects of lingual exercise on swallowing in older adults. *J Am Geriatr Soc* 2005;*53*(9):1483–1489

[153]Robbins J, Kays SA, Gangnon RE, et al. The effects of lingual exercise in stroke patients with dysphagia. *Arch Phys Med Rehabil* 2007;*88*(2):150–158

[154]Juan J, Hind J, Jones C, McCulloch T, Gangnon R, Robbins J. Case study: application of isometric progressive resistance oropharyngeal therapy using the Madison Oral Strengthening Therapeutic device. *Top Stroke Rehabil* 2013;*20*(5):450–470

[155]Crary MA, Carnaby GD, LaGorio LA, Carvajal PJ. Functional and physiological outcomes from an exercise-based dysphagia therapy: a pilot investigation of the McNeill Dysphagia Therapy Program. *Arch Phys Med Rehabil* 2012;*93*(7):1173–1178

[156]Lan Y, Ohkubo M, Berretin-Felix G, Sia I, Carnaby-Mann GD, Crary MA. Normalization of temporal aspects of swallowing physiology after the McNeill dysphagia therapy program. *Ann Otol Rhinol Laryngol* 2012;*121*(8):525–532

[157]Carnaby GD, LaGorio L, Miller D, et al. A randomized double blind trial of neuromuscular electrical stimulation + McNeill Dysphagia Therapy (MDTP) after stroke (ANSRS). Presentation to the Dysphagia Research Society Annual Meeting; March, 2012; Toronto, Canada

[158]Huckabee ML, Cannito MP. Outcomes of swallowing rehabilitation in chronic brainstem dysphagia: A retrospective evaluation. *Dysphagia* 1999;*14*(2):93–109

[159]Crary MA, Carnaby Mann GD, Groher ME. Identification of swallowing events from sEMG Signals Obtained from Healthy Adults. *Dysphagia* 2007;*22*(2):94–99

[160]Stepp CE. Surface electromyography for speech and swallowing systems: measurement, analysis, and interpretation. *J Speech Lang Hear Res* 2012;*55*(4):1232–1246

[161]Crary MA, Carnaby Mann GD, Groher ME. Biomechanical correlates of surface electromyography signals obtained during swallowing by healthy adults. *J Speech Lang Hear Res* 2006;*49*(1):186–193

[162]Huckabee ML, Doeltgen S. Emerging modalities in dysphagia rehabilitation: neuromuscular electrical stimulation. *N Z Med J* 2007;*120*(1263):U2744

[163]Clark H, Lazarus C, Arvedson J, Schooling T, Frymark T. Evidence-based systematic review: effects of neuromuscular electrical stimulation on swallowing and neural activation. *Am J Speech Lang Pathol* 2009;*18*(4):361–375

[164]Gallas S, Marie JP, Leroi AM, Verin E. Sensory transcutaneous electrical stimulation improves post-stroke dysphagic patients. *Dysphagia* 2010;*25*(4):291–297

[165]Kushner DS, Peters K, Eroglu ST, Perless-Carroll M, Johnson-Greene D. Neuromuscular electrical stimulation efficacy in acute stroke feeding tube-dependent dysphagia during inpatient rehabilitation. *Am J Phys Med Rehabil* 2013;*92*(6):486–495

[166]Suiter DM, Leder SB, Ruark JL. Effects of neuromuscular electrical stimulation on submental muscle activity. *Dysphagia* 2006;*21*(1):56–60

[167]Humbert IA, Michou E, MacRae PR, Crujido L. Electrical stimulation and swallowing: how much do we know? *Semin Speech Lang* 2012;*33*(3):203–216

[168]Ludlow CL. Electrical neuromuscular stimulation in dysphagia: current status. *Curr Opin Otolaryngol Head Neck Surg* 2010;*18*(3):159–164

[169]Berretin-Felix G, Sia I, Barikroo A, Carnaby GD, Crary MA. Immediate effects of transcutaneous electrical stimulation on physiological swallowing effort in older versus young adults. *Gerodontology* 2016;*33*(3):348–355

[170]Park JW, Oh JC, Lee HJ, Park SJ, Yoon TS, Kwon BS. Effortful swallowing training coupled with electrical stimulation leads to an increase in hyoid elevation during swallowing. *Dysphagia* 2009;*24*(3):296–301

[171]Lim KB, Lee HJ, Lim SS, Choi YI. Neuromuscular electrical and thermal-tactile stimulation for dysphagia caused by stroke: a randomized controlled trial. *J Rehabil Med* 2009;*41*(3):174–178

[172]Permsirivanich W, Tipchatyotin S, Wongchai M, et al. Comparing the effects of rehabilitation swallowing therapy vs. neuromuscular electrical stimulation therapy among stroke patients with persistent pharyngeal dysphagia: a randomized controlled study. *J Med Assoc Thai* 2009;*92*(2):259–265

[173]Bülow M, Speyer R, Baijens L, Woisard V, Ekberg O. Neuromuscular electrical stimulation (NMES) in stroke patients with oral and pharyngeal dysfunction. *Dysphagia* 2008;*23*(3):302–309

[174]Tan C, Liu Y, Li W, Liu J, Chen L. Transcutaneous neuromuscular electrical stimulation can improve swallowing function in patients with dysphagia caused by non-stroke diseases: a meta-analysis. *J Oral Rehabil* 2013;*40*(6):472–480

[175]Hamdy S. Dysphagia recovery by electrical stimulation. U.S. Patent No. 8,092,433. January 10, 2012

[176] Michou E, Mistry S, Jefferson S, Singh S, Rothwell J, Hamdy S. Targeting unlesioned pharyngeal motor cortex improves swallowing in healthy individuals and after dysphagic stroke. *Gastroenterology* 2012;*142*(1):29–38

[177] Yang EJ, Baek SR, Shin J, et al. Effects of transcranial direct current stimulation (tDCS) on post-stroke dysphagia. *Restor Neurol Neurosci* 2012;*30*(4):303–311

[178] Macrae PR, Jones RD, Huckabee ML. The effect of swallowing treatments on corticobulbar excitability: a review of transcranial magnetic stimulation induced motor evoked potentials. *J Neurosci Methods* 2014;*233*:89–98

[179] DePippo KL, Holas MA, Reding MJ, Mandel FS, Lesser ML. Dysphagia therapy following stroke: a controlled trial. *Neurology* 1994;*44*(9):1655–1660

[180] Dennis M. Dysphagia in acute stroke: a long-awaited trial. *Lancet Neurol* 2006;*5*(1):16–17

[181] Brown M, Glassenberg M. Mortality factors in patients with acute stroke. *JAMA* 1973;*224*(11):1493–1495

## Suggested Reading

[1] Butler S, Pelletier C, Steele C. Compensatory strategies and techniques. In: Shaker R, Easterling K, Belafsky P, Postma G, eds. Manual of Diagnostic and Therapeutic Techniques for Disorders of Deglutition. New York, NY: Springer; 2013:219–316

[2] Crary MA, Carnaby GD. Adoption into clinical practice of two therapies to manage swallowing disorders: exercise-based swallowing rehabilitation and electrical stimulation. *Curr Opin Otolaryngol Head Neck Surg* 2014;*22*(3):172–180

[3] Clark HM. Neuromuscular treatments for speech and swallowing: a tutorial. *Am J Speech Lang Pathol* 2003;*12*(4):400–415

# 21 Dysphagia in Traumatic Brain Injury

*Paras M. Bhattarai*

## Summary

Overall, patients with traumatic brain injury can present with a variable pattern of swallow functioning, ranging from very mild to very severe. Clinicians who work with patients with traumatic brain injury must be mindful of the influence that accompanying cognitive-linguistic deficits may have on the patient's ability to safely tolerate an oral diet. Multiple factors, including severity of injury, length of ventilation, and patient age, influence patient outcomes.

## Keywords

cerebrovascular accident, diffuse axonal injury, epidural hematoma, Glasgow Coma Scale (GCS), Rancho Los Amigos Scale (RLAS), subarachnoid hemorrhage, subdural hematoma

### Learning Objectives

- To understand the incidence and prevalence of traumatic brain injury (TBI) and understand dysphagia as one of the major complications
- To understand the differences in the pathophysiology and presentation of different types of TBI
- To understand TBI as a distinct entity among other causes of neurogenic dysphagia in terms of presentation, evaluation, and management
- To understand the clinical presentation, complications, and outcome of dysphagia in TBI
- To understand the basic principles of evaluation and management of dysphagia in TBI

## 21.1 Introduction

Traumatic brain injury (TBI) is one of the major causes of death and disability in the United States, contributing to almost one-third (30%) of all injury-related deaths.[1] It results from both blunt and penetrating injury to the head leading to primary and secondary injury to the brain. Major causes include motor vehicle accidents, falls, assaults, and unintentional blunt trauma. Despite variability in presentation based on the type of insult and its severity, common presentation in cases of TBI includes changes in level of consciousness, memory disturbances, confusion, and neurologic signs.[2] Dysphagia is a common problem following TBI, the frequency of which depends on a variety of factors, including the severity of injury, Glasgow Coma Scale (GCS) and Rancho Los Amigos Scale (RLAS) scores, presence of tracheostomy, duration of ventilation, underlying neuropathology, and computed tomographic (CT) scan findings.[3] Cognitive,

behavioral, and communicative disorders are common in TBI, which makes the evaluation and management of dysphagia a challenging task.[4] Presence of dysphagia is a major determinant of increased morbidity, including longer inpatient length of stay.[5]

Evaluation of swallowing function in a brain-injured patient starts at the acute care hospital when the patient is consistently awake and alert.[6] Clinical findings alone tend to miss a significant proportion of patients with aspiration.[7,8] Videofluoroscopy, which is considered to be the gold standard, and fiberoptic endoscopic evaluation of swallowing (FEES) are the most commonly used procedures.[9,10,11]

There is no specific treatment for TBI-related dysphagia. The multifaceted nature of post-TBI dysphagia requires patient-specific treatment, taking into consideration neuromuscular, cognitive-communicative, and behavioral presentation. Despite this, common treatment and management strategies for dysphagia related to other etiologies, in general, work for patients with TBI.[12] Mealtime low-risk strategies are followed, targeting cognitive-behavioral and communicative issues.[5] As in other types of neurogenic dysphagia, compensatory treatment and therapy techniques are followed.[13] Swallowing outcomes are affected by several factors, the most important of which include admitting GCS score, RLAS score, CT scan findings, and ventilation time.[3,14]

The definition of TBI has not been consistent over the years. It tends to vary based on specialties and circumstances. TBI is a suddenly acquired and nondegenerative injury to the cranium and the intracranial contents from an external mechanical force, possibly leading to permanent or temporary impairment of cognitive, physical, and psychosocial functions with an associated diminished or altered state of consciousness.[16,17,18] TBI can result when the head suddenly and violently hits an object or when an object pierces the skull and enters the brain tissue. The term *brain injury* is used synonymously with *head injury*. TBI encompasses both primary and secondary injury to the brain after trauma. The physical, cognitive, and behavioral sequelae of TBI constitute a major cause of death and disability in all ages and are often devastating to the family and society. The economic costs of TBI in terms of medical cost include both acute care and continuous ambulatory and rehabilitative care. Additionally, lost productivity of the patient and of the individuals who become the patient's caretakers is also substantial. The early age at which TBI occurs, combined with medical advances improving initial survival and increasing the life span, stand to increase this socioeconomic burden.[19]

*Neurogenic dysphagia* is a loose term that encompasses dysphagia resulting from damage to the central nervous system. Neurogenic dysphagia has various causes, including TBI, cerebrovascular accident, neurologic cancers, and degenerative neurologic conditions, among others.[13] As with other causes of neurogenic dysphagia, many people who develop dysphagia from TBI survive the injury and are subsequently treated in rehabilitation centers.

## 21.2 Case Presentation Part 1

JS is a 14-year-old boy who was brought to the emergency department after being hit by a baseball bat on his right temporal area about half an hour earlier. He complained of headache at the site of impact but appeared to be alert and oriented to time, place, and person. Emergency department records show a Glasgow Coma Scale (GCS) score of 15 at arrival. No imaging was ordered, but the patient was observed closely. Two hours after the impact, his GCS score dropped to 6. He was intubated and got a stat CT scan of the head that showed a right epidural hematoma with mass effect and mild midline shift (**Fig. 21.1**). The hematoma was evacuated through craniotomy. He developed weakness of the left upper and lower extremities. He was kept in the pediatric intensive care unit and extubated after 2 days. Speech-language pathology was consulted 2 days after extubation, as the patient's awareness and ability to follow commands improved.

## 21.3 Incidence and Prevalence of Traumatic Brain Injury

The annual incidence of TBI in developed countries is approximately 200 per 100,000.[13] In children, the incidence has been reported to be as high as 280 per 100,000. TBI results in 1.7 million emergency room visits every year. More than 80% of patients are treated and released from the emergency department, but approximately 52,000 deaths and 275,000 hospitalizations result.

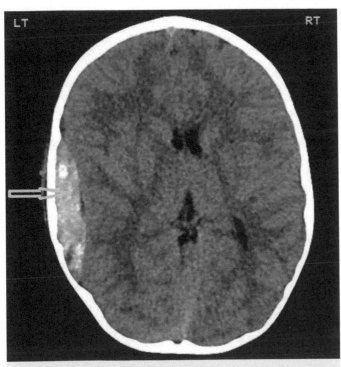

**Fig. 21.1** Computed tomographic (CT) scan of the head with right epidural hematoma (with arrow pointing at the lesion). No fracture was noticed. There is resultant mass effect on surrounding brain parenchyma.

Based on reports from the Centers for Disease Control and Prevention in 2011, it is estimated that between 3.2 and 5.3 million people, or 1.1–1.7% of the US population, are living with a long-term disability as a result of brain injury.[17,20,21] TBI is a major cause of mortality in the United States. Overall, it is responsible for almost one-third (30.5%) of all injury-related deaths. Children aged from birth to 4 years, older adolescents aged 15 to 19 years, and adults aged 65 years and older are most likely to sustain a TBI. Children between the ages of 0 and 14 years account for nearly half a million (473,947) emergency department visits for TBI annually. Adults aged 75 years and older have the highest rates of TBI-related hospitalization and death. In every age group, TBI rates are higher for males than for females. Overall, approximately 1.4 times as many TBIs occur among males as among females. Males between the ages of birth and 4 years have the highest rates for TBI-related emergency department visits, hospitalizations, and deaths combined. Falls are the leading cause of TBI overall. Rates are highest for children ages 0 to 4 years and for adults aged 75 years and older. Falls result in the greatest number of TBI-related emergency department visits (523,043) and hospitalizations (62,334). On the other hand, motor vehicle–traffic injury is the leading cause of TBI-related death. Rates are highest for adults aged 20 to 24 years.[1] Injuries are the leading cause of death in persons 1 and 19 years of age, accounting for 62% of all deaths in this population, with up to 50% of injury-related deaths being attributed to TBIs (**Box 21.1**).

### Box 21.1

**TBI in the United States by the Numbers: Years 2002–2006 (CDC Reports)**

- Total cases: 1.7 million (estimated)
- Emergency room visits: 1,365,000
- Hospitalizations: 275,000
- Deaths: 52,000(3%) or 137 deaths/d

## 21.4 Pathophysiology of Traumatic Brain Injury

TBI is the result of an external mechanical force applied to the cranium and the intracranial contents. Severity ranges widely, from mild concussion to coma and death.[22] The GCS (**Box 21.2**) and RLAS (**Box 21.3**)[23,24] are used within the first 48 hours of injury to assess the severity of TBI, with the former being more commonly used. On the GCS, a score of above 12 is considered mild, scores between 9 and 12 are moderate, and scores of 3 to 8 are severe. Statistically, about 75% of the TBIs that occur each year are mild, otherwise known as concussions. However, the true incidence of mild TBI is difficult to determine because of the number of individuals with symptoms attributable to TBI who do not seek medical care. Approximately 16 to 25% of patients with TBI do not seek medical care after sustaining an injury.[25]

## Box 21.2

**Assessment of Severity of Brain Injury by Glasgow Coma Scale[23,24]**

The GCS is the most commonly used scoring system to describe the level of consciousness in a person following traumatic brain injury. The scoring system seeks scores from (1) eye opening (E), (2) verbal response (V), and (3) motor response (M). GCS is the sum of all the responses: E + V + M.

A modified version of GCS is used in infants and children less than 5 years old.

GCS is commonly used to define or classify severity of TBI as follows:

- Mild: GCS score 13–15
- Moderate: GCS score 9–12
- Severe: GCS score 3–8

Duration of loss of consciousness (LOC) is another measure of the severity of TBI. It is usually classified as follows:

- Mild: LOC less than 30 minutes
- Moderate: LOC 30 minutes to 6 hours
- Severe: LOC more than 6 hours

## Box 21.3

**Ranchos Los Amigos Scale of Cognitive Functioning**

- Level I: No response
- Level II: Generalized response
- Level III: Localized response
- Level IV: Confused-agitated
- Level V: Confused-inappropriate
- Level VI: Confused-appropriate
- Level VII: Automatic-appropriate
- Level VIII: Purposeful-appropriate

Injury in TBI is divided into primary injury, which occurs at the moment of trauma, and secondary injury, which starts at the time of trauma but produces effects that continue for a long time. Primary injury occurs due to collision and sudden motion and involves tissue compression, stretching, and distortion. Depending on the insult, there may be focal injury, such as skull fracture, intracranial hemorrhage, coup and countercoup contusions, and penetrating head injuries, or there can be diffuse damage, such as diffuse axonal injury. In patients sustaining TBI, it is often a secondary insult causing global cerebral hypoxia or hypoperfusion that markedly increases morbidity and mortality. A well-recognized complication of TBI is posttraumatic cerebral infarction, which occurs in approximately 2% of TBIs.[26] This more localized insult may occur secondary to focal mass effect, vascular impingement usually caused by herniation, cerebral vasospasm, thromboembolism, cerebrovascular injury, or venous congestion at craniectomy sites. Other types of secondary injury include cerebral edema and herniation, which may develop acutely, and

hydrocephalus due to blood products blocking the flow of cerebrospinal fluid. The details of primary and secondary injuries are beyond the scope of this chapter.[27]

## 21.5 Etiology of Traumatic Brain Injury

Though they vary according to age, the major causes of TBI include falls, motor vehicle collision (MVC), assault, and other unintentional injuries. Major causes across different age groups are illustrated in **Table 21.1** and **Fig. 21.2**.

The National Health Interview Survey, which focused on mild to moderate brain injury (1991), found the risk of medically attended brain injury to be highest in teens and young adults, males, and persons of low income who reside by themselves.[28]

**Table 21.1** Causes of traumatic brain injury: variation according to age of an individual

| Age range | Major causes of TBI |
| --- | --- |
| Infants | Abusive head trauma |
| Children below 5 years | Falls |
| Preadolescent children | Falls, pedestrian injury, motor vehicle injury |
| Adolescents and young adults | Motor vehicle injury |
| Adults | Motor vehicle injury, falls |

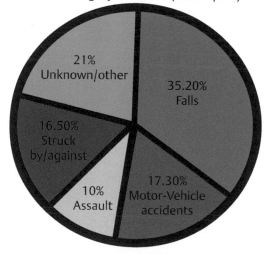

Overall incidence of TBI based on broad category of causes (CDC report)

- 21% Unknown/other
- 35.20% Falls
- 16.50% Struck by/against
- 17.30% Motor-Vehicle accidents
- 10% Assault

**Fig. 21.2** Causes of traumatic brain injury in the United States. These data are based on a Centers for Disease Control and Prevention report and are for the United States only. Data are comparable to those for other developed countries.

## 21.6 Assessment of Severity of Traumatic Brain Injury

TBI is a heterogeneous group of conditions with variable clinical presentations, severity, and outcomes. Because of this, various methods for measuring severity of TBI have been devised. In the acute setting, such as a trauma center, the GCS is used (**Box 21.2**). During long-term management and especially while one is managing complications, such as dysphagia, other types of severity rating scales are used to assess cognitive functioning and disability. These include the RLAS (**Box 21.3**).

## 21.7 Patterns of Trauma in Traumatic Brain Injury

As mentioned previously, TBI can result in focal injury or diffuse injury. Examples of focal injuries include scalp injury, skull fracture, cerebral contusions, and epidural or subdural hematomas. Injuries caused by rapid acceleration and deceleration, such as diffuse axonal injury and diffuse hypoxic-ischemic injury, are examples of diffuse injury. A patient may have both types of injuries.

Patient presentation in the acute care setting depends on both primary and secondary injuries. Primary injury is induced by the mechanical force and occurs at the moment of injury because of either contact or rapid acceleration-deceleration. Examples include contusions, diffuse axonal injury, different types of intracranial hematoma (**epidural** and **subdural hematoma**), **subarachnoid hemorrhage**, diffuse vascular injury, and injury to the cranial nerves and pituitary stalk. Primary injury can be either focal or diffuse. Secondary injury is a superimposed injury on an injured brain that may occur hours or days after insult and results from decline in cerebral blood flow related to a combination of local edema, hemorrhage, and increased intracranial pressure.[29]

## 21.8 Dysphagia in Traumatic Brain Injury

Dysphagia is common following TBI. Individuals with dysphagia resulting from TBI are placed into the broad category of nonspecific neurogenic dysphagia, along with cerebrovascular accident, degenerative neurologic disease, and neurologic cancers. However, unlike other neurogenic dysphagia, dysphagia following TBI has different pathophysiology and hence needs to be considered separately. To better understand the etiology of dysphagia in TBI, a basic understanding of anatomy and pathophysiology is required.

### 21.8.1 Anatomical Structures Involved in Dysphagia

Swallowing difficulty can occur from impaired function at the level of the mouth, pharynx, upper esophageal sphincter, and esophagus. Neurogenic dysphagia results from neurological insult leading to abnormal function of the aforementioned structures.

For most people, swallowing is a simple and effortless act that takes around 750 milliseconds. Despite its ease, it is a complex and dynamic sensorimotor activity that involves 26 muscles and five pairs of cranial nerves (V, VII, IX, X, and XII). Neuroregulation of swallowing occurs as a result of a complex interplay of cortical, medullary, and subcortical structures. Swallowing enables the safe delivery of ingested food, as a bolus, from the mouth to the stomach, while ensuring protection of intact airway.[30]

### 21.8.2 Neurological Control of Swallowing

Neurological control of swallowing is multidimensional in nature, involving multiple levels of the nervous system. The brainstem swallowing center is a nondiscrete area located in the upper medulla and pons and is bilaterally distributed within the reticular formation, a network of neurons in the brainstem involved in consciousness, breathing, and the transmission of sensory stimuli to higher brain centers. This network of neurons is made up of an afferent component, an efferent component, and a complex organizing system of interneurons known as the central pattern generator (CPG). Although the cerebral cortex is thought to be responsible for the initiation of swallowing, the CPG organizes the sequential activation of motor neurons controlling the swallowing muscles.

Although CPGs of the brainstem control the timing of the phases of swallowing, the peripheral manifestation of these phases depends on sensory feedback through reflexes of the pharynx and esophagus.[31] Subcortical structures, such as the basal ganglia, hypothalamus, amygdala, and tegmental area of the brain, represent the second level of the swallowing control mechanism. Representing a third level of control are the suprabulbar cortical swallowing centers.[30]

### 21.8.3 Incidence of Dysphagia in Traumatic Brain Injury

The incidence of dysphagia has been reported in some studies to be as high as 93% in patients with severe traumatic brain injury.[32] Few studies have examined the incidence of dysphagia in children with TBI. Morgan et al found an average incidence of 5.3% across all pediatric head injury admissions, with a higher incidence in more severe cases as noted in **Fig. 21.3**.[3]

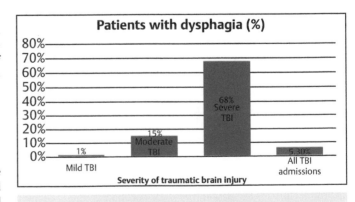

**Fig. 21.3** Incidence of dysphagia based on severity of traumatic brain injury in children. (Based on data from Morgan et al.[3])

**Table 21.2** Control of swallowing function: different stages

|  | Involvement of brain structure | Voluntary or involuntary |
| --- | --- | --- |
| Oral | Cerebral cortex (frontal lobe along with insula, hypothalamus, and cerebellum) | Voluntary |
| Pharyngeal | Brainstem swallowing center | Semireflexive |
| Esophageal | No direct brain involvement | Reflexive |

The unique aspect of dysphagia in TBI is its variable presentation from one person to the next because of diffuse and differential patterns of neurological damage. Unlike other forms of neurogenic dysphagia, such as stroke, it may not involve contiguous areas of the brain. Hence dysphagia will have variable characteristics and severity. Because the diagnosis of head injury actually represents many diverse diagnoses with different grades of severity, the association between dysphagia and TBI has been poorly delineated. Coexisting cognitive and behavioral deficits may also compromise swallowing in patients with TBI, something that is less commonly encountered in other types of neurogenic dysphagia.

## 21.8.4 Etiology of Dysphagia in Traumatic Brain Injury

As discussed in other chapters of this book, swallowing is typically divided into three phases under volitional and reflexive control, the oral, pharyngeal, and esophageal phases. The oral phase comprises the volitional transfer of ingested material, as a prepared bolus, from the mouth into the oropharynx. This phase is controlled by discrete areas in the cerebral cortex, specifically the frontal lobe. The pharyngeal phase is the first semireflexive component triggered by activation of cortical and subcortical brain regions, mainly the CPG in the brainstem, which subsequently controls muscles in the oropharynx to deliver the bolus from the oropharynx to the relaxed cricopharyngeus muscle. The third and final phase, the esophageal phase, begins following the closure of the upper esophageal sphincter. This later reflexive component serves the primary function of transporting food to the stomach by sequential peristaltic contraction initiated in the pharynx and relaxation of the lower esophageal sphincter. Because swallowing is influenced by several tiers of afferent and efferent limbs of the nervous system, any disturbance in one or more levels of this process would likely result in dysphagia (**Table 21.2**).

Dysphagia in TBI has a triad of deficits, namely motor, sensory, and cognitive. A person with TBI, especially if the TBI is severe, may exhibit abnormal muscle tone, reflexes, and sensation. Poor sensory input results in poor motor response to bolus presentation in the oral cavity. The end result is prolonged oral transit, delayed swallowing response, and reduced oropharyngeal peristalsis. Apart from sensory and motor deficits, cognitive impairment plays a significant role in swallowing impairments. TBI that involves cortical and subcortical centers and their connections results in cognitive impairments, including decreased alertness, attention, and memory. Cognitive deficits coupled with sensory and motor impairments result in significant swallowing impairment. An RLAS score of IV (confused and agitated) is thought to be the minimum requirement to begin eating.[33]

Because of the variable injuries that occur during TBI, from focal to diffuse injury and from mild to severe, the presentation of dysphagia may vary from patient to patient. TBI has a wide variety of clinical (and radiological) presentations as illustrated in **Fig. 21.4**.

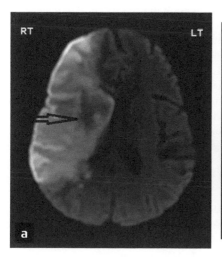
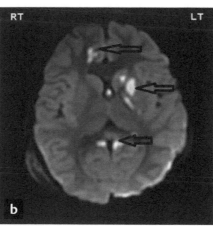
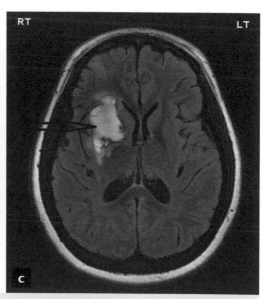

**Fig. 21.4 (a)** Cerebrovascular accident (ischemic stroke) with involvement of right middle artery territory distribution. **(b)** Diffusion-weighted magnetic resonance imaging (MRI) scans of a 6-year-old boy who sustained diffuse axonal injury as a result of a high-speed motor vehicle collision (MVC). **(c)** T2-weighted fluid-attenuated inversion recovery images of a 13-year-old girl who was a victim of a pedestrian versus motor vehicle accident.

Why do we need to address TBI-related dysphagia separately from other types of neurogenic dysphagia? The short answer is because the dysphagia associated with TBI differs significantly from other types of neurogenic dysphagia, especially dysphagia following cerebrovascular accident, in a variety of important ways. The important differences between the two predominant types of neurogenic dysphagia are outlined in **Table 21.3**. [13,34]

## 21.8.5 Factors That Predict the Occurrence of Dysphagia in Traumatic Brain Injury

Historically, predictive factors indicating which patients with TBI will develop dysphagia are not well understood, especially in children. This is because TBI represents many different diagnoses with variable degrees of severity, and studies investigating dysphagia in TBI have had different inclusion and exclusion criteria. However, research is continuing to define the factors that can predict the presence and severity of dysphagia in TBI. [35]

### Extent of Injury

Extent or severity of injury is not only the most important factor that predicts the occurrence of dysphagia; it is also intertwined with other factors that result in dysphagia. The extent or severity of injury would likely determine the GCS (**Box 21.2**) and RLAS scores (**Box 21.3**). Duration of coma is one of the determinants of the extent of head injury, and the severity of swallowing impairment increases as duration of coma increases. Patients in coma for more than 24 hours are more likely to exhibit severe swallowing problems than those in coma for less than 24 hours. [35] Individuals with a lower GCS score on admission (scores of 3, 4, or 5) have a significantly longer duration until the initiation of oral feeding, a longer duration until achieving total oral intake, and almost three times the duration between the initial oral trials and achieving total oral feeding. The relationship is not always linear, however; many patients who have no or short duration of coma are found to have dysphagia (**Box 21.4**).

### Box 21.4

**Factors Increasing the Incidence of Dysphagia in Traumatic Brain Injury**

- Severe injury
- Physical trauma to the oral, pharyngeal, laryngeal structures
- Other underlying disorders of oral, pharyngeal, and laryngeal structures
- Underlying etiology

Severity of injury in TBI, which can be assessed by a number of discrete and nondiscrete ways, is an important consideration in dysphagia. Patients with more severe CT scan or magnetic resonance imaging (MRI) findings are more likely to have dysphagia than are those with less severe ones. Important findings in imaging include midline shift, presence of brainstem injury, and intracranial bleeds requiring emergent surgical intervention. Brainstem injury that may appear relatively small is likely to result in dysphagia

because the swallowing center and cranial nerve nuclei involved in swallowing are found in the brainstem (**Fig. 21.5**). [14]

## Need for Endotracheal Intubation and Tracheostomy

Patients with TBI often need airway control and mechanical ventilation. Many of them require intubation because of the nature and extent of brain injury. [36] Paralytics are used commonly during this process and can result in a loss of glottic protective function, protective cough reflex, as well as a lack of spontaneous breathing and swallowing. Many factors likely result in swallowing dysfunction in TBI. These are summarized in **Box 21.5**.

### Box 21.5

**Factors Complicating Swallowing Dysfunction in Traumatic Brain Injury**

- Nature of medical or surgical illness (e.g., brainstem injury)
- Prolonged disuse of swallowing muscles (deconditioning)
- Medications blunting the swallowing mechanism (paralytics, sedatives)
- Localized injury around the glottis due to translaryngeal intubation or tracheostomy

Though the need for intubation and tracheostomy may indicate the severity of TBI resulting in dysphagia, increased duration of ventilation, endotracheal intubation, and the presence of a tracheostomy can adversely affect swallowing. Among patients with severe TBI, ventilation lasting more than 15 days resulted in a significantly higher risk of having dysphagia and aspiration (90%), compared to ventilation duration of 8–14 days (75%) and ventilation lasting 7 days or less (42.9%). [14]

### Sites of Injury

As discussed elsewhere in this book, injury to vital parts of the brain as well as certain cranial nerves involved in swallowing function can result in dysphagia. Injury to the brainstem, which houses both the swallowing center and the respiratory control centers, is a perfect example (see **Fig. 21.5**). Involvement of the corticospinal tract, insula (especially if bilateral), cerebellar pathways, and extrapyramidal pathways may cause dysphagia. [37] The most common brain injury lesions associated with aspiration are brainstem or multilobe injuries, usually with more than three injury sites. [7] Trauma-related indicators that predict dysphagia are listed in **Box 21.6**.

### Box 21.6

**Dysphagia in Traumatic Brain Injury: Trauma-Related Indicators**

- Low GCS score (3, 4, or 5)
- Low admitting cognitive (RLAS) assessment scores
- Presence of a tracheostomy
- Need for and longer duration of ventilation
- Longer stay in the hospital
- Severe CT scan findings

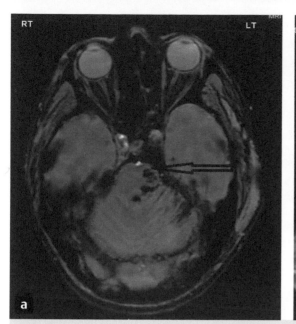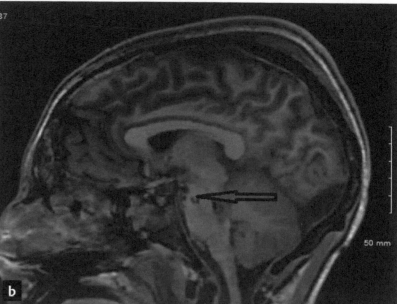

**Fig. 21.5** **(a)** Axial T1-weighted MRI scan of the head of a patient with traumatic brain injury because of an MVC. Axial susceptibility-weighted imaging (MRI series sensitive to detect blood) showing areas of hypointense signal in the left half of the pons, consistent with petechial hemorrhages. The patient was a victim of an MVC and presented with respiratory failure and dysphagia. The arrow points to petechial hemorrhages in the upper pons, where the swallowing center is located. Though the injury appeared to be minor, it led to respiratory failure and dysphagia. **(b)** MRI scan of the head of the same patient on sagittal T1-weighted image showing hypointense areas (arrow) within the pons corresponding to the hemorrhages.

**Table 21.3** Differences in dysphagia related to cerebrovascular accident and traumatic brain injury[13,34]

| | Cerebrovascular accident | Traumatic brain injury |
|---|---|---|
| Patient demographics | Elderly; multiple premorbid degenerative comorbidities | Relatively young and healthy; statistically more common in males |
| Brain involvement | Usually focal; one major artery distribution | Diffuse involvement; complex of focal injury with diffuse axonal injury ± hypoxic injury |
| Neurologic deficit | One or two major deficits (e.g., motor, sensory) | Variety of neuromuscular and sensory deficits likely; clinically heterogeneous |
| Oropharyngeal deficits | Reduced tongue control more problematic | Reduced pharyngeal peristalsis |

## Cognitive and Behavioral Impairment

Apart from obvious physiological deficits leading to swallowing impairment, cognitive and behavioral as well as communicative problems can also influence swallow function. Depending on the injury, there may be deficits in sensory reception and perception, attention, memory, organization, problem solving, judgment, and reasoning. Based on a study by Cherney and Halper, such deficits occur more commonly in patients with severe dysphagia (**Fig. 21.6**).[5]

Behavioral problems such as agitation, impulsivity, and apathy often preclude oral intake or increase the risk of aspiration if oral intake is attempted. The details of cognitive and behavioral impairment are listed and explained in **Table 21.4**.

## 21.8.6 Complications of Dysphagia in Patients with Traumatic Brain Injury

Patients with TBI are at risk for malnutrition secondary to trauma, dysphagia, and other complications. Malnutrition is very common with TBI, with an incidence of 68% at 2 months postinjury.[38] Malnutrition is a common occurrence in TBI because of a hypermetabolic state and hypercatabolism that result from additional injuries (quite common in TBI) and decreased levels of consciousness. Compared to patients with other types of trauma, patients with brain injuries have a mean increase in resting metabolic expenditure of 40%, leading to negative nitrogen balance and muscle wasting.[39] Loss of consciousness results in the inability to protect the airways due to the lack of protective pharyngeal reflexes, increasing the risk of aspiration. Additional risk of aspiration occurs at the time of intubation, either at the scene or in the acute care setting. Pneumonia is a major aspiration-related pulmonary complication and, by far, the most common clinically significant complication in a patient with TBI.[36] Aspiration pneumonia is a factor that complicates hospitalization and delays oral feeding, increases the cost of care, and at times results in death.[40] Based on multiple studies, the length of hospitalization increases significantly if the patient has dysphagia as an additional complication, with additional morbidity and cost.[5] The various complications of dysphagia in TBI can be remembered with the mnemonic AIMS, as summarized in **Box 21.7**.

**Table 21.4** Cognitive-communicative and behavioral deficits impairing swallowing function in traumatic brain injury

| Deficit | Potential impact on oral intake |
| --- | --- |
| Agitation or anxiety | • Low tolerance level for oral stimulation<br>• Respond to stimulation with physical/verbal abuse<br>• Chance for aspiration increased<br>• Extreme agitation precludes oral intake |
| Apathy (lethargy) | • Reduced participation<br>• Reduced initiation of oral feeding/swallowing |
| Attention | • May preclude oral intake<br>• Increased time spent on meals<br>• Reduced use of compensatory strategies for swallowing |
| Executive function (e.g., planning) | • Less likely to be independent in total feeding process<br>• Reduced use of compensated strategies |
| High-level cognitive function (organization, reasoning, and problem solving) | • Difficulty learning a sequence of steps |
| Impulsivity/disinhibition | • Increased risk of aspiration due to rapid intake of large amount of food |
| Memory | • Decreased comprehension and retention of instructions<br>• Difficulty learning new strategies |
| Sensory reception and perception | • Reduced recognition of food smells, textures, and tastes<br>• Lack of appetite |

*Source:* Modified from Halper et al.[4]

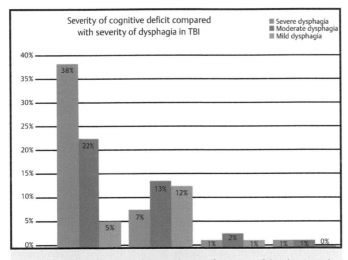

**Fig. 21.6** Graph depicting the correlation of severity of dysphagia and cognitive deficits in patients with traumatic brain injury. (Modified from Cherney and Halper.[5])

## Box 21.7

**Complications of Dysphagia in Traumatic Brain Injury (mnemonic: AIMS)**

• Aspiration pneumonia
• Increased hospital stay: costs, associated morbidity, and complications
• Malnutrition, weight loss, and dehydration
• Social and economic impact

## 21.8.7 Outcome and Prognosis in Patients with Dysphagia with Traumatic Brain Injury

Swallowing impairment in TBI has a multitude of complications, including aspiration pneumonia and malnutrition, with increased morbidity and mortality. Outcomes appear to be dependent upon a number of factors, including severity of injury, patient age, tracheostomy tube placement, and duration of ventilation.[3,34] Winstein completed a retrospective study of 201 patients with neurological disease or injury, including TBI, to determine the frequency, progression, and outcome of dysphagia and found a swallowing problem in 25%. At discharge from the rehabilitation, 84% of patients with dysphagia became oral feeders, and on follow-up, that number rose to 94%. On admission, cognitive problems were identified as the most common interfering factor in 96% of patients recommended for nonoral means of nutrition. The average time of injury to the successful completion of oral feeding was 13 weeks.[41]

Length of stay for TBI patients with swallowing dysfunction is significantly higher than for those without dysphagia (126.7 days vs. 52.3 days).[42] Increased incidence of medical complications, namely aspiration, malnutrition, and subsequent poor wound healing, resulted in prolonged hospitalization.[42]

Few studies have assessed how cognitive function affects swallowing impairment. Terré and Mearin found a correlation between cognitive impairment, evaluated by RLAS, and the presence of swallowing impairment, determined by the Modified Barium Swallow (MBS).[12] Additionally, feeding mode at discharge (oral vs. nonoral diet) correlated strongly with RLAS level at admission and both RLAS score and disability rating scale at discharge. Hansen et al also found the chance of returning to oral intake depended on the severity of brain injury and could be predicted from GCS score, RLAS score, and functional oral intake at the time of admission.[32]

## 21.9 Questions

1. Dysphagia is one of the complications of traumatic brain injury (TBI) in adults and children. Which one of the following statements about the incidence of dysphagia in TBI is false?

A. The incidence varies widely depending on the level of severity of injury.
B. Timing of assessment may influence the incidence rate..
C. The incidence rate increases steadily from arrival at the hospital to outpatient clinics.
D. Different methods of assessment give variable results.
E. Studies done in different parts of the world have similar results.

2. TBI is a leading cause of death and disability in the United States. Which one of the following statements is true regarding TBI?

A. In children, TBI is most common between the age of 5 and 10 years.
B. Recent data show that the numbers of fall-related TBIs among children aged 0–4 years and adults older than 75 years are decreasing.
C. Children are more susceptible to diffuse axonal injuries, and adults are more likely to have focal injuries, such as subdural hematoma.
D. There is no gender difference in the incidence of TBI.
E. People above the age of 65 have a low incidence of TBI-related hospitalization.

3. Regarding malnutrition in TBI, which one of the following statements is true?

A. TBI, especially severe TBI, results in a hyperanabolic state.
B. There is a substantial increase of counterregulatory hormones during the first few months post-TBI.
C. Hypertonia that may develop during ensuing weeks helps to preserve energy.
D. The prevalence of malnutrition after 2 months of TBI is around 10–12%.
E. The nitrogen balance is positive substantially during the rehabilitation phase of TBI.

4. Dysphagia in TBI is influenced by many factors, including neuromuscular problems, sensory deficits, and cognitive-communicative and behavioral problems, among others. Which of the statements is correct regarding the pathophysiology of dysphagia in TBI?

A. Decreased elevation of the larynx is the most frequently seen deficit.

B. Hypertonia preserves swallowing function, whereas muscle hypotonia is associated with a higher chance of dysphagia and aspiration.
C. Prolonged endotracheal intubation increases the risk of dysphagia, whereas tracheostomy decreases the risk of dysphagia.
D. Despite differences in etiology, the oropharyngeal deficits in TBI and cerebrovascular accident (stroke) are identical.
E. The RLAS score is the most important independent predictor of the time to return to oral feeding.

5. Which one of the following situations is the most likely risk factor for the prediction of dysphagia in a patient with TBI?

A. GCS score of 13 in a 4-year-old child
B. RLAS of cognitive functioning score of VIII
C. MRI scan of the head showing contusion of the left occipital pole with areas of restricted diffusion
D. Loss of consciousness lasting 5 minutes at the scene of the head injury
E. CT scan findings of injury in the brainstem and insula

## 21.10 Answers and Explanations

1. **Correct: incidence rate increases steadily from arrival to hospital to outpatient clinics (C).**
   The incidence of dysphagia following TBI is quite high based on studies; swallowing function improves over time. The reported incidence of dysphagia in TBI varies between 26 and 70%. When one is specifically looking at the incidence rate at rehabilitation, the rate goes down to one-third (26–42%). At the time of discharge from rehabilitation centers, more than 75% of individuals with TBI are tolerating an oral diet. At follow-up in the outpatient clinic, this number goes up to more than 90%. In a prospective cohort study involving 48 patients with severe TBI who were admitted to a rehabilitation center, Terré et al found that, at the time of discharge from rehabilitation, 72% were on an oral diet (45% on a normal and 27% on a modified oral diet), 14% were on combined oral intake and gastrostomy feeding, and 14% were fed exclusively by gastrostomy.[12]

   (**A**) The incidence of dysphagia in TBI increased sharply with the higher level of severity. Lower GCS and RLAS scores, increased rates of mechanical ventilation, increased rates of tracheostomy, and significant CT scan findings are indicators of severity in TBI. (**B**) Reported incidence of dysphagia following TBI varies based on timing of the assessment. Studies from data available from different groups of patients (hospital, rehab facilities) may show variable incidences. (**D**) Assessment of dysphagia with different clinical and diagnostic techniques in different studies has shown variable results. (**E**) Though not available from every part of the world, the incidences of dysphagia in TBI is comparable.

**2. Correct: children are more susceptible to diffuse axonal injuries, and adults are more likely to have focal injuries, such as subdural hematoma (C).**

Studies suggest that children more frequently present with diffuse brain injury and cerebral swelling (44%) with resultant intracranial hypertension when compared with adults who experienced severe TBI. Children are more susceptible to diffuse axonal injury as a result of rotational acceleration and deceleration because of their relatively higher head-to-body ratio, weak neck musculature, and lack of myelination (in children younger than 3 years) (**Fig. 21.6**). In cases of nonaccidental trauma in children, diffuse injury is the typical presentation, with diffuse anoxia and hypotension representing secondary injuries, often associated with delay in medical care. Additionally, children have a higher incidence of immediate seizures than do adults, which may also account for a higher incidence of hypoxia/anoxia. On the other hand, focal injuries, such as subdural, epidural, and intracranial hematoma, are more common in adults (30–40%) than in children (15–20%).[43] (**A**) There are two peaks of TBI in children: early childhood (< 5 years) and mid to late adolescence. In early childhood, nonaccidental trauma is the major cause of severe TBI, representing up to two-thirds of cases. Young children are injured in pedestrian or bicycle-related injuries, whereas adolescents are likely to be injured as passengers in MVCs.[43,44,45] (**B**) According to the CDC, falls are the leading cause of TBI in children 0–4 years of age and people above the age of 75 years. However, MVCs and traffic-related deaths account for the largest percentage of TBI-related deaths (31.8%).[46] (**D**) For each year from 2001 to 2010, men had higher TBI-related emergency department visits compared to women, based on CDC reports. Men are three times more likely to die from TBI.[47] (**E**) According to statistics from the CDC, people over the age of 65 years have the highest TBI-related hospitalizations and deaths.

**3. Correct: there is a substantial increase of counterregulatory hormones during the first few months post-TBI (B).**

TBI, as with any other type of injury, is associated with excessive production of counterregulatory hormones, such as epinephrine, norepinephrine, and cortisol. (**A**) TBI, like any other injury, is a hypermetabolic or hypercatabolic state, not an anabolic state, because of excessive increase of counterregulatory hormones and a negative nitrogen balance.[48]

(**C**) Hypertonia leads to excessive energy consumption rather than preservation. (**D**) Because of inconsistent inclusion criteria used in studies, the incidence of malnutrition in TBI patients is difficult to estimate. Based on a study by French and Merriman, approximately 68% of patients showed signs of malnutrition in the early phase of rehabilitation (2 months post-TBI).[38]

(**E**) Because of excessive muscle breakdown and production of counterregulatory hormones, there is a negative nitrogen balance during post-TBI and rehabilitation phases.[41]

**4. Correct: the Ranchos Los Amigos Scale score is the most important independent predictor of the time to return to oral feeding (E).**

Based on studies, a low admitting RLAS level is a strong predictor of resumption of oral intake. In a study by Mackay et al, patients with lower RLA levels (I/II) took longer to initiate and achieve total oral feeding. The chance of returning to a total unrestricted oral diet was found to be dependent on the severity of the brain injury and could be predicted by the RLAS level at admission as well as the GCS score, Functional Independence Measure (FIM) score, and functional oral intake at admission.[32] (**A**) The most common swallowing problems in patients with TBI include prolonged oral transit times (87.5%), vallecular residue (62.5%), and piriform sinus residue (62.5%).[42] Mackay et al also reported other swallowing deficits, including poor bolus control in 79%, reduced lingual control in 79%, and decreased tongue base retraction in 61% of patients. Among the least common abnormalities are delayed initiation of the swallowing response (48%), reduced laryngeal closure (45%), and reduced laryngeal elevation (36%). The most common factor impacting swallowing problems was cognitive problems.[49] (**B**) Both hypotonia and hypertonia are detrimental in terms of ability to swallow. Hypertonia resulting from upper motor neuron injury is quite common and is found to limit range of motion. This is usually associated with weakness, ataxia, apraxia, and extrapyramidal movement disorders. These impairments commonly occur in combination because selective injury of a particular neural tract is rare.[50] (**C**) Both prolonged endotracheal intubation and tracheostomy are risk factors for swallowing impairment. Both may cause injuries to the surrounding tissues. Intubation may cause supraglottic/glottic edema, laryngospasm, oropharyngeal injury, vocal cord paresis, tracheomalacia, and tracheal stenosis. Incidence is variable from 1 to 20%. In the prospective study by Stauffer et al, patients with prolonged endotracheal intubation followed by tracheostomy had a higher incidence of laryngeal injury at autopsy ($p = 0.05$) than patients with short-term endotracheal intubation followed by tracheostomy.[49] (**D**) The oropharyngeal deficits in cerebrovascular accident (CVA) are different from those of TBI. Patients with TBI have demonstrated more frequent and severe tongue control, whereas pharyngeal contraction pressures are less severely affected. On the other hand, dysphagia due to CVA results in less severe tongue control deficits, whereas pharyngeal peristalsis is compromised more often.[8] See **Table 21.3** for important differences between the dysphagia related to CVA and TBI.

**5. Correct: CT scan findings of injury in the brainstem and insula (E).**

CT scan showing significant abnormality is predictive of swallowing dysfunction. Trauma to the brainstem (which contains the swallowing center) and insula (area of the temporal lobe) are critical areas of the brain involved in swallowing dysfunction. Injury to cranial nerves V, VII, IX, X, and XII is very likely with injury to the brainstem, which has either sensory input to the oropharyngeal structures or gives motor output to the muscles involved in the swallowing process.[30] (**A**) GCS is used to assess the severity of TBI. GCS is modified to be used in infants and small children. A GCS score of 13 denotes mild TBI, and only 1% patients with mild TBI was likely to have dysphagia.[3] (**B**) An RLAS of cognitive functioning score of VIII is a purposeful-appropriate state. An

RLAS score of at least IV is needed to start oral feeding. (**C**) Major trauma to the cerebral cortex as well as the brainstem is likely to cause dysphagia. However, the occipital pole, which is primarily involved in vision, is unlikely to cause swallowing dysfunction. The area of restricted diffusion in an MRI scan of the head is most likely posttraumatic infarction, which is a secondary injury and is being increasingly recognized with the advent of improved MRI techniques.[27] (**D**) Duration of consciousness is used to assess the severity of TBI. Loss of consciousness of less than 30 minutes is considered mild TBI and would have less likelihood of causing swallowing dysfunction.[44]

# References

[1] US Department of Health and Human Services Centers for Disease Control and Prevention. National Center for Injury Prevention and Control; 2010. http://www.cdc.gov/traumaticbraininjury/pdf/blue_book.pdf.

[2] American Psychiatric Assocation. Diagnostic and Statistical Manual of Mental Disorders. 5th ed. Arlington, VA: American Psychiatric Publishing; 2013

[3] Morgan A, Ward E, Murdoch B, Kennedy B, Murison R. Incidence, characteristics, and predictive factors for dysphagia after pediatric traumatic brain injury. *J Head Trauma Rehabil* 2003;*18*(3):239–251

[4] Halper AS, Cherney LR, Cichowski K, Zhang M. Dysphagia after head trauma: the effect of head trauma: the effect of cognitive-communicative impairments in functional outcomes. *J Head Trauma Rehabil* 1999;*14*(5):486–496

[5] Cherney LR, Halper AS. Swallowing problems in adults with traumatic brain injury. *Semin Neurol* 1996;*16*(4):349–353

[6] Zafonte RD, Katz DI, Zasler ND. Brain Injury Medicine: Principles and Practice. New York, NY: Demos Medical Publishers; 2013

[7] Splaingard ML, Hutchins B, Sulton LD, Chaudhuri G. Aspiration in rehabilitation patients: videofluoroscopy vs bedside clinical assessment. *Arch Phys Med Rehabil* 1988;*69*(8):637–640

[8] Lazarus C, Logemann JA. Swallowing disorders in closed head trauma patients. *Arch Phys Med Rehabil* 1987;*68*(2):79–84

[9] Alhashemi HH. Dysphagia in severe traumatic brain injury. *Neurosciences (Riyadh)* 2010;*15*(4):231–236

[10] Hoppers P, Holm SE. The role of fiberoptic endoscopy in dysphagia rehabilitation. *J Head Trauma Rehabil* 1999;*14*(5):475–485

[11] Kang SH, Kim DK, Seo KM, Seo JH. Usefulness of videofluoroscopic swallow study with mixed consistency food for patients with stroke or other brain injuries. *J Korean Med Sci* 2011;*26*(3):425–430

[12] Terré R, Mearin F. Prospective evaluation of oro-pharyngeal dysphagia after severe traumatic brain injury. *Brain Inj* 2007;*21*(13-14):1411–1417

[13] Howle AA, Baguley IJ, Brown L. Management of dysphagia following traumatic brain injury. *Curr Phys Med Rehabil Rep* 2014;*2*(4):219–230

[14] Mackay LE, Morgan AS, Bernstein BA. Factors affecting oral feeding with severe traumatic brain injury. *J Head Trauma Rehabil* 1999;*14*(5):435–447

[15] Steyerberg EW, Mushkudiani N, Perel P, et al. Predicting outcome after traumatic brain injury: development and international validation of prognostic scores based on admission characteristics. *PLoS Med* 2008;*5*(8):e165, discussion e165 doi: 10.1371/journal.pmed.0050165

[16] Niedzwecki CM, Marwitz JH, Ketchum JM, Cifu DX, Dillard CM, Monasterio EA. Traumatic brain injury: a comparison of inpatient functional outcomes between children and adults. *J Head Trauma Rehabil* 2008;*23*(4):209–219

[17] Dawodu ST. Traumatic Brain Injury - Definition and Pathophysiology. http://emedicine.medscape.com/article/326510-overview. Updated Sept, 2015. Accessed Feb, 2016

[18] Dombovy ML. Traumatic brain injury. *Continuum (Minneap Minn)* 2011;*17*(3 Neurorehabilitation):584–605

[19] Morgan AT. Dysphagia in childhood traumatic brain injury: a reflection on the evidence and its implications for practice. *Dev Neurorehabil* 2010;*13*(3):192–203

[20] Coronado VG, Xu L, Basavaraju SV, et al; Centers for Disease Control and Prevention (CDC). Surveillance for traumatic brain injury-related deaths—United States, 1997-2007. *MMWR Surveill Summ* 2011;*60*(5):1–32

[21] Zaloshnja E, Miller T, Langlois JA, Selassie AW. Prevalence of long-term disability from traumatic brain injury in the civilian population of the United States, 2005. *J Head Trauma Rehabil* 2008;*23*(6):394–400

[22] Centers for Disease Control and Prevention, National Center for Injury Prevention and Control. Report to Congress on mild traumatic brain injury in the United States: steps to prevent a serious public health problem. 2003. www.cdc.gov/ncipc/pub-res/mtbi/mtbireport.pdf

[23] Teasdale G, Jennett B. Assessment of coma and impaired consciousness. A practical scale. *Lancet* 1974;*2*(7872):81–84

[24] Pangilinam PH. Classification and Complications of Traumatic Brain Injury. https://emedicine.medscape.com/article/326643-overview. Published Sept 2015. Accessed Feb, 2016

[25] Mirvis SE, Wolf AL, Numaguchi Y, Corradino G, Joslyn JN. Posttraumatic cerebral infarction diagnosed by CT: prevalence, origin, and outcome. *AJR Am J Roentgenol* 1990;*154*(6):1293–1298

[26] Tawil I, Stein DM, Mirvis SE and Scalea TM. Posttraumatic cerebral infarction: incidence, outcome, and risk factors. *J Trauma* 2008;*64*(4):849–853

[27] Chesnut RM, Marshall LF, Klauber MR, et al. The role of secondary brain injury in determining outcome from severe head injury. *J Trauma* 1993;*34*(2):216–222

[28] Sosin DM, Sniezek JE, Thurman DJ. Incidence of mild and moderate brain injury in the United States, 1991. *Brain Inj* 1996;*10*(1):47–54

[29] Lang IM. Brain stem control of the phases of swallowing. *Dysphagia* 2009;*24*(3):333–348

[30] Hansen TS, Engberg AW, Larsen K. Functional oral intake and time to reach unrestricted dieting for patients with traumatic brain injury. *Arch Phys Med Rehabil* 2008;*89*(8):1556–1562

[31] Mackay L, Morgan AS. Early swallowing disorders with severe head injuries: relationship between the RLA and the progression of oral intake. *Dysphagia* 1993;*8*:161

[32] Smith DH, Meaney DF, Shull WH. Diffuse axonal injury in head trauma. *J Head Trauma Rehabil* 2003;*18*(4):307–316

[33] Mandaville A, Ray A, Robertson H, Foster C, Jesser C. A retrospective review of swallow dysfunction in patients with severe traumatic brain injury. *Dysphagia* 2014;*29*(3):310–318

[34] Morgan AS, Mackay LE. Causes and complications associated with swallowing disorders in traumatic brain injury. *J Head Trauma Rehabil* 1999;*14*(5):454–461

[35] Wiles CM. Neurogenic dysphagia. *J Neurol Neurosurg Psychiatry* 1991;*54*(12):1037–1039

[36] French A, Merriman S. Nutritional status of a brain-injured population in a long-stay rehabilitation unit: pilot study. *J Hum Nutr Diet* 1999;*12*(1):35–42

[37] Young B, Ott L, Phillips R, McClain C. Metabolic management of the patient with head injury. *Neurosurg Clin N Am* 1991;*2*(2):301–320

[38] Langmore SE, Terpenning MS, Schork A, et al. Predictors of aspiration pneumonia: how important is dysphagia? *Dysphagia* 1998;*13*(2):69–81

[39] Gedeit R. Head injury. *Pediatr Rev* 2001;*22*(4):118–124

[40] Greenwald BD, Burnett DM, Miller MA. Congenital and acquired brain injury. 1. Brain injury: epidemiology and pathophysiology. *Arch Phys Med Rehabil* 2003;*84*(3, Suppl 1):S3–S7

[41] Winstein CJ. Neurogenic dysphagia. Frequency, progression, and outcome in adults following head injury. *Phys Ther* 1983;*63*(12):1992–1997

[42] O'Suilleabhain P, Dewey RB Jr. Movement disorders after head injury: diagnosis and management. *J Head Trauma Rehabil* 2004;*19*(4):305–313

[43] Adelson PD, Kochanek PM. Head injury in children. *J Child Neurol* 1998;*13*(1):2–15

[44] Center for Disease Control and Prevention. Severe TBI. 2016. http://www.cdc.gov/TraumaticBrainInjury/severe.html

[45] Center for Disease Control and Prevention. Rates of TBI-related Emergency Department Visits by Sex — United States, 2001–2010. 2016. http://www.cdc.gov/traumaticbraininjury/data/rates_ed_bysex.html

[46] Loan T. Metabolic/nutritional alterations of traumatic brain injury. *Nutrition* 1999;*15*(10):809–812

[47] Pepe JL, Barba CA. The metabolic response to acute traumatic brain injury and implications for nutritional support. *J Head Trauma Rehabil* 1999;*14*(5):462–474

[48] Field LH, Weiss CJ. Dysphagia with head injury. *Brain Inj* 1989;*3*(1):19–26

[49] Stauffer JL, Olson DE, Petty TL. Complications and consequences of endotracheal intubation and tracheotomy. A prospective study of 150 critically ill adult patients. *Am J Med* 1981;*70*(1):65–76

[50] ERABI Research Group. Evidence-based Review of Moderate to Severe Acquired Brain Injury. 2015. www.abiebr.com

## Suggested Reading

[1] Centers for Disease Control and Prevention (CDC), National Center for Injury Prevention and Control. Guide to Writing about Traumatic Brain Injury in News and Social Media. Atlanta (GA): Centers for Disease Control and Prevention; 2015. http://www.cdc.gov/traumaticbraininjury/get_the_facts.html

[2] Faul M, Xu L, Wald MM, Coronado VG. Traumatic brain injury in the United States: emergency department visits, hospitalizations, and deaths, 2002–2006

[3] Logemann JA. Evaluation and treatment of swallowing problems. In: Zafonte RD, Katz DI, Zasler ND. Brain Injury Medicine: Principles and Practice. New York, NY: Demos Medical; 2013:1111–1118

[4] Morgan AT, Ward EC. Swallowing disorders following traumatic brain injury. Section III. In: Murdoch BE, Theodoros DG, eds. Traumatic Brain Injury: Associated Speech, Language and Swallowing Disorders. New York, NY: Delmar Cengage Learning; 2001:313–401

# 22 Head and Neck Cancer

*Heather M. Starmer*

## Summary

Dysphagia is commonly associated with head and neck cancer and its treatment. Speech-language pathologists are very important members of the head and neck care team and should be well versed in the potential swallowing difficulties their patients may experience. Treatment may encompass dietary modification, use of compensatory strategies, and direct/indirect swallowing interventions. Preventive therapy should be provided prior to radiation-based treatment to prevent radiation-associated dysphagia.

## Keywords

head and neck cancer, laryngectomy, glossectomy, radiation therapy, chemoradiation, radiation fibrosis, human papilloma virus, dysphagia management

### Learning Objectives
- List the causes of dysphagia in patients with head and neck cancer
- Explain the characteristics of dysphagia following surgical and nonsurgical management of head and neck cancer
- Use evidence-based research in evaluating and managing dysphagia in patients with head and neck cancers

## 22.1 Introduction

In the last 10 years, the incidence of head and neck cancer has increased, largely due to the rise in oropharyngeal cancers related to the human papilloma virus (HPV).[1] Whether treatment consists of surgical or nonsurgical intervention, patients with head and neck cancers are at elevated risk for short- and long-term dysphagia. It is incumbent on speech-language pathologists to understand the pathophysiology of, as well as the evidence-based strategies to minimize the risk for and impact of, such dysphagia. This chapter provides an introduction to swallowing difficulties associated with head and neck cancer and evidence to support treatment planning for these patients.

## 22.2 Epidemiology

Head and neck cancers largely arise from the mucosal lining of the upper aerodigestive tract and are typically referred to as squamous cell carcinomas, referring to the squamous cells of origin. Although other pathologies are seen in the head and neck region (adenoid cystic carcinoma, sinonasal undifferentiated carcinoma, nasopharyngeal carcinoma, etc.), the vast majority of head and neck cancers are categorized as squamous cell carcinomas.[2] Head and neck cancers account for 3–5% of new cancers diagnosed in the United States each year.[3] Head and neck cancers include cancers that arise from the oral cavity, oropharynx (soft palate, palatine tonsils, lingual tonsils/base of tongue), nasopharynx, nasal cavity/paranasal sinuses, salivary glands, hypopharynx, and larynx. Some consider cancers of the thyroid gland as arising from the head and neck region as well, although pathology and outcomes are quite different from squamous cell cancers. Head and neck cancers have traditionally been linked to tobacco and alcohol consumption, with most cancers arising in the sixth and seventh decades of life. The 5-year overall survival rate for head and neck cancers is ~ 40–50%.[3]

Over the past several decades, a significant change in the demographics of patients with head and neck cancer has become evident in the United States. A new profile of head and neck cancers has become increasingly apparent and has been related to the rise in oropharyngeal carcinomas related to the human papilloma virus (HPV). Although the incidence of head and neck cancers (aside from thyroid cancer) has been steadily declining due to educational campaigns regarding smoking hazards, the incidence of oropharyngeal carcinoma has been on the rise, and this increase is attributed directly to HPV.[4] HPV-associated disease is typically seen in younger, healthier, nonsmoking patients.[5] Additionally, because these individuals remain active in the workforce following their diagnosis and treatment, there is a much greater emphasis on quality of life than has been noted in past decades. HPV status is strongly correlated with favorable oncological outcomes, with a 2-year survival rate of 85–90% (compared to 50–65% in those with HPV-negative disease).[6] Thus we see two unique profiles of patients diagnosed with head and neck cancer: those associated with older age and tobacco use and those associated with younger age and virus exposure (**Box 22.1**).

### Box 22.1

**Human Papilloma Virus**

The human papilloma virus (HPV), also responsible for all cervical cancers, is the most common cause of oropharyngeal squamous cell cancers in the United States. This virus can be prevented by vaccination prior to sexual debut.

Dysphagia is not uncommon prior to head and neck cancer treatment.[7,8] Patient-reported changes may include difficulty with swallowing certain foods, feeling like some foods cause them to choke, a need to alter their diet, and increased time to consume meals. Interestingly, as tumors are typically slow growing, patients often adapt to the slow changes in their swallowing and underestimate the degree of dysphagia. Patient report and clinical examination underreport dysphagia compared to what is noted on instrumental, objective measures of swallowing.[9,10]

In addition to pretreatment alteration of swallowing, dysphagia is very common following treatment for head and neck cancer. Incidence of dysphagia depends heavily on the details of the tumor size and location as well as type and combination of oncological treatment. Data consistently show that advanced tumor stage as well as primary tumors in the hypopharynx, larynx, and base of tongue are associated with a higher potential for dysphagia.[11] In general, more extensive surgeries yield higher rates of postoperative dysphagia than do minimally invasive surgeries.[12,13] Likewise, the addition of chemotherapy to radiation therapy is associated with greater potential for dysphagia.[11]

## 22.3 Etiology

Dysphagia related to head and neck cancer can be divided into three categories: anatomical, physiological, and a combination of the two. These deficits arise due to insults to the muscles and nerves as well as to the vascular and lymphatic systems. Typically, anatomical dysphagia arises following surgical interventions, whereas physiological dysphagia is more common after nonoperative treatment modalities. Head and neck cancers are primarily treated with surgery or radiation therapy, with chemotherapy typically used as a radiation sensitizer or to manage disease that has spread systemically to other parts of the body. Smaller tumors are more likely to be treated with a single modality of treatment (e.g., surgery alone or radiation alone). Larger tumors are more likely to require a combination of two or three modalities (e.g., surgery followed by radiation or concurrent chemoradiation). Because patients may require a combination of treatments to cure their cancer, they may experience both anatomical and physiological changes to their swallowing function.

## 22.4 Surgical Procedures

Head and neck cancer surgery may be described as open or minimally invasive. Open surgeries require more extensive and morbid approaches to the region of concern and may require transcervical or transmandibular approaches. Recent advances to surgical access have led to techniques such as laser and robotically assisted procedures, with less functional morbidity resulting.[14] It is critical for the speech-language pathologist to review operative reports prior to assessing the swallow of patients with head and neck cancers to fully appreciate the extent of tissue resection as well as the impact on the cranial nerves. Additionally, understanding of reconstruction techniques is important in determining expectations of function. A review of common surgical procedures and how they may impact swallow function is warranted.

### 22.4.1 Glossectomies

*Glossectomy* refers to surgical removal of portions of or all of the tongue. Glossectomies may be referred to as partial (< 50%), hemi (50%), subtotal (> 50% but < 90%), or total (> 90% of oral and tongue base). Surgeons aim to achieve a 2 mm margin of healthy tissue around the tumor during surgery, therefore leading to a larger surgical defect than initial tumor imaging would suggest. When thinking about the impact of glossectomy on swallowing,

it is important to consider the region of the tongue resected (**Table 22.1**). The major functional regions of the tongue include the tongue tip, tongue body, and tongue base. Surgeries involving the tongue tip are likely to result in oral-stage difficulties with bolus containment, mastication, and oral clearance, whereas surgeries including the body of the tongue will result in issues with bolus containment and posterior propulsion. If surgery extends to the tongue base, issues with pharyngeal clearance will also be observed. Aspiration is a common finding following subtotal and total glossectomy due to reduced bolus clearance and reduced hyolaryngeal excursion due to removal of the suprahyoid muscles.[15]

In addition to considering the extent of resection, we must also consider the type of reconstruction after surgery. The primary functional purpose of reconstruction is to provide bulk within the oral cavity to assist with speech and swallowing function. If the degree of resection is limited, the surgical field is typically closed through primary closure or through suturing remaining structures together. Research has shown that primary closure yields better functional outcomes than tissue transfer when the extent of surgical resection is limited to less than 25% of the tongue.[16] Larger resections may require reconstruction using skin grafts or tissue transfer. Reconstructions can be considered local if adjacent tissues are used and distant if tissue from areas distant from the resection is required. Skin flaps involve transportation of skin and underlying subcutaneous tissue from one region to another while maintaining a pedicle to the original site. Myocutaneous flaps also include underlying muscle and are used for more extensive reconstructions. Examples of myocutaneous flaps include the pectoralis major flap and the platysma flap. The platysma flap is used for smaller reconstructions and is based on the platysmal branch of the facial artery, whereas the pectoralis flap is more bulky and useful for larger reconstructions. More recently, microvascular advances have allowed for transfer of muscle and tissue from a remote area of the body to the surgical site due to the ability to reconnect the blood supply from regional sources to maintain the viability of the tissue. A primary advantage of this type of flap is the ability to be more selective about the amount of tissue harvested/transplanted. This prevents both inadequate and excessive bulk, both of which may negatively impact swallowing outcomes. Additionally, anastomosis of nerves in the graft to regional nerves may enable sensory innervation of flaps. There is evidence that patients undergoing hemi and subtotal glossectomy have more favorable swallowing outcomes if they receive innervated flaps.[17] These "free flaps" are commonly utilized for reconstruction of larger tongue resections. Examples of free flaps include the radial forearm free flap, which is a thinner option, and the anterolateral thigh flap.

**Table 22.1** Types of swallowing problems associated with tongue region resection

| | |
|---|---|
| Tongue tip | Bolus containment issues<br>Difficulty masticating<br>Reduced oral clearance |
| Tongue body | Bolus containment issues<br>Difficulty with posterior propulsion |
| Tongue base | Pharyngeal clearance<br>Laryngeal elevation<br>Aspiration |

## 22.4.2 Oral Composite Resections

Composite resections involve removal of more than one component structure of the oral cavity and may include excision of the floor of the mouth, mandible, maxilla, and tongue. As with glossectomy, the amount and location of resection have significant implications for function. Resection of the floor of the mouth will commonly result in anchoring or tethering of the anterior tongue, leading to issues with anterior bolus loss, bolus manipulation for mastication, and oral clearance. Floor of mouth and alveolar ridge resection will also commonly lead to removal of dentition, impacting bite and mastication. Laryngeal elevation may be impacted due to removal of suprahyoid musculature, thus increasing the risk of aspiration if compensatory strategies are not employed. With extended mandibular resection, reconstruction plays a significant role in preserving function. Osseocutaneous flaps have been shown to improve speech and swallowing outcomes after mandibular resection.[18]

## 22.4.3 Maxillary Resections

Tumors arising from the palate will result in resection of the maxilla and potentially the soft palate as well. Because the palate serves as the barrier between the oral and nasal cavities, the primary concern with maxillary resection is the potential for nasal regurgitation. Additionally, if velopharyngeal incompetence results from palatal resection, the ability to generate adequate driving pressures behind the bolus may be impaired, leading to reduced pharyngeal clearance. Finally, loss of maxillary teeth can impact mastication.

## 22.4.4 Oropharyngeal Resections

Oropharyngeal resections have benefited significantly from recent surgical advancements. Whereas surgical access to the tonsils has traditionally been transoral, approaches to the tongue base have traditionally required splitting the mandible, resulting in substantial swallowing-related morbidity.[19,20] More recently, minimally invasive approaches have been introduced, including use of transoral robotic surgery (TORS). With this approach, surgeons are able to use articulated surgical instruments to access the tongue base through the oral cavity, thus negating the need for splitting the mandible. As a result, oropharyngeal resection now results in substantially less swallowing dysfunction than noted with more traditional approaches. Despite these advancements, changes to swallowing can be anticipated based on the region of resection. Resections limited to the palatine tonsils will result in significant odynophagia (pain on swallowing) for the first 1–2 weeks following surgery but will otherwise result in unimpaired swallowing function. However, when resection extends to the soft palate, issues with velopharyngeal insufficiency may lead to nasal regurgitation and difficulty generating pressure behind the bolus. Surgery at the tongue base may lead to issues with bolus propulsion and clearance in the pharynx. Sensory deficits may also contribute to postoperative dysphagia. More extensive tongue base resections may also result in disruption of laryngeal elevation due to involvement of the suprahyoid musculature. Although TORS has less morbidity than traditional approaches,[21] its impact on swallowing function remains somewhat nebulous.

The majority of data available regarding functional outcomes after TORS evaluates surrogate measures for swallowing, such as feeding-tube dependence.[22] Though available evidence suggests relatively positive outcomes after TORS, information regarding the physiological impact of this technique are currently lacking.

## 22.4.5 Laryngeal Surgeries/ Laryngectomies

As with glossectomies, laryngectomy outcomes vary significantly based on the extent and location of resection. The larynx can be divided into the supraglottic, glottic, and subglottic levels. Cancers arising from the supraglottic larynx are surgically managed through either the supraglottic or the supracricoid laryngectomy. The supraglottic region is instrumental in ensuring laryngeal vestibular closure; hence surgery in this region may impact airway protection, leading to aspiration. The supraglottic laryngectomy may include resection of parts of the hyoid bone, epiglottis, aryepiglottic folds, and false vocal folds. As was discussed regarding oropharyngeal resection, advances in technology have led to less morbid approaches to resecting the supraglottic larynx. With traditional open supraglottic laryngectomy, recovery is protracted, and it may take up to 3 months for the patient to return to a full oral diet.[23,24] Extension inferiorly or superiorly can further prolong recovery, and dysphagia tends to be more severe, commonly lasting 2–6 months and up to 2 years for some patients.[23,25] Size and extent of tumor are directly related to subjective swallowing-related quality of life judgments after supraglottic laryngectomy.[26]

In contrast, endoscopic laser resection of supraglottic tumors results in less dysphagia with more rapid return to normal swallowing, sometimes as rapidly as 2–7 days postoperatively.[27,28] One possible reason for improved outcomes in patients undergoing endoscopic procedures is the preservation of the superior laryngeal nerve. Sasaki and colleagues[28] report an intact glottic closure reflex in six patients within 72 hours of surgery as demonstrated by testing with fiberoptic endoscopic evaluation of swallowing (FEES) with sensory testing. In contrast, the majority of patients following open supraglottic laryngectomy had persistent loss of glottic closure reflex up to 12 years following surgery.

If the supraglottic laryngectomy is extended to include part or all of the hyoid bone, laryngeal elevation may be affected, compounding airway protection concerns from removal of the epiglottis and false vocal folds. If the base of the tongue is involved, impaired bolus propulsion may result in residue after the swallow and increase the risk of penetration and aspiration after the swallow.[23,29] Both cricopharyngeal myotomy and pharyngeal plexus neurectomy at the time of partial laryngectomy have been shown to reduce dysphagia related to cricopharyngeal muscle spasm in supraglottic laryngectomy patients.[30]

The supracricoid laryngectomy is based on the concept that the cricoarytenoid unit (arytenoid cartilage, cricoarytenoid joint, posterior and lateral cricoarytenoid muscles, and recurrent and superior laryngeal nerves) is the functional anatomical unit of the larynx.[31] This procedure includes the removal of the true and false vocal folds bilaterally, the bilateral paraglottic space, the entire thyroid cartilage, and at times the epiglottis and one arytenoid. Given that airway protection is compromised at the most inferior level of the larynx by the removal of the true and false vocal folds and potentially the epiglottis, aspiration is one of the greatest concerns following this procedure. Despite poor airway protection following surgery, studies consistently show that, with mindful patient selection, return to full oral diets and functional swallowing is possible for the majority of patients.[32,33] Characteristics of dysphagia following supracricoid laryngectomy include premature spillage, reduced bolus propulsion/clearance, laryngeal penetration/aspiration, and inability to clear aspirated material by coughing.[34]

Unlike partial laryngeal surgeries, safety (aspiration) is not a typical concern after total laryngectomy. However, swallowing efficiency can be substantially compromised by structural abnormalities and pharyngoesophageal motility issues.[23] During laryngectomy there is disruption of pharyngeal musculature and innervation, leading to poor pharyngeal propulsion through the neopharynx. This often leads to effortful swallowing and prolonged mealtimes. A pseudoepiglottis/pseudovallecula may form at the base of the tongue, leading to residue and potential backflow into the oro- or nasopharynx.[23] Stricture or narrowing of the pharyngoesophageal segment or esophagus can cause difficulty clearing solids and occasionally liquids. Incidence of stricture after total laryngectomy may be as high as 39%[35] and has been cited as more common with more extensive surgeries, such as laryngopharyngectomy with primary tracheal esophageal puncture.[36] Performing a cricopharyngeal myotomy at the time of total laryngectomy may limit problems due to spasm at this site and retention of foods in the upper esophagus.[37] Though safety is relatively preserved following total laryngectomy, the majority of patients report some change in swallowing after surgery, and those changes may lead to reduced social participation.[38]

### 22.4.6 Hypopharyngeal Resection

Disease arising from the hypopharynx is typically surgically managed with total laryngectomy in order to achieve adequate margins of healthy tissue around the tumor. Limited resections of small tumors arising from the piriform sinus region may result in scarring or obliteration of the piriform sinus space.

### 22.4.7 Thyroidectomy

The most common cause of dysphagia following thyroid surgery is related to disruption of the recurrent or superior laryngeal nerves. Recurrent laryngeal nerve injury may lead to vocal fold paralysis and difficulty achieving glottic closure during swallowing. The external branch of the superior laryngeal nerve is responsible for supraglottic sensation; thus, injury to this nerve may reduce patient sensitivity to penetration/aspiration (**Box 22.2**).

### Box 22.2

**Surgery and the Risk of Dysphasia**

In general, more extensive surgeries result in higher potential for development of dysphagia.

## 22.5 Nonsurgical Treatments

In addition to surgical procedures, nonoperative treatments may impact swallowing function. Although the structures of swallowing largely remain intact, their function may not. A common misconception when nonsurgical approaches were popularized was that preservation of structure would equate to preservation of function. It has become clear in recent years that functional preservation relies on more than just preservation of normal anatomical structures. A substantial body of evidence suggests that patients receiving nonsurgical treatment for head and neck cancer are at risk for both acute toxicities and long-term alteration of swallow function.[39,40,41,42] Such alterations may contribute to long-term decrements in health status and quality of life.[43,44,45] As with surgery, the larger the tumor, the larger the field of treatment, and therefore the greater the potential for dysphagia.[7,8] Radiation therapy may impact swallowing function in three distinct ways. First, during the course of treatment, patients typically swallow less frequently due to acute treatment toxicities, such as pain and dry mouth (**Box 22.3**). Disuse atrophy may develop, leading to weakening of the swallowing musculature.

### Box 22.3

**Acute Treatment Toxicities**
- Xerostomia—dry mouth
- Dysgeusia—taste change
- Mucositis—painful ulcers of the mouth and throat
- Loss of appetite/weight loss

Second, radiation fibrosis may develop later in treatment and during the months and years following completion of treatment. Fibrosis results from a maladaptive healing response where excessive collagen deposition in a region of inflammation leads to scar formation, resulting in restricted mobility and range of motion. Fibrosis in the head and neck can lead to long-term and permanent dysphagia. Finally, in a small subset of patients, lower cranial nerve neuropathies may develop in the years following treatment completion.[46] Because chemotherapy is used as a radiation sensitizer to help the radiation work better, it also amplifies the negative effects of treatment, leading to higher potential for dysphagia during and after treatment.

## 22.6 Postradiation Swallowing

Dysphagia and resultant diet modifications are well documented in those receiving nonsurgical treatment, although patient-reported functional status and quality of life improve over time.[47,48,49] Many individuals receiving primary nonsurgical intervention report that eating returns to normal or near-normal levels[50,51] and that quality of life approximates pretreatment levels several months following treatment.[52,53] What these patient-reported outcome measures fail to account for is the tendency for individuals to adapt to change over time with acceptance of a "new normal" for swallowing and diet. It has been shown that Penetration-Aspiration Scale (PAS) scores do not correlate well with patient-reported outcomes following radiation-based interventions.[43] RTOG 91-11 is a clinical trial that showed a laryngectomy-free survival benefit when chemotherapy was added concurrently to radiation therapy compared to induction chemotherapy and radiation alone.[54] A recent follow-up to this trial showed that, although long-term (10-year) cancer-related death rates were similar between the three groups, noncancer-related deaths were significantly higher in the group receiving chemoradiation.[55] Because it is well established that dysphagia risk is significantly higher in individuals receiving concurrent chemoradiotherapy, it has been postulated that these noncancer-related deaths may be due, in part, to aspiration pneumonia. Aspiration pneumonia has been documented as occurring in ~ 20–25% of patients undergoing chemoradiotherapy, with advanced tumor stage, hypopharyngeal or nasopharyngeal primary, older age, increased comorbidity, patient-reported dysphagia, and aspiration on videofluoroscopy being most associated with pneumonia.[56,57] Further, aspiration pneumonia leads to a 42% increase in risk of death when controlling for other variables.[57] Hence it is critical not to rely solely on patient-reported outcomes in this population but rather to consider actual physiological functioning.

Patterns of physiological dysfunction following radiation and chemoradiation have been well described in the literature. Common decompensations include laryngeal penetration and aspiration, reduced tongue base retraction, reduced pharyngeal constriction, lack of epiglottic retroflexion, reduced laryngeal elevation, and need for multiple swallows to clear pharyngeal residue.[38,40,42,58] Physiological swallowing abnormalities have been shown to increase over the first year following treatment in some patients, likely reflecting the insidious nature of fibrosis.[59] Aspiration events typically occur after the swallow in this population due to poor bolus propulsion and clearance.[58,60] Stricture, or failure of opening of the upper esophagus due to fibrosis, can be seen in 20–35% of patients receiving radiation therapy and is most commonly seen in women and patients with larynx and hypopharyngeal primary tumors.[60,61,62] Strictures typically arise more than 30 days following treatment completion and recur frequently after they are surgically addressed.[63]

Additional long-term side effects of radiation-based interventions can further exacerbate dysphagia. Complications associated with radiotherapy include dysgeusia, trismus, and xerostomia.[64,65] Dysgeusia, or taste changes, are experienced by the majority of patients by the third week of radiation.[66] Significant improvement in taste occurs during the first year following treatment, but dysgeusia may persist past the 1-year mark, leading to changes in diet and enjoyment of foods.[67] Trismus, or limited mouth opening, has been reported as a common issue following head and neck cancer treatment in approximately one-third of patients.[68] Operational definitions of trismus vary; however, it is generally agreed upon that the distance between the incisors should measure at least 35–40 mm.[65] Trismus may impact oral intake by preventing entry of selected items into the mouth and by impacting mastication.[65] Xerostomia, or dry mouth, is one of the most bothersome long-term toxicities reported by patients. Radiation doses as low as 30 Gy can lead to permanent damage to the salivary glands, leading to a high prevalence of xerostomia following radiation to the head and neck region.[69,70] Reduced salivary flow interferes with mastication, particularly with drier foods, such as breads and meats, often requiring dietary adaptations or compensations, such as increased fluid intake with meals. Further, because saliva provides a protective role for the teeth, xerostomia raises the risk of dental caries, which can, in turn, lead to additional issues with mastication. Another toxicity to consider that may impact long-term swallowing outcomes is lymphedema. Lymphedema is a condition where damage to the lymphatic system during surgery or radiation leads to collection of lymphatic fluid rather than typical drainage. This may result in fibrosis and impaired range of motion of involved and adjacent structures and thereby contribute to dysphagia.

## 22.7 Management of Head and Neck Cancer Patients

Diagnosis of dysphagia in head and neck cancer patients should consider anatomical and physiological changes as measured during instrumental swallowing assessments, impact on oral diet, tube-feeding reliance, and patient perceived swallowing function. This global assessment will provide the most comprehensive picture of how the patient is experiencing swallowing.

Due to the elevated risk of silent dysphagia in head and neck cancer, instrumental assessment is essential prior to oncological therapy, particularly for those individuals at greatest risk for dysfunction.[71] Pretreatment dysphagia may lead to adverse outcomes during treatment, such as aspiration pneumonia, dehydration, and malnutrition. Such events may compromise oncological outcomes due to treatment breaks. Determining aspiration risk prior to treatment may assist in ensuring optimal intervention by the speech-language pathologist through application of compensatory maneuvers, dietary modifications, and rehabilitative interventions. Understanding which patients are at highest risk for dysphagia prior to treatment may assist in efficient, cost-effective allocation of resources. Further, understanding pretreatment organ function may influence determination of the most appropriate oncological treatment approach in order to maximize overall function and quality of life posttreatment. For instance, in patients determined at baseline to have poor laryngeal function, application of organ-sparing treatments is unlikely to restore adequate function for safe and efficient swallowing.

Instrumental swallowing evaluation can be accomplished through a videofluoroscopic swallow study (VFSS) or FEES. These tools are complementary, and both have an important role in the assessment of dysphagia in patients with head and neck cancer. VFSS is generally considered the gold standard for assessment of oropharyngeal disorders due to its ability to provide visualization of the coordinated stages of swallowing as well as specific physiology. In addition, use of VFSS allows for evaluation of the oral and esophageal aspects of swallowing. In contrast, FEES provides the benefits of avoiding radiation exposure, a flexible service delivery model, and direct visualization of relevant anatomy. Investigation of the comparability of these tools has revealed high levels of agreement, sensitivity, specificity, and positive and negative predictive values.[72] The FEES evaluation has also been shown to demonstrate greater sensitivity to laryngeal penetration and aspiration compared with VFSS.[73] A thorough FEES evaluation conducted by an experienced speech-language pathologist can provide anatomical and physiological information, assessment of swallowing abilities across viscosities and textures, and implementation of compensatory postures and strategies when dysfunction is identified. When necessary, a VFSS can be performed to answer additional questions regarding issues such as physiological, oral, or esophageal dysfunction. VFSS may also be required in cases where significant alteration of anatomy due to tumor precludes adequate visualization of structures of interest for swallowing. Based on a systematic review of the literature, Mlynarek and colleagues[74] proposed that instrumental swallowing evaluation, assessment of speech intelligibility, supplemental speech evaluation when indicated, and patient-reported swallowing outcomes should be measured prior to, during, and following treatment for oral and oropharyngeal cancers.

## 22.7.1 Postsurgical Management

Management of dysphagia arising from surgical treatments is heavily influenced by the type and extent of the surgical procedure performed. In general, rehabilitation may encompass use of compensatory strategies, dietary modifications, and range of motion and strengthening exercises. The goal of intervention should be to facilitate a safe and efficient swallow with the least restrictions or adaptations required. When possible, adaptations should be selected to mimic more normal eating behaviors that the patient will be more apt to adhere to in social settings. Compensatory maneuvers have been shown to eliminate aspiration in up to 81% of patients following head and neck surgery.[29]

Resections limited to the oral cavity will primarily impact bolus control, propulsion, and clearance. Thus strategies should be chosen to optimize each. Anterior bolus loss due to facial palsy can often be overcome by tilting the head to the intact side during mastication and by use of a straw to the better side during drinking. When patients experience issues with bolus containment due to intraoral resections, strategies such as a head tilt to the unaffected side or a head tilt back may allow for better bolus control. Patients with oral bolus control issues typically do best with thicker viscosities. Preferential bolus placement to the posterior aspect of the better side paired with a head tilt back may be of benefit when patients have difficulty with posterior bolus propulsion.[75] For patients with posterior bolus loss, a chin tuck may be beneficial for bolus containment.[76] If a significant portion of the tongue has been resected, a palatal drop prosthesis may provide additional benefit by narrowing the oral cavity, thus resulting in an easier target for tongue apposition.[77] When oral bolus clearance deficits result from restricted propulsion, use of a liquid wash can facilitate bolus clearance. In general, patients experiencing issues with bolus propulsion and clearance do better with thinner viscosities. For patients with inability to propel the bolus due to subtotal/total glossectomy, gavage feeding can be used to bypass the oral phase. A red-rubber catheter can be affixed to a syringe, and liquids and thinner purees can be piped directly into the pharynx. Patients undergoing maxillary resection without primary reconstruction may experience nasal regurgitation. A palatal obturator can be fashioned by a maxillofacial prosthodontist to fill the defect. Trismus, or restricted mouth opening, can create significant issues for getting the food into the mouth. Use of shallow dish spoons (e.g., infant spoons) can help with oral entry, though in severe cases a straw may be the only implement for oral delivery. Jaw stretches and use of a TheraBite trismus device (Atos Medical) can contribute to improved oral aperture.[78,79] Therapeutic exercises for oral resection may include lingual range of motion and strengthening exercises. Range of motion exercises applied for the first 3 months following surgery result in better long-term outcomes.[80] **Table 22.2** lists strategies and exercises for surgical patients.

Resections in the pharynx typically result in more issues with pharyngeal clearance; therefore, strategies should be chosen to increase the efficiency of pharyngeal bolus transport. A head turn to the affected side may narrow the pharynx in the region of the resection and increase the upper esophageal sphincter opening, thus allowing the intact musculature to clear the bolus better.[81] Additionally, a head tilt to the intact side may preferentially shunt the bolus to the stronger side.[82] Patients with pharyngeal resection should be encouraged to swallow with additional effort and may require multiple swallows and liquid wash strategies.[82] For patients with velopharyngeal insufficiency from palatal resection, a head tilt back can minimize nasal regurgitation. The Mendelsohn maneuver can be utilized to improve laryngeal elevation and cricopharyngeal opening.[83] Typically, patients with pharyngeal resections do better with thinner viscosities due to ease of clearance, unless laryngeal elevation is diminished. Swallowing exercises after pharyngeal resection should include strengthening of the tongue, pharynx, and muscles of laryngeal elevation using exercises such as the Masako, Mendelsohn, effortful swallow, effortful pitch glide, and Shaker.

As previously discussed, patients undergoing laryngeal resection typically have the greatest deficits in airway protection. Following a supraglottic laryngectomy, efforts should focus on optimizing glottic airway closure and narrowing the vestibular entrance. The supraglottic swallow and super-supraglottic swallow are commonly used for this purpose. The supraglottic swallow focuses on achieving airway closure prior to the bolus entering

**Table 22.2** Strategies and exercises for surgical patients

|  | Strategies | Exercises |
|---|---|---|
| Oral resection | Tilt to the good side<br>Head tilt back<br>Preferential bolus placement<br>Liquid wash<br>Gavage | Range of motion stretches<br>Strengthening exercises |
| Pharyngeal resection | Head turn to bad side<br>Head tilt to good side<br>Chin tuck<br>Hard swallow<br>Head tilt back | Effortful swallow<br>Masako<br>Effortful pitch glide<br>Mendelsohn maneuver<br>Shaker exercises |
| Laryngeal resection | Supraglottic swallow<br>Super-supraglottic swallow<br>Breath hold<br>Chin tuck<br>Effortful swallow<br>Head turn to bad side | Supraglottic swallow<br>Super-supraglottic swallow<br>Effortful swallow<br>Effortful pitch glide<br>Mendelsohn maneuver<br>Shaker exercises<br>Laryngeal adduction exercises |

the pharynx and maintaining closure until the completion of the swallow.[84] The cough prior to inspiration serves to clear any residual material in the laryngeal inlet. The super-supraglottic swallow further enhances airway protection through apposition of the tongue base to the laryngeal inlet, thus narrowing the entry into the laryngeal vestibule.[84] Surgery focused at the level of the glottis will typically require strategies that enhance narrowing of the laryngeal vestibular entrance, such as a chin tuck or an effortful swallow. A head turn to the affected side can improve the extent of glottic closure. For patients undergoing total laryngectomy, bolus clearance is the primary issue due to lack of pharyngeal propulsion. In these individuals, a liquid wash is often beneficial, particularly when paired with increased effort. Typically, patients can better tolerate thicker items following partial laryngeal resections. Following total laryngectomy, thinner viscosities are easier to clear. Therapeutic exercises that may be beneficial after laryngeal surgery include the effortful swallow, Mendelsohn maneuver, effortful pitch glide, supraglottic and super-supraglottic swallow, Shaker, and laryngeal adduction exercises.

Direct exercises to work on range of motion and strength typically require clearance by the surgeon and do not begin until ~ 2 weeks following surgery. This allows ample time for healing to take place for most patients, though for patients with complex reconstructions or delayed healing, exercises may be deferred for a greater duration. Exercises should target intact musculature to improve the safety and efficiency of swallowing. Swallowing therapy also often includes diet progression from least to most difficult using appropriate strategies, as outlined earlier. It is important to note that patients frequently have complicated resections involving one or more of the regions already discussed. Additionally, patients frequently receive a combination of therapies (e.g., chemoradiation followed by salvage surgery) and thus may require a combination of strategies to achieve safe and efficient swallowing.

## 22.7.2 Nonsurgical Treatment

The importance of prophylactic swallowing therapy during nonoperative head and neck cancer treatments is increasingly appreciated and acknowledged. A retrospective case control study by Carroll and colleagues[85] demonstrated the value of initiating prophylactic therapy prior to chemoradiation. Individuals performing exercises prior to and during chemoradiation demonstrated more normal tongue base apposition to the posterior pharyngeal wall during swallowing as well as more normal epiglottic inversion. A randomized controlled trial by Kotz and colleagues[86] further demonstrated that those patients receiving prophylactic swallowing therapy had more favorable diet levels 3–6 months following completion of treatment. These two papers together demonstrated that both physiology and function are optimized with application of preventive dysphagia exercises. A study by van der Molen and colleagues[87] demonstrated the feasibility of initiating prophylactic swallowing therapy during chemoradiation and patient adherence to treatment recommendations. In their series, 69% of subjects were able to implement therapeutic exercises immediately following training, and an additional 31% were able to follow through within the first week of treatment.

Carnaby-Mann and colleagues[88] provided objective data regarding the clinical impact of preventive swallowing therapy in patients with head and neck cancer undergoing chemoradiation. Six-month posttreatment muscle size/composition on magnetic resonance imaging was the primary outcome for their investigation. In the active treatment arm where patients performed swallowing exercises twice daily over the duration of treatment, there was less structural change in the genioglossus, hyoglossus, and mylohyoid muscles than in the other two treatment groups. Individuals in the active treatment group were more likely to continue an oral diet during treatment. A composite measure was designed to designate a favorable swallowing-related outcome and included weight loss < 10%, maintenance of an oral diet, and a change of < 10 points on the Mann Assessment of Swallowing Ability. In the active treatment arm, 86% of patients achieved this desirable outcome, whereas only 47% of those who were not actively engaged in swallowing treatment achieved this. Their data revealed a 36% absolute risk reduction for loss of swallowing ability when participating in preventive exercise. These positive results serve as strong evidence that patients receiving nonoperative head and neck cancer treatment should be engaged in swallowing therapy prior to the start of radiation treatment.

Speech-language pathologists working with patients with head and neck cancer need to have a solid understanding of swallowing physiology and the structures impacted by treatment in order to devise an appropriate treatment plan. In the absence of clinical trials demonstrating superiority of particular exercises, therapists must use their knowledge to select the most appropriate exercises. Adherence to treatment recommendations is often limited,[89] therefore, the therapist should be mindful to provide an efficient, feasible therapy plan. Swallowing exercises frequently used in this population include the Masako maneuver, effortful swallow, effortful pitch glide, Mendelsohn maneuver, and Shaker exercises. Additionally, jaw range of motion exercises and the TheraBite trismus device have shown value for preventing and treating trismus.[78] Finally, although evidence of a direct link between decreasing lymphedema and improving swallowing does not currently exist, it is possible that submental lymphedema may inhibit range of motion of the muscles involved in laryngeal elevation. Because there is evidence of benefit from decongestive therapies on lymphedema,[90] this may be another factor of treatment worth consideration.

In addition to performance of swallowing exercises for prevention of dysphagia, there is evidence that maintenance of oral intake during treatment has a positive impact on swallowing outcomes. Posttreatment diet level has been significantly associated with oral intake during treatment in that those who maintained at least some oral intake had significantly more advanced diet levels following treatment.[91] Additional evidence concerning oral intake and posttreatment diet level was provided by Hutcheson et al.[92] This study demonstrated that eating and exercising swallowing musculature during radiation-based treatments provide protective benefit for maintenance of diet following treatment. For individuals not eating and not exercising, return to a normal diet was enjoyed by only 65% of patients. For those who both ate and exercised during treatment, 92% returned to a normal oral diet after treatment completion. Thus it is clear that the speech-language pathologist should be involved in the care of patients prior to the start of radiation therapy to provide prophylactic swallowing exercises and encourage continued oral intake.

## 22.8 Case Presentation

### Case Presentation Part 1

Mr. J is a 54-year-old man diagnosed with a T2N2b squamous cell carcinoma of the right base of the tongue. He was treated with concurrent chemoradiotherapy with a posttreatment neck dissection. Prior to treatment he complained of dysphagia characterized by a sense of food sticking in his throat and the need for a liquid wash. He had no complaints of aspiration. Following chemoradiotherapy, Mr. J complained of xerostomia (dry mouth), taste changes (dysgeusia), and difficulty swallowing solids, with foods frequently sticking in his throat. His past medical history was otherwise remarkable only for hypertension. He is a non-smoker, and his alcohol intake is social. He is married with two grown children and works as a project manager in a technology firm.

### Case Presentation Part 2— Discussion of Diagnosis

Mr. J completed a pretreatment swallowing evaluation, which included clinical and instrumental assessment using fiberoptic endoscopic evaluation of swallowing (FEES). Clinical examination revealed normal oromotor function and maximal interincisor distance of 42 mm (normal is > 40 mm, functional cutoff is 30 mm). These findings are important because they suggest a lack of tumor invasion into the deep tongue musculature as well as the masseter and lateral pterygoid muscles. His diet was reportedly mildly restricted with avoidance of nuts and rice, which he felt were more likely to get stuck. Using the Functional Oral Intake Scale (FOIS), his diet score was 6, indicating limited diet restriction. He completed the MD Anderson Dysphagia Inventory (MDADI), a quality of life tool that reveals patients' perception of swallowing-related handicap. His overall score was 82/100, indicating a mild self-perceived swallowing handicap. The FEES examination revealed a large, exophytic mass of the right tongue base, which extended into the vallecular space. When swallowing purees and solids, residual material was noted to cling to the tumor, requiring multiple swallows and/or liquid wash to clear. No laryngeal penetration or aspiration was detected and his Penetration-Aspiration Scale score was 1.

Two months after completion of radiation, Mr. J repeated a comprehensive assessment of swallowing. Clinical examination revealed mild restriction in tongue mobility as evidenced by reduced range of motion. Maximal interincisor distance was slightly lower than at baseline (35 mm) but remained within functional limits. Diet restriction was greater than at baseline, with the patient reporting avoidance of starchy foods like breads and crackers and reliance on foods that were either pureed or liquid, with minimal intake of soft foods. His FOIS score was 5, indicating special preparation of foods was required. His immediate posttreatment MDADI had declined to 68/100, indicating a more moderate self-perceived swallowing handicap. A modified barium swallow study revealed a thickened epiglottis that did not

tilt, reduced tongue base retraction, reduced superior and middle constrictor function, and reduced anterior hyoid excursion. These physiological findings led to moderate vallecular residue and transient supraglottic penetration of purees and liquids after the swallow without aspiration (Penetration-Aspiration Scale score = 2).

Prior to the onset of radiation therapy, Mr. J met with the speech-language pathologist to discuss expectations during and following treatment as well as for administration of a prophylactic swallowing exercise protocol. Initial education included a review of normal swallowing anatomy and physiology and the mechanism for his baseline swallowing changes. He was informed about treatment toxicities during radiation (pain, dry mouth, changes in mucus, taste changes) and how these toxicities impact the patient's desire to eat. The importance of adherence to team treatment recommendations to minimize the impact of typical treatment toxicities was reviewed. The mechanisms of physiological swallowing dysfunction from disuse atrophy and fibrosis were discussed, and the importance of maintaining oral intake and completing swallowing exercises was reviewed. The patient was trained in a series of exercises (Masako maneuver, Mendelsohn maneuver, effortful swallow, and effortful pitch glide) and asked to perform three sets of 10 repetitions of each exercise twice daily. In addition, he was provided with a series of jaw stretches to be performed two to three times each day to minimize the risk of trismus.

### Case Presentation Part 3— Discussion of Management

During the course of treatment, Mr. J was seen on three additional occasions: week 2, week 4, and week 7. At those visits exercise adherence and accuracy were assessed and the importance of continuing exercises despite toxicities was emphasized. At each visit the patient was counseled on strategies for managing the toxicities that were impacting his oral intake. He was informed that reassessment of his swallowing function would occur 2–3 months following treatment completion in order to allow for resolution of the acute toxicities of treatment. Further, it was reinforced that swallowing exercises should be considered a lifelong part of his daily routine.

## 22.9 Questions

Based on what you have read, answer the following questions regarding what you might anticipate for Mr. J.

1. What kinds of eating and swallowing issues might you predict prior to treatment based on Mr. J's diagnosis?

A. Tending toward a soft diet
B. Avoidance of hard, crunchy foods
C. Reduced pharyngeal clearance
D. A, B, and C
E. A and B only

**2.** What physiological swallowing outcomes might you anticipate following treatment for Mr. J?

A. Reduced epiglottic tilt
B. Lower esophageal stricture
C. Reduced pharyngeal constriction
D. Reduced laryngeal elevation
E. A, C, and D

**3.** Aside from physiological swallowing abnormalities, what other treatment-related effects might interfere with Mr. J returning to a normal oral diet?

A. Skin burn on neck
B. Trismus
C. Xerostomia
D. No teeth
E. Both B and C

**4.** At what point of treatment should Mr. J consult with a speech-language pathologist?

A. Before treatment starts
B. In the middle of treatment
C. Right after treatment ends
D. Only if he complains of dysphagia
E. Never

**5.** What information should the speech-language pathologist focus on in educating Mr. J?

A. The rationale for prophylactic swallowing exercises
B. Toxicities that may occur during treatment
C. Signs and symptoms of true dysphagia
D. The role of the speech-language pathologist on the treatment team
E. All of the above

**6.** What specific treatment recommendations and plan of care would you recommend?

A. VitalStim
B. Percutaneous endoscopic gastrostomy tube reliance
C. Pharyngeal swallowing exercises
D. Oral motor exercises using whistles, bubbles, and kazoos
E. None of the above

## 22.10 Answers and Explanations

**1. Correct: A, B, and C (D).**
Prior to treatment it is common for patients with tongue-base tumors to have some pain with swallowing or a sense of solid foods sticking in the throat due to the tumor and/or reduced pharyngeal clearance. As a result, they often alter their diets toward more soft foods that are easier to clear.

**2. Correct: A, C, and D (E).**
Though upper esophageal strictures are seen in patients with head and neck cancer, radiation does not reach the lower esophagus to cause stricture at that level. Reduced epiglottic tilt, reduced pharyngeal constriction, and diminished laryngeal elevation are very common after radiation for oropharyngeal cancer.

**3. Correct: both B and C (E).**
Though burns on the skin are common during treatment and may be painful, they rarely impact eating or swallowing. Patients with head and neck cancer may be prone to dental issues due to dry mouth, but these are long-term effects not likely to impact recovery right after radiation. Both trismus (reduced mouth opening) and xerostomia (dry mouth) can lead to dietary modifications and are seen in the early days following radiation.

**4. Correct: before treatment starts (A).**
The key to managing radiation-associated dysphagia is to prevent it from happening. So the best time to consult with a speech-language pathologist is prior to the start of radiation.

**5. Correct: all of the above (E).**
It is important for the patient to understand the difference between acute treatment toxicities and physiological dysphagia and to know what is anticipated versus unusual and requiring further attention. Additionally, for patients to follow through with exercises during radiation, it is important for them to understand the rationale for the exercises.

**6. Correct: pharyngeal swallowing exercises (C).**
There is no evidence supporting the role of either VitalStim or oral motor exercises in this population. Percutaneous endoscopic gastrostomy tubes are associated with increased dysphagia risk and hence should be used as a backup or for support. Pharyngeal swallowing exercises are a well-established treatment modality during radiation.

## References

[1] Chaturvedi AK, Engels EA, Anderson WF, Gillison ML. Incidence trends for human papillomavirus-related and -unrelated oral squamous cell carcinomas in the United States. *J Clin Oncol* 2008;*26*(4):612–619

[2] Licitra L, Locati LD, Bossi P, Cantù G. Head and neck tumors other than squamous cell carcinoma. *Curr Opin Oncol* 2004;*16*(3):236–241

[3] Howlander N, Noone AM, Krapcho M, et al. SEER Cancer Statistics Review (CSR) 1975–2011. Bethesda, MD: National Cancer Institute; 2014

[4] Chaturvedi AK, Engels EA, Pfeiffer RM, et al. Human papillomavirus and rising oropharyngeal cancer incidence in the United States. *J Clin Oncol* 2011;*29*(32):4294–4301

[5] Gillison ML, D'Souza G, Westra W, et al. Distinct risk factor profiles for human papillomavirus type 16-positive and human papillomavirus type 16-negative head and neck cancers. *J Natl Cancer Inst* 2008;*100*(6):407–420

[6] Fakhry C, Westra WH, Li S, et al. Improved survival of patients with human papillomavirus-positive head and neck squamous cell carcinoma in a prospective clinical trial. *J Natl Cancer Inst* 2008;*100*(4):261–269

[7] van der Molen L, van Rossum MA, Ackerstaff AH, Smeele LE, Rasch CR, Hilgers FJ. Pretreatment organ function in patients with advanced head and neck cancer: clinical outcome measures and patients' views. *BMC Ear Nose Throat Disord* 2009;9:1–9

[8] Pauloski BR, Rademaker AW, Logemann JA, et al. Pretreatment swallowing function in patients with head and neck cancer. *Head Neck* 2000;*22*(5):474–482

[9] Starmer H, Gourin C, Lua LL, Burkhead L. Pretreatment swallowing assessment in head and neck cancer patients. *Laryngoscope* 2011;*121*(6):1208–1211

[10] Rosen A, Rhee TH, Kaufman R. Prediction of aspiration in patients with newly diagnosed untreated advanced head and neck cancer. *Arch Otolaryngol Head Neck Surg* 2001;*127*(8):975–979

[11] Jiang N, Zhang LJ, Li LY, Zhao Y. Risk factors for late dysphagia after (chemo) radiotherapy for head and neck cancer: a systematic methodological review. *Head Neck* 2014

[12] Karatzanis AD, Psychogios G, Zenk J, et al. Evaluation of available surgical management options for early supraglottic cancer. *Head Neck* 2010;*32*(8):1048–1055

[13] Silver CE, Beitler JJ, Shaha AR, Rinaldo A, Ferlito A. Current trends in initial management of laryngeal cancer: the declining use of open surgery. *Eur Arch Otorhinolaryngol* 2009;*266*(9):1333–1352

[14] Brickman D, Gross ND. Robotic approaches to the pharynx: tonsil cancer. *Otolaryngol Clin North Am* 2014;*47*(3):359–372

[15] Hirano M, Kuroiwa Y, Tanaka S, Matsuoka H, Sato K, Yoshida T. Dysphagia following various degrees of surgical resection for oral cancer. *Ann Otol Rhinol Laryngol* 1992;*101*(2 Pt 1):138–141

[16] McConnel FM, Pauloski BR, Logemann JA, et al. Functional results of primary closure vs flaps in oropharyngeal reconstruction: a prospective study of speech and swallowing. *Arch Otolaryngol Head Neck Surg* 1998;*124*(6):625–630

[17] Chang EI, Yu P, Skoracki RJ, Liu J, Hanasono MM. Comprehensive analysis of functional outcomes and survival after microvascular reconstruction of glossectomy defects. *Ann Surg Oncol* 2015;*22*(9):3061–3069

[18] Buchbinder D, Urken ML, Vickery C, Weinberg H, Sheiner A, Biller H. Functional mandibular reconstruction of patients with oral cancer. *Oral Surg Oral Med Oral Pathol* 1989;*68*(4 Pt 2):499–503, discussion 503–504

[19] Babin R, Calcaterra TC. The lip-splitting approach to resection of oropharyngeal cancer. *J Surg Oncol* 1976;*8*(5):433–436

[20] Sessions DG. Surgical resection and reconstruction for cancer of the base of the tongue. *Otolaryngol Clin North Am* 1983;*16*(2):309–329

[21] Lee SY, Park YM, Byeon HK, Choi EC, Kim SH. Comparison of oncologic and functional outcomes after transoral robotic lateral oropharyngectomy versus conventional surgery for T1 to T3 tonsillar cancer. *Head Neck* 2014;*36*(8):1138–1145

[22] Hutcheson KA, Holsinger FC, Kupferman ME, Lewin JS. Functional outcomes after TORS for oropharyngeal cancer: a systematic review. *Eur Arch Otorhinolaryngol* 2015;*272*(2):463–471

[23] Lazarus CL. Management of swallowing disorders in head and neck cancer patients: optimal patterns of care. *Semin Speech Lang* 2000;*21*(4):293–309

[24] Logemann JA, Gibbons P, Rademaker AW, et al. Mechanisms of recovery of swallow after supraglottic laryngectomy. *J Speech Hear Res* 1994;*37*(5):965–974

[25] Wasserman T, Murry T, Johnson JT, Myers EN. Management of swallowing in supraglottic and extended supraglottic laryngectomy patients. *Head Neck* 2001;*23*(12):1043–1048

[26] Strek P, Hydzik-Sobocińska K, Składzień J, et al. Self-assessment of the effect of dysphagia on the quality of life in patients after partial laryngectomy for cancer initially located in the supraglottic area [in Polish]. *Pol Merkuriusz Lek* 2005;*19*(111):362–364

[27] Jepsen MC, Gurushanthaiah D, Roy N, Smith ME, Gray SD, Davis RK. Voice, speech, and swallowing outcomes in laser-treated laryngeal cancer. *Laryngoscope* 2003;*113*(6):923–928

[28] Sasaki CT, Leder SB, Acton LM, Maune S. Comparison of the glottic closure reflex in traditional "open" versus endoscopic laser supraglottic laryngectomy. *Ann Otol Rhinol Laryngol* 2006;*115*(2):93–96

[29] Logemann JA, Rademaker AW, Pauloski BR, Kahrilas PJ. Effects of postural change on aspiration in head and neck surgical patients. *Otolaryngol Head Neck Surg* 1994;*110*(2):222–227

[30] Ceylan A, Köybaşioğlu A, Asal K, Kizil Y, Inal E. The effects of pharyngeal neurectomy and cricopharyngeal myotomy on postoperative deglutition in patients undergoing horizontal supraglottic laryngectomy [in Turkish]. *Kulak Burun Bogaz Ihtis Derg* 2003;*11*(6):170–174

[31] Tufano RP. Organ preservation surgery for laryngeal cancer. *Otolaryngol Clin North Am* 2002;*35*(5):1067–1080

[32] Zacharek MA, Pasha R, Meleca RJ, et al. Functional outcomes after supracricoid laryngectomy. *Laryngoscope* 2001;*111*(9):1558–1564

[33] Farrag TY, Koch WM, Cummings CW, et al. Supracricoid laryngectomy outcomes: the Johns Hopkins experience. *Laryngoscope* 2007;*117*(1):129–132

[34] Schindler A, Favero E, Nudo S, Albera R, Schindler O, Cavalot AL. Long-term voice and swallowing modifications after supracricoid laryngectomy: objective, subjective, and self-assessment data. *Am J Otolaryngol* 2006;*27*(6):378–383

[35] Davis RK, Vincent ME, Shapshay SM, Strong MS. The anatomy and complications of "T" versus vertical closure of the hypopharynx after laryngectomy. *Laryngoscope* 1982;*92*(1):16–22

[36] Nyquist GG, Hier MP, Dionisopoulos T, Black MJ. Stricture associated with primary tracheoesophageal puncture after pharyngolaryngectomy and free jejunal interposition. *Head Neck* 2006;*28*(3):205–209

[37] Horowitz JB, Sasaki CT. Effect of cricopharyngeus myotomy on postlaryngectomy pharyngeal contraction pressures. *Laryngoscope* 1993;*103*(2):138–140

[38] Maclean J, Cotton S, Perry A. Dysphagia following a total laryngectomy: the effect on quality of life, functioning, and psychological well-being. *Dysphagia* 2009;*24*(3):314–321

[39] Kotz T, Costello R, Li Y, Posner MR. Swallowing dysfunction after chemoradiation for advanced squamous cell carcinoma of the head and neck. *Head Neck* 2004;*26*(4):365–372

[40] Graner DE, Foote RL, Kasperbauer JL, et al. Swallow function in patients before and after intra-arterial chemoradiation. *Laryngoscope* 2003;*113*(3):573–579

[41] Lazarus C. Tongue strength and exercise in healthy individuals and in head and neck cancer patients. *Semin Speech Lang* 2006;*27*(4):260–267

[42] Starmer HM, Tippett D, Webster K, et al. Swallowing outcomes in patients with oropharyngeal cancer undergoing organ-preservation treatment. *Head Neck* 2014;*36*(10):1392–1397

[43] Gillespie MB, Brodsky MB, Day TA, Sharma AK, Lee FS, Martin-Harris B. Laryngeal penetration and aspiration during swallowing after the treatment of advanced oropharyngeal cancer. *Arch Otolaryngol Head Neck Surg* 2005;*131*(7):615–619

[44] Eisbruch A, Kim HM, Feng FY, et al. Chemo-IMRT of oropharyngeal cancer aiming to reduce dysphagia: swallowing organs late complication probabilities and dosimetric correlates. *Int J Radiat Oncol Biol Phys* 2011;*81*(3):e93–e99

[45] Hutcheson KA, Lewin JS, Barringer DA, et al. Late dysphagia after radiotherapy-based treatment of head and neck cancer. *Cancer* 2012;*118*(23):5793–5799

[46] Awan MJ, Mohamed AS, Lewin JS, et al. Late radiation-associated dysphagia (late-RAD) with lower cranial neuropathy after oropharyngeal radiotherapy: a preliminary dosimetric comparison. *Oral Oncol* 2014;*50*(8):746–752

[47] Newman LA, Robbins KT, Logemann JA, et al. Swallowing and speech ability after treatment for head and neck cancer with targeted intraarterial versus intravenous chemoradiation. *Head Neck* 2002;*24*(1):68–77

[48] Fung K, Lyden TH, Lee J, et al. Voice and swallowing outcomes of an organ-preservation trial for advanced laryngeal cancer. *Int J Radiat Oncol Biol Phys* 2005;*63*(5):1395–1399

[49] Goguen LA, Posner MR, Norris CM, et al. Dysphagia after sequential chemoradiation therapy for advanced head and neck cancer. *Otolaryngol Head Neck Surg* 2006;*134*(6):916–922

[50] Meleca RJ, Dworkin JP, Kewson DT, Stachler RJ, Hill SL. Functional outcomes following nonsurgical treatment for advanced-stage laryngeal carcinoma. *Laryngoscope* 2003;*113*(4):720–728

[51] Newman LA, Vieira F, Schwiezer V, et al. Eating and weight changes following chemoradiation therapy for advanced head and neck cancer. *Arch Otolaryngol Head Neck Surg* 1998;*124*(5):589–592

[52] Murry T, Madasu R, Martin A, Robbins KT. Acute and chronic changes in swallowing and quality of life following intraarterial chemoradiation for organ preservation in patients with advanced head and neck cancer. *Head Neck* 1998;*20*(1):31–37

[53] Mowry SE, LoTempio MM, Sadeghi A, Wang KH, Wang MB. Quality of life outcomes in laryngeal and oropharyngeal cancer patients after chemoradiation. *Otolaryngol Head Neck Surg* 2006;*135*(4):565–570

[54] Weber RS, Berkey BA, Forastiere A, et al. Outcome of salvage total laryngectomy following organ preservation therapy: the Radiation Therapy Oncology Group trial 91-11. *Arch Otolaryngol Head Neck Surg* 2003;*129*(1):44–49

[55] Forastiere AA, Zhang Q, Weber RS, et al. Long-term results of RTOG 91-11: a comparison of three nonsurgical treatment strategies to preserve the larynx in patients with locally advanced larynx cancer. *J Clin Oncol* 2013;*31*(7):845–852

[56] Hunter KU, Lee OE, Lyden TH, et al. Aspiration pneumonia after chemo-intensity-modulated radiation therapy of oropharyngeal carcinoma and its clinical and dysphagia-related predictors. *Head Neck* 2014;*36*(1):120–125

[57] Xu B, Boero IJ, Hwang L, et al. Aspiration pneumonia after concurrent chemoradiotherapy for head and neck cancer. *Cancer* 2015;*121*(8):1303–1311

[58] Lazarus CL, Logemann JA, Pauloski BR, et al. Swallowing disorders in head and neck cancer patients treated with radiotherapy and adjuvant chemotherapy. *Laryngoscope* 1996;*106*(9 Pt 1):1157–1166

[59] Eisbruch A, Lyden T, Bradford CR, et al. Objective assessment of swallowing dysfunction and aspiration after radiation concurrent with chemotherapy for head-and-neck cancer. *Int J Radiat Oncol Biol Phys* 2002;*53*(1):23–28

[60] Lee WT, Akst LM, Adelstein DJ, et al. Risk factors for hypopharyngeal/upper esophageal stricture formation after concurrent chemoradiation. *Head Neck* 2006;28(9):808–812

[61] Caudell JJ, Schaner PE, Desmond RA, Meredith RF, Spencer SA, Bonner JA. Dosimetric factors associated with long-term dysphagia after definitive radiotherapy for squamous cell carcinoma of the head and neck. *Int J Radiat Oncol Biol Phys* 2010;76(2):403–409

[62] Best SR, Ha PK, Blanco RG, et al. Factors associated with pharyngoesophageal stricture in patients treated with concurrent chemotherapy and radiation therapy for oropharyngeal squamous cell carcinoma. *Head Neck* 2011;33(12):1727–1734

[63] Agarwalla A, Small AJ, Mendelson AH, Scott FI, Kochman ML. Risk of recurrent or refractory strictures and outcome of endoscopic dilation for radiation-induced esophageal strictures. *Surg Endosc* 2015; 29(7): 1903–1912

[64] Jham BC, da Silva Freire AR. Oral complications of radiotherapy in the head and neck. *Rev Bras Otorrinolaringol (Engl Ed)* 2006;72(5):704–708

[65] Dijkstra PU, Kalk WW, Roodenburg JLN. Trismus in head and neck oncology: a systematic review. *Oral Oncol* 2004;40(9):879–889

[66] Mossman K, Shatzman A, Chencharick J. Long-term effects of radiotherapy on taste and salivary function in man. *Int J Radiat Oncol Biol Phys* 1982;8(6):991–997

[67] Irune E, Dwivedi RC, Nutting CM, Harrington KJ. Treatment-related dysgeusia in head and neck cancer patients. *Cancer Treat Rev* 2014;40(9):1106–1117

[68] Bensadoun RJ, Riesenbeck D, Lockhart PB, Elting LS, Spijkervet FK, Brennan MT; Trismus Section, Oral Care Study Group, Multinational Association for Supportive Care in Cancer (MASCC)/International Society of Oral Oncology (ISOO). A systematic review of trismus induced by cancer therapies in head and neck cancer patients. *Support Care Cancer* 2010;18(8):1033–1038

[69] Cassolato SF, Turnbull RS. Xerostomia: clinical aspects and treatment. *Gerodontology* 2003;20(2):64–77

[70] Haisfield-Wolfe ME, McGuire DB, Soeken K, Geiger-Brown J, De Forge B, Suntharalingam M. Prevalence and correlates of symptoms and uncertainty in illness among head and neck cancer patients receiving definitive radiation with or without chemotherapy. *Support Care Cancer* 2012;20(8):1885–1893

[71] Simental AA, Carrau RL. Assessment of swallowing function in patients with head and neck cancer. *Curr Oncol Rep* 2004;6(2):162–165

[72] Langmore SE, Schatz K, Olson N. Endoscopic and videofluoroscopic evaluations of swallowing and aspiration. *Ann Otol Rhinol Laryngol* 1991;100(8):678–681

[73] Wu CH, Hsiao TY, Chen JC, Chang YC, Lee SY. Evaluation of swallowing safety with fiberoptic endoscope: comparison with videofluoroscopic technique. *Laryngoscope* 1997;107(3):396–401

[74] Mlynarek AM, Rieger JM, Harris JR, et al. Methods of functional outcomes assessment following treatment of oral and oropharyngeal cancer: review of the literature. *J Otolaryngol Head Neck Surg* 2008;37(1):2–10

[75] Furia CL, Carrara-de Angelis E, Martins NM, Barros AP, Carneiro B, Kowalski LP. Video fluoroscopic evaluation after glossectomy. *Arch Otolaryngol Head Neck Surg* 2000;126(3):378–383

[76] Welch MV, Logemann JA, Rademaker AW, Kahrilas PJ. Changes in pharyngeal dimensions effected by chin tuck. *Arch Phys Med Rehabil* 1993;74(2):178–181

[77] Toyoshita Y, Koshino H, Hirai T, Matsumi T. Effect of wearing a palatal plate on swallowing function. *J Prosthodont Res* 2009;53(4):172–175

[78] Kamstra JI, Roodenburg JL, Beurskens CH, Reintsema H, Dijkstra PU. TheraBite exercises to treat trismus secondary to head and neck cancer. *Support Care Cancer* 2013;21(4):951–957

[79] Dijkstra PU, Sterken MW, Pater R, Spijkervet FK, Roodenburg JL. Exercise therapy for trismus in head and neck cancer. *Oral Oncol* 2007;43(4):389–394

[80] Logemann JA, Pauloski BR, Rademaker AW, Colangelo LA. Speech and swallowing rehabilitation for head and neck cancer patients. *Oncology (Williston Park)* 1997;11(5):651–656, 659, discussion 659, 663–664

[81] Logemann JA, Kahrilas PJ, Kobara M, Vakil NB. The benefit of head rotation on pharyngoesophageal dysphagia. *Arch Phys Med Rehabil* 1989;70(10):767–771

[82] Lazarus C, Logemann JA, Song CW, Rademaker AW, Kahrilas PJ. Effects of voluntary maneuvers on tongue base function for swallowing. *Folia Phoniatr Logop* 2002;54(4):171–176

[83] Kahrilas PJ, Logemann JA, Krugler C, Flanagan E. Volitional augmentation of upper esophageal sphincter opening during swallowing. *Am J Physiol* 1991;260(3 Pt 1):G450–G456

[84] Ohmae Y, Logemann JA, Kaiser P, Hanson DG, Kahrilas PJ. Effects of two breath-holding maneuvers on oropharyngeal swallow. *Ann Otol Rhinol Laryngol* 1996;105(2):123–131

[85] Carroll WR, Locher JL, Canon CL, Bohannon IA, McColloch NL, Magnuson JS. Pretreatment swallowing exercises improve swallow function after chemoradiation. *Laryngoscope* 2008;118(1):39–43

[86] Kotz T, Federman AD, Kao J, et al. Prophylactic swallowing exercises in patients with head and neck cancer undergoing chemoradiation: a randomized trial. *Arch Otolaryngol Head Neck Surg* 2012;138(4):376–382

[87] van der Molen L, van Rossum MA, Burkhead LM, Smeele LE, Rasch CR, Hilgers FJ. A randomized preventive rehabilitation trial in advanced head and neck cancer patients treated with chemoradiotherapy: feasibility, compliance, and short-term effects. *Dysphagia* 2011;26(2):155–170

[88] Carnaby-Mann G, Crary MA, Schmalfuss I, Amdur R. "Pharyngocise": randomized controlled trial of preventative exercises to maintain muscle structure and swallowing function during head-and-neck chemoradiotherapy. *Int J Radiat Oncol Biol Phys* 2012;83(1):210–219

[89] Shinn EH, Basen-Engquist K, Baum G, et al. Adherence to preventive exercises and self-reported swallowing outcomes in post-radiation head and neck cancer patients. *Head Neck* 2013;35(12):1707–1712

[90] Smith BG, Hutcheson KA, Little LG, et al. Lymphedema outcomes in patients with head and neck cancer. *Otolaryngol Head Neck Surg* 2015;152(2):284–291

[91] Langmore S, Krisciunas GP, Miloro KV, Evans SR, Cheng DM. Does PEG use cause dysphagia in head and neck cancer patients? *Dysphagia* 2012;27(2):251–259

[92] Hutcheson KA, Bhayani MK, Beadle BM, et al. Eat and exercise during radiotherapy or chemoradiotherapy for pharyngeal cancers: use it or lose it. *JAMA Otolaryngol Head Neck Surg* 2013;139(11):1127–1134

# 23 Artificial Airways and Swallowing

*Debra M. Suiter and Martin B. Brodsky*

## Summary

Artificial airways, including endotracheal tubes and tracheostomy tubes, have the potential to impact swallow function negatively. However, it remains unclear whether it is the illness necessitating placement of the artificial airway rather than the artificial airway itself that affects swallowing. This chapter reviews information regarding assessment and treatment options for individuals with artificial airways. Endotracheal intubation and postextubation dysphagia are discussed in detail, including how and when to assess individuals postextubation. This is followed by a discussion regarding tracheostomy tubes and the potential impact they may have on swallow function. Current research evidence regarding assessment and treatment options is presented.

## Keywords

intubation, extubation, endotracheal tube, tracheotomy, tracheostomy

### Learning Objectives
- Explain why an artificial airway would be placed
- Understand the impact an endotracheal or tracheostomy tube may have on swallow function
- Discuss how and when swallow function should be assessed in individuals postextubation
- Discuss optimal means of swallow assessment in individuals with a tracheostomy tube
- Explain research findings regarding the impact, or lack thereof, an inflated tracheostomy tube cuff has on swallow function

## 23.1 Introduction

Endotracheal tubes and tracheostomy tubes are two types of artificial airways that may be placed in individuals with compromised respiratory function. An endotracheal tube is placed through the nose or mouth, through the pharynx, and ultimately positioned between the vocal folds to maintain airway patency and facilitate mechanical ventilation. Damage to the structures of the pharynx or larynx can occur at the time of intubation (i.e., when the endotracheal tube is placed), while the patient is intubated, or when the patient is extubated (i.e., when the endotracheal tube is removed). Swallow function can be impacted negatively if structural damage occurs. Accurate assessment and management are critical for individuals at risk for dysphagia postextubation. This chapter discusses the optimal timing and means of assessing these individuals.

Tracheostomy tubes are often placed following a period of prolonged intubation, usually at least 2 weeks. These tubes are placed between the second and third tracheal rings, and the tube remains within the trachea. Although a tracheostomy tube does not traverse the same structures as those involved in swallowing, namely the structures of the pharynx, there is a significant body of research investigating the potential impact these tubes have on swallowing. This information will be discussed at length, along with optimal means of assessing and treating individuals with a tracheostomy tube who present with oropharyngeal dysphagia.

A detailed discussion of endotracheal and tracheostomy tubes includes the following key topics:

- Indications for endotracheal intubation
- Impact of endotracheal tubes on swallow function
- Optimal timing and means of assessing swallow function postextubation
- Indications for tracheostomy tube placement
- Impact of tracheostomy tubes on swallow function
- Optimal means of assessing and treating swallow dysfunction in individuals with a tracheostomy tube

## 23.2 Breathing and Swallowing

It is noteworthy that breathing and swallowing share the same conduit—the pharynx—thus establishing a basis for concerns related to safe swallowing. Regardless of age, breathing and swallowing are well coordinated in healthy humans and mammals throughout the animal kingdom.[1,2,3] Breathing stops at approximately the time of swallowing initiation and resumes after swallowing has completed; that is, healthy individuals *never* breathe while swallowing and *never* swallow while breathing. But what happens when this coordination of breathing and swallowing becomes uncoordinated? We've all experienced it. At some point, you were drinking when you laughed at the very moment someone said something funny or you were scared by a sudden sound or someone's gesture and water spurted out of your mouth (or out of your nose). Effectively, this was the body's way of saying to you, "I choose safety over nutrition." But what if circumstances changed quickly, and instead of safety versus nutrition the choice were life versus death? In fact, this decision is at the core of the very set of circumstances leading to endotracheal intubation.

## 23.3 Endotracheal Intubation

In the United States, approximately 1 million (20%) of the 5 million people admitted to the intensive care unit (ICU) are intubated annually.[4,5] Across the world the number of endotracheal intubations climbs to 13–20 million annually.[4] Once intubated, U.S. patients can expect a mortality rate of nearly

35%, and hospital bills of $600–$1,500 per day for mechanical ventilation, with 39% remaining intubated for 4 days or more.[5] Although the neuromuscular block wears off rather quickly, patients are often sedated and bedridden for lengthier periods of time, predisposing the patient to what is known as ICU-acquired weakness, and its aftermath postdischarge from the ICU, known as post–intensive care syndrome (PICS). PICS consists of a set of new or worsening impairments in mental, cognitive, and/or physical health domains that began in the ICU and continued through hospital discharge.[6] Swallowing dysfunction, germane to the *physical* health difficulties associated with PICS, currently is realized only after the endotracheal tube has been removed and the patient is at least screened. At the time of the writing of this chapter, there is a considerable knowledge gap between what is known about the larynx, voice, and swallowing after extubation and their long-term impairments and outcomes.[6,7]

Individuals who have compromised breathing, such as those who have reduced airway safety (e.g., external injury, bleeding), are in respiratory distress (i.e., difficulty/labored breathing), or worse, respiratory failure (i.e., absence of breathing function). To maintain the body's oxygen requirements, placement of an artificial airway may be necessary. This artificial airway, once placed, is then connected to a mechanical ventilator for automated assistance in maintaining the delivery of oxygen. Patients undergoing certain surgical procedures with general anesthesia delivered via the airway are also intubated, with or without the need for supplemental oxygen. For these purposes, the endotracheal tube has shifted from a life-sustaining method to an airway maintenance and anesthesia delivery system.

Patients requiring an emergent airway with the goal of being placed on a mechanical ventilator undergo a procedure called rapid sequence intubation.[8] In short, a quick-acting anesthetic is followed by a quick-acting neuromuscular block to allow for the passage of an endotracheal tube using a laryngoscope, typically orally (nasal is an alternate route), through the pharynx, past the vocal folds, and stopping short of the carina in the mainstem bronchus (**Fig. 23.1**). During rapid sequence intubation, care must be exercised with manipulation of the laryngoscope so as to avoid chipping teeth (i.e., typically the incisors) and accidental esophageal intubation.

In average adults, the journey of the endotracheal tube is approximately 21–24 cm (8.25–9.5 in) with a tube that is 10–13 mm in diameter. At the distal end of the endotracheal tube is an inflatable cuff that, when inflated, allows for a positive pressure of air to enter the lungs without escape superiorly via the upper airway (**Fig. 23.2**). In order to determine whether the cuff is inflated, a pilot balloon is connected to the outer hub of the endotracheal tube. When the pilot balloon is inflated and "puffy," this indicates that the cuff is also inflated; likewise, when the pilot balloon is "flat," the cuff is deflated. Although the endotracheal tube comes in a variety of sizes, from very small and appropriate for neonates to large and appropriate for adults, the hub of the endotracheal tube is a standard 15 mm in the United States for connections to respiratory equipment. Patients may be nasally or orally intubated for very short periods (i.e., hours), as in the case of surgery, or for prolonged periods (generally up to 2 weeks). Currently debated, and without much resolution at the time of this book's printing, is when patients should be converted from an oral (or nasal) endotracheal tube to a tracheostomy for durations

longer than 10–14 days.[9,10,11] Arguments are related to increased comorbidities, infection, and anticipated need (i.e., predictions based on clinical course). This debate and its controversies, however, are beyond the scope of this chapter.

Although the oral (and sometimes the nasal) cavity is the initial pathway for the endotracheal tube, the pharynx, larynx, and trachea are the most affected by the tube and the apparatus. Endotracheal tubes traverse the vocal folds, creating opportunity for complications affecting voice and swallowing functions.[12] Even if the patient were awake during oral (or nasal) intubation, phonation is immediately compromised because the endotracheal tube prevents complete glottic closure. Concurrent with a patient's inability to adduct the vocal folds is also the inability to close—and thus protect—the airway, ultimately leading to potential complications (e.g., aspiration pneumonia, ventilator-associated pneumonia) arising from aspiration of saliva and other secretions. As has been addressed previously in this text, the coordination of breathing and swallowing is most evident at the level of the larynx, where protection of the upper and lower airways takes place. Anything that disrupts the ability to coordinate bolus flow with airway closure can lead to airway compromise and ultimately aspiration. To this point, in patients who have been intubated, whether through an oral or nasal endotracheal tube or by a tracheostomy tube (see the "Tracheostomy Tubes" section this chapter), it is a common misconception that aspiration takes place once secretions have fallen *below* the level of the cuff. In fact, by the time secretions have reached the level of the cuff, they have *already been* aspirated. Recall that the definition of aspiration is anything that has passed inferiorly through the vocal folds. Recall also that the endotracheal tube—and its cuff—were passed through the vocal folds; that is, the cuff is inferior to the larynx and resides in the mid to distal trachea.

There are at least two opportunities for injury to occur to the oropharynx, larynx, and trachea related to intubation—*at the* time of endotracheal tube placement and *during* the time of intubation. Additional injuries may occur during unplanned (i.e.,

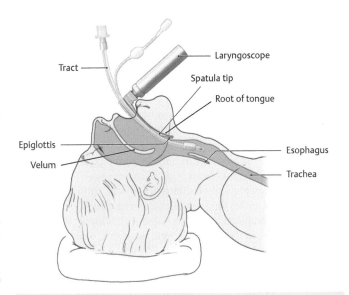

**Fig. 23.1** Intubation.

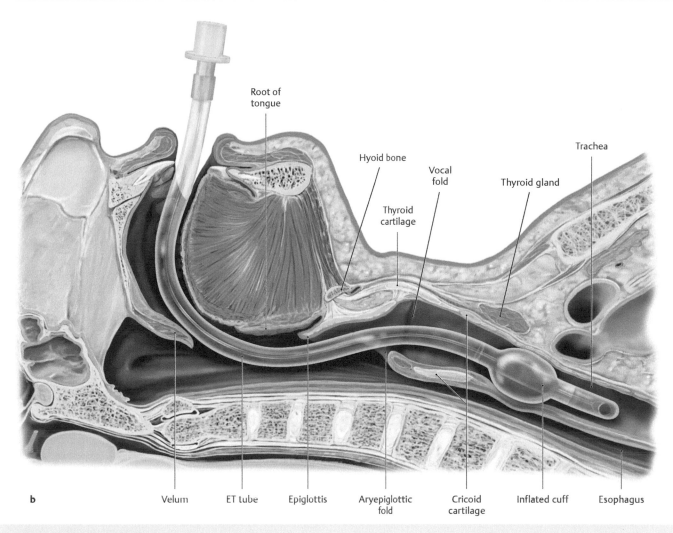

Root of tongue

Hyoid bone

Vocal fold

Trachea

Thyroid gland

Thyroid cartilage

b  Velum  ET tube  Epiglottis  Aryepiglottic fold  Cricoid cartilage  Inflated cuff  Esophagus

**Fig. 23.2** Endotracheal tube in place.

self-, accidental) extubations. Duration of intubation, patient sex, and endotracheal tube size have been associated with comorbidities to the pharynx and larynx. Among these complications are edema, tissue damage (e.g., hematomas, lacerations), infection, subluxation of the arytenoid cartilages, and weakness/paralysis of vocal fold movement.[13,14] Specific to the larynx, corniculate and arytenoid cartilage damage is reported in 85% of ICU patients after extubation, and in severe cases can lead to permanent vocal fold damage and dysphagia resulting in aspiration. Prolonged intubation can lead to further complications, including tracheal stenosis, formation of granulation tissue, epithelial/mucosal abrasions, and formation of tracheoesophageal fistulas.[14,15,16,17] Apart from weakness or paralysis of vocal fold closure, what is not yet understood well is which patients are most at risk for these injuries, and specifically those that will result in dysphagia.[12] Research addressing these clinical issues is under way.

Individuals who are endotracheally intubated are unable to take oral nutrition for a number of reasons that are mechanical to swallowing. You are already aware that airway closure at the level of the glottis cannot occur due to placement of the endotracheal tube between the vocal folds. Oral and nasal endotracheal tubes

are fastened by tape to the patient's lips and/or nose, providing stabilization and security of placement, and ultimately preventing the tube from abrupt and inadvertent movements, either by the patient or by the clinical staff. Because the oral tube passes over the tongue blade, and both oral and nasal tubes cross the tongue base, the tube obstructs oral tongue elevation and posterior movement of the tongue blade and tongue base during the swallow, theoretically impairing transport and clearance of the bolus. (The term *theoretically* is used because it is unethical to attempt to feed patients while they are orally intubated. Thus this statement considers the literature and what is known about swallowing physiology to imply that the primary functions of the tongue—to propel the bolus from the oral cavity, through the pharynx, and finally into the esophagus—are likely impaired due to restricted movement of the tongue from the exogenous forces of the oral [and nasal] endotracheal tube.) Placement of a nasal endotracheal tube further restricts elevation of the soft palate during swallowing, a compromise similar to the restriction the endotracheal tube places on closure of the vocal folds. Moreover, the epiglottis is prevented from inverting, and the larynx is tethered by the inflated endotracheal tube cuff, preventing contraction of the pharynx, laryngeal elevation, and approximation of the arytenoids to the base of the epiglottis, effectively eliminating the remaining defenses for airway protection during swallowing. A patient's level of alertness aside, it is, therefore, evident that placement of a tube capable of delivering an alternative means of nutrition, generally either a nasogastric, orogastric, or percutaneous gastric tube, is necessary while the patient is intubated. Placement of these tubes is generally completed at approximately the same time as placement of the artificial airway such that the chest X-ray following the intubation and feeding tube placement can verify both in the same film.

Dysphagia following prolonged endotracheal intubation (generally defined as ≥ 48 hours) has been reported in 3 to 62% of adult patients,[18,19,20,21,22] with most of these studies indicating prevalence based on referred subject sampling. Physician practice and referral patterns are varied, a likely reason for wide reported prevalence.[23,24] It is unclear whether dysphagia occurs as a result of intubation/extubation, the critical care delivered during intubation, or the underlying illness necessitating placement of an artificial airway. Several studies have described alterations in swallow physiology following extubation, including decreased laryngeal sensation, resulting in silent aspiration.[19,21] Others have noted decreased laryngeal elevation, presence of residue in the valleculae and piriform sinuses, and premature spillage of the bolus.[18]

Duration of intubation appears to be a factor affecting response to intubation.[7,21,25] In fact, the odds of patient-reported symptoms of dysphagia increase 80% *each day* while a patient is intubated; after which, no additional increased odds of dysphagia were noted.[26] Most studies report an increased incidence of dysphagia and/or aspiration with increased duration of intubation. This is possibly due to increased likelihood of laryngeal injury and its sequelae. Additionally, although age may appear to affect incidence of dysphagia postextubation, specifically with individuals 65 years or older having a greater incidence and prolonged period in which they experience dysphagia symptoms compared to younger individuals, this finding continues to be debated.[7,26,27] Regardless of age, approximately 75% of patients will recover from dysphagia in 3–6 months postextubation, whereas others may take as long as 5 years for their recovery.[28]

## 23.4 Swallowing Evaluation Postextubation

Not all patients who are intubated will experience postextubation swallowing difficulty, and not all will require swallow evaluation. However, because dysphagia with prandial aspiration can have significant morbidity and mortality in the critically ill ICU patient, including pneumonia, respiratory failure, and death, it is especially important to evaluate these individuals postextubation. However, there is no consensus regarding either *when* or *how* to perform swallow testing postextubation.[24]

There is no consensus for *when* to evaluate a patient's swallowing postextubation among speech-language pathologists. In clinical practice, speech-language pathologists wait a median of 24 hours prior to completing a swallow evaluation postextubation.[24] Waiting for this amount of time presumably allows the patient to stabilize medically and, according to some research, improve initiation of the pharyngeal swallow.[22] However, there is no empirical

evidence supporting the need to wait for an extended period. Leder and colleagues[29] administered the Yale Swallow Protocol[30] to 202 individuals postextubation. Initial administration of the Yale Swallow Protocol was at 1 hour postextubation. Patients who passed were started on a diet. For those who failed, the Yale Swallow Protocol was readministered at 4 hours postextubation. Again, if they passed, the patients were started on an oral diet. If they failed, the Yale Swallow Protocol was readministered at 24 hours postextubation. Individuals who failed the protocol at all three time points were then referred for further testing, such as endoscopic evaluation of swallowing, as appropriate. A total of 166/202 (82.2%) of participants pass the Yale Swallow Protocol at 1 hour postextubation, with an additional 11 participants passing at 4 hours postextubation and 8 additional individuals passing at 24 hours postextubation. Participants who passed the protocol and were started on an oral diet were followed for an average of 8.9 days postevaluation, and 87% were tolerating their diet. The remaining 13% were recommended nonoral nutrition after initially passing the Yale Swallow Protocol due to either unstable medical status or altered neurologic status. Based on the results of this study, there is no need to wait for 24 hours postextubation to evaluate swallow function. Clinicians are encouraged to complete a swallow evaluation once the patient is deemed medically and neurologically stable enough to be considered for an oral diet.

Regarding the *how* to evaluate swallowing function postextubation, there is variability in clinical practice. Options to consider are screening for dysphagia risk, clinical swallow evaluation, endoscopic evaluation of swallowing, and videofluoroscopic swallow evaluation. Because of the risk of laryngeal injury associated with intubation, there is concern that individuals are more likely to aspirate silently if aspiration occurs. Reports of incidence of silent aspiration postextubation are variable[12,20,21,25,31] and range from 20 to 69%.[31] Because of the possibility of increased incidence of silent aspiration, some clinicians advocate for an instrumental assessment for all patients postextubation, although whether to use endoscopy or videofluoroscopy is debatable. Endoscopic evaluation is often suggested because a direct view of the laryngeal structures can be obtained, and any effect of laryngeal injury on swallow function can be observed.[12] Second, as with any swallow assessment, clinicians must consider the medical stability of their patient when choosing when and how to assess swallow function. In some facilities, there are restrictions on transporting patients out of ICUs for a swallow evaluation, such as usually occurs for videofluoroscopic swallow studies. On general medical floors, transferring a patient may be accomplished by someone from the transport assistance team, a nursing assistant, or a nurse. Transporting a patient in the ICU often requires a critical care nurse and/or an individual trained in advanced cardiac life support. Providing coverage for the patients in ICU while covering the patient being transported then becomes a very real staffing issue. Thus clinicians may be limited by logistics to either noninstrumental assessment of swallowing or endoscopic evaluation.

## 23.5 Tracheostomy Tubes

Tracheotomy is one of the most common surgical procedures performed in the United States each year, averaging 100,000 annually.[32] The terms *tracheotomy* and *tracheostomy* are often used interchangeably in clinical practice. However, they are

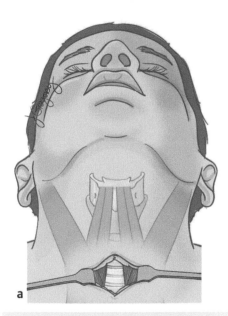
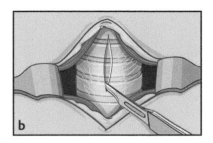
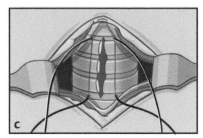
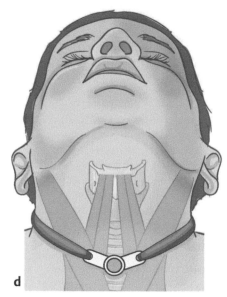

**Fig. 23.3** Tracheotomy.

two distinct terms. A tracheotomy is a surgical procedure, during which an opening into an individual's trachea is created. Typically, the incision is positioned between the second and third tracheal rings. A tracheostomy is the surgically created hole in the patient's neck; thus a tracheostomy tube is then inserted through the tracheostomy to create an airway (**Fig. 23.3**).

Tracheotomy is often performed after a person has been endotracheally intubated for a period of time. The length of time physicians wait before transitioning from an endotracheal tube to a tracheostomy tube is variable, ranging from as little as 1 day to 2 weeks, and the timing depends on the underlying reason for intubation, the likelihood of weaning from mechanical ventilation, and the patient's response to weaning efforts. In addition to prolonged intubation or need for mechanical ventilation, indications for tracheotomy include the need for pulmonary hygiene (e.g., managing secretions), upper airway obstruction (e.g., a neoplasm), stenosis, obstructive sleep apnea, or a difficult-to-maintain airway.[33]

There are a number of different manufacturers of tracheostomy tubes, and each company's product varies with regard to material from which the tube is made, sizing, and other factors. Tracheostomy tubes are most often made of either polyvinyl chloride (PVC), silicone, or, less commonly, metal (stainless steel or silver). PVC and silicone tracheostomy tubes are generally more comfortable for patients because the material is more pliable than metal, and plastic tubes may include a cuff (which cannot be used with a metal tube). Metal tubes are often used for individuals who require prolonged tracheal intubation because they are more durable and more resistant to bacterial contamination than PVC tubes.

Tracheostomy tubes consist of several parts (**Fig. 23.4**). Most tracheostomy tubes have a 15 mm hub to which ventilator tubing may be connected. The neck flange rests against the skin of the neck, and ties or fabric adhesive strips can be placed through holes on either side of the flange to secure the tracheostomy tube. The size of the tracheostomy tube is indicated on the neck

flange. Tracheostomy tube sizes vary by the diameter of the outer cannula, or the outer wall of the tracheostomy tube. Size of the tracheostomy tube is selected based on the patient's age, weight, and height. The inner cannula fits within the outer cannula and can be removed for cleaning. Tracheostomy tubes may be cuffed or uncuffed. The cuff, similar to that of an endotracheal tube, is an air- or foam-filled balloon that encircles the outer cannula and serves to seal off the upper airway, preventing air from flowing into the upper airway. Patients who are on mechanical ventilation will have tracheostomy tubes with cuffs that are inflated. The cuff may be deflated to allow for suctioning and restoration of some airflow through the upper airway. Cuffless tracheostomy tubes are often used as part of the tracheostomy weaning process because they restore airflow through the upper airway. They are also used with pediatrics and in metal tracheostomy tubes.

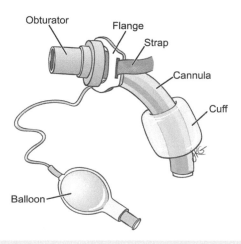

**Fig. 23.4** Tracheostomy tube.

# 23.6 Tracheostomy Tubes and Swallowing

The presence of a tracheostomy tube alters the airway such that the individual inhales and exhales through the tracheostomy tube rather than through the mouth and nose; thus taste and smell may be diminished.[34,35] Because this airway is below the level of the true vocal folds, airflow through the vocal folds is diminished, and the ability to phonate is virtually eliminated (**Fig. 23.5**). Additionally, some have questioned whether the presence of a tracheostomy tube affects swallow function. Prolonged lack of airflow through the upper airway has been found to result in diminished adductor vocal fold reflexes in individuals following prolonged tracheal intubation (e.g., 6 months or more).[36] The adductor vocal fold response is a protective reflex that prevents unwanted material, such as food or liquid, from entering the lower airway.[37] Individuals with diminished laryngeal adductor responses, including those with prolonged tracheal intubation, are thus less likely to cough in response to aspiration of material; in other words, they aspirate silently.[25]

Tracheostomy tubes also affect swallowing by altering the coupling of breathing and respiration. Typical patterns of breathe-swallow coordination involve an exhalation–swallow–exhalation pattern most frequently or a less frequently observed inhalation–swallow–exhalation pattern. The postswallow exhalation is believed to be a protective mechanism that assists with clearing any material that may have entered the laryngeal vestibule during the swallow.[1,2,3,38,39] This pattern is often altered in individuals with a tracheostomy tube, and as many as half of individuals with neuromuscular disease and tracheostomy tubes exhibited a postswallow inhalation rather than exhalation.[40] This postswallow inhalation places the patient at increased risk of aspiration.[1]

The open respiratory system created by the tracheostomy tube also results in a reduction in subglottal air pressure.[41,42,43] A number of studies have observed that individuals who aspirate when the tracheostomy tube is open do not aspirate when the tracheostomy tube is occluded, either digitally or with a speaking valve or tracheostomy cap or plug.[30,44,45,46,47,48] It has been suggested that these differences in aspiration status can be attributed to restoration of subglottal air pressure when the tracheostomy tube is occluded.[43] The role of subglottal air pressure in swallowing was first evaluated by Eibling and Gross[41,49] and colleagues, who observed peak subglottal air pressures occurring concurrent with laryngeal elevation during the swallow. They suggested that subglottal air pressure serves to stimulate mechanoreceptors in the trachea, and stimulation of these mechanoreceptors results in inhibition of inhalation during the swallow. Loss of subglottal air pressure with an open tracheostomy tube would, in theory, lead to a lack of mechanoreceptors in the trachea and interrupt the coordination between swallowing and respiration, thus placing the patient at increased risk of aspiration during or after the pharyngeal phase of swallowing.

Because the tracheostomy tubing adds weight to the neck, some have postulated that the presence of a tracheostomy tube negatively impacts hyolaryngeal excursion. Additionally, if the tracheostomy tube is cuffed, and if the cuff remains inflated when the patient swallows, some have suggested that this further contributes to tethering of the larynx and reduced hyolaryngeal

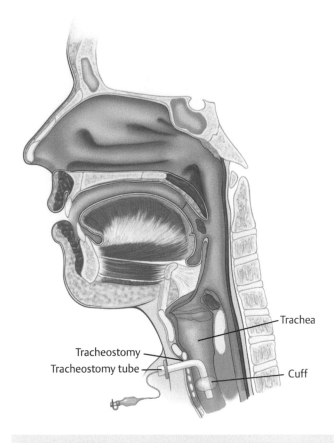

**Fig. 23.5** Tracheostomy Tube in situ.

excursion.[50] However, these postulations are not supported by the research literature. Studies in which the impact of a tracheostomy cuff on hyolaryngeal excursion has been examined within the same patient (i.e., swallowing assessed with and without the cuff inflated within the same individual) have found no causal relationship between the presence of a tracheostomy tube and decreased hyolaryngeal movement.[48,51]

Others have suggested that the tracheostomy tube cuff itself can lead to swallowing impairment. Overinflation of the tracheostomy cuff can cause significant complications, including tracheal necrosis, tracheal stenosis, laryngeal nerve palsy, or tracheoesophageal fistula. Additionally, an overinflated tracheostomy tube cuff can impede the flow of food or liquid through the esophagus. Care should be taken by medical staff involved in caring for the patient's tracheostomy tube, and a pressure manometer can be used to measure cuff pressures to ensure the cuff is not overinflated.

Evidence in the research literature suggests that the presence of a tracheostomy tube can result in alterations in swallowing. It is important to remember that many individuals with a tracheostomy tube have underlying medical conditions that could predispose them to development of dysphagia and aspiration. Thus it can be difficult to discern whether swallow problems that occur in patients with tracheostomy tubes are due to the tubes themselves. Additionally, most studies in which a causal relationship has been suggested have examined a patient's swallow status only after the tracheostomy tube was placed, not *both* before and after placement. In most cases, this is not possible because the patient is being converted from an endotracheal tube where there is no possibility of swallowing. Thus one cannot definitively determine whether swallow function was impacted negatively by placement of the tracheostomy tube. When swallow function was assessed pre- and posttracheotomy within the same individual, no significant change in swallow function was found as a result of tracheostomy tube placement.[52,53]

## 23.7 Swallowing Assessment in Individuals with a Tracheostomy Tube

Information regarding screening and clinical swallow evaluation is discussed in Chapter 4. Clinical swallow evaluation in individuals with a tracheostomy tube poses a challenge to the clinician. As previously discussed in this chapter, prolonged tracheal intubation leads to diminished laryngeal adductor response. Because of this, individuals with a tracheostomy tube are less likely to cough in response to aspiration.[25] Additionally, because phonation is interrupted in individuals with open tracheostomy tubes, voicing changes in response to aspiration (e.g., wet vocal quality) may not be readily observable if penetration or aspiration occurs. Thus the clinical signs or symptoms that are used to identify aspiration risk in patients without tracheostomy tubes may not be evident in patients with tracheostomy tubes.

To improve accuracy of the clinical swallow evaluation for individuals with a tracheostomy tube, the modified Evans blue dye test was developed.[54] As described originally, drops of Evans blue dye were placed on the patient's tongue every 4 hours over a period of 48 hours, and patients were suctioned at set intervals. The presence of blue-tinged secretions, because they were suctioned from below the vocal folds via the tracheostomy tube, confirmed aspiration of secretions. The modified Evans blue dye test (MEBDT) is an extension of the original. During the MEBDT, blue dye is added to various foods and liquids that the patient then ingests. Patients are then suctioned. If blue dye is detected in suctioned secretions (or secretions the patient expectorates through the tracheostomy tube), aspiration is confirmed. Accuracy of the MEBDT for detecting aspiration has been questioned, and reported findings are equivocal.[55,56,57,58,59] In studies that have examined accuracy of the MEBDT by simultaneously completing the test with instrumental assessment (videofluoroscopy or endoscopy), a high rate of false-negative responses was found for the MEBDT (50%), and when individuals aspirated trace amounts, the MEBDT failed to detect aspiration.[56,57] Accuracy of the MEBDT for detecting aspiration improved only when gross aspiration was present.[56,57] Clinicians are thus urged to use caution when interpreting results of the MEBDT, and, at best, this tool should be considered a screening tool for gross aspiration only.

Because of the increased risk of aspiration being silent when it occurs in patients with tracheostomy tubes, and because of the lack of sufficient evidence to support the use of currently available screening tools, such as the MEBDT, to detect aspiration in patients with tracheostomy, instrumental assessment is advised when concerns regarding swallow function arise in the patient population. Choice of instrumentation, either videofluoroscopy or endoscopy, should be based on the clinical considerations involving videofluoroscopy and endoscopy discussed elsewhere in this book.

Some clinicians have expressed concerns over possible deleterious effects of an inflated tracheostomy cuff, including reduced hyolaryngeal excursion, impingement on the esophagus, and the lack of airflow through the upper airway. Because of this some authors have advised deflating the tracheostomy tube cuff prior to completing a swallow evaluation.[60] As discussed earlier in this chapter, there is no empirical evidence to support the notion that an inflated tracheostomy tube cuff hampers hyolaryngeal excursion.[48,51] Thus there is no contraindication to swallow assessment in individuals who are unable to tolerate tracheostomy cuff deflation. Clinicians are advised to assess swallow function under the conditions in which their patient will be eating, the cuff inflated or cuff deflated, and with or without a speaking valve in place.

## 23.8 Swallowing Treatment in Individuals with a Tracheostomy Tube

Swallowing treatments for individuals with a tracheostomy tube do not vary greatly from swallowing treatments used for individuals without tracheostomy tubes. Traditional compensatory and rehabilitative therapy strategies may be used with patients with a tracheostomy tube, although there are some cautions. It is generally accepted that the Shaker exercise, in which the head is lifted toward the chest, should not be recommended for patients with a tracheostomy tube because there is a possibility of the tube becoming displaced. Use of compensatory strategies that require breath holding, such as the super-supraglottic swallow, which requires occlusion (i.e., digital, one-way speaking valve, cap), may also prove challenging for individuals with a tracheostomy tube and provide an additional strain on an already compromised respiratory system. It is important to note that there is no empirical research investigating the use of any of these techniques specifically in patients with a tracheostomy tube. Thus, effectiveness of these techniques should be evaluated on a case-by-case basis.

There is a significant body of literature that has evaluated the effects of tracheostomy tube occlusion, either by speaking valve placement or capping, on swallow function and aspiration status in individuals with a tracheostomy tube.[43,47,48,61,62,63,64] It is important to note that there are many manufacturers of tracheostomy speaking valves, but research has almost exclusively focused on use of the Passy-Muir Tracheostomy Speaking Valve. It is unclear whether similar results would be found with other speaking valves. With the exception of Leder,[62,64] results indicate improved swallow function (lowered prevalence of aspiration) when the tracheostomy tube is occluded. When aspiration status has been examined for speaking valve on versus off conditions within the same individual, results have been equivocal (aspiration was reduced for some individuals who aspirated thin liquids but not for individuals who aspirated pureed textures).[48] Because tracheostomy tube occlusion necessitates cuff deflation, any possible effects the tracheostomy cuff may have on swallow function are eliminated. Additionally, deflating the cuff restores airflow through the upper airway and allows air to stimulate the laryngeal and subglottal sensory receptors. Occluding the tracheostomy tube restores subglottal air pressure that may improve swallow safety.[43] Clinicians are encouraged to evaluate swallow function with and without the speaking valve in place for patients who are able to tolerate valve placement.

In summary, empirical evidence does not support the notion that tracheostomy tubes in and of themselves affect swallow function adversely. Many individuals with a tracheostomy tube have underlying medical conditions that could predispose them to swallowing difficulty, and it is likely the underlying condition, not the tracheostomy tube, results in any alterations in swallowing that may be observed. When dysphagia is suspected in an individual with a tracheostomy tube, clinicians are encouraged to utilize instrumental swallow assessment and complete the assessment in a manner similar to that in which the individual will eat (i.e., tracheostomy cuff inflated or deflated; speaking valve in place or not).

## 23.9 Questions

1. For which of the following reasons should an individual who is presently intubated not be fed orally?

A. The inflated endotracheal tube cuff inhibits hyolaryngeal excursion.

B. The intubated patient is typically too somnolent to participate in an evaluation.

C. The endotracheal tube is positioned between the true vocal folds, thus preventing airway protection at this level during the swallow.

D. The inflated endotracheal tube cuff inhibits vocal fold adduction.

E. All of the above are reasons for not feeding a patient who is intubated.

2. Why do many clinicians choose to postpone assessment of swallow function in patients until 24 hours postextubation?

A. There is empirical evidence indicating that hyolaryngeal excursion does not return fully in most individuals until they have been extubated for at least 24 hours.

B. There is empirical evidence indicating that laryngeal sensation does not return fully in most individuals until they have been extubated for at least 24 hours.

C. There is empirical evidence indicating that epiglottic retroflexion does not return fully in most individuals until they have been extubated for at least 24 hours.

D. There is empirical evidence indicating that tongue base retraction does not return fully in most individuals until they have been extubated for at least 24 hours.

E. Anecdotal evidence from other clinicians suggests that it is a reasonable approach.

3. Which of the following commonly held beliefs regarding tracheostomy tube effects on swallow function is *not* true?

A. The tracheostomy tube alters the coupling of breathing and respiration so patients are more likely to inhale post-swallow.

B. The tracheostomy tube tethers the larynx and thus reduces hyolaryngeal excursion.

C. The tracheostomy tube reduces subglottal air pressure, which serves to stimulate the mechanoreceptors in the trachea.

D. The tracheostomy tube diminishes the adductor vocal fold reflexes following periods of prolonged intubation.

E. None of the above are true. The tracheostomy tube does not affect swallow function.

4. During a clinical evaluation of swallowing in individuals with a tracheostomy tube, clinicians should:

A. Be aware that typical signs and symptoms of aspiration, such as changes in vocal quality or cough responses, may not be present.

B. Ask the patient to phonate following the swallow in order to assess changes in vocal quality.

C. Add blue dye to the boluses they are presenting because blue dye testing has been found to identify aspiration reliably.

D. Make sure the tracheostomy tube cuff is deflated or refuse to do the evaluation.

E. Administer the 3-ounce water swallow challenge.

5. The most effective treatment for dysphagia for individuals with a tracheostomy tube is

A. Thermal-tactile application

B. Neuromuscular electrical stimulation

C. The super-supraglottic swallow

D. Shaker exercises

E. None of the above

## 23.10 Answers and Explanations

1. **Correct: all of the above are reasons for not feeding a patient who is intubated (E).**
Whether placed orally or nasally, and endotracheal tube traverses the base of the tongue, pharynx, and endolarynx, ultimately being positioned between the true vocal folds. Because of this, the patient is unable to protect the airway at the level of the true vocal folds during the swallow. This, and the inhibition of epiglottic movement that occurs when an endotracheal tube is present, places the patient at significant risk for aspiration. Thus an alternative means of nutrition, such as an orogastric or nasogastric feeding tube, is recommended for patients who are intubated.

**2. Correct: anecdotal evidence from other clinicians suggests that it is a reasonable approach (E).**

In clinical practice, speech-language pathologists wait a median of 24 hours prior to completing a swallow evaluation postextubation. Waiting for 24 hours to assess is thought to allow patients to stabilize medically and improve the timeliness of pharyngeal swallow initiation. However, there is no empirical evidence to support the need to wait 24 hours postextubation to assess patients. Leder and colleagues examined 202 patients within an hour of extubation and found the majority, 82.2%, were able to pass the Yale Swallow Protocol and resume an oral diet safely.

**3. Correct: the tracheostomy tube tethers the larynx and thus reduces hyolaryngeal excursion (B).**

Because of the weight of a tracheostomy tube and the possible presence of an inflated tracheostomy tube cuff, some have speculated that hyolaryngeal excursion is reduced in individuals with a tracheostomy tube; however, empirical evidence does not support this. Studies in which the impact of a tracheostomy tube itself or a tracheostomy tube with an inflated cuff was examined within the same patient have found no causal relationship between the presence of a tracheostomy tube and decreased hyolaryngeal excursion. Current best practice requires the use of an instrumental evaluation with all patients who have a tracheostomy tube.

**4. Correct: be aware that typical signs and symptoms of aspiration such as changes in vocal quality or cough responses may not be present (A).**

The presence of a tracheostomy tube, particularly for a prolonged period of time, results in diminished adductor reflex responses. This means a patient with a tracheostomy tube is more likely to aspirate silently if aspiration occurs. Additionally, changes in vocal quality may occur in patients with a tracheostomy tube because of damage done to the larynx during intubation or extubation. Blue dye testing has not been found to be sensitive for determining the presence of aspiration.

**5. Correct: none of the above (E).**

There are currently no available studies in which effectiveness of any dysphagia intervention has been examined specifically in patients with a tracheostomy tube. Use of the Shaker exercise is contraindicated for patients with a tracheostomy tube because the tube may become displaced. The super-supraglottic swallow would be difficult for an individual with a tracheostomy tube to complete successfully because of the inclusion of a hard breath hold.

## References

[1] Martin-Harris B, Brodsky MB, Michel Y, Ford CL, Walters B, Heffner J. Breathing and swallowing dynamics across the adult lifespan. *Arch Otolaryngol Head Neck Surg* 2005;131(9):762–770

[2] Martin-Harris B, Brodsky MB, Price CC, Michel Y, Walters B. Temporal coordination of pharyngeal and laryngeal dynamics with breathing during swallowing: single liquid swallows. *J Appl Physiol (1985)* 2003;94(5):1735–1743

[3] Pitts T, Rose MJ, Poliacek I, Condrey J, Davenport PW, Bolser DC. Effect of laparotomy on the swallow-breathing relationship in the cat. *Lung* 2015;193(1):129–133

[4] Adhikari NKJ, Fowler RA, Bhagwanjee S, Rubenfeld GD. Critical care and the global burden of critical illness in adults. *Lancet* 2010;376(9749):1339–1346

[5] Wunsch H, Linde-Zwirble WT, Angus DC, Hartman ME, Milbrandt EB, Kahn JM. The epidemiology of mechanical ventilation use in the United States. *Crit Care Med* 2010;38(10):1947–1953

[6] Needham DM, Davidson J, Cohen H, et al. Improving long-term outcomes after discharge from intensive care unit: report from a stakeholders' conference. *Crit Care Med* 2012;40(2):502–509

[7] Skoretz SA, Flowers HL, Martino R. The incidence of dysphagia following endotracheal intubation: a systematic review. *Chest* 2010;137(3):665–673

[8] Reynolds SF, Heffner J. Airway management of the critically ill patient: rapid-sequence intubation. *Chest* 2005;127(4):1397–1412

[9] Liu CC, Livingstone D, Dixon E, Dort JC. Early versus late tracheostomy: a systematic review and meta-analysis. *Otolaryngol Head Neck Surg* 2015;152(2):219–227

[10] Siempos II, Ntaidou TK, Filippidis FT, Choi AMK. Effect of early versus late or no tracheostomy on mortality and pneumonia of critically ill patients receiving mechanical ventilation: a systematic review and meta-analysis. *Lancet Respir Med* 2015;3(2):150–158

[11] Keeping A. Early versus late tracheostomy for critically ill patients: a clinical evidence synopsis of a recent Cochrane Review. *Can J Respir Ther* 2016;52(1):27–28

[12] Scheel R, Pisegna JM, McNally E, Noordzij JP, Langmore SE. Endoscopic assessment of swallowing after prolonged intubation in the ICU setting. *Ann Otol Rhinol Laryngol* 2016;125(1):43–52

[13] Alessi DM, Hanson DG, Berci G. Bedside videolaryngoscopic assessment of intubation trauma. *Ann Otol Rhinol Laryngol* 1989;98(8 Pt 1):586–590

[14] Whited RE. A prospective study of laryngotracheal sequelae in long-term intubation. *Laryngoscope* 1984;94(3):367–377

[15] Sue RD, Susanto I. Long-term complications of artificial airways. *Clin Chest Med* 2003;24(3):457–471

[16] Skoretz SA, Flowers HL, Martino R. The incidence of dysphagia following endotracheal intubation: a systematic review. *Chest* 2010;137(3):665–673

[17] Hillel AT, Karatayli-Ozgursoy S, Samad I, et al; North American Airway Collaborative (NoAAC). Predictors of posterior glottic stenosis: A multi-institutional case-control study. *Ann Otol Rhinol Laryngol* 2016;125(3):257–263

[18] Tolep K, Getch CL, Criner GJ. Swallowing dysfunction in patients receiving prolonged mechanical ventilation. *Chest* 1996;109(1):167–172

[19] Barquist E, Brown M, Cohn S, Lundy D, Jackowski J. Postextubation fiberoptic endoscopic evaluation of swallowing after prolonged endotracheal intubation: a randomized, prospective trial. *Crit Care Med* 2001;29(9):1710–1713

[20] El Solh A, Okada M, Bhat A, Pietrantoni C. Swallowing disorders post orotracheal intubation in the elderly. *Intensive Care Med* 2003;29(9):1451–1455

[21] Ajemian MS, Nirmul GB, Anderson MT, Zirlen DM, Kwasnik EM. Routine fiberoptic endoscopic evaluation of swallowing following prolonged intubation: implications for management. *Arch Surg* 2001;136(4):434–437

[22] de Larminat V, Montravers P, Dureuil B, Desmonts JM. Alteration in swallowing reflex after extubation in intensive care unit patients. *Crit Care Med* 1995;23(3):486–490

[23] Brodsky MB, González-Fernández M, Mendez-Tellez PA, Shanholtz C, Palmer JB, Needham DM. Factors associated with swallowing assessment after oral endotracheal intubation and mechanical ventilation for acute lung injury. *Ann Am Thorac Soc* 2014;11(10):1545–1552

[24] Macht M, Wimbish T, Clark BJ, et al. Diagnosis and treatment of post-extubation dysphagia: results from a national survey. *J Crit Care* 2012;27(6):578–586

[25] Leder SB, Cohn SM, Moller BA. Fiberoptic endoscopic documentation of the high incidence of aspiration following extubation in critically ill trauma patients. *Dysphagia* 1998;13(4):208–212

[26] Brodsky MB, Gellar JE, Dinglas VD, et al. Duration of oral endotracheal intubation is associated with dysphagia symptoms in acute lung injury patients. *J Crit Care* 2014;29(4):574–579

[27] Macht M, King CJ, Wimbish T, et al. Post-extubation dysphagia is associated with longer hospitalization in survivors of critical illness with neurologic impairment. *Crit Care* 2013;17(3):R119

[28] Brodsky MB, Huang M, Shanholtz C, et al. Recovery from dysphagia symptoms after oral endotracheal intubation in acute respiratory distress syndrome survivors. A 5-year longitudinal study. *Ann Am Thorac Soc* 2017;14(3):376–383

[29] Leder SB, Warner HL, Suiter DM, et al. Evaluation of swallow post-extubation: Is it necessary to wait 24 hours? *Ann Otol Rhinol Laryngol* 2019 Mar 6:3489419836115. [Epub ahead of print]

[30] Leder SB, Suiter DM. The Yale Swallow Protocol: An Evidence-Based Approach to Decision Making. New York, NY: Springer; 2014

[31] Hafner G, Neuhuber A, Hirtenfelder S, Schmedler B, Eckel HE. Fiberoptic endoscopic evaluation of swallowing in intensive care unit patients. *Eur Arch Otorhinolaryngol* 2008;*265*(4):441–446

[32] Yu M. Tracheostomy patients on the ward: multiple benefits from a multidisciplinary team? *Crit Care* 2010;*14*(1):109

[33] Cheung NH, Napolitano LM. Tracheostomy: epidemiology, indications, timing, technique, and outcomes. *Respir Care* 2014;*59*(6):895–915, discussion 916–919

[34] Lichtman SW, Birnbaum IL, Sanfilippo MR, Pellicone JT, Damon WJ, King ML. Effect of a tracheostomy speaking valve on secretions, arterial oxygenation, and olfaction: a quantitative evaluation. *J Speech Hear Res* 1995;*38*(3):549–555

[35] Tsikoudas A, Barnes ML, White P. The impact of tracheostomy on the nose. *Eur Arch Otorhinolaryngol* 2011;*268*(7):1005–1008

[36] Sasaki CT, Suzuki M, Horiuchi M, Kirchner JA. The effect of tracheostomy on the laryngeal closure reflex. *Laryngoscope* 1977;*87*(9 Pt 1):1428–1433

[37] Domer AS, Kuhn MA, Belafsky PC. Neurophysiology and clinical implications of the laryngeal adductor reflex. *Curr Otorhinolaryngol Rep* 2013;*1*(3):178–182

[38] Nishino T, Yonezawa T, Honda Y. Effects of swallowing on the pattern of continuous respiration in human adults. *Am Rev Respir Dis* 1985;*132*(6):1219–1222

[39] Paydarfar D, Gilbert RJ, Poppel CS, Nassab PF. Respiratory phase resetting and airflow changes induced by swallowing in humans. *J Physiol* 1995;*483*(Pt 1):273–288

[40] Terzi N, Orlikowski D, Aegerter P, et al. Breathing-swallowing interaction in neuromuscular patients: a physiological evaluation. *Am J Respir Crit Care Med* 2007;*175*(3):269–276

[41] Eibling DE, Gross RD. Subglottic air pressure: a key component of swallowing efficiency. *Ann Otol Rhinol Laryngol* 1996;*105*(4):253–258

[42] Gross RD, Atwood CW Jr, Grayhack JP, Shaiman S. Lung volume effects on pharyngeal swallowing physiology. *J Appl Physiol (1985)* 2003;*95*(6):2211–2217

[43] Gross RD, Mahlmann J, Grayhack JP. Physiologic effects of open and closed tracheostomy tubes on the pharyngeal swallow. *Ann Otol Rhinol Laryngol* 2003;*112*(2):143–152

[44] Muz J, Mathog RH, Nelson R, Jones LA Jr. Aspiration in patients with head and neck cancer and tracheostomy. *Am J Otolaryngol* 1989;*10*(4):282–286

[45] Muz J, Hamlet S, Mathog R, Farris R. Scintigraphic assessment of aspiration in head and neck cancer patients with tracheostomy. *Head Neck* 1994;*16*(1):17–20

[46] Logemann JA, Pauloski BR, Colangelo L. Light digital occlusion of the tracheostomy tube: a pilot study of effects on aspiration and biomechanics of the swallow. *Head Neck* 1998;*20*(1):52–57

[47] Dettelbach MA, Gross RD, Mahlmann J, Eibling DE. Effect of the Passy-Muir valve on aspiration in patients with tracheostomy. *Head Neck* 1995;*17*(4):297–302

[48] Suiter DM, McCullough GH, Powell PW. Effects of cuff deflation and one-way tracheostomy speaking valve placement on swallow physiology. *Dysphagia* 2003;*18*(4):284–292

[49] Gross R, Dettelbach M, Eibling D, Zajac D. Measurement of subglottic air pressure during swallowing in a patient with tracheostomy. *Otolaryngol Head Neck Surg* 1994;*111*(2):133

[50] Bonanno PC. Swallowing dysfunction after tracheostomy. *Ann Surg* 1971;*174*(1):29–33

[51] Terk AR, Leder SB, Burrell MI. Hyoid bone and laryngeal movement dependent upon presence of a tracheotomy tube. *Dysphagia* 2007;*22*(2):89–93

[52] Leder SB, Ross DA. Confirmation of no causal relationship between tracheotomy and aspiration status: a direct replication study. *Dysphagia* 2010;*25*(1):35–39

[53] Leder SB, Ross DA. Investigation of the causal relationship between tracheotomy and aspiration in the acute care setting. *Laryngoscope* 2000;*110*(4):641–644

[54] Cameron JL, Reynolds J, Zuidema GD. Aspiration in patients with tracheostomies. *Surg Gynecol Obstet* 1973;*136*(1):68–70

[55] Thompson-Henry S, Braddock B. The modified Evan's blue dye procedure fails to detect aspiration in the tracheostomized patient: five case reports. *Dysphagia* 1995;*10*(3):172–174

[56] Donzelli J, Brady S, Wesling M, Craney M. Simultaneous modified Evans blue dye procedure and video nasal endoscopic evaluation of the swallow. *Laryngoscope* 2001;*111*(10):1746–1750

[57] Brady SL, Hildner CD, Hutchins BF. Simultaneous videofluoroscopic swallow study and modified Evans blue dye procedure: An evaluation of blue dye visualization in cases of known aspiration. *Dysphagia* 1999;*14*(3):146–149

[58] Belafsky PC, Blumenfeld L, LePage A, Nahrstedt K. The accuracy of the modified Evan's blue dye test in predicting aspiration. *Laryngoscope* 2003;*113*(11):1969–1972

[59] Winklmaier U, Wüst K, Plinkert PK, Wallner F. The accuracy of the modified Evans blue dye test in detecting aspiration in head and neck cancer patients. *Eur Arch Otorhinolaryngol* 2007;*264*(9):1059–1064

[60] Leder SB. Incidence and type of aspiration in acute care patients requiring mechanical ventilation via a new tracheotomy. *Chest* 2002;*122*(5):1721–1726

[61] Elpern EH, Borkgren Okonek M, Bacon M, Gerstung C, Skrzynski M. Effect of the Passy-Muir tracheostomy speaking valve on pulmonary aspiration in adults. *Heart Lung* 2000;*29*(4):287–293

[62] Leder SB. Effect of a one-way tracheotomy speaking valve on the incidence of aspiration in previously aspirating patients with tracheotomy. *Dysphagia* 1999;*14*(2):73–77

[63] Stachler RJ, Hamlet SL, Choi J, Fleming S. Scintigraphic quantification of aspiration reduction with the Passy-Muir valve. *Laryngoscope* 1996;*106*(2 Pt 1):231–234

[64] Leder SB, Tarro JM, Burrell MI. Effect of occlusion of a tracheotomy tube on aspiration. *Dysphagia* 1996;*11*(4):254–258

# 24 Dysphagia in Esophageal Disease

*Caryn Easterling and Reza Shaker*

## Summary

This chapter covers information related to esophageal structure and function, as well as common disorders of the esophagus and tools that are used to assess esophageal function. Although speech-language pathologists are not directly involved in the treatment of esophageal diseases or dysfunction, knowledge about the esophagus and its functions/dysfunctions is important. Food and liquid boluses traverse the oral cavity and pharynx before entering the esophagus. Because of the anatomical connection of the pharynx to the esophagus, dysfunction in the esophagus has the potential to impact pharyngeal function and vice versa. The American Speech-Language-Hearing Association (ASHA) "Guidelines for Speech-Language Pathologists Performing Videofluoroscopic Swallowing Studies" (ASHA, 2004) states, "Clinicians should be aware that oropharyngeal swallowing function is often altered in patients with esophageal motility disorders and dysphagia. Speech-language pathologists (SLPs) have knowledge and skills to recognize patient signs and symptoms associated with esophageal phase dysphagia." The purpose of a swallow evaluation is to relate the patient's symptoms to function. When the patient's symptoms do not correlate to findings on assessment of oropharyngeal swallow function, it is important to consider esophageal dysfunction as a possible culprit. Speech-language pathologists should possess sufficient knowledge about the esophagus to recognize when referral for further assessment is indicated.

## Keywords

esophageal disorders, esophageal dysphagia, esophageal evaluation, esophageal testing, 24-hour pH probe, multichannel intraluminal impedance

### Learning Objectives

- Understand successful esophageal bolus transit as well as how a bolus may be impeded through the esophagus in health and disease
- Understand the dynamic mechanism of the upper and lower esophageal sphincters and how each sphincter interacts with changes that occur in the esophageal body, pharynx, and larynx
- Understand why specific instrumentation is used in differential diagnosis of esophageal disorders

## 24.1 Introduction

This chapter provides the reader with a basic understanding of esophageal anatomy and physiology and an introduction to some of the many reflexes that enable coordination of esophageal function with that of the pharynx, larynx, upper esophageal sphincter, and lower esophageal sphincter during deglutition. Common disorders of the esophagus and the treatments used for the disorders are discussed. The chapter also describes several instrumental techniques currently used to differentially diagnose esophageal disorders and discusses the diagnostic yield to be expected from each technique.

A swallowing specialist should be aware of dysphagia symptoms that are a result of oropharyngeal disorders as well as those resulting from esophageal disorders. This chapter provides an understanding of why the patient's history, symptoms, and instrumental examination are crucial in determining a differential diagnosis of an oropharyngeal or esophageal disorder. Oropharyngeal and esophageal disorders may coexist, which can confound diagnosis, treatment, and management. During the course of evaluation of a patient with dysphagia, the speech-language pathologist (SLP) may uncover evidence of an esophageal disorder and be in a position to recommend appropriate referrals. Certain treatments for oropharyngeal conditions can exacerbate problems of esophageal dysphagia; the converse is also possible. Finally, recognition of the presence of an esophageal problem may help lead to the diagnosis of a previously unsuspected systemic disease, which may have implications for oropharyngeal functions. These reasons support the swallowing specialist's use of a team approach for this multifactorial problem involving many physical systems.

## 24.2 Anatomy and Physiology of the Esophagus

The esophagus is a muscular tube that is collapsed when not swallowing. During swallowing, the esophagus moves a bolus from the upper esophageal sphincter (UES) to the lower esophageal sphincter (LES) via peristalsis. Primary peristalsis is initiated by a swallow, whereas secondary peristalsis is initiated by esophageal distension, resulting in esophageal clearance. The esophagus is 18 to 26 centimeters in length depending on the size of the individual. During a swallow, the esophageal lumen is able to expand to 2 cm in diameter to accommodate food boluses. The esophageal wall is 2–4 mm thick at rest[1] and consists of four layers: mucosa, submucosa, muscularis propria, and adventitia.[2] The proximal one-fourth of the esophagus, including the UES, is composed of striated muscle, whereas the distal half is smooth muscle. The midportion of the esophageal body is composed of both striated and smooth muscle that, when evaluated manometrically, produces lower peristaltic pressure amplitudes than the proximal and mid- to distal portions of the esophageal body.[3] The esophageal musculature consists of external longitudinal muscle fibers, whereas the inner layer consists of circular muscle fibers. These fibers course from the inferior pharyngeal constrictor to the LES.[2] The contraction of the longitudinal and circular muscles produces the peristaltic pressure wave that moves the bolus from the proximal to the distal esophagus. Primary peristaltic pressure contraction is influenced by bolus size, viscosity, temperature, and body position, produces pressure amplitude ranging from 30 to 150 mm HG, and lasts from 3 to 7 seconds.[4,5,6] The esophagus sensory capacity is maintained by vagal and spinal sensory innervations.[6] The vagus nerve supports motor innervations of the esophagus and allows primary peristaltic pressure waves.[7]

## 24.3 The Upper and Lower Esophageal Sphincters

The upper and lower esophageal sphincters are distinguished from the esophageal body by their manometrically defined high-pressure zone, which is appreciated through manometric evaluation and analysis. These sphincters protect the esophageal body from air and bolus flow in and out of the esophagus.

The UES is bounded by the posterior surface of the thyroid and cricoid cartilages. The sphincter is composed of the cricopharyngeus (CP), the inferior pharyngeal constrictor (IPC), and the cranial cervical esophagus. The CP is striated muscle that arises from the inferior part of the dorsolateral aspect of the cricoid cartilage and forms a horizontal loop to attach to the cricoid cartilage on the opposite side. The CP is made up of predominantly type 1 slow-twitch muscle fibers. Additionally, the CP includes some fast-twitch type 2 glycolytic muscle fibers and connective tissue. The combination of muscle fibers and connective tissue may enable the UES to maintain contractile tone over prolonged periods as well as exhibit rapid contraction following swallowing.[8] These muscles maintain UES tone; however, only the CP contracts and relaxes with the UES during all physiological states.[9] The UES high-pressure zone is 2–4 cm in length and is located at the juncture of the hypopharynx and the cervical esophagus, or about 1 cm below the level of the vocal cords and adjacent to the C5–C6 vertebrae.[10] Motor innervation to the UES is provided by the pharyngeal plexus and the recurrent laryngeal nerve. The glossopharyngeal nerve and superior laryngeal nerve provide sensory innervation. Motor neuron control of the cricopharyngeus muscle is ipsilateral within the nucleus ambiguus of the medulla, and the excitatory neurotransmitter is acetylcholine.

The UES at rest sustains high pressure to maintain closure and prevent retrograde entry of digestive tract refluxate or air from entering the airway. The UES pressure varies and is changed by speech, emotion, neck position, sleep, and medications.[10] The UES, unlike the LES, is not affected postprandially.[11] Focal distension of the esophagus can result in UES contraction, and diffuse distension of the esophageal body can cause UES relaxation. Body posture has been found to affect UES response to esophageal distension; that is, UES contraction is the predominant response to water distension if a person is in the supine position, whereas air distension of the esophagus will produce UES relaxation.[12]

During a swallow, the UES opens for approximately 300–600 ms. The UES opens because of a combination of relaxation or inhibition of tone, anterior traction force, distensibility of the sphincter, and intrabolus pressure. The UES relaxation begins during UES elevation, achieves maximum sphincter opening, and finally reaches maximum relaxation in less than 0.1 second.[13]

The LES and the crural diaphragm are attached by the phrenoesophageal ligament. Because of this attachment, the LES and crural diaphragm move together with inspiration and expiration. The movement of the two structures separates when the longitudinal muscle of the esophagus contracts during peristalsis and transient LES relaxation.[14]

The high-pressure zone, or the intraluminal pressure at the esophagogastric junction (EGJ), is a measure of the strength or pressure of the sphincter mechanism. This high-pressure zone results from a combination of the strength of the smooth muscles of the LES and the skeletal muscles of the crural diaphragm. The length of the high-pressure zone is 3.5–4 cm. The crural diaphragm is about 2 cm in length and encircles the proximal 2 cm of the high-pressure zone.[15]

The vagus nerve is the major motor nerve of the esophagus and the LES. The afferent innervation is supplied by vagal and spinal afferents.

## 24.4 Esophageal Reflexes

There are several reflex mechanisms that allow coordination of the esophageal function with that of the pharynx, larynx, UES, and LES. The reflexes are stimulated by esophageal distension and result in clearance of the esophagus as well as act as protection for the respiratory tract from effects of gastric contents. Primary esophageal reflexes include secondary peristalsis, esophago-LES relaxation, esophago-UES contraction, esophago-UES relaxation, and esophagoglottal closure reflexes.[16] These reflexes are activated in response to certain stimuli, such as distention or surface contact. There are nine response mechanisms resulting in clearance of the pharynx and esophagus, such as the reflexive pharyngeal swallow and secondary esophageal peristalsis. There are also response mechanism reflexes that accentuate upper esophageal pressure, thus enhancing the barrier between the upper aerodigestive tract and the esophagus: the esophago-UES, pharyngo-UES, and laryngo-UES contractile reflexes. Additionally, response mechanisms induce glottal closure, such as the esophagoglottal closure reflex, pharyngoglottal closure reflex, and laryngolaryngeal reflex. The effects of combinations of these mechanisms help to prevent pharyngeal reflux and laryngeal aspiration of swallowed and reflux materials.[17]

## 24.5 Disorders of the Esophagus

Disruption of bolus transport from the proximal to the distal esophagus can occur because of motor abnormalities or structural changes of the esophageal body, the UES, and/or the LES.

Motor disorders characteristically present as intermittent, slow but progressive difficulty swallowing liquids and solids. Motor abnormalities include achalasia, diffuse esophageal spasm, scleroderma esophagus, and nonspecific motility disorders.

*Achalasia* means "failure to relax," which describes the primary characteristic of this disorder, that is, inconsistent and incomplete relaxation of the LES accompanied by aperistalsis of the esophagus (**Fig. 24.1**). A characteristic "bird beak" appearance of the LES is seen when one is evaluating achalasia with a barium esophagogram (**Fig. 24.2**). The lack of relaxation of the LES creates

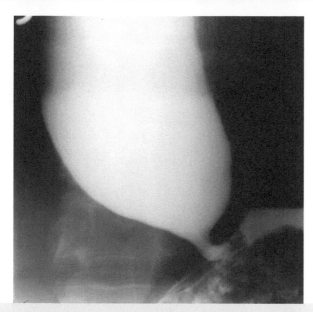

**Fig. 24.1** An example of the aperistaltic esophageal body dilatation, commonly seen in long-standing idiopathic achalasia.

a functional outflow obstruction. Three classifications have been established by the Northwestern Group: type I, classic achalasia (impaired relaxation with esophageal dilation and negligible esophageal pressurization); type II, esophageal pressurization; and type III, vigorous achalasia with spastic contractions of the distal esophageal segment.[18] Dysphagia gradually worsens and is ever present with liquids and solids (**Fig. 24.3**).

Therapy to relieve patient symptoms, improve esophageal emptying, and prevent development of megaesophagus includes dilation of the LES and myotomy. Pharmacological agents, including calcium channel blockers and botulinum toxin, are also used but with less effective elimination of patient symptoms. The most successful outcomes have been when multiple modalities have been employed.[19]

*Diffuse esophageal spasm* includes several manometrically identified classifications of abnormal esophageal peristaltic pressure waves. The pressure waves can be simultaneous intermittent contractions of greater than 3 mm Hg amplitude, representing at least 20% of all swallows with a normal LES profile.[20] Manometric findings do not always correspond with the patient's dysphagia symptoms. Radiographic findings may show a normal esophagram with some disruption of peristalsis and an appearance of "corkscrew" esophagus.[21] Medications can be used in conjunction with behavioral therapy to diminish patient symptoms.

Nutcracker esophagus (NE) is characterized by increased mean distal esophageal amplitude greater than 180 mm Hg and greater than 6 seconds' duration with normal peristalsis and normal LES profile in most patients. However, incomplete LES relaxation can occur in NE.[20] If gastroesophageal reflux disease (GERD) is present, medications are prescribed to alleviate acid exposure. Myotomy may also be performed with successful patient outcomes.[22]

GERD has been associated with spastic esophageal disorders. Therefore, patients with spastic esophageal disorders may also benefit from a pH probe evaluation for GERD.[23]

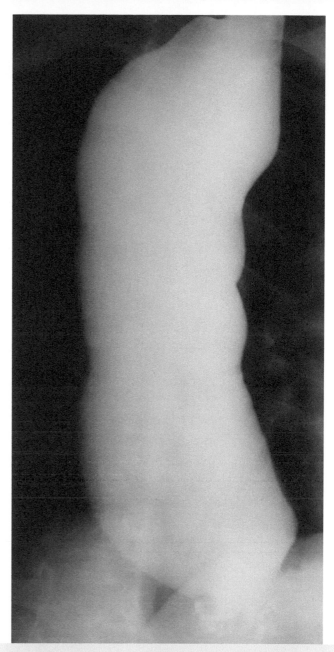

**Fig. 24.2** An example of the bird beak narrowing representing the spastic lower esophageal sphincter in achalasia. Note aperistaltic esophageal body dilatation, commonly seen in long-standing idiopathic achalasia.

*Scleroderma*, a systemic disease without known cause, is characterized by functional and structural changes in small blood vessels and development of fibrosis of the skin and internal organs. Dysphagia is common is patients with scleroderma. The disease can result in changes to salivary gland function, voice changes, limited mouth opening, and limitations in mastication.[24] Esophageal dysphagia is common and is characterized by a dilated esophagus and patulous but narrow LES, resulting in frequent reflux events[25] (**Fig. 24.4**). Treatment is focused on relieving the patient's symptoms with medications.

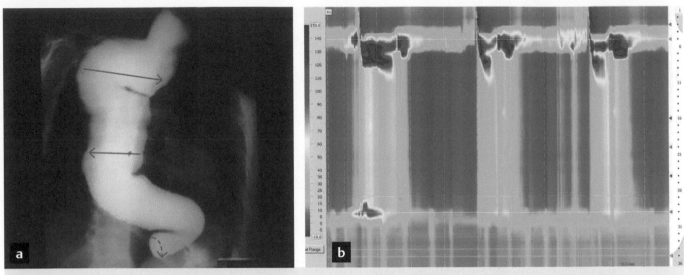

**Fig. 24.3** Examples of **(a)** radiographic and **(b)** manometric features of idiopathic achalasia. Note the dilatation of the esophageal body (straight arrow) and bird beak narrowing of the lower esophageal sphincter (LES, broken arrow) in the radiographic image, and the absence of LES relaxation and esophageal peristalsis in the manometric recording displayed as a contour plot of the pressures.

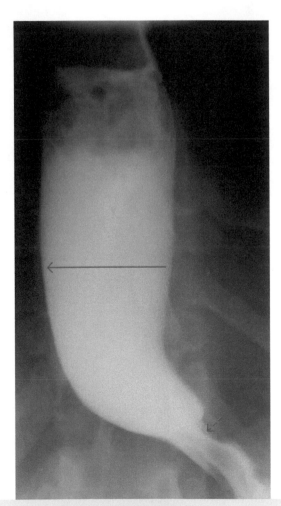

**Fig. 24.4** An example of scleroderma esophagus. Note dilated aperistaltic distal esophagus (straight arrow) and fixed mild stricture of lower esophageal sphincter (broken arrow).

Structural lesions of the esophagus usually cause solid food dysphagia. Structural abnormalities include strictures, rings, and webs; esophageal carcinoma; and extrinsic compression of the esophagus.

## 24.5.1 Strictures

Strictures are most commonly related to reflux but can be caused by radiation, pill impaction, ingestion of caustic chemicals, and malignancy.

Peptic esophageal strictures are the most common type of stricture, accounting for 70–80% of strictures. They are found in the distal esophagus at the squamocolumnar junction, the junction between the squamous epithelium and the columnar epithelium at the gastroesophageal junction. They are caused by exposure to refluxate. Peptic strictures are smooth on the mucosal surface and are less than 1–8 cm in length.[26] Conditions predisposing to peptic strictures include untreated GERD; scleroderma; nonsteroidal anti-inflammatory drugs (NSAIDs, e.g., ibuprofen or aspirin); and prolonged nasogastric-tube feeding.[27] There is an association. Strictures form when peptic acid exposure causes injury or inflammation of the mucosal lining of the esophagus (**Fig. 24.5**). The changes that occur to the esophageal mucosa result in esophageal narrowing. Over time, without the use of acid-suppressing medications, the mucosa, muscle, and eventually the intrinsic innervations to the esophagus undergo permanent changes, that is, esophageal narrowing and esophageal wall thickening, shortening, and fibrosis.[28] Treatment of strictures may include lifestyle modifications and medication for control of GERD. The main treatments to improve dysphagia are dilation and corticosteroid injection to the stricture.[29] Although less prevalent than peptic strictures, strictures may also be caused by caustic injection and radiation injury (**Fig. 24.6**). Treatment of all types of strictures is dilation with bougies or balloon dilators. Strictures caused by radiation may be longer, tortuous, and of small diameter. These

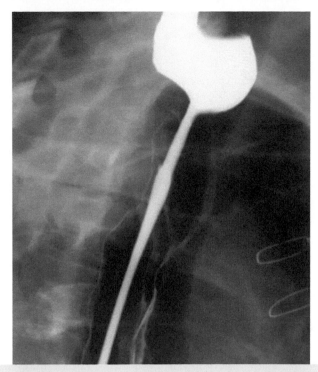

**Fig. 24.6** Long esophageal caustic stricture developed after ingestion of drain cleaner containing sodium hydroxide.

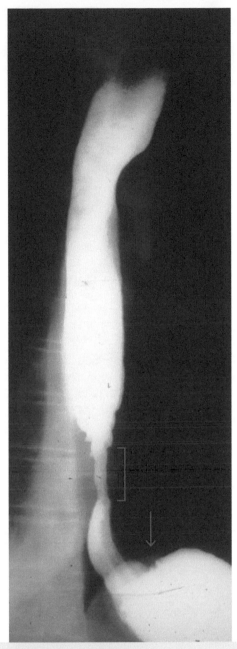

**Fig. 24.5** An example of distal esophageal peptic stricture (bracket) in the presence of a hiatal hernia (arrow).

types of strictures have had favorable outcomes after the placement of self-expanding stents.[30]

## 24.5.2 Rings

Esophageal rings are composed of squamous mucosa and columnar epithelium and are located in the distal esophagus at the gastroesophageal junction. They are smooth and thin in structure and are less than 4 mm in length. The etiology of rings, such as the Schatzki or B ring, is unknown; however, there does appear to be an association between GERD and the development of rings. The Schatzki ring composition does not include muscle tissue and, therefore, will not alter esophageal peristalsis. The A ring, which is less commonly found, does involve the muscular layer of the esophagus and is characterized by muscle hypertrophy and will thus alter esophageal peristalsis. The A ring changes occur 2 cm above the gastroesophageal junction.[31,32] Patients who are symptomatic with esophageal dysphagia typically complain of intermittent and inconsistent solid food dysphagia (**Fig. 24.7**). They report symptoms in the neck area, sternal notch, and midchest area[33] Treatment for esophageal rings is dilation and acid suppression medications. Patients with rings need to be monitored for recurrence of symptoms and may require repeated dilations.

## 24.5.3 Webs

Webs that occur in the esophagus are membranous structures that are not circumferential but do narrow the esophageal lumen. Esophageal webs are thin and superficial and are found in the proximal esophagus, commonly on the anterior wall of the post-cricoid area (**Fig. 24.8**). However, webs can be found throughout the esophagus as in Plummer–Vinson's syndrome, which is a condition that occurs in individuals with chronic iron deficiency anemia resulting in formation of multiple esophageal webs. Webs can be symptomatic but are often asymptomatic findings during a videofluoroscopic swallow study or esophagram. A patient who has a symptomatic web may complain of solid food sticking in the cervical area or have symptoms of nasopharyngeal reflux or oropharyngeal regurgitation. Treatment of symptomatic webs includes dilation and laser therapy.[34]

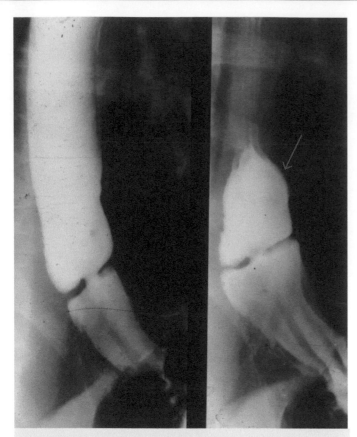

**Fig. 24.7** Impacted marshmallow (arrow) in a Schatzki ring during a marshmallow challenge.

## 24.6 Eosinophilic Esophagitis

Eosinophilic esophagitis (EoE) affects all ages but is more prevalent in males than females. EoE presents as a chronic, immune, antigen-mediated esophageal disease with eosinophilic inflammation.[35] The exact pathogenesis is poorly understood. Eosinophils are white blood cells that are typically not present in the esophagus. In EoE, large numbers of eosinophils are found in the esophageal tissue. EoE is thought to be multifaceted because it involves exposure to food or aero allergens and genetic factors.[36,37] The inflammation that occurs in the esophageal lining causes swelling and luminal compromise, resulting in esophageal solid food dysphagia. Over time, if the condition is undiagnosed and untreated, it will lead to fibrosis and permanent esophageal narrowing, with possible stricturing and ring formation.[38] Food impaction is common in EoE patients with esophageal narrowing and ring formation. Patients may also complain of heartburn and retrosternal pain, especially when consuming liquids with high acidity.[39] Diagnosis requires esophageal endoscopy (esophagoduodenoscopy [EGD]) with biopsies of the esophagus showing excessive eosinophil-mediated inflammation (**Fig. 24.9**). Typical EGD findings may include corrugated rings, furrows, white exudates, and friability of the esophageal mucosa. However, some individuals with

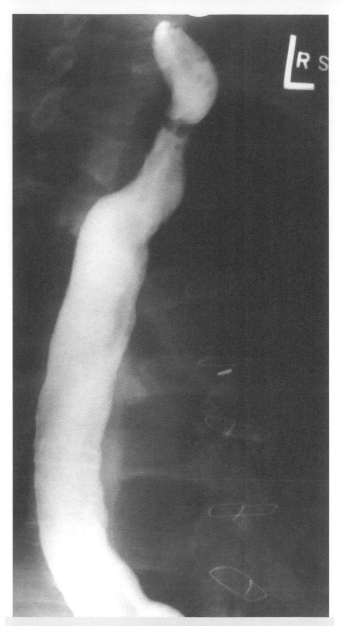

**Fig. 24.8** Esophageal webs are thin and superficial located in the proximal esophagus commonly on the anterior wall of the postcricoid area.

EoE may have a normal-appearing esophagus and require a biopsy pathology report to confirm the diagnosis.[36] A contrast esophagogram is seldom helpful to diagnose EoE unless there has been significant luminal narrowing and compromise.[40] Treatment for solid dysphagia may require successive dilations[41] and treatment with empirical acid suppression trials.[42] The condition has demonstrated treatment response to dietary exclusion and topical aerosolized steroids to treat the inflammatory component accompanied with dilation treating the structural change to improve dysphagia.

## 24.7 Instrumental Evaluation of Esophageal Disorders

Common instrumental modalities employed to diagnose esophageal dysphagia include EGD, barium esophagram, esophageal manometry, pH monitoring, and multichannel intraluminal impedance testing.

## 24.8 Esophagoduodenoscopy

EGD is performed under conscious sedation to evaluate the mucosa, structure, and function of the esophagus, stomach, and duodenum. The EGD employs a flexible videoendoscope 9–10 mm in diameter that allows the clinician to biopsy and perform dilations. When the stomach and duodenum do not need to be examined, a transnasal esophagoscopy (TNE) can be performed. Both the EGD and the TNE are performed to evaluate patients with reflux, dysphagia, head and neck cancer, and esophageal pathology. The TNE does not require conscious sedation and enables the clinician to acquire biopsies when appropriate as well as evaluate supraesophageal regions.[43,44] The TNE is done in the office, reducing the patient's procedure cost and time from daily responsibilities.

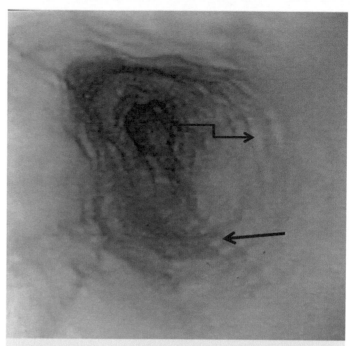

**Fig. 24.9** Diagnosis of eosiniphillic esophagitis requires esophageal endoscopy (esophagoduodensocopy [EGD]) with biopsies of the esophagus showing excessive eosinophil-mediated inflammation.

## 24.9 Esophagogram

The barium esophagogram is the radiographic technique used to evaluate patients with dysphagia, symptoms of obstructive structural disorders, gastroesophageal reflux, motility disorders, esophageal spasm, achalasia, and other esophageal diseases. The esophagogram is most useful in identifying anatomical alterations of the esophagus, such as strictures, webs, and rings, as well as hiatal hernias and in evaluation of esophageal motor function and esophageal clearance. An esophagogram is performed with the patient in upright, prone, upright oblique, and recumbent positions. The patient is given high-density barium and low-density barium to define the mucosal relief of the esophagus. The patient also ingests effervescent crystals followed by high-density barium in order to distend the esophagus. The distended view allows the radiologist to appreciate the contour and profile of the esophagus while the collapsed or partially collapsed views show the longitudinal folds and structure. The radiologist then is able to examine the gastric cardia, which is identified by three or four stellate folds radiating to the central point at the gastroesophageal junction. The patient is given low-density barium and observed in the right anterior oblique position while taking single swallows in order to observe esophageal motility. The esophagus is then imaged while the patient is on the right lateral position in order to observe spontaneous gastroesophageal reflux while performing a Valsalva maneuver.[45]

## 24.10 Manometry

Esophageal manometry measures pressure phenomena at multiple sites in the esophagus, interpretation of which provides assessment of esophageal sphincters, esophageal muscle function, and peristalsis. What is now termed high-resolution manometry (HRM) was introduced in the 1990s by Clouse and colleagues as a 21-sensor system (with sensors 1 cm apart) that recorded pressures via circumferentially oriented transducers on the perimeter of the catheter. The pressures were interpreted by a dedicated software program that generated three-dimensional topographic contour plots that represented esophageal motor function.[46] Today, this technique uses as many as 96 high-fidelity circumferential solid-state sensors incorporated into a flexible motility catheter producing topographic contour plots.

The use of water-perfused manometry and solid-state unidirectional sensor catheters to measure UES pressure has been unsuccessful due to less than adequate fidelity and inability to capture the radial asymmetry of the UES and the superior excursion during the swallow.[47] The catheter pressure recordings are captured by software that displays in vivid color the pressure data as topographic plots of distance and time on vertical and horizontal axes. Manometry may be used in the pharynx, UES, and LES to determine the location of the sphincters for placement of pH probes; determine intrabolus pressure values; determine UES resting and relaxation pressure; correlate UES pressure and patient symptoms in response to stimuli; and determine effectiveness of therapeutic interventions on pharyngeal response and UES. The use of HRM to measure UES pressure should be approached cautiously at this time because there are no gold standards or consensus criteria to correlate UES pressures determined by HRM with a particular diagnosis. Databases of UES pressures for all age groups need to be established in order to determine abnormal pressure representation. UES pressure is affected by age,[48] and the largest reported data set available contains data for individuals under age 50 years.[3] UES pressure can be affected by changes in neck position,[49] and duration of UES relaxation is altered by bolus size swallowed. The HRM catheters are unable to determine a unilateral defect in UES function because of the radially arranged sensors yielding a single pressure reading that averages the values from the sensors at a particular location.[50] This sensor design is appropriate for the esophagus and LES versus the asymmetrical UES, which moves during swallowing. The parameters most evaluated are baseline UES pressure, UES relaxation time, nadir pressure during UES relaxation, UES coordination with pharyngeal contraction, amplitude of pharyngeal contraction, and intrabolus pressure.

Esophageal HRM is used to evaluate esophageal peristalsis by providing the shape, amplitude, and duration of esophageal contractions. Esophageal manometry can also provide the UES and LES resting and nadir pressure and the timing of sphincter relaxation in relation to pharyngeal and esophageal contractions. The manometric catheter is placed transnasally and measures the esophageal contractions shown as pressure values in vivid colors. The Chicago Classification of esophageal motility disorders uses an algorithmic scheme to analyze clinical high-resolution manometry studies. The Chicago Classification is an updated analysis scheme for clinical esophageal HRM recordings developed by the International HRM Working Group. This group uses a hierarchical approach sequentially prioritizing the following: disorders of esophagogastric junction (EGJ) outflow; major disorders of peristalsis, such as absent contractility, distal esophageal spasm, hypercontractile esophagus; and minor disorders of peristalsis characterized by impaired bolus transit. The group has also defined the evaluation of the EGJ at rest morphology and contractility, "fragmented contractions," and ineffective esophageal motility.[51]

Manometry is used to define the location of the UES and LES in order to place pH probes for 24-hour monitoring. Additionally, manometry is used prior to antireflux surgery to document esophageal peristalsis.[52]

## 24.11 24-Hour pH Probe

pH monitoring is commonly used for patients who have symptoms of GERD that have not responded to antisecretory therapy, and as a medical follow-up to assess the efficacy of a prescribed treatment or surgery. pH monitoring results can enhance the clinician's understanding of reflux events and their correlation with patient symptoms and can direct further care. The results of 24-hour probe placement will quantitatively discern whether there is partial acid suppression and the presence of non–acid reflux as well as whether there is no acid reflux present.

## 24.12 Multichannel Intraluminal Impedance

Impedance devices measure the changes in resistance to electrical current across electrodes. Silny described the use of the multichannel intraluminal impedance device and procedure designed to measure changes in resistance to bolus presentation within the esophageal lumen.[53] The impedance system is able to recognize the transit of different bolus types (gas, liquid, or mixed) because each produces a signature current resistance as it passes the electrodes placed 2 cm apart on the transnasally placed catheter. In addition, when combined with concurrent pH monitoring, the impedance device can distinguish acid from nonacid events and improve the sensitivity of the evaluation. Use of combined pH and impedance testing for reflux events quantifies these events and enables the clinician to categorize the events for analysis into acid, weakly acid, and weakly alkaline reflux events.[54,55] Combined multichannel intraluminal impedance and pH probe testing is thought to be the most sensitive tool to measure reflux events[56,57,58] and correlate with patient symptoms.[55]

Multichannel intraluminal impedance has been used to describe bolus transit patterns in healthy subjects and in patients with mild esophagitis,[59,60] and when combined with manometry it provides monitoring of bolus transit patterns, esophageal clearance, and relaxation of the LES without use of radiographic imaging.[61]

## 24.13 Questions

1. The upper esophageal sphincter

A. resting pressure is affected after a meal like the lower esophageal sphincter.

B. resting pressure is unchanged by speech, neck position, sleep, medications, and emotion.

C. opens because of a combination of relaxation, anterior traction force, dispensability of the sphincter, and intrabolus pressure.

D. is a high-pressure zone that is maintained by hyolaryngeal elevation during the swallow.

E. receives sensory and motor innervation from the glossopharyngeal nerve.

2. The primary esophageal reflexes that coordinate the esophageal and pharyngeal, laryngeal, UES, and lower esophageal sphincter (LES) function are

A. not activated by surface esophageal mechanoreceptors sensitive to surface contact and distention.

B. those that decrease UES pressure enhancing the barrier between the upper aerodigestive tract and the esophagus.

C. mechanisms that allow refluxate into the pharynx.

D. stimulated by esophageal distension and result in clearance of the esophagus as well as protect the respiratory tract from the effects of the presence of gastric contents.

E. apt to disrupt the safe and successful transport of a swallowed bolus.

**3.** Esophageal motor disorders characteristically

A. include esophageal strictures.
B. present as intermittent, slow but progressive difficulty swallowing liquids and solids, with abnormality in peristaltic pressure wave profile.
C. appear as a "bird beak" shape at the LES.
D. are strictures, webs, and rings.
E. appear the same when using radiographic imaging or manometry for differential diagnosis.

**4.** Differential diagnosis of esophageal disorders is

A. best achieved with a combination of radiographic imaging and pH monitoring techniques.
B. best achieved using multichannel intraluminal impedance (MII).
C. best achieved using a barium esophagogram.
D. an evaluation of the UES pressure, relaxation time, nadir pressure during relaxation, and the coordination of relaxation with pharyngeal contraction and intrabolus pressure.
E. inclusive of one or several of the following instrumental diagnostic tools: barium esophagogram, manometry, 24-hour pH monitoring, MII.

## 24.14 Answers and Explanations

**1. Correct: opens because of a combination of relaxation, anterior traction force, dispensability of the sphincter and intrabolus pressure (C).**
(A) The lower esophageal sphincter pressure is changed postprandially, or after a meal. The pressure changes at that sphincter are protective and rise to protect from reflux of gas, liquid, or solid from entering the esophagus. The upper esophageal sphincter (UES) pressure does not change after a meal. (B) When we speak, change neck position, sleep, become emotional, or take certain medications, the resting pressure of the UES is altered. (D) Sphincteric pressure decreases with hyolaryngeal elevation. UES relaxation begins during UES elevation, achieves maximum sphincteric opening, and reaches maximum relaxation in less than 0.1 second during this period. (E) Sensory innervation is provided by the glossopharyngeal nerve and the superior laryngeal nerve. The pharyngeal plexus and the recurrent laryngeal nerve provide motor innervation.

**2. Correct: stimulated by esophageal distension and result in clearance of the esophagus as well as protect the respiratory tract from the effects of the presence of gastric contents (D).**
This describes the action of the primary esophageal reflexes, which include secondary peristalsis, esophago-LES relaxation, esophago-UES contraction, esophago-UES relaxation, and esophagoglottal closure reflexes. (A) In fact these reflexes are stimulated by esophageal distention and contact with the

esophageal mucosa and react, for example, with a secondary peristaltic wave to clear the esophageal body without activation of a pharyngeal clearing swallow. (B) These reflexes actually increase the upper esophageal pressure to protect or enhance the barrier between the upper aerodigestive tract and the esophagus. (C) These reflexes, in conjunction with the reflexes that enhance glottal closure, such as the esophagoglottal closure reflex, pharyngoglottal closure reflex, and laryngolaryngeal reflex, help to prevent pharyngeal reflux and aspiration of swallowed and reflux materials. (E) These reflexes are protective and stimulate clearance and protective glottal closure if/when a bolus transport is not efficient. The result is that the bolus has a greater chance to reach the stomach without aerodigestive tract misdirection or harm.

**3. Correct: present as intermittent, slow but progressive difficulty swallowing liquids and solids, with abnormality in peristaltic pressure wave profile (B).**
This causes a disruption from the proximal to distal esophagus and can occur because of a motor or bolus movement inefficiency from the proximal to the distal esophagus. (A) Esophageal strictures are classified as structural esophageal disorders because strictures are a result of a change in the structural integrity of the esophageal body from exposure to peptic acid or other irritants over an extended period of time. The stricture causes narrowing and change in the shape and function of the esophagus. (C) The "bird beak" appearance of the LES is a classic presentation of achalasia. The LES has this appearance as the sphincter fails to relax and thus has an appearance of the narrow beak where the LES should be open and relaxed, allowing the bolus to transit to the stomach. Achalasia is only one of many esophageal motor disorders. (D) Strictures, webs, and rings are classified as structural changes of the esophagus. (E) Each of the esophageal motor disorders has a different presentation on radiographic imaging and a distinct manometric pressure profile. Therefore manometry is an appropriate and accurate differential diagnostic tool to use in determining the specific esophageal motor disorder and begin to be able to medically manage and treat the specific disorder.

**4. Correct: inclusive of one or several of the following instrumental diagnostic tools; barium esophagogram, manometry, 24-hour pH monitoring, MII (E).**
(A) Radiographic imaging is used to observe bolus transit and can be used to rule out moderate to advanced motor and structural disorders. The differential confirmation of the diagnosis for motor disorders may be confirmed by following up with a manometric evaluation or, for suspected structural disorders, esophagoduodenoscopy (EGD). pH monitoring is used to quantitatively discern the presence of acid in the esophageal body or pharynx. (B) MII measures changes in resistance to electrical current across electrodes placed within a space, in this case within the esophageal body. Impedance recognizes different bolus consistencies, that is, gas, liquid, or solid, passing through in an antegrade or retrograde direction within the esophagus. Combined MII with pH probe is thought to be the most sensitive diagnostic tool for detecting reflux events and correlating

with a patient's symptoms, so this instrument is best used to define refluxate. (**C**) The barium esophagogram is used to evaluate patients with symptoms of dysphagia, obstructive symptoms, reflux, motility symptoms, suspected esophageal spasm, achalasia, and other esophageal diseases. Although the barium esophagogram is usually the initial examination ordered, it is not sensitive to mild or moderate motility or structural disorders and therefore is coupled with other instrumental examinations, such as EGD or manometry, for a differential diagnosis. (**D**) An evaluation of esophageal disorders includes both the UES and the LES as well as the motor and structural integrity of the esophageal body.

# References

[1] Xia F, Mao J, Ding J, Yang H. Observation of normal appearance and wall thickness of esophagus on CT images. *Eur J Radiol* 2009;72(3):406–411

[2] Sleisenger M, et al. Sleinger and Fordtran's Gastrointestinal and Liver Disease: Pathophysiology, Diagnosis, Management. Philadelphia, PA: Saunders/Elsevier; 2010

[3] Ghosh SK, Janiak P, Schwizer W, Hebbard GS, Brasseur JG. Physiology of the esophageal pressure transition zone: separate contraction waves above and below. *Am J Physiol Gastrointest Liver Physiol* 2006;290(3):G568–G576

[4] Hollis JB, Castell DO. Effect of dry swallows and wet swallows of different volumes on esophageal peristalsis. *J Appl Physiol* 1975;38(6):1161–1164

[5] Dooley CP, Schlossmacher B, Valenzuela JE. Effects of alterations in bolus viscosity on esophageal peristalsis in humans. *Am J Physiol* 1988;254(1 Pt 1):G8–G11

[6] Richter JE, Castell DO. The Esophagus. Oxford, UK: Wiley-Blackwell; 2012

[7] Sengupta JN, Kauvar D, Goyal RK. Characteristics of vagal esophageal tension-sensitive afferent fibers in the opossum. *J Neurophysiol* 1989;61(5):1001–1010

[8] Bonington A, Mahon M, Whitmore I. A histological and histochemical study of the cricopharyngeus muscle in man. *J Anat* 1988;156:27–37

[9] Lang IM, Shaker R. An overview of the upper esophageal sphincter. *Curr Gastroenterol Rep* 2000;2(3):185–190

[10] Massey B. Physiology of oral cavity, pharynx and upper esophageal sphincter. GI Motility Online; 2006

[11] Kahrilas PJ, Dodds WJ, Dent J, Haeberle B, Hogan WJ, Arndorfer RC. Effect of sleep, spontaneous gastroesophageal reflux, and a meal on upper esophageal sphincter pressure in normal human volunteers. *Gastroenterology* 1987;92(2):466–471

[12] Babaei A, Dua K, Naini SR, et al. Response of the upper esophageal sphincter to esophageal distension is affected by posture, velocity, volume, and composition of the infusate. *Gastroenterology* 2012;142(4):734–743.e7

[13] Kahrilas PJ, Dodds WJ, Dent J, Logemann JA, Shaker R. Upper esophageal sphincter function during deglutition. *Gastroenterology* 1988;95(1):52–62

[14] Pandolfino JE, Zhang QG, Ghosh SK, Han A, Boniquit C, Kahrilas PJ. Transient lower esophageal sphincter relaxations and reflux: mechanistic analysis using concurrent fluoroscopy and high-resolution manometry. *Gastroenterology* 2006;131(6):1725–1733

[15] Heine KJ, Mittal RK. Lower esophageal sphincter: how to quantitate? *Gastroenterology* 1992;103(1):346–347

[16] Lang IM, Medda BK, Shaker R. Mechanisms of reflexes induced by esophageal distension. *Am J Physiol Gastrointest Liver Physiol* 2001;281(5):G1246–G1263

[17] Shaker A, Shaker R. Airway protective mechanisms, reciprocal physiology of the deglutitive axis. In: Shaker R, Belafsky PC, Postma N, Easterling C, eds. Principles of Deglutition. New York, NY: Springer; 2013

[18] Pandolfino JE, Kwiatek MA, Nealis T, Bulsiewicz W, Post J, Kahrilas PJ. Achalasia: a new clinically relevant classification by high-resolution manometry. *Gastroenterology* 2008;135(5):1526–1533

[19] Vela MF, Richter JE, Wachsberger D, Connor J, Rice TW. Complexities of managing achalasia at a tertiary referral center: use of pneumatic dilatation, Heller myotomy, and botulinum toxin injection. *Am J Gastroenterol* 2004;99(6):1029–1036

[20] Hoppo T, Jobe B. Surgical treatment of achalasia and spastic esophageal disorders. In: Shaker R, Belafsky PC, Postma N, Easterling C, eds. Principles of Deglutition. New York, NY: Springer; 2013

[21] Hewson EG, Ott DJ, Dalton CB, Chen YM, Wu WC, Richter JE. Manometry and radiology. Complementary studies in the assessment of esophageal motility disorders. *Gastroenterology* 1990;98(3):626–632

[22] Leconte M, Douard R, Gaudric M, Dumontier I, Chaussade S, Dousset B. Functional results after extended myotomy for diffuse oesophageal spasm. *Br J Surg* 2007;94(9):1113–1118

[23] Herbella FA, Raz DJ, Nipomnick I, Patti MG. Primary versus secondary esophageal motility disorders: diagnosis and implications for treatment. *J Laparoendosc Adv Surg Tech A* 2009;19(2):195–198

[24] Rout PG, Hamburger J, Potts AJ. Orofacial radiological manifestations of systemic sclerosis. *Dentomaxillofac Radiol* 1996;25(4):193–196

[25] Ntoumazios SK, Voulgari PV, Potsis K, Koutis E, Tsifetaki N, Assimakopoulos DA. Esophageal involvement in scleroderma: gastroesophageal reflux, the common problem. *Semin Arthritis Rheum* 2006;36(3):173–181

[26] Richter JE. Long-term management of gastroesophageal reflux disease and its complications. *Am J Gastroenterol* 1997;92(4, Suppl)30S–34S, discussion 34S–35S

[27] El-Serag HB, Sonnenberg A. Association of esophagitis and esophageal strictures with diseases treated with nonsteroidal anti-inflammatory drugs. *Am J Gastroenterol* 1997;92(1):52–56

[28] Jeyasingham K. What is the histology of an esophageal stricture before and after dilatation? In: Giuli R, Tytgat G, DeMeester T, eds. The Esophageal Mucosa. Amsterdam, Netherlands: Elsevier Science BB; 1994:335

[29] Altintas E, Kacar S, Tunc B, et al. Intralesional steroid injection in benign esophageal strictures resistant to bougie dilation. *J Gastroenterol Hepatol* 2004;19(12):1388–1391

[30] Oh YS, Kochman ML, Ahmad NA, Ginsberg GG. Clinical outcomes after self-expanding plastic stent placement for refractory benign esophageal strictures. *Dig Dis Sci* 2010;55(5):1344–1348

[31] DeVault KR. Lower esophageal (Schatzki's) ring: pathogenesis, diagnosis and therapy. *Dig Dis* 1996;14(5):323–329

[32] Schatzki R. The lower esophageal ring. Long term follow-up of symptomatic and asymptomatic rings. *Am J Roentgenol Radium Ther Nucl Med* 1963;90:805–810

[33] Smith DF, Ott DJ, Gelfand DW, Chen MY. Lower esophageal mucosal ring: correlation of referred symptoms with radiographic findings using a marshmallow bolus. *AJR Am J Roentgenol* 1998;171(5):1361–1365

[34] Lindgren S. Endoscopic dilatation and surgical myectomy of symptomatic cervical esophageal webs. *Dysphagia* 1991;6(4):235–238

[35] Liacouras CA, Spergel JM, Ruchelli E, et al. Eosinophilic esophagitis: a 10-year experience in 381 children. *Clin Gastroenterol Hepatol* 2005;3(12):1198–1206

[36] Furuta GT, Straumann A. Review article: the pathogenesis and management of eosinophilic oesophagitis. *Aliment Pharmacol Ther* 2006;24(2):173–182

[37] Rothenberg ME. Biology and treatment of eosinophilic esophagitis. *Gastroenterology* 2009;137(4):1238–1249

[38] Lucendo AJ, Arias A, De Rezende LC, et al. Subepithelial collagen deposition, profibrogenic cytokine gene expression, and changes after prolonged fluticasone propionate treatment in adult eosinophilic esophagitis: a prospective study. *J Allergy Clin Immunol* 2011;128(5):1037–1046

[39] Straumann A, Bussmann C, Zuber M, Vannini S, Simon HU, Schoepfer A. Eosinophilic esophagitis: analysis of food impaction and perforation in 251 adolescent and adult patients. *Clin Gastroenterol Hepatol* 2008;6(5):598–600

[40] Shastri N, Vijayapal A, Antonik SJ, et al. Is there a difference when eosinophilic esophagitis (EE) strikes at a later onset in adult life? *Gastro* 2009;136(5):A-282

[41] Vasilopoulos S, Murphy P, Auerbach A, et al. The small-caliber esophagus: an unappreciated cause of dysphagia for solids in patients with eosinophilic esophagitis. *Gastrointest Endosc* 2002;55(1):99–106

[42] Molina-Infante J, Ferrando-Lamana L, Ripoll C, et al. Esophageal eosinophilic infiltration responds to proton pump inhibition in most adults. *Clin Gastroenterol Hepatol* 2011;9(2):110–117

[43] Kumar VV, Amin MR. Evaluation of middle and distal esophageal diverticuli with transnasal esophagoscopy. *Ann Otol Rhinol Laryngol* 2005;114(4):276–278

[44] Shaker R. Unsedated trans-nasal pharyngoesophagogastroduodenoscopy (T-EGD): technique. *Gastrointest Endosc* 1994;40(3):346–348

[45] Laufer I, Levine M. Baruim studies of the upper gastrointestinal tract. In: Gore R, Levine M, eds. Textbook of Gastrointestinal Radiology. Philadelphia, PA: WB Saunders; 2008:311–322

[46] Clouse RE, Staiano A. Topography of the esophageal peristaltic pressure wave. *Am J Physiol* 1991;261(4 Pt 1):G677–G684

[47] Massey BT. The use of intraluminal manometry to assess upper esophageal sphincter function. *Dysphagia* 1993;8(4):339–344

[48] Shaker R, Ren J, Podvrsan B, et al. Effect of aging and bolus variables on pharyngeal and upper esophageal sphincter motor function. *Am J Physiol* 1993;264(3 Pt 1):G427–G432

[49] Takasaki K, Umeki H, Kumagami H, Takahashi H. Influence of head rotation on upper esophageal sphincter pressure evaluated by high-resolution manometry system. *Otolaryngol Head Neck Surg* 2010;*142*(2):214–217

[50] Bardan E, Kern M, Torrico S, Arndorfer RC, Massey BT, Shaker R. Radial asymmetry of the upper oesophageal sphincter pressure profile: fact or artefact. *Neurogastroenterol Motil* 2006;*18*(6):418–424

[51] Kahrilas PJ, Bredenoord AJ, Fox M, et al; International High Resolution Manometry Working Group. The Chicago Classification of esophageal motility disorders, v3.0. *Neurogastroenterol Motil* 2015;*27*(2):160–174

[52] Waring JP, Hunter JG, Oddsdottir M, Wo J, Katz E. The preoperative evaluation of patients considered for laparoscopic antireflux surgery. *Am J Gastroenterol* 1995;*90*(1):35–38

[53] Silny J. Intraluminal multiple electric impedance procedure for measurement of gastrointestinal motility. *J Gastrointest Motil* 1991;*3*:151–162

[54] Sifrim D, Castell D, Dent J, Kahrilas PJ. Gastro-oesophageal reflux monitoring: review and consensus report on detection and definitions of acid, non-acid, and gas reflux. *Gut* 2004;*53*(7):1024–1031

[55] Bredenoord AJ, Weusten BL, Timmer R, Conchillo JM, Smout AJ. Addition of esophageal impedance monitoring to pH monitoring increases the yield of symptom association analysis in patients off PPI therapy. *Am J Gastroenterol* 2006;*101*(3):453–459

[56] Park W, Vaezi MF. Esophageal impedance recording: clinical utility and limitations. *Curr Gastroenterol Rep* 2005;*7*(3):182–189

[57] Sifrim D, Blondeau K. Technology insight: The role of impedance testing for esophageal disorders. *Nat Clin Pract Gastroenterol Hepatol* 2006;*3*(4):210–219

[58] Tutuian R, Castell DO. Review article: complete gastro-oesophageal reflux monitoring - combined pH and impedance. *Aliment Pharmacol Ther* 2006;*24*(Suppl 2):27–37

[59] Imam H, Shay S, Ali A, Baker M. Bolus transit patterns in healthy subjects: a study using simultaneous impedance monitoring, videoesophagram, and esophageal manometry. *Am J Physiol Gastrointest Liver Physiol* 2005;*288*(5):G1000–G1006

[60] Sifrim D, Tutuian R. Oesophageal intraluminal impedance can identify subtle bolus transit abnormalities in patients with mild oesophagitis. *Eur J Gastroenterol Hepatol* 2005;*17*(3):303–305

[61] Savarino E, Tutuian R. Combined multichannel intraluminal impedance and manometry testing. *Dig Liver Dis* 2008;*40*(3):167–173

## Suggested Reading

[1] Babaei A, Venu M, Naini SR, et al. Impaired upper esophageal sphincter reflexes in patients with supraesophageal reflux disease. *Gastroenterology* 2015;*149*(6):1381–1391

[2] Dua KS, Surapaneni SN, Kuribayashi S, Hafeezullah M, Shaker R. Effect of aging on hypopharyngeal safe volume and the aerodigestive reflexes protecting the airways. *Laryngoscope* 2014;*124*(8):1862–1868

[3] Easterling C, Shaker R. UES opening muscle dysfunction. In: Shaker R, Belafsky PC, Postma GN, Easterling C, eds. Principles of Deglutition: A Multidisciplinary Text for Swallowing and Its Disorders. New York, NY: Springer; 2013:529–538

[4] Jadcherla SR. Nascent eophagus, sensory-motor physiology during maturation. In: Shaker R, Belafsky PC, Postma GN, Easterling C, eds. Principles of Deglutition: A Multidisciplinary Text for Swallowing and Its Disorders. New York, NY: Springer; 2013:295–302

[5] Lacy BE, Weiser K, Chertoff J, et al. The diagnosis of gastroesophageal reflux disease. *Am J Med* 2010;*123*(7):583–592

[6] Lang IM, Medda BK, Babaei A, Shaker R. Role of peripheral reflexes in the initiation of the esophageal phase of swallowing. *Am J Physiol Gastrointest Liver Physiol* 2014;*306*(8):G728–G737

[7] Menard-Katcher P, Falk GW. Normal aging and the esophagus. In: Shaker R, Belafsky PC, Postma GN, Easterling C, eds. Principles of Deglutition: A Multidisciplinary Text for Swallowing and Its Disorders. New York, NY: Springer; 2013:287–294

[8] Richter JE. High-resolution manometry in diagnosis and treatment of achalasia: help or hype. *Curr Gastroenterol Rep* 2014;*16*(12):420

[9] Samuel EA, Shaker R. Deglutitive pharyngeal and UES pressure phenomena. In: Shaker R, Belafsky PC, Postma GN, Easterling C, eds. Principles of Deglutition: A Multidisciplinary Text for Swallowing and Its Disorders. New York, NY: Springer; 2013:269–287

[10] Yadlapati R, Gawron AJ, Keswani RN, et al. Identification of quality measures for performance of and interpretation of data from esophageal manometry. *Clin Gastroenterol Hepatol* 2016;*14*(4):526–534.e1

# 25 Dysphagia in Pediatric Pulmonary Disease

*James D. Tutor*

## Summary

Aspiration is a significant cause of respiratory morbidity and occasionally mortality in children. It occurs when airway protective reflexes fail, especially if dysphagia is also present. Clinical symptoms and physical findings of dysphagia and aspiration can be nonspecific, often slowing early diagnosis. However, new therapeutic advances can significantly improve outcome and prognosis. This chapter reviews the anatomy and physiology involved in normal swallowing in children from the newborn period through adolescence. Next the protective reflexes that help to prevent aspiration and the pathophysiological events that occur after an aspiration event are discussed, followed by the respiratory sequelae of dysphagia and aspiration in children. Finally, the various methods of treatment of dysphagia, aspiration, and the respiratory sequelae in children are reviewed.

## Keywords

cough, wheezing, dysphagia, PFT, aspiration, pediatrics, pulmonary, bronchiectasis, pneumonia, abscess

### Learning Objectives

- Describe the development of swallowing and the anatomical changes in the infant swallowing mechanism (compared to the adult mechanism) that increase the risk of aspiration in the infant
- Understand the protective airway reflexes that help to prevent aspiration
- Understand the pathophysiological events associated with aspiration
- Understand the respiratory sequelae of aspiration in children with dysphagia
- Understand the modalities of treatment available for dysphagia, aspiration, and the respiratory sequelae

## 25.1 Introduction

Dysphagia can lead to aspiration, the inhalation of foreign material into the lower airways. Dysphagia affects approximately 1% of children annually.[1] Aspiration can be an acute event or a chronic syndrome. When it is chronic and recurrent in children, the effects on lung development can be devastating and can lead to significant respiratory problems that severely impair lung function and cause pulmonary scarring. These problems cause significant morbidity and can occasionally lead to death. Thus the diagnosis of dysphagia and aspiration in children needs to be made as soon as possible to prevent lung damage. Unfortunately, it frequently goes unrecognized by primary care physicians or caregivers as a cause of chronic respiratory symptoms.[2]

This chapter reviews the respiratory problems associated with dysphagia and aspiration in children. First, the development of swallowing is briefly reviewed, along with the anatomical changes that increase the risk of aspiration as the infant swallowing mechanism changes to resemble that of an adult. Next the airway protective reflexes that help to prevent aspiration are reviewed, followed by the pathophysiological events that occur with aspiration. The chapter then discusses the various respiratory problems that can occur in children due to recurrent aspiration. Finally, the treatment modalities for dysphagia, aspiration, and the associated respiratory problems in children are described.

## 25.2 Case Presentation Part 1

The patient was a 9-week-old Caucasian boy who was seen in consultation by the pediatric pulmonology service after his admission to a children's hospital. He had a loud, lingering cough since 2 days of age. At age 5 weeks, the cough frequency increased and was accompanied by wheezing, nasal congestion, and posttussive emesis (vomiting after coughing). His pediatrician started him on an oral steroid (**Box 25.1**) and albuterol by nebulization (**Box 25.2**). This therapy produced equivocal results to improve his respiratory symptoms. He was then placed on oral lansoprazole (**Box 25.3**), which did not improve his respiratory symptoms. At the age of 9 weeks, he was admitted to a children's hospital after he developed respiratory distress, a need for supplemental oxygen, and poor oral intake. There was no fever.

### Box 25.1

**Clinical Note**

Steroids are hormones that occur naturally in the human body. They have many functions, which include decreasing inflammation and blocking histamine, to name just two. Steroid medications are manufactured but are designed to imitate the functions of naturally occurring steroids. Corticosteroids are used to treat diseases and are different from anabolic steroids, which are sometimes used to enhance muscle development in athletes and body builders. Corticosteroids are prescribed to treat various conditions, including ulcerative colitis, arthritis, allergies, and asthma.

### Box 25.2

**Albuterol**

Albuterol belongs to a class of drugs known as bronchodilators. A nebulizer is a machine that changes the albuterol solution to a fine mist for inhalation. After inhalation the albuterol provides quick relief to the patient as it helps to open the respiratory passageways and relaxes muscles.

## Box 25.3

**Lansoprazole**

Lansoprazole is a proton pump inhibitor. These types of drugs work to decrease acid production by the stomach and are used to treat gastroesophageal reflux disease. Lansoprazole is sold under the common brand name of Prevacid, among others.

The patient was born at a weight of 8 lb, 3 oz at 39 weeks gestation by spontaneous vaginal delivery. He was subsequently discharged to home with his mother after an uneventful course in the nursery. The family history revealed that the mother had asthma and allergies. There was also a family history of eczema. There were two dogs present in the home. There were no smokers present in the home. A 3-year-old sibling attended a daycare center. The patient's review of systems was negative except for the respiratory symptoms.

The only abnormality noted on the physical examination at admission was the presence of coarse breath sounds and coarse expiratory wheezes on auscultation of the lungs. A chest radiograph done at admission revealed the presence of mild bilateral peribronchial thickening (**Box 25.4**) and bilateral hyperexpansion of the lungs. The aortic arch was on the left.

## Box 25.4

**Bilateral Peribronchial Thickening**

Mild bilateral peribronchial thickening, also known as peribronchial cuffing, is a radiological sign that is present when there is excess fluid or mucus in the small airway passages. It causes patches of atelectasis (closure of a part of the lung) and resulting reductions in gas exchange.

## 25.3 Development of Swallowing

Development of swallowing begins early in fetal development, and development of the aerodigestive tract develops integrated with the development of the respiratory centers in the brainstem. Control and coordination movements of mastication, respiration, and swallowing occur within the nucleus ambiguus and nucleus tractus solitarii.[3,4] Cortical input facilitates the oral phase and the initiation of the pharyngeal phase of swallowing. Sensory afferent feedback transmitted via cranial nerves V, VII, IX, and X (trigeminal, facial, glossopharyngeal, and vagus, respectively). Primary efferent activity for swallowing is provided by cranial nerves V, VII, IX, XII (trigeminal, facial, glossopharyngeal, and hypoglossal nerves, respectively), and cervical nerves C1 to C3. Pharyngeal swallowing is noted to occur by 10 to 14 weeks of gestation, nonnutritive sucking and swallowing at 15 weeks, and suckling with anterior to posterior tongue movements between 19 and 24 weeks. At 26 to 29 weeks of gestation, reflexes between taste buds and facial muscles occur. Some infants can feed by mouth at 32 to 33 weeks, although 34 weeks is the earliest that infants can sustain full nutrition and hydration orally.[5]

The upper aerodigestive tract of the infant provides the optimal arrangement for safe, effective nipple feeding.[6] The anatomy of the newborn swallowing mechanism gradually changes over the first months of life as the larynx descends in the pharynx, and the upper aerodigestive tract begins to resemble that of the adult by age 5 months. Laryngeal descent allows for tidal breathing in the infant and coincides with the peak incidence of sudden infant death syndrome.[7] The more caudal positioning of the larynx as it descends sacrifices the aspiration protection believed to be afforded to the young infant by the intranaral positioning of the epiglottis during swallowing. Intranaral epiglottic positioning is only possible with the most cephalic positioning of the larynx with the tip of the epiglottis at the level of the cervical vertebrae C2 to C3.[8]

## 25.4 Airway Protective Reflexes

The airway is protected from aspiration by a series of reflexes with mechanoreceptors and chemoreceptors located in the pharynx, larynx, and esophagus.[9,10] Laryngeal chemoreceptors in the newborn are the primary defense against aspiration of liquids. As the infant matures, the laryngeal cough reflex becomes more prominent. In adults, the chemoreflexive responses of the larynx continue to provide the primary source of airway protection.[11] The nature of the protective reflex response varies as a function of the age of the individual and the region of the pharynx or larynx that is stimulated. In infants, mechanical stimulation of the larynx invokes reflex swallowing and apnea, whereas in older children laryngeal closure and cough are predominant reflexes.[5] Viral respiratory infections can cause the adult response, coughing and swallowing, to revert to the immature pattern in which apnea predominates.[12] This tendency may explain why prone infants with respiratory syncytial virus have an increased incidence of apnea and sudden infant death syndrome, particularly when lying face downward.[13,14,15] Failure of the airway protective reflexes allows aspiration to occur from swallowed boluses. In fact, decreased laryngeal sensation correlates very highly with aspiration.[16,17,18]

## 25.5 Pathophysiology Events Associated with Aspiration

Aspiration can potentially cause permanent damage to the developing lungs of infants and children. Aspiration of large particles can cause acute airway obstruction and severe hypoventilation. Smaller particle or liquid aspirates may induce hypoxemia by a variety of mechanisms including reflex airway closure, hemorrhagic pneumonitis, destruction and dilution of surfactant with secondary atelectasis, and pulmonary edema from leakage of intravascular fluids and protein.[19] Lung injury increases as the pH of aspirated materials drops below 2.5 (**Box 25.5**), with maximal lung injury occurring at a pH of 1.5.[20] The volume of the aspirated material also plays a major role in lung injury. In dogs, 1 mL/kg of acid aspiration produces only mild effects, whereas 2 mL/kg of acid aspirate causes serious effects, usually death.[21] Histological findings of aspiration include degeneration of bronchiolar epithelium, pulmonary edema and hemorrhage, focal atelectasis, exudation of fibrin, and acute inflammatory cell infiltrate. Later findings include regeneration of bronchiolar epithelium, proliferation of fibroblasts, and fibrosis.[22] Gastric contents instilled into the trachea of dogs appear on the lung surface within 12 to 18 seconds. Extensive atelectasis develops within 3 minutes. Changes of acute pneumonia occur within hours, and granulomatous changes develop within 48 hours.[23,24] Chronic pulmonary aspiration can ultimately lead to the development of bronchiectasis in children.[25]

## Box 25.5

**pH Value**
A pH value is a measurement of the hydrogen (H) ion concentration in an aqueous solution, expressed as a (negative) power ("p") of 10. The pH scale ranges from 1 to 14, with 7 being neutral. A pH below 7 is acidic and a pH above 7 is alkaline or basic.

Aspiration is most commonly the result of dysphagia, gastroesophageal reflux disease, or insufficient management of nasal/oral secretions.[26] As described in other chapters in this book, children can have several medical conditions that predispose them to aspiration.

## 25.6 Symptoms of Dysphagia/Aspiration

Infants and children with dysphagia and aspiration may present to the clinician with several symptoms: chronic cough, recurrent wheezing that is poorly responsive to appropriate therapies, failure to thrive, stridor, or recurrent laryngitis and hoarseness. They may also come to the clinician with a history of recurrent pneumonias, atelectasis, bronchiectasis, pulmonary abscess, pulmonary fibrosis, bronchiolitis obliterans, or acute life-threatening events/recurrent apnea and bradycardia episodes. In addition, young infants who develop viral respiratory illnesses, such as respiratory syncytial virus bronchiolitis, may develop silent aspiration.[23] This can lead to unexpected acute respiratory deterioration if these infants continue to eat by mouth. Providing thickened oral feedings to these infants during the course of their bronchiolitis has been suggested.[27] Also, acute episodes of aspiration can occur when infants or children swallow volatile or oily liquids, such as mineral oil, medium-chain triglycerides, furniture polish, or other hydrocarbon-containing liquids.[28,29] Liquids cause extensive airway mucosal and lung parenchymal inflammation and injury, resulting in pneumonia with the possibility of acute respiratory distress syndrome[30] and pulmonary parenchymal fibrosis.[19]

Infants and children with an absent or ineffective reflex may have silent aspiration and have findings of only increased respiratory mucus, congestion, and chronic wheeze or rhonchi, recurrent bronchitis, or recurrent pneumonia.[31,32]

## 25.7 Physical Evaluation for Aspiration

It is important that the clinician observe the infant or child eating and auscultate the chest and back both before and after feeding for crackles, wheezes, "wet" upper airway noises, and wet voice quality. Attention should be given to nasopharyngeal reflux, difficulty when sucking or swallowing, and associated coughing and choking. Drooling or excessive accumulation of secretions in the mouth suggests dysphagia.[33]

## 25.8 Diagnosis of Aspiration in Children with Dysphagia

As mentioned in previous chapters, any child with suspected dysphagia needs to be evaluated by a speech-language pathologist trained in assessment of swallowing in children. Most of these children will also need an instrumental assessment using the videofluoroscopic swallowing study (VFSS) and/or fiberoptic endoscopic evaluation of swallowing (FEES).[34]

The initial test for a child with chronic or recurrent respiratory symptoms who is suspected of having recurrent aspiration is the chest radiograph. In these children, the chest radiograph can reveal the presence of bronchial wall thickening, hyperinflation, or diffuse or localized infiltrates. About 14% of radiographs can be normal. In infants with recurrent aspiration, infiltrates can be in dependent areas, such as the upper lobes and the posterior areas of the lower lobes.[22] Chest radiographs are largely insensitive to early changes of lung injury.[35]

Computed tomographic (CT) scans, particularly high-resolution images, are more sensitive in the detection of early airway and parenchymal disease in children who aspirate, particularly in those with lipoid pneumonia.[36] In children who chronically aspirate, CT findings (**Fig. 25.1**) can include bronchial wall thickening, air trapping, bronchiectasis, ground-glass opacities, and centrilobular opacities ("tree in bud").[26]

The salivagram has been used to try to detect salivary aspiration in patients who have dysphagia. Though it has been reported to be a sensitive test for salivary aspiration, three retrospective studies found there was only a 26–28% presence of positive salivagrams in children suspected of aspiration.[37,38,39] Also, salivagrams have poor correlation with other tests of aspiration, such as VFSS and milk scans.[40]

There are several other tests available that may complement VFSS and FEES to determine if a child with dysphagia is also aspirating. Biomarkers obtained from the lungs during a bronchoalveolar lavage have been sought and evaluated in order to identify children with significant aspiration. The most extensively studied biomarker is the calculation of a quantitative index of lipid-laden macrophages (LLMs). Theoretically, an increased prevalence of lipid-filled macrophages in the lower airway suggests aspiration of food during swallowing or following reflux from the stomach.[5] However, the results of several studies of the prevalence of LLMs in the bronchoalveolar lavage of children with chronic aspiration have been inconsistent.[41,42,43,44] Elevated LLM indexes have been found in children not suspected of aspirating who have various diseases, including cystic fibrosis; those receiving intravenous lipid

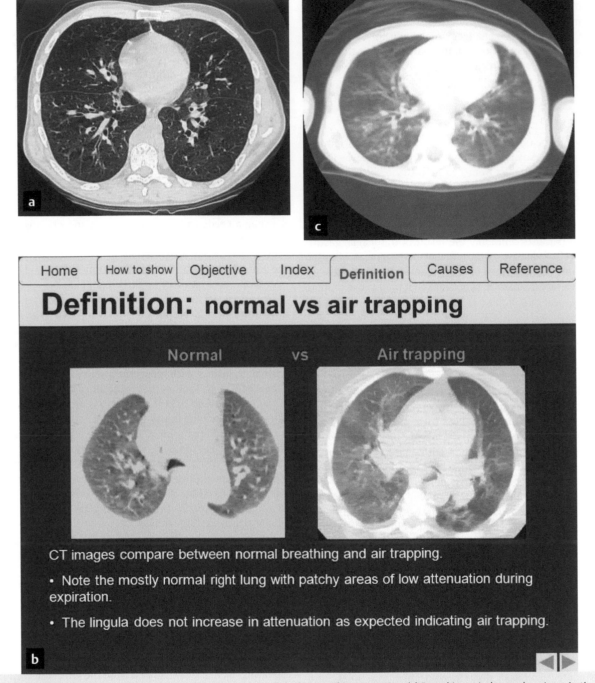

**Fig. 25.1** Computed tomographic (CT) images. **(a)** Mild bronchial wall thickening. **(b)** Air trapping. **(c)** Bronchiectasis due to chronic aspiration.

preparations; those with pulmonary fat embolism in sickle cell disease; and those with endogenous lipoid pneumonia from bronchial obstruction.[45,46,47,48,49] Despite all of these limitations, an LLM index may provide supporting evidence of aspiration in select patients.[50]

Besides the LLM index, other potential biomarkers that have been studied as indicators of aspiration include pepsin, bile acids, and milk protein.[51] Pepsin has been evaluated as a biomarker of aspiration in intubated premature infants, pediatric critical care patients, and lung transplant recipients.[52,53,54,55,56,57] Farhath et al[52] found pepsin in 92% of samples from 45 preterm babies. It has been suggested that the finding of high levels of pepsin in tracheal aspirates of preterm infants was correlated with the development of severe bronchopulmonary dysplasia.[52,53] These studies, with their high incidence of positive pepsin from lung secretions, along with other studies showing positive pepsin and bile acids in normal control subjects, seem to suggest these assays may be overly sensitive.[58,59] Detection of milk protein in tracheal aspirates by various methods has been utilized, but there is little published replicative work.[60,61] All of these tests—pepsin, bile acids, and milk proteins—lack standardization, and they may be applicable only for detecting recent aspiration events.[51]

## 25.9 Pulmonary Function Tests in Infants with Dysphagia

One of the tools now available for monitoring the chronic respiratory problems caused by dysphagia and chronic aspiration in infants is pulmonary function tests (PFTs). Tutor and Gosa[2] reported on a group of 38 neurologically normal infants, born at term, each with a history of recurrent cough and wheezing and who had dysphagia newly diagnosed using VFSS. These infants had PFTs performed within 2 weeks of their diagnosis of dysphagia. Twenty-five of them had abnormal spirometric values, 18 had abnormal plethysmographic values, and 15 demonstrated evidence of bronchodilator responsiveness (BDR). Seventeen of the 38 infants underwent repeat PFTs 6 months later after receiving therapy for their dysphagia. Ten of the infants continued to have abnormal spirometric values, two infants' spirometric values remained normal, three infants' abnormal spirometric values had normalized, and two infants' previously normal spirometric values had become abnormal. Eight of the 17 infants had continued abnormal plethysmographic values, six had continued normal plethysmographic values, and three infants' previously normal plethysmographic values had become abnormal. Eight of the 17 infants demonstrated BDR, of which 5 continued to demonstrate BDR after 6 months of therapy for dysphagia, and 3 infants developed BDR. The remainder continued not to have BDR (2 infants) or lost BDR (3 infants). The authors concluded that 6 months of therapy for dysphagia did not significantly improve pulmonary function in these infants. Future long-term studies will be necessary to determine if these PFT abnormalities persist into later childhood or even adulthood.

## 25.10 Case Presentation Part 2

During the hospitalization, the pediatric pulmonologist felt that the patient's chronic cough and need for oxygen supplementation could be consistent with a congenital lesion, such as a vascular ring or H-type tracheoesophageal fistula (TEF), or the presence of cystic fibrosis. Subsequently, a sweat chloride test was normal. A barium esophagogram was interpreted by the radiologist as the possible presence of a TEF with connection of the distal trachea to the esophagus just above the origin of the left mainstem bronchus. The patient underwent bronchoscopy by an otorhinolaryngologist but no TEF was found. A VFSS demonstrated the presence of mild dysphagia characterized by a slight delay in the pharyngeal swallow response and shallow laryngeal penetration by swallowed thin liquids. The laryngeal penetration improved when the patient was fed oral liquids thickened to nectar consistency during the VFSS. The patient's dysphagia improved in the hospital with thickening of oral liquids to nectar consistency and the use of an Avent stage 3 nipple. The patient also had a gastric

scintiscan performed that revealed the presence of three episodes of gastroesophageal reflux to the proximal esophagus but no aspiration. The gastric emptying was also slightly delayed. The patient was placed on oral lansoprazole. With the therapies for dysphagia and gastroesophageal reflux, the patient progressively weaned off his supplemental oxygen. He was discharged from the hospital 2 weeks after his admission on these therapies along with nebulized albuterol to use as needed to treat wheezing.

The patient was subsequently seen in the pediatric pulmonologist's clinic for follow-up of his wheezing, dysphagia, and gastroesophageal reflux. Subsequent VFSS done 3 months later and again 10 months later continued to demonstrate the same findings as the first VFSS. Other tests of significance performed on an outpatient basis included CT of the chest done about 2 months after his discharge from the hospital. It revealed the presence of scattered airspace disease with volume loss, atelectasis of the right lower lung lobe, left lower lung lobe, and some of the segments of the right upper lung lobe. There was also evidence of aspiration pneumonia in the right lower lung lobe (**Fig. 25.2**). Infant PFTs performed about 2 weeks after hospital discharge and again 3 months later revealed the presence of mild to moderate obstruction of the small airways on spirometry and the presence of mild air trapping on plethysmography. No BDR was present. The patient continued to receive oral liquids thickened to nectar consistency and lansoprazole. Four months later, the infant PFT was repeated and revealed that the spirometric and plethysmographic values had normalized. The patient was lost to follow-up by the pediatric pulmonologist about 6 months later.

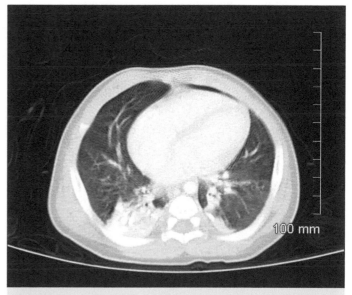

**Fig. 25.2** CT scan of the chest with intravenous contrast of the patient presented in the case study. There is airspace disease with volume loss. There is atelectasis of the right lower lobe, segments of the right upper lobe, and the left lower lobe. There is an air bronchogram and aspirated barium in the right lower lobe, resulting in aspiration pneumonitis. The heart size is at the upper limits of normal.

## 25.11 Respiratory Conditions Associated with Dysphagia and Chronic Aspiration

As mentioned in the section on symptoms of dysphagia and aspiration and as demonstrated in the case presentation, children can have recurrent wheezing that is poorly responsive to appropriate therapies as well as a chronic cough. Stridor and voice abnormalities can also be present in children with dysphagia and chronic aspiration. The pharyngeal phase of swallowing can be affected by airway compromise by laryngomalacia and vocal cord paralysis.[62] Thus, if the otorhinolaryngologist suspects ongoing aspiration, if surgery will involve the glottis, or if surgery will repair a subglottic stenosis that may be preventing aspiration, a swallowing evaluation involving VFSS or FEES will often be performed preoperatively.[63] After supraglottoplasty for treatment of severe laryngomalacia, children may develop transient dysphagia requiring dietary modifications, positioning alterations, and antireflux medications.[64] **Fig. 25.3** illustrates the effects of chronic aspiration.

Reflexes originating in the laryngeal chemoreceptors, including laryngeal chemoreflexes and nonnutritive swallowing, contribute to the occurrence of apnea, bradycardia, and hypoxemia in early life. Immaturity of the preterm newborn impairs the coordination between swallowing and breathing. This may lead to apnea, especially in preterm infants. Nonnutritive swallowing has been reported with central, obstructive, or mixed apneas in human newborns.[65] Apneas also occur in patients with dysphagia who are past the newborn period. Dysphagia was found to be present in about half of a group of 72 patients with obstructive sleep apnea in one study, leading the authors to conclude that questions about swallowing should be part of the medical history in the management of these patients.[66]

Dysphagia resulting in acute or chronic pulmonary aspiration can lead to the development of infections in the lungs, such as pneumonia or an abscess. In a report from 2007, in a group of 150 children with VFSS-proven dysphagia, the odds ratio for pneumonia was significantly increased in children with postswallow residue or aspiration of thin fluids, but not thick fluids or purees. In multilogistic regression, pneumonia was associated with diagnosis of asthma, Down syndrome, gastroesophageal reflux

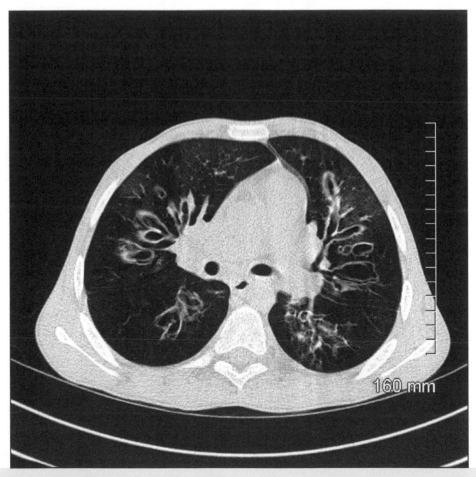

**Fig. 25.3** CT scan of the chest without intravenous contrast from an 18-year-old with chronic aspiration. There is bilateral diffuse tubular bronchiectasis. A few of the dilated bronchi in the left lower lobe contain fluid. There is bilateral mosaic perfusion of both lungs that represents air trapping.

disease, history of lower respiratory tract infection, moist cough, and oxygen supplementation.[67]

In neonates, swallowing incoordination can lead to aspiration, which in turn can lead to physical obstruction of the airway. This can lead to atelectasis (collapse of one or more areas of the lung) and/or consolidation (swelling and/or hardening of the lung caused by fluid in the alveoli) and predispose to infection. The infant may develop cyanosis, apnea, or gasping, and crepitations (crackling or rattling sound) and rhonchi (continuous, low-pitched, lung sounds resembling snoring) on auscultation will be heard. A new area of consolidation or infiltrate on the chest radiograph, particularly in the upper lobes and the posterior areas of the lower lobes, are suggestive of aspiration. Following the episode of aspiration, the airway should be cleared, and the infant may require supplementary oxygen or even ventilator support. Broad-spectrum antimicrobial coverage should be given, such as flucloxacillin (antibiotic derived from penicillin) and an aminoglycoside (antibiotic that inhibits protein synthesis) for at least 5 days.[22,68]

Aspiration pneumonia can also occur in children past the neonatal period who have dysphagia. It may be accompanied by fever, coughing, wheezing, leukocytosis (increased number of white cells in the blood, which often occurs during an infection), and infiltrates seen radiologically. There are several conditions predisposing to infectious complications of aspiration: gingivitis, decayed teeth, gastric outlet or intestinal obstruction, enteral tube feeding, prolonged hospitalization, endotracheal intubation, prone positioning without elevation of the head, and use of antacids or acid blockers. Multiple bacterial pathogens found in the oropharynx can cause aspiration pneumonia in children with dysphagia. Aerobic and facultative bacteria found included *Streptococcus pneumoniae*, group A streptococci, *Staphylococcus aureus*, *Proteus* species, *Pseudomonas aeruginosa*, *Klebsiella pneumoniae*, *Escherichia coli*, *Aerobacter* species, *Haemophilus influenzae*, and others. Anaerobic organisms in adults with ventilator-associated aspiration pneumonia predominate in the oropharynx with a ratio between 3:1 and 10:1. When aspiration occurs in the hospitalized patient, or in a patient receiving broad-spectrum antibiotic therapy, nosocomial and facultative organisms predominate. Most commonly these include *E. coli*, *Proteus* species, and *P. aeruginosa*.[19] There is a role for flexible bronchoscopy with bronchoalveolar lavage or using protected specimen brushes early in the pneumonia to help to identify the bacterial organism. If the child has very limited reserve (pulmonary or immunological) or highly infectious aspirate is suspected, early empirical antibiotics may be warranted. In the previously healthy individual, in whom anaerobic bacteria are most likely to predominate, initial therapy with penicillin, ampicillin, or clindamycin is recommended. In the treatment of pneumonia in children with underlying chronic lung disease, institutionalized patients, and those having received broad-spectrum antibiotic therapy, a second- or third-generation cephalosporin should be considered. In immunocompromised patients, a combination of an aminoglycoside and a synthetic penicillin or cephalosporin, such as ceftazidime, might be initiated until culture results are available to guide more specific therapy. Culture results should be used to discontinue or narrow antibiotic therapy. Treatment with antibiotics for 7 to 10 days is reasonable for patients who respond promptly.[19]

The development of a lung abscess is another infectious process that can occur as a result of aspiration in children with dysphagia.

A lung abscess is a localized area composed of thick-walled purulent material formed as a result of lung infection that leads to destruction of lung parenchyma, cavitation, and central necrosis.[69] Aspiration is the most important cause leading to development of a lung abscess. Children who have dysphagia, gastroesophageal reflux disease, TEFs, and a variety of neurologic conditions are at increased risk. It is likely that the number of aspirations, the volume of the aspirated material, and any impairment of normal respiratory tract clearance mechanisms of aspirated material contribute to the likelihood of abscess formation.[70] If the aspiration event occurred while the child was recumbent, the right and left upper lobes and apical segment of the right lower lobe are the dependent areas most likely to be affected. In a child who was upright, the posterior segments of the upper lobes were dependent and therefore are the most likely to be affected.[69] The organisms that lead to development of a lung abscess are the same ones seen in aspiration pneumonia. Symptoms of lung abscess are fever (84%), cough (53%), dyspnea (35%), chest pain (24%), anorexia (20%), production of purulent sputum (18%), rhinorrhea (16%), and malaise and lethargy (11%). Weight loss may also occur. The physical findings include tachypnea, localized decreased air entry, dullness to percussion, and localized crackles on auscultation. The diagnosis is often suggested by the presence of a thick-walled cavity containing an air-fluid level on chest radiograph.[70] Ultrasound can help differentiate an abscess from a loculated empyema. Contrast-enhanced chest CT is considered the investigation of choice, showing a cavity with thick walls and central mobile fluid. The mainstay of treatment is the use of parenteral antibiotics for 2–3 weeks followed by 4–8 weeks of oral antibiotics. Penicillin, with or without clindamycin, or metronidazole is the usual choice to cover the most prevalent pathogens due to aspiration.[71] The routine use of CT-guided aspiration for abscess and the more recent use of CT-guided pigtail drainage catheters at the time of presentation have been associated with a decrease in the length of hospital stay, but this needs to be confirmed by additional studies.[72] Complications of lung abscess include empyema, pyothorax, pneumothorax, bronchopleural fistula, and bronchiectasis. The prognosis is usually good if effective therapy and close follow-up are provided and the predisposing cause can be eliminated. Complete radiologic resolution may take up to 6 months.[70]

Bronchiolitis obliterans (BO) syndrome is a rare, irreversible obstructive lung disease resulting from bronchiolar obstruction and luminal obliteration. It has gained prominence as the major cause of lung transplant failure beyond the immediate posttransplant period (40% of pediatric deaths). It is also a significant cause of morbidity after bone marrow transplants. Fatal progression can occur, particularly in posttransplant patients. Gastroesophageal reflux is very common in transplant patients (73% in one retrospective study), and aspiration of the refluxed material may contribute to BO.[73] In two recent studies, Atkins et al[74,75] reported that, in a group of 263 lung transplant patients, 70.5% had postoperative dysphagia when examined by FEES or VFSS, and 63.8% demonstrated aspiration. Preoperative tobacco abuse, gastroesophageal reflux, and cardiopulmonary bypass predicted dysphagia. Peak forced expiratory volume in the first second of expiration ($FEV_1$) predicted BO, and mortality was predicted by ventilator dependence and peak $FEV_1$. A normal swallowing evaluation was associated with improved survival in these patients. The authors recommended that identifying unrecognized dysphagia and the use of aggressive pulmonary toilet may improve results of pulmonary transplantation.

The clinical onset of BO is often insidious. Symptoms include cough (94%), wheezing (87%), exercise intolerance (87%), tachypnea (77%), and frequent respiratory illnesses (77%). Physical findings include the presence of crackles (87%), wheezing (71%), and tachypnea (61%). There is the presence of irreversible relentless decline in $FEV_1$ on spirometry. High-resolution chest CT demonstrates a mosaic pattern of hypolucencies due to air trapping, which is more prominent in the expiratory phase CT views. The definitive diagnosis requires a lung biopsy specimen. There is circumferential bronchiolar thickening of the submucosa from collagenous scarring. This results in distortion of the airway architecture and narrowing of the lumen. The presence of lymphocytic bronchiolitis in post–lung transplant patients is a significant risk factor for the development of BO. Treatment options for BO are limited, with most therapies having limited evidence supporting their use. However, there is evidence that the use of tacrolimus and mycophenolate mofetil may provide superior prevention and treatment of BO in lung transplant patients.[73]

Bronchiectasis is the abnormal dilatation of bronchi and bronchioles that results from damage to the airways caused by infection and inflammation.[76] It can lead to considerable morbidity, including chronic cough, recurrent infections, and impaired lung function.[77] When bronchiectasis develops during childhood, it may become irreversible and lead to chronic disease into adulthood, with increased risk for mortality due to respiratory failure.[78,79]

Usually a chronic or an intense insult, such as chronic or acute aspiration, causes the initial lung damage, eventually leading to the emergence of bronchiectasis. Damage to the mucociliary clearance system evolves, leading to stasis of pulmonary secretions and further lung injury. There is a change in the epithelium from ciliated to cuboidal and squamous, reserve cell hyperplasia, and mucosal thickening. With progression, there is damage to the muscular and elastic layers and eventual bronchial wall destruction with erosion of bronchial cartilage. Once secondary infection is present, a cycle of infection and inflammation predisposes to further mucosal and bronchial wall injury. In chronic cases, there may be vascular proliferation of the adjacent bronchial arteries that anastomose with pulmonary arteries and predispose the child to hemoptysis.[80] The shape of the bronchiectasis is variable. The classic Reid classification divides bronchiectasis into three different patterns: (1) cylindrical, where a uniform dilation is found; (2) varicose, with constrictions superimposed on cylindrical bronchiectasis; and (3) cystic or saccular, where progressive dilation occurs, usually associated with more advanced disruption of lung architecture.[81]

The natural history of bronchiectasis is varied, ranging from mild respiratory morbidity to death from airway obstruction, pulmonary infection, and respiratory failure with hypercapnia.[82] Cor pulmonale and right heart failure are now uncommon complications of advanced bronchiectasis.[83] Wheeze and asthma symptoms are common in people with bronchiectasis, although reported prevalence varies from 11 to 46%.[84,85] Unfavorable prognostic factors for patients with bronchiectasis include presence of asthma, bilateral lung involvement, and saccular bronchiectasis.[86,87]

Chronic pulmonary aspiration is a well-known cause of bronchiectasis in children. In a study by Piccione et al,[25] a group of 100 children, age 6 months to 19 years, with swallow study- or airway endoscopy-confirmed aspiration identified over a 21-month period of time, underwent rigid and flexible bronchoscopy and high-resolution chest CT. Overall 66% had bronchiectasis, including 51% of those less than 2 years old. The youngest was 8 months old. Severe neurologic impairment and a history of gastroesophageal reflux were identified as risk factors.

Chronic respiratory complaints are the usual clinical findings in children with bronchiectasis. A productive cough is frequently present, which may be associated with wheezing or dyspnea. Fetid sputum may be present. Hemoptysis may be present in the more severely affected children. Crackles and rhonchi are the usual auscultatory findings. Digital clubbing is a variable finding, being reported in up to half of patients. Malnutrition is frequently present in patients.[80]

The goals of evaluating children with suspected bronchiectasis are (1) to confirm the diagnosis, (2) to define the distribution and severity of airway involvement, (3) to characterize extrapulmonary organ involvement associated with bronchiectasis (such as cor pulmonale), and (4) to identify familial and treatable underlying causes of bronchiectasis and contributors to its progression.[82]

High-resolution chest CT is the gold standard for diagnosis of bronchiectasis, and plain chest radiographs are insensitive.[25] The characteristic finding in bronchiectasis on high-resolution CT is the presence of a "signet ring," where the diameter of a dilated bronchus is greater than that of the accompanying blood vessel in cross section.[88,89] In children with bronchiectasis, the bronchoarterial ratio (defined as the diameter of the bronchial lumen divided by the diameter of its accompanying artery) is at least 0.8 or greater.[90] Chest high-resolution CT signs of bronchiectasis include air-fluid levels in distended bronchi, a linear array or cluster of cysts, dilated bronchi in the periphery of the lung, parallel bronchi that do not taper, the tram line appearance, and bronchial wall thickening due to peribronchial fibrosis. Aspiration typically causes lower lobe bronchiectasis.[80,91] (**Fig. 25.4**).

Common respiratory pathogens in children with bronchiectasis are *Haemophilus influenzae*, *Streptococcus pneumoniae*, *Moraxella catarrhalis*, *H. parainfluenzae*, *Staphylococcus aureus*, and

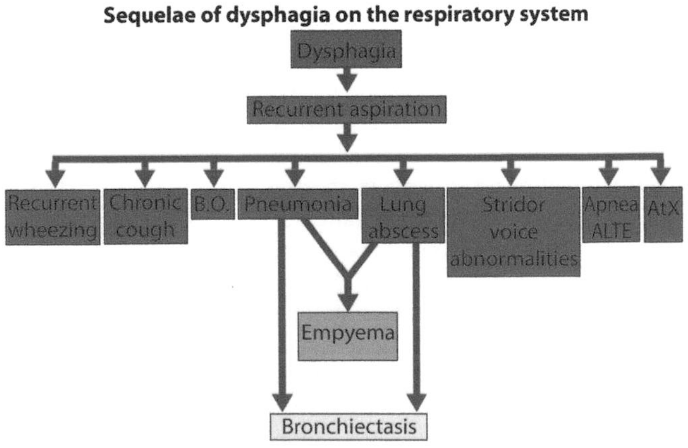

**Sequelae of dysphagia on the respiratory system**

**Fig. 25.4** Aspiration and bronchiectasis. Abbreviations: ALTE, apparent life-threatening event; AtX, atelectasis; B.O., bronchiolitis obliterans

*Pseudo-monas* species.[80] In pediatric bronchiectasis, the pathogen isolation rate from sputum or bronchoalveolar lavage is between 53 and 67%.[92] Persistent *Pseudomonas* endobronchial infection is associated with more severe and progressive bronchiectasis and poorer quality of life.[77]

The management of bronchiectasis should focus on the care of the underlying condition and the management of the suppurative lung injury itself.[80] This includes aggressive management of infections with antimicrobials; regular use of airway clearance methods; and attention to nutrition, coupled with a vigilant monitoring of long-term clinical trends. Proactive care has led to improved survival and preservation of lung function.[93,94] The aims of regular review include optimal postnatal lung growth, prevention of premature respiratory decline, maximal quality of life, and prevention of complications due to bronchiectasis.[82]

Symptomatic exacerbations of bronchiectasis assumed to be infectious in nature are characterized by increased sputum expectoration; cough severity; change in cough quality (dry to wet); or sputum purulence, with or without reduction in exercise tolerance and energy.[92] Infectious exacerbations should be treated with appropriate antibiotics selected by antibiotic sensitivities of the organisms cultured from the patient's respiratory secretions.

Macrolides are used in patients with cystic fibrosis for their anti-inflammatory and mucoregulatory effects. In an uncontrolled study in adults with non–cystic fibrosis bronchiectasis who received azithromycin for a median period of 20 months, a decrease in pulmonary exacerbations and improvement in lung function was demonstrated.[80] Nonsteroidal anti-inflammatory drugs have a major effect on peripheral neutrophil function, significantly reducing neutrophil chemotaxis and fibronectin degradation by resting and stimulated neutrophils, but they have no effect on bacterial colonization of the airways or superoxide anion generation by neutrophils.[95] Tamaoki et al reported a significant reduction in sputum production over 14 days in the treatment group (4 days of inhaled indomethacin) compared with placebo, and a significant improvement in a dyspnea score. There was no significant difference between groups in lung function or blood indices.[96]

Mucoactive agents are treatments that enhance mucus clearance from the respiratory tract in conditions where mucus clearance is impaired.[97] Several types of mucoactive agents that work by various mechanisms are used in children. Recombinant deoxyribonuclease, which lyses DNA originating from bacteria and neutrophils in respiratory mucus, is efficacious in cystic fibrosis but contraindicated in non–cystic fibrosis bronchiectasis because it resulted in higher exacerbation and hospitalization rates and more rapid pulmonary decline in patients with non–cystic fibrosis bronchiectasis when studied.[98] Inhaled osmotic agents, such as 7% hypertonic saline, improve airway clearance and lung function and reduce exacerbation frequency in people with suppurative lung disease (cystic fibrosis and non–cystic fibrosis). Pretreatment with a short-acting bronchodilator is recommended to avoid bronchospasm, which occurs in some patients.[99,100] Chest physiotherapy is beneficial with improved quality of life and exercise capacity and reduced cough and sputum volumes.[101,102]

Asthma in children with bronchiectasis should be treated on its own merits. Inhaled corticosteroids have, at best, a modest benefit in those with severe bronchiectasis and those with *Pseudomonas aeruginosa*.[103] Short- and long-acting $\beta_2$ agonists also have an indeterminate role in the management of bronchiectasis, and their use must be individualized.[104,105]

Surgery is considered most often when bronchiectasis is focal and medical therapy has failed. In several reviews of surgical therapy for bronchiectasis, the compiled group of adults and pediatric patients experienced 1% mortality and an operative complication rate of 8.5%. Complications included empyema, bronchopulmonary fistulas, hypotension, and bleeding. Surgical treatment was more effective in patients with localized disease.[106,107]

## 25.12 Conclusion

Chronic aspiration can occur in children with dysphagia when there is failure of the airway protective reflexes to prevent it. There are several tests currently available to demonstrate the presence of pulmonary aspiration. Pulmonary function tests in infants demonstrate that significant impairment occurs in the lungs when there is chronic aspiration. Chronic aspiration in children with dysphagia can lead to the development of several pulmonary disease processes, which can cause significant morbidity and possibly mortality for the patients. The early involvement of a pediatric pulmonologist in the evaluation and treatment of these children is strongly recommended.

## 25.13 Questions

1. Which of the following is a false statement regarding the airway protective reflexes?

A. The laryngeal chemoreceptors are the primary defense against aspiration in newborns.
B. Infants with respiratory syncytial virus bronchiolitis respond with coughing and swallowing when the laryngeal receptors are stimulated.
C. The reflexes of the larynx are the primary source of airway protection in adults.
D. Decreased laryngeal sensation correlates with the occurrence of aspiration.
E. The receptors of the airway protective reflexes are located in the pharynx, larynx, and esophagus.

2. Which of the following is a true statement regarding the pathophysiological events associated with aspiration?

A. Maximal lung injury occurs if the aspirated material has a pH of 3.
B. Gastric contents aspirated into the trachea appear on the lung surface in 60 seconds.
C. Acid aspiration of 2 mL/kg results in serious effects, usually death.
D. Changes of acute pneumonia occur in the lung at least 24 hours after the aspiration event.
E. Aspiration injury is quickly repaired by the lung and does not cause permanent damage.

**3.** Which of the following is true regarding the diagnosis of aspiration?

A. The salivagram is a highly sensitive test for salivary aspiration.
B. The results of salivagrams correlate well with the results of videofluoroscopic swallow studies (VFSSs) and milk scans.
C. Elevated lipid-laden-macrophage indexes have been found in children not suspected of aspirating.
D. Elevated levels of pepsin in tracheal aspirates from preterm infants do not correlate with the development of severe bronchopulmonary dysplasia.
E. The right middle lobe is the most frequently affected lobe on chest radiographs in children who aspirate.

**4.** Which of the following is true regarding bronchiolitis obliterans (BO)?

A. BO is a reversible obstructive lung disease resulting from bronchiolar obstruction and luminal obliteration.
B. The forced expiratory volume during the middle half of expiration ($FEF_{25-75\%}$) predicted the development of BO in a group of lung transplant patients.
C. The definitive diagnosis of BO can be made by a high-resolution chest computed tomography (CT).
D. The use of tacrolimus and mycophenolate mofetil may provide superior prevention and treatment of BO in lung transplant patients.
E. Preoperative tobacco abuse, dysphagia, and cardiopulmonary bypass predicted gastroesophageal reflux in a group of lung transplant patients.

**5.** Which of the following is true regarding bronchiectasis in children?

A. In one study, up to 66% of children with chronic aspiration had bronchiectasis present on bronchoscopy and chest CT.
B. A bronchoarterial ratio of at least 1 to 1.5 on chest CT is needed to diagnose bronchiectasis in children.
C. In pediatric bronchiectasis, the pathogen isolation rate from sputum or bronchoalveolar lavage is < 50%.
D. Use of DNase is a standard of care for children with non–cystic fibrosis bronchiectasis.
E. Plain chest radiographs are the recommended radiological modality to diagnose bronchiectasis.

## 25.14 Answers and Explanations

**1. Correct: infants with respiratory syncytial virus bronchiolitis respond with coughing and swallowing when the laryngeal receptors are stimulated (B).**
Viral respiratory infections, such as respiratory syncytial virus bronchiolitis, cause the mature response, coughing and swallowing, to revert to the immature response, apnea, when the laryngeal receptors are stimulated. (**A, C, D, E**) are all true.

**2. Correct: acid aspiration of 2 mL/kg results in serious effects, usually death (C).**
(**A**) Maximal lung injury occurs if aspirated material has a pH < 2.5. (**B**) Gastric contents aspirated into the airway appear on the lung surface within 12 to 18 seconds. (**D**) Changes of acute pneumonia occur within < 24 hours after the aspiration event. (**E**) Aspiration injury can cause permanent damage to the lungs.

**3. Correct: elevated lipid-laden-macrophage indexes have been found in children not suspected of aspirating (C).**
Elevated lipid-laden-macrophage indexes have been found in children with fat embolism who have sickle cell disease, cystic fibrosis, children receiving intravenous lipid preparations, and children with endogenous lipoid pneumonia with bronchial obstruction. (**A**) The sensitivity of the salivagram is only 26 to 27% positive in children with suspected aspiration. (**B**) The results of salivagrams do not correlate well with the results of VFSS and milk scans. (**D**) Elevated pepsin levels in tracheal aspirates from preterm infants seem to correlate with the development of severe bronchopulmonary dysplasia. (**E**) The upper lobes and the posterior parts of the lower lobes are the most affected areas on chest radiographs from children who aspirate.

**4. Correct: the use of tacrolimus and mycophenolate mofetil may provide superior prevention and treatment of BO in lung transplant patients (D).**
(**A**) BO is an irreversible obstructive lung disease. (**B**) The peak $FEV_1$ predicted the development of BO in a group of lung transplant patients. (**C**) The definitive diagnosis of BO requires a lung biopsy. (**E**) Preoperative tobacco abuse, gastroesophageal reflux, and cardiopulmonary bypass predicted dysphagia in a group of lung transplant patients.

**5. Correct: in one study, up to 66% of children with chronic aspiration had bronchiectasis present on bronchoscopy and chest CT (A).**
(**B**) A bronchoarterial ratio of 0.8 or greater on chest CT is required to diagnose bronchiectasis in children. (**C**) In pediatric bronchiectasis, the pathogen isolation rate from sputum or bronchoalveolar lavage is 53 to 67%. (**D**) Use of DNase in children with non–cystic fibrosis bronchiectasis is contraindicated. (**E**) High-resolution chest CT is the gold standard for the diagnosis of bronchiectasis; plain chest radiographs are insensitive.

### References

[1] Bhattacharyya N. The prevalence of pediatric voice and swallowing problems in the United States. *Laryngoscope* 2015;*125*(3):746–750
[2] Tutor JD, Gosa MM. Dysphagia and aspiration in children. *Pediatr Pulmonol* 2012;*47*(4):321–337
[3] Delaney AL, Arvedson JC. Development of swallowing and feeding: prenatal through first year of life. *Dev Disabil Res Rev* 2008;*14*(2):105–117
[4] Barlow SM. Central pattern generation involved in oral and respiratory control for feeding in the term infant. *Curr Opin Otolaryngol Head Neck Surg* 2009;*17*(3):187–193
[5] Boesch AP, Wood RE. Aspiration. In: Wilmott RW, Boat TF, Bush A, Chernick V, Deterding RR, Ratjen F, eds. Kendig and Chernick's Disorders of the Respiratory Tract in Children. 8th ed. Philadelphia, PA: Elsevier Saunders; 2012:947–956

[6] Newman LA. Anatomy and physiology of the infant swallow. *Perspectives on Swallowing Disorders* 2001;*10*:3–4

[7] Sasaki CT, Levine PA, Laitman JT, Crelin ES Jr, Crelin ES. Postnatal descent of the epiglottis in man. A preliminary report. *Arch Otolaryngol* 1977;*103*(3):169–171

[8] Sasaki CT, Isaacson G. Functional anatomy of the larynx. *Otolaryngol Clin North Am* 1988;*21*(4):595–612

[9] Harding R, Johnson P, McClelland ME. Liquid-sensitive laryngeal receptors in the developing sheep, cat and monkey. *J Physiol* 1978;*277*:409–422

[10] Storey AT. A functional analysis of sensory units innervating epiglottis and larynx. *Exp Neurol* 1968;*20*(3):366–383

[11] Thach BT. Maturation of cough and other reflexes that protect the fetal and neonatal airway. *Pulm Pharmacol Ther* 2007;*20*(4):365–370

[12] Sessle B, Lucier G. Functional aspects of the upper respiratory tract and larynx: a review. In: Tilden JT, Roeder LM, Steinschneider A, eds. Sudden Infant Death Syndrome. New York, NY: Academic Press; 1983

[13] Gilbert R, Rudd P, Berry PJ, et al. Combined effect of infection and heavy wrapping on the risk of sudden unexpected infant death. *Arch Dis Child* 1992;*67*(2):171–177

[14] Anas N, Boettrich C, Hall CB, Brooks JG. The association of apnea and respiratory syncytial virus infection in infants. *J Pediatr* 1982;*101*(1):65–68

[15] Pickens DL, Schefft GL, Storch GA, Thach BT. Characterization of prolonged apneic episodes associated with respiratory syncytial virus infection. *Pediatr Pulmonol* 1989;*6*(3):195–201

[16] Murray J, Langmore SE, Ginsberg S, Dostie A. The significance of accumulated oropharyngeal secretions and swallowing frequency in predicting aspiration. *Dysphagia* 1996;*11*(2):99–103

[17] Link DT, Willging JP, Miller CK, Cotton RT, Rudolph CD. Pediatric laryngopharyngeal sensory testing during flexible endoscopic evaluation of swallowing: feasible and correlative. *Ann Otol Rhinol Laryngol* 2000;*109*(10 Pt 1):899–905

[18] Thompson DM. Laryngopharyngeal sensory testing and assessment of airway protection in pediatric patients. *Am J Med* 2003;*115*(Suppl 3A):166S–168S

[19] Colombo JL, Thomas HM. Aspiration syndromes. In: Taussig LM, Landau LI, Le-Souëf PN, Morgan WJ, Martinez FD, Sly PD, eds. Pediatric Respiratory Medicine. 2nd ed. Philadelphia, PA: Mosby Elsevier; 2008:337–345

[20] Teabeaut JR II. Aspiration of gastric contents; an experimental study. *Am J Pathol* 1952;*28*(1):51–67

[21] Greenfield LJ, Singleton RP, McCaffree DR, Coalson JJ. Pulmonary effects of experimental graded aspiration of hydrochloric acid. *Ann Surg* 1969;*170*(1):78–86

[22] Colombo JL. Pulmonary aspiration. In: Hilman BC, ed. Pediatric Respiratory Disease: Diagnosis and Treatment. Philadelphia, PA: WB Saunders;1993:429–436

[23] Moran TJ. Experimental food-aspiration pneumonia. *AMA Arch Pathol* 1951;*52*(4):350–354

[24] Hamelberg W, Bosomworth PP. Aspiration pneumonitis: experimental studies and clinical observations. *Anesth Analg* 1964;*43*:669–676

[25] Piccione JC, McPhail GL, Fenchel MC, Brody AS, Boesch RP. Bronchiectasis in chronic pulmonary aspiration: risk factors and clinical implications. *Pediatr Pulmonol* 2012;*47*(5):447–452

[26] de Benedictis FM, Carnielli VP, de Benedictis D. Aspiration lung disease. *Pediatr Clin North Am* 2009;*56*(1):173–190

[27] Khoshoo V, Ross G, Kelly B, Edell D, Brown S. Benefits of thickened feeds in previously healthy infants with respiratory syncytial viral bronchiolitis. *Pediatr Pulmonol* 2001;*31*(4):301–302

[28] Arena JM. Hydrocarbon poisoning—current management. *Pediatr Ann* 1987;*16*(11):879–883

[29] Bysani GK, Rucoba RJ, Noah ZL. Treatment of hydrocarbon pneumonitis. High frequency jet ventilation as an alternative to extracorporeal membrane oxygenation. *Chest* 1994;*106*(1):200–203

[30] Gurwitz D, Kattan M, Levison H, Culham JAG. Pulmonary function abnormalities in asymptomatic children after hydrocarbon pneumonitis. *Pediatrics* 1978;*62*(5):789–794

[31] Platzer ACG. Gastroesophageal reflux and aspiration syndromes. In: Chernick V, Boat TF, Wilmott RW, Bush A, eds. Kendig's Disorders of the Respiratory Tract in Children. 7th ed. Philadelphia, PA: Saunders Elsevier; 2006:592–609

[32] Lefton-Greif MA, Carroll JL, Loughlin GM. Long-term follow-up of oropharyngeal dysphagia in children without apparent risk factors. *Pediatr Pulmonol* 2006;*41*(11):1040–1048

[33] Colombo JL. Chronic recurrent aspiration. In: Kliegman RM, Stanton BF St. Geme JW III, Schor NF, Behrman RE, eds. Nelson Textbook of Pediatrics. 19th ed. Philadelphia, PA: Saunders Elsevier; 2011:1471–1473

[34] Lefton-Greif MA, McGrath-Morrow SA. Deglutition and respiration: development, coordination, and practical implications. *Semin Speech Lang* 2007;*28*(3):166–179

[35] Boesch RP, Daines C, Willging JP, et al. Advances in the diagnosis and management of chronic pulmonary aspiration in children. *Eur Respir J* 2006;*28*(4):847–861

[36] Zanetti G, Marchiori E, Gasparetto TD, Escuissato DL, Soares Souza A Jr. Lipoid pneumonia in children following aspiration of mineral oil used in the treatment of constipation: high-resolution CT findings in 17 patients. *Pediatr Radiol* 2007;*37*(11):1135–1139

[37] Heyman S, Respondek M. Detection of pulmonary aspiration in children by radionuclide "salivagram". *J Nucl Med* 1989;*30*(5):697–699

[38] Bar-Sever Z, Connolly LP, Treves ST. The radionuclide salivagram in children with pulmonary disease and a high risk of aspiration. *Pediatr Radiol* 1995;*25*(Suppl 1):S180–S183

[39] Levin K, Colon A, DiPalma J, Fitzpatrick S. Using the radionuclide salivagram to detect pulmonary aspiration and esophageal dysmotility. *Clin Nucl Med* 1993;*18*(2):110–114

[40] Baikie G, South MJ, Reddihough DS, et al. Agreement of aspiration tests using barium videofluoroscopy, salivagram, and milk scan in children with cerebral palsy. *Dev Med Child Neurol* 2005;*47*(2):86–93

[41] Colombo JL, Hallberg TK. Recurrent aspiration in children: lipid-laden alveolar macrophage quantitation. *Pediatr Pulmonol* 1987;*3*:86–89

[42] Furuya ME, Moreno-Córdova V, Ramírez-Figueroa JL, Vargas MH, Ramón-García G, Ramírez-San Juan DH. Cutoff value of lipid-laden alveolar macrophages for diagnosing aspiration in infants and children. *Pediatr Pulmonol* 2007;*42*(5):452–457

[43] Bauer ML, Lyrene RK. Chronic aspiration in children: evaluation of the lipid-laden macrophage index. *Pediatr Pulmonol* 1999;*28*(2):79–82

[44] Ding Y, Simpson PM, Schellhase DE, Tryka AF, Ding L, Parham DM. Limited reliability of lipid-laden macrophage index restricts its use as a test for pulmonary aspiration: comparison with a simple semiquantitative assay. *Pediatr Dev Pathol* 2002;*5*(6):551–558

[45] Knauer-Fischer S, Ratjen F. Lipid-laden macrophages in bronchoalveolar lavage fluid as a marker for pulmonary aspiration. *Pediatr Pulmonol* 1999;*27*(6):419–422

[46] Kazahkov MY, Muhlbach MS, Livasy CA, Noah TC. Lipid-laden macrophage index and inflammation in bronchoalveolar lavage fluid in children. *Eur Respir J* 2001;*18*:790–795

[47] Kajetanowicz A, Stinson D, Laybolt KS, Resch L. Lipid-laden macrophages in the tracheal aspirate of ventilated neonates receiving Intralipid: A pilot study. *Pediatr Pulmonol* 1999;*28*(2):101–108

[48] Wang JY, Kuo PH. Jan Is, Lee LN, Yang PC. Serial analaysis of fat-containing macrophages in bronchoalveolar lavage fluid in a patient with fat embolism. *J Formos Med Assoc* 2001;*100*:557–560

[49] Wright BA, Jeffrey PH. Lipoid pneumonia. *Semin Respir Infect* 1990;*5*(4):314–321

[50] Ahrens P, Noll C, Kitz R, Willigens P, Zielen S, Hofmann D. Lipid-laden alveolar macrophages (LLAM): a useful marker of silent aspiration in children. *Pediatr Pulmonol* 1999;*28*(2):83–88

[51] Colombo JL, Hallberg TK. Aspiration: a common event and a clinical challenge. *Pediatr Pulmonol* 2012;*47*(3):317–320

[52] Farhath S, Aghai ZH, Nakhla T, et al. Pepsin, a reliable marker of gastric aspiration, is frequently detected in tracheal aspirates from premature ventilated neonates: relationship with feeding and methylxanthine therapy. *J Pediatr Gastroenterol Nutr* 2006;*43*(3):336–341

[53] Farhath S, He Z, Nakhla T, et al. Pepsin, a marker of gastric contents, is increased in tracheal aspirates from preterm infants who develop bronchopulmonary dysplasia. *Pediatrics* 2008;*121*(2):e253–e259

[54] Meert KL, Daphtary KM, Metheny NA. Gastric vs small-bowel feeding in critically ill children receiving mechanical ventilation: a randomized controlled trial. *Chest* 2004;*126*(3):872–878

[55] Gopalareddy V, He Z, Soundar S, et al. Assessment of the prevalence of microaspiration by gastric pepsin in the airway of ventilated children. *Acta Paediatr* 2008;*97*(1):55–60

[56] Ward C, Forrest IA, Brownlee IA, et al. Pepsin like activity in bronchoalveolar lavage fluid is suggestive of gastric aspiration in lung allografts. *Thorax* 2005;*60*(10):872–874

[57] Stovold R, Forrest IA, Corris PA, et al. Pepsin, a biomarker of gastric aspiration in lung allografts: a putative association with rejection. *Am J Respir Crit Care Med* 2007;*175*(12):1298–1303

[58] Grabowski M, Kasran A, Seys S, et al. Pepsin and bile acids in induced sputum of chronic cough patients. *Respir Med* 2011;*105*(8):1257–1261

[59] Ervine E, McMaster C, McCallion W, Shields MD. Pepsin measured in induced sputum—a test for pulmonary aspiration in children? *J Pediatr Surg* 2009;*44*(10):1938–1941

[60] Miller J, Colasurdo GN, Khan AM, et al. Immunocytochemical detection of milk proteins in tracheal aspirates of ventilated infants: a pilot study. *Pediatr Pulmonol* 2002;*34*(5):369–374

[61] De Baets F, Aarts C, Van Daele S, et al. Milk protein and Oil-Red-O staining of alveolar macrophages in chronic respiratory disease of infancy. *Pediatr Pulmonol* 2010;*45*(12):1213–1219

[62] Wilging JP, de Alarcon A, Miller CK, Kelchner LN, Pentuk S. Feeding, swallowing, and voice disorders. In: Wilmott RW, Boat TF, Bush A, Chernick V, Deterding RR, Ratjen F, eds. Kendig and Chernick's Disorders of the Respiratory Tract in Children. 8th ed. Philadelphia, PA: Elsevier Saunders; 2012:957–965

[63] de Alarcon A, Cotton RT, Rutter MJ. Laryngeal and tracheal airway disorders. In: Wilmott RW, Boat TF, Bush A, Chernick V, Deterding RR, Ratjen F, eds. Kendig and Chernick's Disorders of the Respiratory Tract in Children. 8th ed. Philadelphia, PA: Elsevier Saunders; 2012:969–975

[64] Chun RH, Wittkopf M, Sulman C, Arvedson J. Transient swallowing dysfunction in typically developing children following supraglottoplasty for laryngomalacia. *Int J Pediatr Otorhinolaryngol* 2014;*78*(11):1883–1885

[65] Gaultier C, Denjean A. Developmental anatomy and physiology of the respiratory system. In: Taussig LM, Landau LI, LeSouëf PN, Martinez FD, Morgan WJ, Sly PD, eds. Pediatric Respiratory Medicine. 2nd ed. Philadelphia, PA: Mosby Elsevier; 2008:15–34

[66] Schindler A, Mozzanica F, Sonzini G, et al. Oropharyngeal dysphagia in patients with obstructive sleep apnea syndrome. *Dysphagia* 2014;*29*(1):44–51

[67] Weir K, McMahon S, Barry L, Ware R, Masters IB, Chang AB. Oropharyngeal aspiration and pneumonia in children. *Pediatr Pulmonol* 2007;*42*(11):1024–1031

[68] Greenough A, Murthy V, Milner AD. Respiratory disorders in the newborn. In: Wilmott RW, Boat TF, Bush A, Chernick V, Deterding RR, Ratjen F, eds. Kendig and Chernick's Disorders of the Respiratory Tract in Children. 8th ed. Philadelphia, PA: Elsevier Saunders; 2012:358–385

[69] Lakser O. Pulmonary abscess. In: Kliegman RM, Stanton BF St. Geme JW III, Schor NF, Behrman RE, eds. Nelson Textbook of Pediatrics. 19th ed. Philadelphia, PA: Elsevier Saunders; 2011:1480–1481

[70] Crawford SE, Daum RS. Bacterial pneumonia, lung abscess, and empyema. In: Taussig LM, Landau LI, LeSouëf PN, Martinez FD, Morgan WJ, Sly PD, eds. Pediatric Respiratory Medicine. 2nd ed. Philadelphia, PA: Mosby Elsevier; 2008:501–553

[71] Marostica PJ, Stein RT. Community-acquired bacterial pneumonia. In: Wilmott RW, Boat TF, Bush A, Chernick V, Deterding RR, Ratjen F, eds. Kendig and Chernick's Disorders of the Respiratory Tract in Children. 8th ed. Philadelphia, PA: Elsevier Saunders; 2012:461–472

[72] Nagasawa KK, Johnson SM. Thoracoscopic treatment of pediatric lung abscesses. *J Pediatr Surg* 2010;*45*(3):574–578

[73] Lee RL, White CW. Bronchiolitis obliterans. In: Taussig LM, Landau LI, LeSouëf PN, Martinez FD, Morgan WJ, Sly PD, eds. Pediatric Respiratory Medicine. 2nd ed. Philadelphia, PA: Mosby Elsevier; 2008:1031–1038

[74] Atkins BZ, Trachtenberg MS, Prince-Petersen R, et al. Assessing oropharyngeal dysphagia after lung transplantation: altered swallowing mechanisms and increased morbidity. *J Heart Lung Transplant* 2007;*26*(11):1144–1148

[75] Atkins BZ, Petersen RP, Daneshmand MA, Turek JW, Lin SS, Davis RD Jr. Impact of oropharyngeal dysphagia on long-term outcomes of lung transplantation. *Ann Thorac Surg* 2010;*90*(5):1622–1628

[76] Barker AF. Bronchiectasis. *N Engl J Med* 2002;*346*(18):1383–1393

[77] Martínez-García MA, Soler-Cataluña JJ, Perpiñá-Tordera M, Román-Sánchez P, Soriano J. Factors associated with lung function decline in adult patients with stable non-cystic fibrosis bronchiectasis. *Chest* 2007;*132*(5):1565–1572

[78] O'Donnell AE. Bronchiectasis. *Chest* 2008;*134*(4):815–823

[79] Onen ZP, Gulbay BE, Sen E, et al. Analysis of the factors related to mortality in patients with bronchiectasis. *Respir Med* 2007;*101*(7):1390–1397

[80] Jones MH, Marostica PJC. Bronchiectasis. In: Taussig LM, Landau LI, LeSouëf PN, Martinez FO, Morgan WJ, Sly PD, eds. Pediatric Respiratory Medicine. 2nd ed. Philadelphia, PA: Mosby Elsevier; 2008:999–1003

[81] Reid LM. Reduction in bronchial subdivision in bronchiectasis. *Thorax* 1950;*5*(3):233–247

[82] Chang AB, Redding GJ. Bronchiectasis and chronic suppurative lung disease. In: Wilmott RW, Boat TF, Bush A, Chernick V, Deterding RR, Ratjen F, eds. Kendig and Chernick's Disorders of the Respiratory Tract in Children. 8th ed. Philadelphia, PA: Elsevier Saunders; 2012:473–488

[83] Sanderson JM, Kennedy MC, Johnson MF, Manley DCE. Bronchiectasis: results of surgical and conservative management. A review of 393 cases. *Thorax* 1974;*29*(4):407–416

[84] Doğru D, Nik-Ain A, Kiper N, et al. Bronchiectasis: the consequence of late diagnosis in chronic respiratory symptoms. *J Trop Pediatr* 2005;*51*(6):362–365

[85] Santamaria F, Montella S, Pifferi M, et al. A descriptive study of non-cystic fibrosis bronchiectasis in a pediatric population from central and southern Italy. *Respiration* 2009;*77*(2):160–165

[86] Field CE. Bronchiectasis. A long-term follow-up of medical and surgical cases from childhood. *Arch Dis Child* 1961;*36*:587–603

[87] Perry KMA, King DS. Bronchiectasis: a study of prognosis based on follow-up of 400 patients. *Am Rev Tuberc* 1940;*41*:531–548

[88] Web WR, Muller NI, Naidich DP, eds. Airway Diseases. High-Resolution CT of the Lung. Vol 3. Philadelphia, PA: Williams & Wilkins Lippincott; 2001:467–546

[89] Westcott JL. Bronchiectasis. *Radiol Clin North Am* 1991;*29*(5):1031–1042

[90] Kapur N, Masel JP, Watson D, Masters IB, Chang AB. Bronchoarterial ratio on high-resolution CT scan of the chest in children without pulmonary pathology: need to redefine bronchial dilatation. *Chest* 2011;*139*(6):1445–1450

[91] Naidich DP, McCauley DI, Khouri NF, Stitik FP, Siegelman SS, Siegelman SS. Computed tomography of bronchiectasis. *J Comput Assist Tomogr* 1982;*6*(3):437–444

[92] Kapur N, Masters IB, Chang AB. Exacerbations in noncystic fibrosis bronchiectasis: Clinical features and investigations. *Respir Med* 2009;*103*(11):1681–1687

[93] Ellerman A, Bisgaard H. Longitudinal study of lung function in a cohort of primary ciliary dyskinesia. *Eur Respir J* 1997;*10*(10):2376–2379

[94] Frederiksen B, Lanng S, Koch C, Høiby N. Improved survival in the Danish center-treated cystic fibrosis patients: results of aggressive treatment. *Pediatr Pulmonol* 1996;*21*(3):153–158

[95] Llewellyn-Jones CG, Johnson MM, Mitchell JL, et al. In vivo study of indomethacin in bronchiectasis: effect on neutrophil function and lung secretion. *Eur Respir J* 1995;*8*(9):1479–1487

[96] Tamaoki J, Chiyotani A, Kobayashi K, Sakai N, Kanemura T, Takizawa T. Effect of indomethacin on bronchorrhea in patients with chronic bronchitis, diffuse panbronchiolitis, or bronchiectasis. *Am Rev Respir Dis* 1992;*145*(3):548–552

[97] King M, Rubin BK. Mucus-controlling agents: past and present. *Respir Care Clin N Am* 1999;*5*(4):575–594

[98] O'Donnell AE, Barker AF, Ilowite JS, Fick RB. Treatment of idiopathic bronchiectasis with aerosolized recombinant human DNase I. rhDNase Study Group. *Chest* 1998;*113*(5):1329–1334

[99] Elkins MR, Robinson M, Rose BR, et al; National Hypertonic Saline in Cystic Fibrosis (NHSCF) Study Group. A controlled trial of long-term inhaled hypertonic saline in patients with cystic fibrosis. *N Engl J Med* 2006;*354*(3):229–240

[100] Daviskas E, Anderson SD. Hyperosmolar agents and clearance of mucus in the diseased airway. *J Aerosol Med* 2006;*19*(1):100–109

[101] Murray MP, Pentland JL, Hill AT. A randomised crossover trial of chest physiotherapy in non-cystic fibrosis bronchiectasis. *Eur Respir J* 2009;*34*(5):1086–1092

[102] Mutalithas K, Watkin G, Willig B, Wardlaw A, Pavord ID, Birring SS. Improvement in health status following bronchopulmonary hygiene physical therapy in patients with bronchiectasis. *Respir Med* 2008;*102*(8):1140–1144

[103] Kapur N, Bell S, Kolbe J, Chang AB. Inhaled steroids for bronchiectasis. *Cochrane Database Syst Rev* 2009;*1*(1):CD000996

[104] Sheikh A, Nolan D, Greenstone M. Long-acting beta-2-agonists for bronchiectasis. *Cochrane Database Syst Rev* 2001;*4*(4):CD002155

[105] Franco F, Sheikh A, Greenstone M. Short acting beta-2 agonists for bronchiectasis. *Cochrane Database Syst Rev* 2003;*3*(3):CD003572

[106] Balkanli K, Genç O, Dakak M, et al. Surgical management of bronchiectasis: analysis and short-term results in 238 patients. *Eur J Cardiothorac Surg* 2003;*24*(5):699–702

[107] Kutlay H, Cangir AK, Enön S, et al. Surgical treatment in bronchiectasis: analysis of 166 patients. *Eur J Cardiothorac Surg* 2002;*21*(4):634–637

# 26 Considerations Emerging from the End of Life

*Pamela A. Smith, Mary L. Casper, and Paula Leslie*

## Summary

The considerations emerging at the end of life are no different from those that originate at other points of the life span. Regardless of the stage of life, the clinician must always be aware of regulations, *and* how they apply to patient rights and the ability to make an informed decision about patient care. Clinicians must approach all communication with patients without bias and must be free of paternalism so that the patient's values are respected. Documentation of conversations should clearly and thoroughly summarize the information provided, the questions asked, and the decisions made. Clear evidence should exist as to how the patient (or family) demonstrated their understanding. Health care providers must recognize that all patients across the life span have the right to make choices about their care, and it is our responsibility to ensure that all choices are informed, with costs and benefits of treatment alternatives, including the option of no treatment, fully outlined. We encourage all clinicians and future clinicians to embrace this philosophy of care, which respects human choice at all stages of life and is, very likely, that which clinicians themselves might embrace at the end of their own life.

## *Keywords*

ethics, shared decision-making, autonomy, beneficence, medical paternalism, cost-benefit analysis

### *Learning Objectives*

- Discuss levels of regulation in health care service delivery, and explain the differences between federal statutes, professional association guidelines, and ethical principles
- Discuss resident/patient rights, including rights of self-determination and rights of refusal
- Discuss the historical underpinnings of medical paternalism and how it can affect patient care today
- Describe the influence of clinician communication during patient education on the patient's decision-making process
- Describe three desirable characteristics of the clinical interaction that will lead to shared decision making and reduce instances of disagreement

## 26.1 Introduction

End of life issues are historically thought of as relating to the care of people who have a diagnosis for which there is no cure and that has progressed to the point where rehabilitative efforts are not considered. We tend to associate this with older, frailer patients, perhaps with multiple disease processes. Swallow difficulties are no different in patients approaching the end of life from those in other situations. Guiding medical, legal, and ethical principles have emerged from considerations of end of life issues that are applicable to our decision-making process with any patient. We caution against the perception that things are different, or that rehabilitation is not appropriate, or that people can take more risks at the end of life. Clinicians should support every decision with a patient from the perspective of that person being an individual whose medical condition, available resources, and preferences are unique.

This chapter is structured around two patients who are described in a very general manner. The text returns to these patients throughout the chapter so the reader can apply the concepts discussed to these two patients. Both are older patients, but only one would be more typically viewed as facing the end of life. *Terminal care*, *hospice care*, and *palliative care* are three terms that appear in many handbooks and are often misunderstood with regard to end of life issues. The terms *palliative care* and *hospice care* are often used interchangeably, but they are not identical. Palliative care is an approach to patient care emphasizing management of symptoms and pain relief regardless of the diagnosis. *Hospice* may refer to an organization or type of agency, as well as to a level of care. The term may also be used to describe an array of services that a provider makes available to people (*hospice benefit*). A hospice *agency* provides support to the patient and to the family at the end of life, with the goal of maintaining comfort throughout the dying process and assistance and support to the family after death has occurred. To qualify for hospice, the person's attending physician must document that death is anticipated within a specified period of time (generally 6 months). *Terminal* is often used in conjunction with *hospice*, in that patients in a terminal stage of their disease are not expected to recover from it. Care for terminal patients is generally maintenance of comfort during the final stages of life. There is a myth that hospice services do not cover therapies or that terminal patients cannot receive therapy. Skilled therapy services can be a very important component of maximizing comfort at the end of life.

## 26.2 Our Patients

Carla, age 74, is a resident of a skilled nursing facility. When she was admitted, her diagnoses included cancer that originated in the lung but had metastasized to the brain and bone. Prior to her admission to the facility, she underwent various treatments for her cancer, but her physicians do not believe the treatments will cure the disease. Carla and her family understand the prognosis, and her goal is to be as comfortable as possible with her cancer diagnosis. Her height is 64 inches, and her weight is below 90 pounds. Her appetite is poor.

Nancy is also age 74, and she is a resident of the same skilled nursing facility. She has been admitted with a diagnosis of cerebrovascular accident (CVA) with right-sided hemiparesis, moderate mixed aphasia, and dysphagia. She is currently receiving an altered diet with thick liquids. She has difficulty walking, dressing and feeding herself, communicating with others, and swallowing. She is eager to improve in all the areas affected by her stroke. Her height is 65 inches, and her weight is 145 pounds; she has lost approximately 10 pounds since her stroke.

On the surface these two residents may sound very different— Carla has a cancer diagnosis with a poor chance of recovery, and Nancy has had a stroke with an expectation of improvement. Both are exhibiting problems swallowing, and both have orders for evaluation and treatment by the speech-language pathologist (SLP). Nancy, with a stroke, may be considered to be more of a candidate for rehabilitation, and Carla, with cancer, might be considered to be an end of life case. Thus, by diagnosis, the patients differ, but the process of evaluating, planning care, and carrying out treatment and management does not differ between the two. This chapter examines regulatory, ethical, clinical, and pragmatic issues that might have emerged as clinicians consider end of life situations in their clinical practice. Importantly, these issues pertain to all patients, regardless of their medical prognosis. Federal laws, clinical best practices, and ethical principles mandate that we follow similar procedures across all patient populations regardless of age or medical condition.

## 26.3  Regulatory Background

Practicing SLPs are aware that there are regulations but often fear them rather than appreciate how a knowledge of them supports our work. Familiarity with current national, local, and professional laws, rules, and regulations supports defensible practice, especially when that practice is out of line with standard (or "as it's always been") actions. For many of our complex patients there will be no standard approach because they and their situations are unique. Intervention should be well reasoned and in line with regulatory systems (**Box 26.2**).

### 26.3.1  The Patient Self-Determination Act

The patient is the health care consumer and the recipient of care delivered. Legally, patients are entitled to learn about, think about, and decide about the type and extent of medical care they will receive. This right is outlined by the Patient Self-Determination Act,[1] a document that describes patients' rights to participate in their own care and direct their own health care decisions. This Act requires Medicare and Medicaid providers (including hospitals, nursing homes, hospice programs, home health agencies, and managed care organizations) to give individuals certain information about their rights under state laws governing advance directives.[1] Under this act patients have the right to accept or refuse medical or surgical treatment, to prepare an advance directive, and to receive information about how the provider or institution will implement these rights. If a patient has not signed an advance directive, the provider is not allowed to limit care, make it provisional, or in any way discriminate against the patient. SLPs as providers of care are not exempt from this law. Understanding that patients do in fact have the right to direct their own care should compel the SLPs to consider the opinions, values, and wishes of the patient when preparing any plan of treatment, for any patient, at any stage of life.

### 26.3.2  Medicare Guidelines

Most older Americans are covered under the Medicare system, which is the U.S. health care program established in 1965 to ensure adequate medical care for (primarily) older Americans.[2] The Centers for Medicare and Medicaid Services (CMS) is the government agency that provides oversight for the Medicare program. CMS does not directly pay for care; it establishes contracts with insurance companies called Medicare Administrative Contractors (MACs), which provide the financial administration of the medical program. MACs may issue their own coverage requirements and decisions, which are called Local Coverage Determinations (LCDs). MACs are restricted to ensure that all LCDs are consistent with federal CMS guidelines. MACs may further specify the requirements for payment for particular services. Coverage decisions may vary across the country or within a state: the MAC's LCD may provide or deny coverage regionally.

### 26.3.3  Least Restrictive Dining Guidelines

Patients who require continued inpatient care after a hospitalization may be admitted to a rehabilitation environment, often a skilled nursing facility. Institutionalized patients across all levels of care do not lose their rights of self-determination simply because they have been admitted to a facility. Advocacy efforts on behalf of these patients are growing. One piece of evidence of the expansion of patient advocacy is the emergence of groups such as the Pioneer Network. The Pioneer Network works with CMS to promote efforts in support of culture change in health care settings. It has developed Feeding and Dining Standards[3] that help health care providers caring for older adults in postacute settings to focus on patients' rights and health outcomes. The national guidelines developed by the Pioneer Network acknowledge the risk factors associated with poor nutrition in older people in long-term care (LTC).

Patients in LTC facilities are likely to exhibit one or more of the poor nutrition risk factors described below. Overall risk depends on an individual's specific circumstances, and a number of risk factors should be considered for all newly admitted patients. These are described in **Box 26.1**.

The very intervention that is supposed to improve the problem is identified as increasing the risk: *therapeutic diets*. The New Dining Practice Standards[3] document draws together the professional positions of the range of professionals involved in elder care as well as research evidence regarding nutrition. These standards assist professionals in recognizing that every choice that a patient may make has both potential costs (financial, physical, emotional) and potential benefits.

## Box 26.1

**Health Risk Factors in Long-Term Care Residents[4]**
- History of recent weight loss or change in appetite
- Functional disability (including signs of possible dysphagia)
- Pressure ulcer(s)
- Terminal illness
- Depression
- Medication use
- Therapeutic diets
- Nausea, vomiting, or diarrhea
- Fluid retention and edema
- Underlying infection

## Box 26.2

**Case Review: Regulatory**
1. Carla and Nancy have different medical diagnoses and different prognoses. What should be similar across the processes of evaluating each of them? What might differ?
2. Given what we know about regulatory background, discuss these patients' candidacy for rehabilitation services. Could they both qualify for services under the Medicare program?
3. How do the New Dining Practice Standards potentially impact recommendations for patients with dysphagia, such as Nancy and Carla?

# 26.4 Medicolegal Framework

Clinicians have several *duties* toward their patients as are outlined in the American Speech-Language-Hearing Association (ASHA) Code of Ethics[5] and Scope of Practice.[6] If a case were brought to a court regarding an SLP, it is likely that the laws applying to physicians would be applied to any clinician. Understanding the medicolegal framework helps keep us clear on our duties, and it also helps us to understand and speak a common language with medicine and law. Physicians have two broad duties regarding treatment: *to disclose information* and *to gain informed consent*.

An often forgotten option for treatment is that of *no treatment*. We need to include this in our discussions of our proposed intervention. The costs and benefits associated with *not* taking thickened liquids must be examined in the same light and regarding the same evidence as the option to take them. Thus a clinician must be familiar with the literature showing that altering the consistency of food or liquid results in reduced intake. This is a serious risk that clinicians working in dysphagia must be aware of (**Box 26.3**).

## 26.4.1 Disclosure

In the United States there are two main standards of disclosure that are broadly interpreted as follows:

- The *reasonable physician* standard: comparing a physician's actions to those of his or her professional peers (also called the professional standard)

- The *reasonable patient* standard: what would a reasonable patient find relevant to his or her decision making (also called the lay standard)

Roughly half of U.S. states use each standard. We will replace the word *physician* with *clinician* to help us see how these standards would apply to SLPs. If a malpractice suit is brought against a professional, then the court will look to local jurisdiction, or how cases are reviewed in that state. Courts may also look further afield and apply the findings of specific cases or tort law.

The reasonable clinician standard compares a clinician's actions to those of his or her professional peers. This means that a professional is acting within the scope and manner of the majority of his or her fellow practitioners and makes common sense. We presume that the majority act in an appropriate manner, with up-to-date practice, and aligned with current clinical guidelines.

The reasonable patient standard accepts that what needs to be discussed should map to what the patient needs to know in order to select a treatment, *or no treatment*. This also makes sense. As patients we lean toward the idea that we want all the information that is *relevant* to us or—the term more often used—what is material to us.

The problem is that it is impossible to know exactly what is material. After the fact we are much wiser, and Judge Robinson acknowledged this in his summary of *Canterbury v. Spence*:

> It places the physician in jeopardy of the patient's hindsight and bitterness. It places the fact-finder in the position of deciding whether a speculative answer to a hypothetical question is to be credited. It calls for a subjective determination solely on testimony of a patient-witness shadowed by the occurrence of the undisclosed risk.[7]

This reference to hindsight links to a third standard that is rarely used: the *subjective* standard. This standard is claimed to be at a greater risk of influence from "hindsight" and "bitterness," and so the generally accepted concept of the reasonable patient favors an objective, universal patient.

## 26.4.2 Consent

Informed consent is a process whereby the patient (or surrogate decision maker) gives the clinician permission to perform some assessment or intervention. Required as part of this process is that the patient should be walked through the treatment options, including that of no treatment, by the responsible clinician. A risk analysis of possible costs (financial, physiological, emotional) and benefits should be undertaken so that the patient can make a knowledgeable (*informed*) decision to permit (*consent* to) the clinician to undertake the intervention. The American Medical Association acknowledges that informed consent should be a process that includes the following:

- Disclosure and discussion (risks, benefits, no treatment, diagnosis, etc.)
- An opportunity for the patient to ask questions to understand options better[8]

Unfortunately the *process* of informed consent became an *event* ("did you consent the patient"). At its worst this means "did you get a signature on some form that purports to absolve the health care provider of legal liability."[9] SLPs must understand that their duty is to explore possible interventions with a patient/family and they may make a recommendation—that is why the patient comes to an expert. Patients do not have to give permission for an intervention that they do not like, so the idea of a patient being "noncompliant" with treatment is somewhat troublesome. As long as the *dialogue of discussion* is clearly documented where the SLP can show that there was reasonable disclosure, and that the patient understood the costs and benefits of the options and his or her final choice, then the process of informed consent is satisfactory.

To show that consent was informed we need to demonstrate that certain conditions were satisfied[10]:

- Voluntariness: that the patient was not coerced, whether overtly (e.g., with the threat of termination of care unless an intervention is agreed to), or covertly (e.g., a clinician indicating displeasure by way of subtle verbal or body language)
- Capacity: that the patient was able to weigh the costs and benefits of each option and explain the rationale for a particular choice
- Intent: that the patient intended to choose the option he or she did and that it represents the patient's values and thoughts over a period of time

The requirement of voluntariness speaks directly to the concept of a waiver. A waiver is a document that a patient/family may be required to sign that purports to absolve the facility of responsibility if anything bad happens to the patient as a result of the patient not following clinical recommendations.[11] In the field of swallowing disorders a waiver will not protect a professional or a facility in the absence of clear documentation of the dialogue of discussion to ensure informed consent. And if you have this documentation, then you do not need a waiver.

Capacity differs from competence, which is a legally judged state of a person with regard to all decisions. Capacity is for *a specific decision at that moment in time* as judged by the clinician discussing the decision. A person with cognitive impairment may have the capacity to choose which sweater to wear but not who may have access to their financial documents. Or a person may have more lucid periods of the day, or medications may affect when the family/clinical team should approach them with decisions to be made.

### 26.4.3 Advance Planning

There are various types of advance directives, and their requirements and applicability vary from country to country and state to state.[12] Living wills are documents typically drawn up with a legal professional to say what will happen to a person while the person is still alive but incapable of communicating her wishes. The living will gives instructions to the medical team regarding treatment and may give direction on when/what to discontinue, to suspend, or to maintain. These documents cannot be used to refuse basic nursing care (e.g., simple hygiene), to stop nursing staff offering food and drink by mouth, or to request euthanasia or unreasonable treatment.[13] The issue of being offered food and drink, advance directives, and conditions such as dementia has recently hit the headlines and is by no means clearly settled, but a fuller consideration of this is beyond our remit.[14]

A component of an advance directive often refers to who can make decisions on a patient's behalf, or who has power of attorney. Typically this refers to who has *financial* rights rather than those related to health care. Clinicians must check that the surrogate decision maker has *health care/medical* power of attorney (also referred to as the health care proxy).[12] This is written by a grantor/principal (the patient) and appoints a designee/attorney-in-fact.[15] The appointment of a health care attorney-in-fact can be made independently to writing a living will, but there are still requirements; for example, the appointing document must state clearly that the patient discussed his wishes with the named health care attorney-in-fact. This appointment can be changed by the patient at any time. The health care attorney-in-fact cannot legally override a specific decision that a patient made in his living will.[16] Patients are advised to consult a legal professional because most aspects of advance directives are state specific.

## Box 26.3

**Case Review: Medicolegal Framework**

1. How do Nancy's and Carla's individual circumstances each challenge the clinician with regard to disclosure?
2. What special challenges may be present in terms of consent and participating in care decisions?

## 26.5 Medical Principles

Ethical principles in general are discussed elsewhere in the book. We include a short description of the framework of medical ethical principles because they are inherent to our understanding of many topics in this chapter. For further detail on these principles readers are encouraged to read Beauchamp and Childress, who are credited with the development of this framework.[10] From an understanding of these principles we may gain an understanding of the tension that we face daily with patients and families: the pull between patients being *autonomous* beings, and even us as clinicians trying to enable this in our patients, and the clinician being duty bound to be a *beneficent* being. And then, what if a patient does not follow our "expert" advice?

### 26.5.1 Autonomy

This is regarded by many as the foundational principle: that of respecting another as an individual who has the right to decide what is done to his or her body. This is exemplified by the ruling and comment from Justice Benjamin Cardozo in one of the first cases in US law courts to adjudicate in a claim of malpractice due to lack of informed consent (or battery as it was then). This principle still applies over one hundred years later:

> Every human being of adult years and sound mind has a right to determine what shall be done with his own body; and a surgeon who performs an operation without his

patient's consent commits an assault for which he is liable in damages. This is true except in cases of emergency where the patient is unconscious and where it is necessary to operate before consent can be obtained.[17]

This principle supports both the concept of informed consent and informed refusal of intervention. We must bear in mind that the idea of the individual wielding 100% of the autonomy votes is a Western construct. Many cultures regard the family as being the decision makers or even the broader social grouping. This is extremely relevant for modern clinical practice in many countries and health care systems, where a wide range of cultures make up the patient *and* provider populations.[18]

## 26.5.2 Beneficence

This is the clinical professional's duty to take positive action to do good for others *and* act to prevent or remove harm. Surely we as SLPs would always be driven by our duty to be beneficent. But consider the action whereby an SLP recommends modification to the consistency of a patient's food/drink. If the patient dislikes the recommended foods and liquids, she may refuse intake, which has dire consequences.[19,20,21] Thus our best intention may put a patient in harm's way. SLPs can optimize their beneficent actions by being professionally competent, up to date on clinical guidelines, and aware of the evidence base behind their decisions.

## 26.5.3 Nonmaleficence

Closely related to beneficence is the principle of nonmaleficence: that a clinician would not cause deliberate harm to a patient. Most clinicians would decry any idea that they would ever be maleficent. But consider the previous example of the modification of food texture or the thickening of drinks. There is now research evidence showing the danger of restricting a patient's diet, and this evidence should be known to clinicians practicing evidence-based care in swallow impairment. The argument could be made that placing a patient on a restrictive diet without due consideration of potential consequences is an act of maleficence.

## 26.5.4 Justice

Justice means to provide what patients need in a fair and equitable manner. On the surface this seems straight forward, but how do we really figure out what people *need*? This is not the same as what *we think* they should have. For this we need to develop the skill of listening to our patients and enabling them to ask the questions that they do not even know they need to ask.

## Box 26.4

**Case Review: Medical Principles**

1. If Nancy is a first-generation Taiwanese immigrant, how might the principle of autonomy be interpreted differently than if she is a fifth-generation German immigrant?
2. Compare and contrast how the principle of *justice* might be applied in Carla's and Nancy's cases.

## 26.6 Professional Standards

Federal statutes describe the rights patients have about the types of care they will receive. Outside of these statutes, standards and policies of our professional governing body (ASHA) provide guidance regarding how, in what areas, with what preparation, and with what knowledge base we as clinicians may practice in the United States. Other countries have their own policy documents, and international clinicians must follow the regulations where they practice. The ASHA Certificate of Clinical Competence (CCC) is the single nationally recognized clinical standard required by most employers.

### 26.6.1 Scope of Practice

ASHA policy documents provide resources for clinicians and students to guide them in acquiring the necessary knowledge and skills to enter the profession and guidelines to providing appropriate care to patients across varying diagnoses and complexities. A key document that describes and delineates the activities of our profession's work is the *Scope of Practice in Speech-Language Pathology*.[6] Professional activities include making clinical decisions across the life span, collaborating with others, and counseling and advocating for individuals so that they can fully participate in shared decision making. To engage in these activities clinicians must have a complete understanding of policy documents and legal statutes governing the practice. SLPs are not permitted to engage in activities that are outside their scope of practice.

SLP activities include evaluating and making recommendations that may facilitate effective swallowing, counseling about effects and risks of proposed swallowing-based interventions, and coordinating/serving on interprofessional teams that assist patients with complex decision making.[22,23] The interprofessional team makes specific recommendations about medications, recommending specific alternate routes or types of nutritional supplements.

### 26.6.2 Certification Standards

Entry-level competencies for practice are delineated in the 2014 Certification Standards,[24] which include knowledge and skills that all clinicians must possess in order to qualify for certification. Academic programs are required to provide experiences for students so that all entry-level practitioners meet these standards. Standards include knowledge about normal and disordered swallowing as well as changes across the life span, knowledge of research principles, ethical practice, and contemporary professional issues. Clinical skills include (among many others) the ability to collect and integrate case history information and adapt clinical procedures to meet client needs. Standard IV-H states that individuals making application for initial certification must demonstrate knowledge of regulations at all levels (local, state, national) that relate to professional practice.[24] Thus there is a mandate from our national association that entry-level professionals must follow all levels of statutes and guidelines.

### 26.6.3 Code of Ethics

The ASHA Code of Ethics[5] also provides a framework for thinking about care for patients across levels of care. The Code of Ethics requires that services shall be provided without discrimination on the basis of (among others) age or disability; therefore, patients across the life span and with any medical condition are equally eligible for intervention and for participating in the development of their plan of care. Furthermore, the Code of Ethics mandates the process of informed consent in that individuals shall inform clients of the nature and possible effects of services rendered. Interventions must be described to patients with sufficient clarity to enable a full understanding of potential costs as well as potential benefits of any intervention considered.

### 26.6.4 Additional Resources

ASHA provides a wide range of clinical resources that includes technical reports, position statements, suggested curricula, and evidence-based resources. Clinicians must remain current on evolving knowledge regarding normal and disordered swallowing, aging and swallowing, and regulatory changes affecting practice in order to remain in compliance with ASHA policies that govern professional practice.

---

### Box 26.5

**Case Review: Professional Standards**

1. Assume that Nancy and Carla have been seen for a dysphagia evaluation, and the SLP does not believe that one of the patients will be able to sustain nutrition orally. How should the clinician address recommendations while maintaining the limitations imposed by our scope of practice? Does it matter whether we are discussing one patient or the other?
2. What options might be available for management of dysphagia for each patient? For each option, consider a potential benefit as well as potential risk. In compliance with the Code of Ethics, how might the SLP discuss these options with each patient?
3. A facility has hired a new graduate completing her clinical fellowship. Given the mandates from the standards, what would be the expectations of this clinician's knowledge base regarding federal, state, and local laws that pertain to practice and patient rights?
4. A colleague states, "This patient is terminal. She does not require speech-language pathology services." Consult the Code of Ethics and formulate a response to your colleague.

---

## 26.7 Interacting with Others

SLPs must follow all legal and ethical guidelines when they work with patients but many SLPs have difficulty doing so in individual cases. Clinicians may be reluctant to "permit a known aspirator to eat/drink" out of fear of clinical or personal consequences. Personal difficulty with following regulations about patient choices may stem from changing philosophies on the relationship between medical staff and patients, how those changes inform how we interact, and the role we have in these interactions.

### 26.7.1 The Patient

Many older adults will live with their medical diagnoses for the rest of their lives and will never truly be healed. Regardless of their status as terminal, hospice, rehabilitative, or any combination, patients have the right to make choices about their care, to participate in care planning, and to function as *the* central and most important member of the team. We do not ignore a patient's medical diagnosis, which is important in understanding the big picture of each clinical case. Equally, in a terminal condition we must respect the individual patient's rights, freedoms, and individuality in planning care. When the patient is terminal, and is considered at the end of life, clinicians may find it easier to acknowledge the importance of the patients' right to plan his own care. However, the *nonterminal* patient also has the same rights to plan her own care, to make her own decisions, and to be an active participant in all aspects of her program.

### 26.7.2 Avoiding Paternalism

Patients may not agree with a clinician-derived plan of care, and clinicians may not want to accept the mandates and ethical directives about honoring patient choices with regard to care. Why do such disagreements occur and who is responsible? Can they be avoided? One answer may be found in a form of beneficence known as medical paternalism. Medical paternalism has been described as *benevolent decision making*, usually made in another's best interest.[25] Decision making always involves a cost–benefit analysis, but in medical paternalism, health care professionals apply *their own analysis* to the decision at hand, prioritizing *their* belief system over that of the patient. Thus paternalism is a form of beneficence in that practitioners *believe* they are protecting the best interests of the patient, despite the fact that they have not used the patient's belief system or wishes.[26] This is inappropriate practice despite its historical use.

There is a long-standing tradition in health care that the physician, with the medical knowledge and experience, is the one best equipped to make decisions. The practice may originate from the old Hippocratic oath (which included the text "according to my judgment and means," wording that is absent from the modern oath).[27] Thus the physician assumed responsibility for knowing and doing what was best. The patient who did not know any better was expected to simply follow the doctor's orders or be deemed noncompliant. Similarly, the SLP has more knowledge about normal and disordered swallowing than the patient, has conducted evaluations using medical instrumentation, and has made recommendations. SLPs may be uncomfortable when relationships deviate from the paternalistic tradition and may refuse to treat patients who disagree with recommendations. This is a one-sided decision-making structure and is inappropriate.

Health care providers are not expected to simply do whatever patients wish, with no regard for potential consequences (undermining the knowledge of the provider). But patients are not expected to simply comply with whatever the provider recommends (undermining the wishes of the patient).[26] Ideally, in reconciling autonomy with beneficence there is shared decision making, whereby honest discussions consider potential good and bad outcomes, values, and wishes, so that agreement on a plan can be reached that supports both parties.

## 26.7.3 Avoiding Bias and Coercion

The professional who believes that the patient "should do what we recommend" may provide information in ways that may be biased or leading in nature. Bias in patient education must be identified and minimized/eradicated because it is unethical to provide information to patients that is prejudicial to their decision making. Unintentional communicative bias can result in patients making choices in agreement with their clinician's value system instead of their own. Biased or incomplete information can be considered coercive in nature because its intent is to influence a decision without respecting the patient's own value system.[26,28]

Consider a patient who is aspirating all thin liquids, regardless of the method of introduction, as per documentation from an instrumental assessment. Patient education should include both the known (assessment results) and the unknown (e.g., individual variations, such as immune response, activity level, general health, oral hygiene, all influencing the possible consequences of aspiration). Complete information includes what we know, do not know, and cannot obtain, taking good care not to lead the patient in one direction or another beyond known medical consequences.[28] Biased communication might include statements such as, "Yes, you can refuse thickened liquids, but if you refuse them you will be aspirating all of those thin liquids, and that can lead to pneumonia." This information excludes important factors, such as the patient's current health status (if the patient is currently aspirating without complication), activity level, oral hygiene, and other individual factors.

Other types of beneficence identified as biases include an inappropriate commitment to some course of action (e.g., "People who aspirate or are at risk of aspiration must receive altered-consistency diets") and bias encouraged by others on the team ("Well, of course you'll be putting him on thickened liquids. Isn't he aspirating? My goodness, the last thing he needs is pneumonia.").[29] No one may coerce patients, even unintentionally, by applying their own value systems and biases to the clinical situation.

Discussions must include the potential consequences of doing nothing as well as the consequences of the proposed intervention. A nonbiased statement might include "You can receive all the fluids needed when the liquids are thickened, but many people do not like them. There is a risk of not drinking enough liquid, which can lead to dehydration. Dehydration can be very dangerous, but we cannot know right now how much liquid you will drink." Then patients can make decisions within their belief system and based upon information that is pertinent to their case. Simplistic statements, such as "We're only doing what's best for the patient" are vague at best and fail to define what "best" actually is and whose judgment it is.[26] No one can define what contributes to the welfare of the person served better than that person and his or her family.[25]

## 26.7.4 Families, Physicians, and Team Members

Families can provide important information about history, likes and dislikes, philosophical underpinnings, and religious/spiritual issues that the patient may be unable to provide. If a patient has difficulty making decisions or has lost his decision-making capacity, the family may become the source for information and assent/consent for interventions or diet recommendations. Families do not always know for sure what their loved one would have wanted, and decisions may be subject to a misuse of the family member's own values and wishes as opposed to those of the patient.

Just like patients, families need complete and nonbiased information either to support the patient in her own independent choice or to make that decision on the patient's behalf. Clinicians should not attempt to direct family members toward a decision inconsistent with the patient's values simply because someone else (family, SLP) might be more comfortable or might agree with it. Clinicians should document family conversations as well as specific responses from family members that clearly indicate that information was processed and comprehended prior to decisions being presented.

Our contributions to patient care are limited to the areas within our scope of practice. Objective information from the assessment process must be presented in the context of the entire patient, which will likely entail medical issues that require the physician's expertise to clarify. Physicians, physician assistants, and nurse practitioners (where applicable) are the team members who write care orders, diet orders, and medication orders. They provide education related to medically based issues, such as feeding tubes, whereas our scope of practice is focused on the patient's swallowing status and physical ability to consume sufficient items for adequate nutrition and hydration.

Our communication should be explicit about who might do what. For example, "You might consider ordering a consultation with the dietitian to review this patient's nutritional status; if you look at his lab values, you might find they're a bit off." SLPs should take care with conversations about medically oriented information with patients and families and refer to the physician or designee (attorney-in-fact) where appropriate. Role delineation is important to protect clinicians from any liability that might follow from violations of our scope of practice.

Other facility staff may not be accustomed to interactive shared decision making when developing plans of care for patients, especially if their experience has been more paternalistic. Legal and ethical frameworks, Medicare guidelines, and Residents' Rights are not specific to dysphagia therapy; thus all caregivers' documented interactions supporting informed choice are important. Development of a facility climate that focuses on residents making informed choices will help ensure the facility treats all patients with dignity and respects their autonomy.

## 26.7.5 Problem Solving

What about the "noncompliant" patient? This term has a connotation of subservience as though the patient is not an equal party in the treatment plan. The term is a remnant of paternalism, and it should not be used: it conveys of a lack of respect for the very individuals we are called to serve. The nature of "compliance" with swallowing therapy was examined via a small survey of eight SLPs who found that patients did not comply with treatment recommendations for reasons that included dislike of altered consistencies, denial of a swallowing disorder, acceptance of a calculated risk, minimization, and accommodation.[30] The study made no reference to attempts to shared decision making, and it is not clear to what extent any patient education was free of bias. Open conversations between the patient, clinician, and medical staff will lead to far fewer cases where patients disagree with the plan of care.

Waivers as previously noted are sometimes attempted to "protect" a facility from consequences of the "noncompliant" patient's decisions, but they do not protect a facility from outright negligence in care. Waivers are coercive, signifying that "We know best, and if you choose not to do what we say, you must sign this paper." Instead, nonbiased and honest discussions can lead to shared decision making with full knowledge of potential benefits and risks.[25]

## Box 26.6

**Case Review: Interacting with Others**

1. For Nancy and Carla, consider two possible courses of treatments, and role play the discussions that might be held to reach a mutually agreeable course of treatment regarding management of their swallowing disorders.
2. How do cognitive and linguistic impairments impact these discussions and further challenge our clinical work?
3. Imagine a discussion to be held with a nursing administrator who is accustomed to a paternalistic approach to patient care. She asks, "Why do we need a speech pathologist anyway, if you're just going to do whatever the patient wants?" Formulate responses that would be appropriate for Nancy's case and Carla's case.

## 26.8 Liability, Certification, Writing Goals, and Planning Care

Conversations about patient choices and decision making are often clouded by fear of liability for negative health consequences of those decisions. This section addresses the regulations about medical liability, how our clinical credentials are involved in liability, and the best ways to plan care and document in ways that minimize risks of negative repercussions.

### 26.8.1 Liability

Diagnosis, patient safety, patient rights, security, negligence, sexual assault, falls, patient care—these considerations are among many that may be a basis for litigation in health care. Health care professionals are expected to apply evidence-based practices within current standards of practice and an ethical framework. In the event that a clinician fails to do this, or to accurately document the services provided, the clinician may

be held responsible for any negative outcomes. According to the National Conference of State Legislatures,[31] under state law, a patient may pursue a civil claim against physicians or other health care providers, called medical liability or medical malpractice, if the health care provider causes injury or death to the patient through a negligent act or omission. To recover damages, the patient must establish (1) that the physician (or health care provider) owed a duty to the patient, (2) the standard of care and that the physician (or health care provider) violated that standard, (3) a compensable injury, and (4) that the violation of the standard of care caused harm suffered by the patient.

Let's then consider the SLP who completes a dysphagia assessment and treatment plan with a patient. The SLP will be best served to do so in conjunction with the patient and the patient's legal health care decision maker. The responsibility (or liability) for the outcomes of treatment should be transparent, and the decisions that are made during each point of contact are accurately documented. Liability may be present in an instance where it can be substantiated that the SLP violated the standard of practice, and the violation caused the harm suffered by the patient.

### 26.8.2 Licensure

State licensure is a state-level (as opposed to federal) regulatory process intended to protect the public from personnel who are not qualified or credentialed to provide services. Professionals must hold the appropriate license in the state(s) in which they practice, assuring the public that the professional providing clinical services is properly trained and is conducting his or her practice consistent with state and local laws. State licensure is a mandate about *professional preparation* and adherence to state-level statutes. State licensure is not a credential that is revoked depending on patient progress, lack of progress, or other medical complications experienced by clients served. Trends in state licensure reported by ASHA[32] indicate that 33 of 50 states include a code of ethics in their statutory or regulatory documents, and 48 of 50 states mandate continuing professional education. Professional conduct includes providing patients with current information about their care and following all laws, including permitting patients to make choices and direct their own care. Anecdotally, some SLPs fear that they will "lose their license" if their name is attached to an "inappropriate" recommendation. The SLP's license is safe regardless of the choices made by patients and families. If SLPs follow ethical principles and adhere to ASHA's scope of practice, then collaborative efforts across patients and families will lead to recommendations that are acceptable to the patient, who is the individual affected most directly by any plan of care.

### 26.8.3 Planning Care and Writing Goals

In the health care setting, goals must be written in a manner consistent with reimbursement guidelines. The CMS *Medicare Benefit Policy Manual*[2] describes the general guidelines for reimbursable services in a postacute setting. Documentation of services reimbursed by Medicare must be at a level of complexity that justifies reimbursement, as described in **Box 26.7**.

## Box 26.7

### Guidelines for Documentation

Documentation in postacute settings must clearly indicate the following:

- Skilled services provided
- Medical necessity for those services
- The patient's response to intervention
- The basis for continuing (or discontinuing) the plan of treatment[2]

More specifically related to dysphagia, Chapter 15, Section 230.3, D.4. of the *Medicare Benefit Policy Manual* states the following:

> Swallowing assessment and rehabilitation are highly specialized services. The professional rendering care must have education, experience and demonstrated competencies. Competencies include but are not limited to: identifying abnormal upper aerodigestive tract structure and function; conducting an oral, pharyngeal, laryngeal and respiratory function examination as it relates to the functional assessment of swallowing; recommending methods of oral intake and risk precautions; and developing a treatment plan employing appropriate compensations and therapy techniques.[2] (p. 207)

In the ASHA Practice Portal,[33] documentation of skilled services is described with the components described in **Box 26.8**.

## Box 26.8

### General Guidelines for Skilled Service Documentation

- Use terminology that reflects the clinician's technical knowledge.
- Indicate the rationale (how the service relates to the functional goal), type, and complexity of activity.
- Report objective data showing progress toward the goal.
  - ○ Accuracy of task performance
  - ○ Speed of response/response latency
  - ○ Frequency/number of responses
  - ○ Decreased number/type of cues
  - ○ Physiological variations in the activity
- Specify feedback provided to the patient/caregiver about performance.
- Explain decision making that results in modifications to treatment activities or the plan of care and how modifications resulted in a functional change.
- Explain advances based on functional change.
- Indicate additional goals or activities.
- Indicate dropped or reduced activities.
- Evaluate the patient's/caregiver's response to training.

Goals for a dysphagia plan of care may include a particular diet consistency, safety, and effectiveness of swallowing. Goals should be functional, meaning that the specific functional target is described in the goal rather than *diet tolerance*. Goals should represent the skills of the SLP; therefore goals measuring food consumption are inadequate. Goals should be measurable and can refer to timing of the swallow, the presence or absence of behaviors, rather than randomly selecting a 90% threshold for performance of a task. Goals should refer to the patient as the actor versus what the clinician or caregiver will do. Note that the structure of goals for patients at the end of life should not differ from goals for any other individuals, and in all cases there should be documentation that the plan of care has been discussed with the patient along with possible options, so that the patient may provide informed consent for care.[23]

Some goal examples include the following:

- Poor: Patient will tolerate least-restrictive diet without s/s of aspiration.
- Better: Through the cues of trained caregivers, the patient will demonstrate (desired behavior) while consuming (diet type, e.g., mechanically altered solids) to support adequate nutritional intake by (date).

This short-term goal is specific and measurable. Diet tolerance is ill-defined and unclear as to the nature of the problem. Least restrictive diet (LRD) is not measurable, and the SLP should specify a diet consistency, as shown in the example. The carrier phrase "through the cues of trained caregivers" demonstrates the skills of the SLP in providing caregiver education.

- Poor: Patient will consume 75% of pureed solids and nectar liquids ×3 meals per day.
- Better: Patient will demonstrate adequate oral bolus clearance with pureed solids as evidenced by no oral residue after swallow in 10/10 trials by (date).

This short-term goal could be addressed through oral strengthening, sensory stimulation, and compensatory strategies, such as tongue sweep. It also reflects the skills of the therapist rather than showing something that nonskilled personnel could monitor (meal consumption).

- Poor: Schedule patient for MBS.

This is something that needs to be addressed in the treatment plan, as appropriate, but the tasks that the therapist performs or facilitates are *not* a short-term goal.

Clinicians must discuss with the patient and the family (if possible) the proposed plan of care, options available, and costs and benefits associated with each. Patient choices must be made with full knowledge of their options, and clinician documentation must reflect that such conversations have taken place. Particularly in cases where the patient has a communication disorder, documentation must reflect the patient's comprehension of options and understanding of costs and benefits. Clinicians should write a progress note that includes a summary of the discussion, statement of the options that were provided, questions that were asked and how they were answered, and a statement of which individuals were present for the discussion.[34] In the discussion, clinicians should avoid the use of professional jargon, using terms like "food and water" rather than "nutrition and hydration," "eating and drinking" rather than "deglutition." Communicatively impaired patients may need picture or written support, extra time to process information, and extra time to formulate responses to make informed decisions.[34] A clearly documented conversation should reflect the use of and response to these supports so that the patient's comprehension is not questioned, as can easily occur with standardized forms sometimes used in place of clear and thorough documentation.[11]

---

### Box 26.9

**Case Review: Planning Care and Documentation**

1. What are some possible goals that could be devised for Nancy and Carla that would be measurable, functional, and require the skilled services of the SLP?
2. How might a plan of treatment be written that specifies the medical necessity of the plan?
3. Plan a discussion with each patient that outlines several options with the costs and benefits for each. How would you document each conversation?

---

## 26.9 Dispelling Common Myths

Clinicians often communicate with well-meaning colleagues through face-to-face communication and social media. Social media permits clinicians around the world to communicate about many different topics, but there is no guarantee that the information will be true, have a basis in regulation, or be applicable to the work setting or location where the clinician is practicing. We will present some of the myths encountered in more informal conversations and provide information that should clarify desired practice patterns and consequences based on the information provided in this chapter.

1. **Myth #1: My primary job is to prevent my patients from aspirating.** It is not possible to prevent aspiration, and even in cases where interventions might possibly reduce prandial aspiration, this might lead to quality of life sacrifices that the patient is not willing to make. Ultimately, decisions about health care are up to the patient, who needs accurate information in order to reach an informed decision. Thus the SLP's primary job is to educate the patient about his or her swallow so that the patient and family can, together with the medical team, decide how they wish to proceed with their care.

2. **Myth #2: If a patient under my care develops complications from pneumonia, I will lose my license.** A license to practice is a statement of meeting state-defined training requirements. It is a credential that indicates one is qualified to practice in the professional area defined by the license. As long as a clinician works within regulatory and ethical standards, the license is safe. The reality is that many of our residents are old and sick with multiple comorbidities that have the potential to contribute to medical complications. The best defense for a clinician who

fears such situations is a well-educated patient and family, who can then make their own care decisions, and ensuring that all conversations are clearly documented in the medical record.

3. **Myth #3: If a patient under my care develops complications from pneumonia, I will be sued.** Legal liability is an unfortunate yet all-too-common fear. In the United States it is not possible to stop someone accusing a professional of malpractice—the important thing is to ensure that the claims will be established as unfounded given appropriate procedure and documentation. There is no liability for providing a patient and the family with the potential benefits and potential costs of any course of treatment and then permitting the patient to choose the care he or she is comfortable pursuing. Real liability is present if the SLP fails to disclose potential costs and benefits before recommending an intervention.

4. **Myth #4. A patient who aspirates must be designated nothing by mouth or be provided altered consistencies.** Such an intervention is one possible alternative among many. All interventions come with potential benefits and potential costs, and the recommendation for nothing by mouth is no different. Its costs include reduced quality of life while not reducing the possibility of aspiration of oral bacteria. An altered consistency may be easier to manage but is of no use if the patient will not eat or drink. It is the clinician's responsibility to provide education about different possible interventions so that an informed choice can be made.

5. **Myth #5. Feeding tubes prevent aspiration, so they should be used when patients aspirate.** The decision to accept any medical procedure belongs to the patient in consultation with the health care team. There are medical risks associated with feeding tubes, and the presence of a feeding tube has been associated with aspiration pneumonia as one possible medical consequence.[35] Tube feeding at the end of life is not supported in the literature; careful hand feeding leads to similar outcomes in terms of health status and quality of life.[36] Patients must have accurate information so that they can make the informed choice of whether or not they wish to accept tube feeding as their medical treatment.

6. **Myth #6. People at the end of life or on hospice services don't need dysphagia therapy.** Current regulations permit skilled speech-language pathology services as part of a program of palliative care and/or hospice care. Goals for patients at this stage in life might be different from those for an acute rehabilitation patient, but patients at the end of life have the right to make choices about their care, including rehabilitation. Such services are no less appropriate as quality of life comfort care and are important in all the interventions and management programs that we provide.

7. **Myth #7. If a patient does not agree with my recommendations about an acceptable diet level, then I cannot work with the patient even to reduce the risk of complications.** Providers must continue to abjure a paternalistic viewpoint where only the clinician's opinion matters and where the clinician knows best. Although the clinician knows about swallowing and dysphagia, the patient has the ability to make choices about care. The clinician still has the responsibility to care for the patient in the best way possible, in ways acceptable to the patient, who is the most important person in this therapeutic relationship.

8. **Myth #8. If a patient does not agree with clinical recommendations, the patient must sign a waiver in order to receive meals.** Waivers are coercive in nature and carry no legal weight. Although they are intended as a substitute for informed consent/refusal,[37] signing a form is not the same as developing a care plan using shared decision making. Even in cases where patients and families have made decisions that seem quite risky, the use of a waiver creates a coercive dynamic that has no place in health care. Rather, a care plan should be developed with discussion among all stakeholders, including the patient, who is ultimately responsible for his or her own care (or the family member or surrogate). These conversations should be documented, but the coercion of signing some kind of release of responsibility has no place in shared decision making or quality medical care.[11,23,34] Similarly, facilities must comply with the patient's right to self-determination and cannot require the family to waive all legal liability. The facility is obligated to work with the patient and family in developing a plan of care and then documenting the results of all discussions.

## 26.10 Questions

1. Patients who are cognitively impaired still have the right to make decisions about their care. This right is specifically described in which of the following?

A. Medicare Benefits Policy Manual
B. Pioneer Network New Dining Standards
C. Clinical Certification Standards
D. Patient Self-Determination Act
E. Affordable Care Act

2. Clinicians may fear that honoring patients' choices about care decisions will lead to risk of their license, when in fact they are obligated to honor patients' choices and provide sufficient information so patients can give informed consent. Which of the following statements best explains why the above is true?

A. Patient rights under the Patient Self Determination Act only apply when the patient is at the end of life.
B. Patients at all stages of life have the right to self-determination and informed consent.
C. Patients need to be provided information only if they are cognitively intact.
D. Cognitively impaired patients do not fall under the Patient Self-Determination Act.
E. Family members may legally change a patient's choices about care when the patient approaches the end of life.

3. Waivers are documents that some clinicians and facilities believe are necessary when a patient disagrees with the proposed plan of care. In reality waivers are ineffective and undesirable documents. Which of the following statements is true about waivers?

A. Waivers provide standard language so they cover all diagnoses and all patient complaints.

B. Waivers are approved by the facility's legal counsel so they should be signed to be in legal compliance with facility regulations.
C. Waivers do not reflect the conversation that should be held with the patient and family and clearly documented to support that patient education and an informed choice have taken place.
D. Waivers do not protect the staff in the event of abuse or neglect, but they are required to protect the staff from the noncompliant patient.
E. Waivers should be used in all cases of patient–clinician disagreement to document the recommended treatment plan.

4. Janice is a patient with a mild cognitive impairment. She does not like altered-consistency foods and liquids and refuses to eat them. She would prefer to have food and drink that is more normal, but the staff will not permit this, saying she is at risk of aspiration and is "noncompliant with recommendations." What is the best response to this scenario?

A. This is a noncompliant patient, and the family should sign a waiver prior to permitting her to have anything but the recommended foods and liquids.
B. This patient is attempting to exercise her right to self-determination, and there should be a meeting to discuss cost and benefit of several possible interventions for her swallowing and her foods and drink so that her choices about her oral intake are made with full information.
C. This patient will likely aspirate and develop complications, so she needs education that will clearly explain these risks to her, encouraging her to agree with the SLP's recommendations.
D. The SLP should discharge the patient from her caseload because the patient does not wish to follow recommendations.
E. If the patient is cognitively impaired, then she does not have the right to refuse clinical recommendations because she is not competent to make her own decisions.

5. Capacity differs from competence, and understanding of this difference is important in ensuring that cognitively impaired patients are respected and are free to make choices about their care. How do they differ?

A. A patient might not be competent to sign legal documents but may have the capacity to decide what she would like to eat for a meal.
B. A patient who is not competent to sign legal documents is also not competent to make decisions about her food and drink.
C. A patient must demonstrate capacity to make decisions at all times in order for her decisions to be respected.
D. A patient who is not competent cannot provide informed consent to any procedure or plan.
E. Cognitively impaired patients neither have capacity to make decisions nor can be deemed competent.

# 26.11 Answers and Explanations

**1. Correct: Patient Self-Determination Act (D).**

The Patient Self-Determination Act describes patients' rights to participate in their own care and direct their own health care decisions.

**2. Correct: patients at all stages of life have the right to self-determination and informed consent (B).**

Despite the fact that many of these issues regarding patient care have emerged as we care for end of life cases, the law is clear that all patients at all stages of life have the right to self-determination and informed consent.

**3. Correct: waivers do not reflect the conversation that should be held with the patient and family and clearly documented to support that patient education and an informed choice have taken place (C).**

Waivers are insufficient documentation, as they do not permit a summary of a conversation where questions have been asked and answered, with shared decision making and mutual agreement on a plan of care.

**4. Correct: this patient is attempting to exercise her right to self-determination, and there should be a meeting to discuss cost and benefit of several possible interventions for her swallowing and her foods and drink so that her choices about her oral intake are made with full information (B).**

The patient has the right to disagree with recommendations and to exercise the right to refuse the treatment plan, but the decision should be made with all the information needed to make a fully informed choice.

**5. Correct: a patient might not be competent to sign legal documents, but may have the capacity to decide what she would like to eat for a meal (A).**

Patients do not relinquish rights to direct their own care due to a cognitive impairment that might limit their ability to make other types of decisions, such as about finances or other such matters.

## References

[1] Patient Self Determination Act § 1395cc (a)(1)(1990)

[2] Center for Medicare and Medicaid Services. Medicare Benefits Policy Manual. 2012. https://www.cms.gov/Regulations-and-Guidance/Guidance/Manuals/Internet-Only-Manuals-Ioms-Items/Cms012673.html. Accessed September 25, 2015.

[3] Pioneer Network and Task Force. New Dining Practice Standards. *J Am Geriatr Soc* 2011;*51*(11):1410–1418

[4] American Medical Directors Assocation. Altered Nutritional Status in Long Term Care Settings: Clinical Practice Guidelines. Columbia, MD: Author; 2010

[5] American Speech-Language-Hearing Association. Code of Ethics. 2016. http://www.asha.org/policy/ET2016-00342/. Accessed February 12, 2016

[6] 6. American Speech-Language-Hearing Association. Scope of Practice in Speech-Language Pathology. 2007. doi: 10.1044/policy.SP2007-00283

[7] Court of Appeals of New York. *Canterbury v. Spence*, 464 F.2d 772 (150 U.S.App.D.C. 263 1972). Court of Appeals of New York (1914)

[8] American Medical Association. Informed Consent. http://www.ama-assn.org/ama/pub/physician-resources/medical-ethics/code-medical-ethics/opinion808.page. Accessed March 1, 2013

[9] Lidz CW, Appelbaum PS, Meisel A. Two models of implementing informed consent. *Arch Intern Med* 1988;*148*(6):1385–1389

[10] Beauchamp T, Childress JF. Principles of Biomedical Ethics. 7th ed. New York, NY: Oxford University Press; 2013

[11] Sharp HM. When patients refuse recommendations for dysphagia treatment. *Perspect Swallowing Swallowing Disord* 2005;*14*(3):3–7

[12] American Bar Association. Living Wills, Health Care Proxies, and Advance Health Care Directives. http://www.americanbar.org/groups/real_property_trust_estate/resources/estate_planning/living_wills_health_care_proxies_advance_health_care_directives.html

[13] Fewing R, Kirk T, Meisel A. Case study. A fading decision. Commentary. *Hastings Cent Rep* 2014;*44*(3):14–15

[14] Span P. Complexities of choosing an end game for dementia. New York Times. http://nyti.ms/1DUWHQ2. Accessed January 20, 2015

[15] Pozgar G. Legal and Ethical Issues for Health Professionals. 3rd ed. Burlington, MA: Jones & Bartlett Learning; 2003

[16] Judson K, Harrison C, Hicks S. Law and Ethics for Medical Careers. 4th ed. New York, NY: McGraw-Hill; 2006

[17] *Schloendorff v. Society of New York Hospital*, 105 N.E. 92 (211 NY 125 1914)

[18] Kleinman A. Illness unto death. In: The Illness Narratives. New York, NY: Basic Books; 1988:146–157

[19] Westergren A, Unosson M, Ohlsson O, Lorefält B, Hallberg IR. Eating difficulties, assisted eating and nutritional status in elderly (> or = 65 years) patients in hospital rehabilitation. *Int J Nurs Stud* 2002;*39*(3):341–351

[20] Wright L, Cotter D, Hickson M, Frost G. Comparison of energy and protein intakes of older people consuming a texture modified diet with a normal hospital diet. *J Hum Nutr Diet* 2005;*18*(3):213–219 doi: 10.1111/j.1365-277X.2005.00605.x

[21] Rowat A, Graham C, Dennis M. Dehydration in hospital-admitted stroke patients: detection, frequency, and association. *Stroke* 2012;*43*(3):857–859 doi: 10.1161/STROKEAHA.111.640821

[22] American Speech-Language-Hearing Association. Roles of speech-language pathologists in swallowing and feeding disorders: technical report. 2001. http://www.asha.org/policy/TR2001-00150/. Accessed September 10, 2015

[23] Sharp H, Genesen L. Ethical decision-making in dysphagia management. *Am J Speech Lang Pathol* 1996;*5*(1):15–22 doi: 10.1044/1058-0360.0501.15

[24] Council for Clinical Certification in Audiology and Speech-Language Pathology of the American Speech-Language-Hearing Association. 2014 SLP Certification Standards. https://www.asha.org/Certification/2020-SLP-Certification-Standards/

[25] Tuckett AG. On paternalism, autonomy and best interests: telling the (competent) aged-care resident what they want to know. *Int J Nurs Pract* 2006;*12*(3):166–173 doi: 10.1111/j.1440-172X.2006.00565.x

[26] Devettere R. Practical Decision Making in Health Care Ethics: Cases and Concepts 3rd ed. Washington, DC: Georgetown University Press; 2010

[27] Johns Hopkins University. Bioethics. 2015. http://guides.library.jhu.edu/bioethics. Accessed January 1, 2015

[28] Aggarwal A, Davies J, Sullivan R. "Nudge" in the clinical consultation—an acceptable form of medical paternalism? *BMC Med Ethics* 2014;*15*(1):31 doi: 10.1186/1472-6939-15-31

[29] Croskerry P. Achieving quality in clinical decision making: cognitive strategies and detection of bias. *Acad Emerg Med* 2002;*9*(11):1184–1204 doi: 10.1111/j.1553-2712.2002.tb01574.x

[30] King J, Ligman K. Patient noncompliance with swallowing recommendations: reports from speech-language pathologists. *Contemp Issues Commun Sci Disord* 2011;*38*:53–60

[31] National Conference of State Legislatures. Medical Liability and Malpractice. http://www.ncsl.org/research/financial-services-and-commerce/medical-liability-and-malpractice.aspx. Accessed October 2, 2016

[32] American Speech-Language-Hearing Association. State Licensure Trends. http://www.asha.org/advocacy/state/StateLicensureTrends/. Accessed September 13, 2015

[33] American Speech-Language-Hearing Association. The Practice Portal. http://www.asha.org/practice-portal/. Accessed October 2, 2016

[34] Sharp HM. Informed consent in clinical and research settings: what do patients and families need to make informed decisions? *Perspect Swallowing Swallowing Disord* 2015;*24*:130–139

[35] Langmore SE, Terpenning MS, Schork A, et al. Predictors of aspiration pneumonia: how important is dysphagia? *Dysphagia* 1998;*13*(2):69–81

[36] Arcand M. End-of-life issues in advanced dementia: Part 2: management of poor nutritional intake, dehydration, and pneumonia. *Can Fam Physician* 2015;*61*(4):337–341

[37] Sharp HM, Wagner LB. Ethics, informed consent, and decisions about nonoral feeding for patients with dysphagia. *Western Michigan University* 2007;*23*(3):240–248

## Suggested Reading

[1] American Speech-Language-Hearing Association. Code of Ethics. 2016. http://www.asha.org/policy/ET2016-00342/

[2] Horner J, Modayil M, Chapman LR, Dinh A. Consent, refusal, and waivers in patient-centered dysphagia care: using law, ethics, and evidence to guide clinical practice. *Am J Speech Lang Pathol* 2016;*25*(4):453–469

# 27 Clinical and Professional Ethics for the Speech-Language Pathologist

*Tammy Wigginton*

## Summary

Principles of ethical reasoning can be applied to professional behavior and clinical care. The American Speech-Language-Hearing Association (ASHA) Code of Ethics can be used as a guide for making day-to-day decisions in the workplace. Ethical breaches can vary in their degree of severity, and consequences are determined accordingly. Ethical breaches related to scope of practice, clinical competence, and current best practice can result in physical harm to patients, particularly those patients with nutrition, feeding, and swallowing issues. Examples of competencies related to swallowing and feeding can be found in ASHA's policy documents.

Effective navigation of clinical ethics requires identification, analysis, and resolution of ethical dilemmas in the context of dynamic patient care. Familiarity with the four principles of medical ethics can help clinicians develop a better understanding of clinical ethics.

## Keywords

professional ethics, clinical ethics, autonomy, beneficence, non-maleficence, justice

### Learning Objectives

- Discuss the differences between professional ethics and clinical ethics
- Discuss the concept of clinical competence with regard to setting, population, and procedures
- Discuss the four principles of medical ethics
- Discuss the concept of net benefits

## 27.1 Introduction

Each year approximately 10 million Americans are evaluated for swallowing difficulties.[1] Feeding and swallowing disorders are associated with high morbidity and mortality[2] as well as significant financial burdens[3] and reduced quality of life.[4] Evaluation and treatment of patients with swallowing disorders can be challenging; issues surrounding nutrition, swallowing, and feeding are often complex. Multiple providers may be involved in a patient's care, and feeding and swallowing issues are often time sensitive and difficult for patients and family members to process. Complex emotions often surround nutrition, feeding, and swallowing issues, and many patients, families, and even other health care providers have preconceived notions or misinformation about these matters. Moreover, several cases involving nutrition, feeding, and swallowing have been sensationalized by the media (Karen Ann Quinlan, Nancy Cruzan, and

Terri Schiavo), resulting in fear and confusion for patients and family members. Under these circumstances, it can be difficult to manage obligations to patients and family members as well as other members of the health care team, institutions, professional organizations, and ourselves in the context of providing optimal patient care. This can be especially true for new clinicians and clinicians who are in the process of acquiring new skills. Given the complex medical and emotional needs of these patients, a functional understanding of ethics is an essential aspect of comprehensive care.

Ethics is a branch of philosophy that explores the nature of moral values and evaluates human actions.[5] The study of moral values and actions as applied to the care of patients is referred to as medical ethics. Principles of ethical reasoning can be applied to professional behavior and clinical care.

## 27.2 Professional Ethics and Management of Patients with Dysphagia

Speech-language pathologists (SLPs), like other health care providers, are credentialed by professional organizations at the national and state level. Professional ethics are typically addressed in the form of a code of ethics or a code of conduct. Codes or guidelines are established to protect patients by ensuring providers are committed to principled reasoning and professional conduct. In the United States, the American Speech-Language-Hearing Association's (ASHA's) Code of Ethics[6] is a framework and focused guide for professionals in support of day-to-day decision making related to professional conduct. ASHA describes the Code as "partially obligatory and disciplinary," addressing issues such as confidentiality, billing, record keeping, scope of practice, clinical competence, and lifelong learning, and "partly aspirational and descriptive" addressing values such as honesty, altruism, and integrity. Speech-language and hearing associations of other countries (Canada, United Kingdom, Australia, Ireland, among others) have similar codes of ethics.

Although ethical infractions regarding confidentiality, billing, and record keeping are very serious, violations of this nature do not typically result in physical harm to patients. In contrast, ethical breaches related to scope of practice, clinical competence, and current best practice can result in physical harm to patients, particularly in the case of patients with nutrition, feeding, and swallowing issues. Therefore, clinicians should provide care only within their area of expertise, setting, and population and should always demonstrate practice patterns that are in keeping with current best evidence.

ASHA requires SLPs to demonstrate competence to evaluate and manage a complex array of communication, feeding, and swallowing disorders, in a variety of settings with diverse patient populations. Competencies are specific to settings, populations, and procedures. A thorough understanding of what constitutes competence should guide professional development and professional behavior.

Clinicians who are reported and proven to be in violation of professional conduct may be sanctioned by their professional organizations at both state and national levels. At the national level, ASHA's Board of Ethics has a range of sanctions it can impose if clinicians are found in violation of one or more provisions of the Code of Ethics. Sanctions range from a reprimand to suspension or withholding of ASHA membership and certification. In addition, the Board of Ethics may also order an individual to cease and desist from any practice or conduct found to be in violation of the Code of Ethics.[7] Generally, more serious violations result in more serious sanctions. Clinicians must also keep in mind that, in addition to sanctions for professional organizations, ethical breaches may result in civil or criminal legal action.

Examples of competencies related to swallowing and feeding can be found in ASHA's policy documents "Knowledge and Skills for Speech-Language Pathologists Providing Services to Individuals with Swallowing and Feeding Disorders"[8] and "Instrumental Diagnostic Procedures for Swallowing"[9] and in a relevant ASHA paper, "Graduate Curriculum on Swallowing and Swallowing Disorders."[10] Competency is typically acquired via a combination of formal course work and a continuing education framework. Appropriate mentorship and a commitment to lifelong learning are essential aspects of competency development and maintenance.

## 27.3 Examples

### Robert

Robert is an SLP who has been working for over 20 years. He specializes in evaluation and treatment of patients with voice disorders, in particular singers. Although he did have training in the evaluation and treatment of patients with dysphagia in graduate school, he has not worked with this population in a number of years and consequently has not remained current regarding treatment trends. Robert is currently treating Mr. Ramirez, an elderly gentleman with presbyphonia. Mr. Ramirez informed Robert that, in addition to voice changes, he is also having difficulty swallowing. Robert discusses his concerns with Mr. Ramirez and with the physician who referred Mr. Ramirez for voice therapy. Robert recommends Mr. Ramirez receive a referral for an evaluation by a clinician with proficiency in swallowing and swallowing disorders and provides the physician with the names of several speech pathologists in the local area who may be able to evaluate Mr. Ramirez. Robert knows it would be unethical to practice outside of his area of expertise.

Can you think of another example of practicing outside one's area of expertise?

### Samantha

Samantha is a relatively new SLP. She completed her clinical fellowship (CF) at a teaching hospital. She was independently evaluating and treating patients with a wide range of communication and swallowing disorders. She and her fiancé have settled in a new town, and she was able to contract with a local rehabilitation

company for a position at a skilled nursing/rehabilitation facility. Samantha is accustomed to having access to instrumentation to evaluate patients with swallowing disorders. She is not sure how she is going to evaluate or treat patients effectively in this setting without instrumentation. She is unclear about the referral process and is also feeling a bit uncomfortable with the billing and record-keeping process in the facility. She realizes she is practicing outside of her previous setting, so she requested mentorship from another speech pathologist who works for the contract company. She also referred to the ASHA website for information regarding billing and record keeping.

Can you think of other strategies Samantha might use to improve her comfort level in this new setting?

### Aubrey

Aubrey has been an SLP for 8 years. She is well on her way to completing requirements for board certification in swallowing and swallowing disorders. Her particular area of expertise is evaluation and treatment of adults with swallowing disorders with a particular focus on head and neck cancer. Aubrey's hospital has opened a new birthing center with a neonatal intensive care unit. The director of the rehabilitation department wants her to begin evaluating and treating neonates; after all she is the department's "dysphagia expert." Aubrey tactfully declines because evaluating and treating neonates without proper knowledge and expertise or mentorship would be practicing outside of her "population" and her area of expertise. Aubrey offers to find out more information about what it would take to get herself up to speed and in the meantime recommends the director of the rehabilitation department either consider hiring a qualified part-time or as-needed clinician with expertise in neonatal swallowing and swallowing disorders or postpone launching the program until she herself is up to speed. Aubrey then speaks to her friend Priyal. Priyal is an SLP colleague who has expertise in neonate and pediatric swallowing disorders. Priyal offers information about continuing education classes she found to be helpful.

What else could Aubrey do to ensure competency prior to undertaking treatment of neonates?

### Scott

Scott has been an SLP for 12 years. He has worked in a wide variety of settings, including home health, skilled nursing, and the public schools. He has taken a 4-year career hiatus to stay home and take care of his young son. Now that his son is in school full time, he has secured a part-time/as-needed position at a local hospital near his son's school. Before returning to work, he has decided to take a few continuing education classes. He is also going to shadow one of the other full-time clinicians for a couple of days to get a feel for the way they do things at this hospital. Michelle is one of Scott's SLP colleagues. She was in the same circumstances a few years ago. She has offered to provide him with support as he returns to work. Scott happily accepts the offer because he knows he needs to update his clinical skills to current best practice in order to provide his patients with competent care.

What other things could Scott do to prepare for his return to work?

## 27.4 Clinical Ethics and Management of Patients with Swallowing Disorders

Although ethical codes may help define professional values and can establish basic rules of practice, ethical codes may not help clinicians identify and resolve dynamic clinical ethical dilemmas.

Clinical ethics involves identification, analysis, and resolution of ethical dilemmas encountered in the context of providing patient care. Competence in clinical ethics depends not only on being able to use a sound method for analysis but also on familiarity with the medical ethics literature. This can be challenging because issues in medical ethics are constantly evolving in response to medical advances and changes in social and cultural values. Clinical ethical issues tend be more challenging to navigate than professional ethical issues because one cannot typically find a solution in a code.

Concerns regarding ethical care of patients can be traced back to the fourth century BC. Hippocrates was a physician and a philosopher, credited with the Hippocratic oath. The Hippocratic oath is considered to be the earliest framework of medical ethics in the Western world. In contemporary times, a common framework used to identify ethical dilemmas is the four principles approach proposed by Beauchamp and Childress.[11] The four principles are respect for autonomy, beneficence, nonmaleficence, and justice.

### 27.4.1 Respect for Autonomy

Medical ethics literature refers to autonomy as the right of a competent patient to make informed decisions about his or her own course of medical care without undue influence by other people or institutions.

Intervention for feeding or swallowing disorders should work toward restoration, improvement, or maintenance of quality of life. Quality of life is the patient's individual idea of health and happiness. Discussion with patients about quality of life should evaluate the effects of the patient's swallowing or feeding disorder in relation to the patient's perception of well-being. To exercise respect for autonomy, we must listen and effectively communicate with patients and caregivers. We must always remember our role is to *educate* patients and caregivers to improve safety while simultaneously respecting patient and caregiver values and choices. This can be challenging when patient choices seem to be unconventional or seem to conflict with recommendations.

### 27.4.2 Beneficence

*Beneficence* refers to "doing good for the patient." According to Beauchamp and Childress,[11] "beneficence goes beyond being good and kind. . . . Healthcare providers are obliged to balance anticipated good versus potential harm which may result from actions or decisions." This can be challenging because an SLP may not be able to perform actions or make recommendations that are potentially beneficial, or prevent harm, without also creating some degree of risk or burden. For example, thickening liquids may successfully eliminate or reduce aspiration volume. However, if patients avoid drinking thickened liquids because they don't like the taste to the extent that they become dehydrated, we have not accomplished the goal of "doing good" for our patients. Not only have we not accomplished doing good; we have actually contributed to the development of a potentially serious medical complication.

When SLPs make recommendations regarding swallowing and feeding interventions, we do so with the intent of producing positive outcomes. Patients, family members, and care team members need to understand that, although there are anticipated benefits of participating in the dysphagia assessment and treatment process, risks may also be present, and positive outcomes cannot be guaranteed. Moreover, the burdens of care (videofluoroscopic swallow study, fiberoptic endoscopic evaluation of swallowing, diet modification, use of postural techniques and therapeutic maneuvers, swallowing exercises, treatment regimens, and enteral feeding) must be examined within the context of the patient's overall medical status, lifestyle, and emotional well-being.

### 27.4.3 Nonmaleficence

*Primum non nocere* is Latin for "first, do no harm." Nonmaleficence involves the avoidance of intentional harm as well as the risk of harm. According to Beauchamp and Childress,[11] "although the principles of beneficence and non-maleficence are not easily separated, they are different because the obligation not to harm a patient is different from, and usually more stringent than, the responsibility to benefit the patient."

Unfortunately, feeding and swallowing interventions can result in harmful outcomes. Although dietary texture modification (pureeing food, using thickening agents and liquid carbonation) is a common recommendation for patients with feeding and swallowing issues, there is evidence that seemingly benign dietary modifications can result in decreased quality of life[12] and may also result in life-threatening medical complications.[13,14]

In 2002, Chaudhuri et al[15] hypothesized that the use of effortful and intentional breath holding and the super-supraglottic swallow may have undesirable cardiac consequences for some patients. Although postural modifications, such as chin tucks, head turns, and head tilts, as well as compensatory maneuvers, such as a supraglottic swallow or a Mendelsohn maneuver, have been shown to improve swallowing safety and efficiency for some patients, other patients continue to exhibit significant aspiration and/or postdeglutitive residue.[16] Despite growing evidence suggesting that the principles of exercise physiology may be applied to the treatment of feeding and swallowing disorders,[17,18,19,20,21,22,23,24] a number of questions remain unanswered. Several other topics, such as the use of neuromuscular electrical stimulation, the utility of thermal tactile stimulation, the safety and utility of free water protocols, and guidelines for appropriate use of enteral feeding support, continue to result in provocative debates.

As clinicians, we should strive to provide our patients with "net benefits," a concept introduced by Gillon.[25] In order to provide our patients with an understanding of net benefits, we must have a clear understanding of anticipated benefits and potential risks associated with nutrition, feeding, and swallowing recommendations and how to functionally communicate this information in the context of patient care. We must also be clear with patients, caregivers, and other team members about potential risks and burdens in relation to the probability of benefit. If the probability of harm is low and the probability of benefit is high, the proposed option may represent a good choice for the patient. In contrast, if the probability of risk or burden is high and the probability of benefit is low, the proposed option likely does not represent a good choice for the patient. And finally, we must have respect for patient autonomy (right to choose) because what constitutes benefit for one patient may constitute a burden or harm for another.

## 27.4.4 Justice

Of all the moral principles, justice may be the most complex to understand because there are so many theories of justice (Aristotle's principles of justice, libertarian and utilitarian theories, and reward for merit). The principle of justice can be deliberated and applied in a variety of contexts (e.g., individual patient care, interactions within departments, within institutions or on progressively larger scales from state to national to worldwide). For example, as a clinician, do you provide the same quality of care to the patients you see earlier in the day (when you are fresh and have a lot of energy) compared to the patients you see at the end of the day (when you are eager to complete your day and get out the door to pick up your child, walk your pet, or meet your friends for dinner)? Is justice being served if your team received 22 referrals for bedside swallows and your team is short staffed and you were able to see only 18 of the 22 patients? Can you meet the needs of your patients if your institution will allow your team only 10 time slots for videofluoroscopic swallow studies and you have 16 patients who need a videofluoroscopic swallow study? How do you decide which patients will be granted those coveted time slots? On a larger scale, is it fair that patients in some rural areas of the country do not have access to clinicians who are qualified to treat patients with swallowing disorders? Is justice being served if a patient's insurance company will not assist with enteral feeding supplies if the patient is able to take small amounts of liquid or food for pleasure and comfort? Do all people have equal access to medical care?

Gillon[26] subdivided justice into three subcategories: (1) distribution of typical health care resources (funds, materials, facilities, personnel, and time) in a fair and equitable manner, (2) respect for people's rights, and (3) respect for morally acceptable laws. According to Gillon, the right to be treated equally and to have equal access to treatment can be influenced by a wide variety of factors, including age, place of residence, social status, ethnic background, culture, sexual preferences, disability, and legal capacity. Additional information regarding clinical ethics, end-of-life issues, and cultural implications is presented elsewhere in the book.

## 27.5 Questions

**1.** *Primum non nocere* means

A.  First, do no harm.
B.  At all cost, treat the patient.
C.  Before you treat, get permission.
D.  Harm is relative.
E.  No harm, no foul.

**2.** The four core principles of medical ethics are

A.  Respect for autonomy, beneficial, nonmaleficence, and justice
B.  Respect for autonomy, beneficence, nonmaleficence, and justice
C.  Respect for autonomy, beneficence, maleficence, and justice
D.  Respect for autocracy, beneficence, nonmaleficence, and justice
E.  Respect for autonomy, beneficence, nonmaleficence, and judicial

**3.** Mr. Jackson received chemoradiation therapy for treatment of tonsillar cancer 9 years ago. He had a percutaneous endoscopic gastrostomy (PEG) tube for approximately 6 months after completion of his treatment. With intensive dysphagia therapy, he was eventually able to resume a general-consistency diet with some food avoidance of troublesome foods, and his feeding tube was removed. A recent swallow study revealed consistent penetration and intermittent episodes of sensed aspiration. In spite of the difficulties, Mr. Jackson has been maintaining his weight and has not had any signs of aspiration-related pulmonary issues. Mr. Jackson recently underwent a carotid endarterectomy. He had some postoperative complications and required mechanical ventilation for 6 days and was a little confused for several days after the procedure. A Dobhoff nasogastric feeding tube was placed. After his mental status cleared, he was referred to speech pathology for a clinical swallowing evaluation. After reviewing Mr. Jackson's history and performing a thorough clinical evaluation, his speech pathologist recommended a videofluoroscopic swallow study, which revealed consistent episodes of penetration, an isolated episode of sensed aspiration, and decreased swallowing efficiency characterized by mild to moderate postdeglutitive residue. Based on these findings, Mr. Jackson's speech-language pathologist (SLP) recommended he remain nothing by mouth, that PEG tube placement be considered, and that he receive dysphagia therapy. Mr. Jackson feels that, although he is weak, his overall swallowing function is not significantly different from what it was before his surgery and that with a little practice he will be able to get enough to eat and drink. He considers PEG tube placement to be a "big step backward." He understands the risks of eating and drinking and clearly verbalizes that not being able to eat or drink would not represent a good quality of life for him.

What ethical principle(s) is/are represented in this scenario?

A.  Autonomy
B.  Beneficence
C.  Nonmaleficence
D.  Justice
E.  Beneficence, nonmaleficence, and respect for autonomy

**4.** Mrs. Rosenbaum is an 89-year-old woman with a history of Parkinson's disease. Her swallowing function has significantly declined over the past 4 years. She has had multiple swallow studies and has participated in dysphagia therapy on and off for the past 6 years. You have had the pleasure of being Mrs. Rosenbaum's primary SLP for several years. Over the years, she has made it very clear to you and other members of her care team that she does not want a feeding tube. Moreover, she has signed an advanced directive reflecting her wishes, and her family has agreed to honor her choices.

Mrs. Rosenbaum was recently admitted to the hospital with nausea and vomiting. She was subsequently found to have aspiration pneumonia. You have been consulted to evaluate her. The general medicine team has recommended a PEG tube be placed in order to prevent aspiration. You have been asked to "encourage the patient and family to comply with this recommendation so this bed can be freed up."

What ethical principle(s) is/are represented in this scenario?

A.   Respect for autonomy, nonmaleficence, and justice
B.   Beneficence
C.   Nonmaleficence
D.   Justice
E.   Respect for autonomy

**5.** You are working in a large level I trauma center. Unfortunately a number of therapists have resigned, and your department has been short staffed for several months. With limited staffing, you and your other teammates are forced to triage patients every day. In general, all you have been able to do is perform clinical swallow studies and instrumental assessments, make dietary consistency recommendations, and discuss recommendations with staff. You rarely have time to follow up, and you cannot remember the last time you were actually able to provide dysphagia therapy to patients. The physicians and nurses are very frustrated. They think you should be following up with patients on a daily basis. Patients and their families are also frustrated because they have a lot of questions, and they want the therapy their physicians and nurses promised they would receive.

What is the primary ethical principle represented in this scenario?

A.   Respect for autonomy
B.   Beneficence
C.   Nonmaleficence
D.   Justice
E.   Respect for autonomy and beneficence only

# 27.6 Answers and Explanations

**1. Correct: first, do no harm (A).**
The phrases "at all cost, treat the patient," "before you treat, get permission," "harm is relative," and "no harm, no foul" do not literally translate from English to Latin as *primum non nocere. Primum non nocere* is a Latin phrase that means "first or above all, do no harm." In other words, when a medical issues exists, it may actually be better to do nothing than risk causing more harm than good by doing something.

**2. Correct: respect for autonomy, beneficence, nonmaleficence, and justice (B).**
Answers **A**, **C**, **D**, and **E** are incorrect because although the words are spelled or sound similar for example, beneficial rather than beneficence and autocracy rather than autonomy, the incorrect words (beneficial, maleficence, autocracy and judicial) do not represent the four principles of medical ethics. Answer **B** is correct because the four core principles of medical ethics, as outlined by Beauchamp and Childress, are: respect for autonomy, beneficence, nonmaleficence, and justice.

**3. Correct: beneficence, nonmaleficence, and respect for autonomy (E).**
The concept of beneficence is represented because the clinician's intent is to "do good for the patient." The clinician has recommended the patient be nothing by mouth with the intent of reducing the patient's risk for aspiration and aspiration sequelae. The clinician recognizes that a Dobhoff can be uncomfortable and is typically used for short-term enteral support. Therefore, the clinician has recommended consideration of a PEG tube. The clinician has also recommended Mr. Jackson participate in dysphagia therapy with the goal of improving his swallowing safety and efficiency. The concept of nonmaleficence is also represented in that the clinician is not only obliged to "do good for the patient" but also to prevent harm or risk of harm. Mr. Jackson's swallowing function has essentially returned to the level of function he had achieved before the carotid endarterectomy. Given the fact that he was functioning well at that level, a recommendation of nothing by mouth does not seem logical. Although the clinician's intent is to reduce aspiration risk, discouraging oral intake can result in harm as a result of disuse atrophy. In spite of the fact that placement of a PEG tube is typically considered a low-risk procedure, there are risks associated with any surgical procedure. Dysphagia therapy may seem like a fairly benign recommendation to the clinician, but there are potential burdens associated with therapy, including time commitments, issues associated with travel, financial burdens, emotional distress, as well as the fact that outcomes cannot be guaranteed. The concept of respect for autonomy is also represented. Mr. Jackson is cognitively intact. He has a long-term history of dysphagia and understands how this impacts his quality of life on a daily basis. He demonstrates an understanding of the risks associated with oral intake and has made a clear choice about how he wishes to proceed with his care.

**4. Correct: respect for autonomy, nonmaleficence, and justice (A).**
The principle of respect for autonomy is represented because Mrs. Rosenbaum has made it clear to you, her family, and her care team that she does not want to have a PEG tube placed. Moreover, she has signed legal documentation to that affect. The principle of nonmaleficence is also represented. Although Mrs. Rosenbaum was admitted to the hospital and found to have aspiration pneumonia, it is not clear whether the pneumonia is related to aspiration of food or perhaps aspiration that may have occurred when she was vomiting.

The general medicine team's belief that placing a PEG tube, will "prevent aspiration" is incorrect. In spite of the presence of a PEG tube patients can still have issues of aspiration sequelae related to aspiration of secretions. Finally, the principle of justice is represented. The medical team should not request that the clinician essentially coerce a patient and family into agreeing to a surgical procedure in order to "free up a bed."

**5. Correct: justice (D).**

Although you are working very diligently to care for patients, time resources are not being fairly distributed. In addition to assessment services, many of the patients would likely benefit from close follow-up and dysphagia therapy. Lack of follow-up and direct therapy may result in a variety of issues: prolonged recommendations for nothing by mouth, prolonged reliance on restrictive diets, unnoticed changes in functional status that could negatively impact patient safety and nutritional level, lack of progress toward treatment goals, and prolonged hospitalization.

## References

[1] Domenech E, Kelly J. Swallowing disorders. *Med Clin North Am* 1999;*83*(1):97–113, ix

[2] Marik PE, Kaplan D. Aspiration pneumonia and dysphagia in the elderly. *Chest* 2003;*124*(1):328–336

[3] Altman KW, Yu G-P, Schaefer SD. Consequence of dysphagia in the hospitalized patient: impact on prognosis and hospital resources. *Arch Otolaryngol Head Neck Surg* 2010;*136*(8):784–789

[4] Ekberg O, Hamdy S, Woisard V, Wuttge-Hannig A, Ortega P. Social and psychological burden of dysphagia: its impact on diagnosis and treatment. *Dysphagia* 2002;*17*(2):139–146

[5] White TI. Business Ethics: A Philosophical Reader. New York, NY: Macmillan; 1993

[6] American Speech-Language-Hearing Association. Code of Ethics. 2016. https://www.asha.org/Code-of-Ethics/

[7] American Speech-Language-Hearing Association. Practices and Procedures of the Board of Ethics. 2018. https://www.asha.org/policy/et2018-00350/

[8] American Speech-Language-Hearing Association. Knowledge and Skills Needed by Speech-Language Pathologists Providing Services to Individuals with Swallowing and/or Feeding Disorders. 2002. https://www.asha.org/policy/ks2002-00079/

[9] American Speech-Language-Hearing Association. Instrumental Diagnostic Procedures for Swallowing. 1992.

[10] American Speech-Language-Hearing Association. Graduate Curriculum on Swallowing and Swallowing Disorders (Adult and Pediatric Dysphagia). Technical report. 2007. https://www.asha.org/policy/tr2007-00280/

[11] Beauchamp TL, Childress JF. Principles of Biomedical Ethics. New York, NY: Oxford University Press; 2001

[12] Bennett JW, Steele CM. Food for thought: the impact of dysphagia on quality of life. *Dysphagia* 2005;*14*(3):24–27

[13] Finestone HM, Foley NC, Woodbury MG, Greene-Finestone L. Quantifying fluid intake in dysphagic stroke patients: a preliminary comparison of oral and non-oral strategies. *Arch Phys Med Rehabil* 2001;*82*(12):1744–1746

[14] Finestone HM, Greene-Finestone LS, Wilson ES, Teasell RW. Malnutrition in stroke patients on the rehabilitation service and at follow-up: prevalence and predictors. *Arch Phys Med Rehabil* 1995;*76*(4):310–316d

[15] Chaudhuri G, Hildner CD, Brady S, Hutchins B, Aliga N, Abadilla E. Cardiovascular effects of the supraglottic and super-supraglottic swallowing maneuvers in stroke patients with dysphagia. *Dysphagia* 2002;*17*(1):19–23

[16] Shanahan TK, Logemann JA, Rademaker AW, Pauloski BR, Kahrilas PJ. Chin-down posture effect on aspiration in dysphagic patients. *Arch Phys Med Rehabil* 1993;*74*(7):736–739

[17] Easterling C, Grande B, Kern M, Sears K, Shaker R. Attaining and maintaining isometric and isokinetic goals of the Shaker exercise. *Dysphagia* 2005;*20*(2):133–138

[18] Easterling C, Kern M, Nitschke T, et al. Restoration of oral feeding in 17 tube fed patients by the Shaker Exercise. *Dysphagia* 2000;*15*:105

[19] Hind JA, Nicosia MA, Roecker EB, Carnes ML, Robbins J. Comparison of effortful and noneffortful swallows in healthy middle-aged and older adults. *Arch Phys Med Rehabil* 2001;*82*(12):1661–1665

[20] Lazarus C, Logemann JA, Huang C-F, Rademaker AW. Effects of two types of tongue strengthening exercises in young normals. *Folia Phoniatr Logop* 2003;*55*(4):199–205

[21] Robbins J, Gangnon RE, Theis SM, Kays SA, Hewitt AL, Hind JA. The effects of lingual exercise on swallowing in older adults. *J Am Geriatr Soc* 2005;*53*(9):1483–1489

[22] Robbins J, Kays SA, Gangnon RE, et al. The effects of lingual exercise in stroke patients with dysphagia. *Arch Phys Med Rehabil* 2007;*88*(2):150–158

[23] Crary MA, Carnaby Mann GD, Groher ME, Helseth E. Functional benefits of dysphagia therapy using adjunctive sEMG biofeedback. *Dysphagia* 2004;*19*(3):160–164

[24] El Sharkawi A, Ramig L, Logemann JA, et al. Swallowing and voice effects of Lee Silverman Voice Treatment (LSVT): a pilot study. *J Neurol Neurosurg Psychiatry* 2002;*72*(1):31–36

[25] Gillon R. Medical ethics: four principles plus attention to scope. *BMJ* 1994;*309*(6948):184–188

[26] Gillon R. Justice and medical ethics. *Br Med J (Clin Res Ed)* 1985;*291*(6489):201–202

# 28 Ethics: Cultural Considerations

*Luis F. Riquelme*

## Summary

It is up to the professional to initiate an exchange that is as devoid of cultural bias and stereotyping as possible. Awareness of the myriad of factors that impact the exchange between patient and practitioner is of most relevance when striving to provide culturally sensitive services. This lifelong process allows for an environment of collaboration and learning between the practitioner and the patient. Ethically, in order to provide relevant and appropriate dysphagia services that include a good assessment, good treatment approaches, and good overall management, the patient's goals and preferences must be an important aspect in the design of care. Without true communication with the patient, the functional outcomes that are best for the patient will not be achieved.

## Keywords

culture, competence, multicultural, sensitivity, adherence

---

### Learning Objectives

- Provide a broad definition of culture
- Define the concepts of assimilation and acculturation
- Generate a rationale for employing cultural sensitivity
- Present the concept of cultural humility
- Describe the rationale for development of the International Dysphagia Diet Standardization Initiative framework

---

## 28.1 Introduction

The ongoing demographic changes in the United States have presented a challenge to the health care system. No longer are health care practitioners to assume they are in control of every clinical encounter, nor can they assume they are able to "figure it all out." Clinical interactions are human interactions and thus are filled with interpersonal complexities that range from personal perceptions, sometimes stereotyped, to differences in communication styles, even when the same language is used to communicate a message. In essence, the practitioner and the patient both bring many complexities to the table. It is fine for one to assume a certain awareness of differences among people, but our perceptions, and those of the patient, take precedence over any clinical knowledge we may wish to share or access during this encounter. The practitioner needs to gain the patient's trust so as to achieve good follow-up with the practitioner's assessment and recommendations. The process is complex but not impossible.

This perception between two parties might be better understood in the context of culture, cultural differences, cultural awareness, and cultural humility. Culture, as a construct, permeates everything we do professionally and personally. The word *culture* refers to integrated patterns of human behavior that include language, thoughts, communications, actions, customs, beliefs, values, and institutions of racial, ethnic, religious, or social groups.[1] This definition is clearly more inclusive than simply addressing culture as related only to ethnicity or race. So, in essence, this means that every individual, patient or physician, presents with many cultures.[2] It is common for us to focus on ethnicity and race when we hear or use the terms *culture*, *diversity*, or *multicultural*. Today's clinician must accept and fully incorporate the notion that everyone has, or is a part of, a culture, or cultures, in order to provide culturally appropriate and relevant services. Not doing so will result in conflict, misunderstanding, and overall poor service provision in all clinical settings, including poor overall patient outcomes. This places both the patient and the practitioner at risk. It is up to the practitioner to define culture more broadly and include not only ethnicity but also religious beliefs, lifestyles, special interests, and even choice of supermarkets.[3] Hence practitioners have a social responsibility to provide services in a culturally sensitive manner and move beyond the kneejerk definition of *culture* that is based only on race and ethnicity.

The concepts that frame ethical service delivery and decision making have been presented in the prior section and will be reviewed and expanded on in the next section. Joining both sections of this chapter is this discussion on culture. Ethics and culture must coexist in order to achieve the best results for all parties involved. For example, the ethics surrounding end-of-life decisions are intertwined with culture. If we accept a broader definition of culture, then decisions at this point in life, made by the patient or the caregivers, will be culturally based. First would be the overall beliefs typically followed by the family; these are usually the first set of rules to which we are exposed in life. Then there are the religious beliefs the patient may ascribe to. Of final importance is the role of life experiences in having shaped the patient's perceptions and preferences. These factors are all culturally based—parts of different aspects of culture or personal preferences that may be shared with another group of people.

## 28.2 Culture: The Concept

The overall concept of culture is one that anthropologists, bioethicists, clinicians, and others struggle with. The term is widely used to characterize shared ways of world-making and forms of local knowledge.[4] Some uses of the "culture concept" focus on cognition and cultural models, whereas others focus on social practices and everyday social interactions. There are several arguments for and against the use of the culture concept. Some argue that it essentializes heterogeneous modes of understanding, because participants of a particular community or nation are described as having a common, uniform culture.[4] This can be concerning to some because it would follow that being a member of a culture or cultural group would necessitate complete agreement on all matters related to that culture. For example, there is an incorrect assumption that all members of the Hispanic community love eating rice and beans in their many forms. Others argue that the concept of culture obscures tensions and cross-currents within communities, fails to explain significant historical changes in popular understandings, minimizes intragroup differences, and belittles the significance of personal agency.[4] An example here would be not recognizing the common belief between Christians, be they Protestant or not, that Christ was on this earth. So, although Christians are heterogeneous, they all share this common belief. These lines of thinking come from our cognitive predisposition to group individuals as we see fit, based on stereotypes and internalized perceptions. By grouping individuals into these categories, we minimize the importance of individualism and of the fact that everyone is a member of many different groups or cultures. In contrast, it should be understood that grouping individuals is sometimes of benefit to their overall care. For example, although Hispanics/Latinos derive from over 22 different countries, it is of political and social benefit to place all members into one group, as needed. This should not negate the multiple differences between them. For this very reason, it is important to understand and apply the concepts of acculturation and assimilation. As described by Riquelme,[5] assimilation is the process of someone in a new environment totally embracing the host culture, whereas acculturation is the integration of the host culture with the native culture to varying degrees. The United States, a country inhabited by immigrants, has a long history of struggles with assimilation and acculturation. These processes were mostly assimilatory until the middle of the 20th century. Subsequent to that, many immigrant groups began to acculturate, that is, balance their native cultures and beliefs with those of the host culture, or "mainstream America" in this example. This is evidenced by recent trends that highlight the "cultural pride" of different groups. Another benefit of creating groups with a shared commonality is that of linking health trends among different groups. For example, there are certain symptom patterns expected in persons with Parkinson's disease, or other progressive neurogenic disorders. So, the benefit of these groupings is evident; however, it also needs to be flexible, as not everyone in a group shares the same symptom patterns or severity.

## 28.3 Cultural Competence or Cultural Sensitivity?

Several additional notions of culture must be understood in order to answer this question as truthfully as possible. In 1998, Tervalon and Murray-García[6] introduced a concept of culture that encompassed lifelong learning and perspective-taking on the part of the practitioner. According to them, "cultural humility incorporates a lifelong commitment to self-evaluation and critique, to redressing the power imbalances in the physician–patient dynamic, and to developing mutually beneficial and nonpaternalistic partnerships with communities on behalf of individuals and defined populations."[6] The dynamic between provider and patient is often compromised by various sociocultural mismatches, including the provider's lack of knowledge regarding the patient's health beliefs and life experiences and the provider's unintentional

and intentional processes of racism, classism, homophobia, and sexism.[2] Crowley et al[7] argue that cultural humility adds a critical element to the discussion on cultural competence, but that cultural humility is not enough when, for example, an examiner is working to distinguish a language disorder from difference. They further add that, "in many of these situations, a clinician's knowledge of the client's culture and language cannot be separated from a clinician's cultural competence." This is certainly true; thus it follows that it would be impossible for any practitioner to be completely culturally competent in all aspects of a patient's culture(s) or in all aspects of our practice as speech-language pathologists. The question arises when someone believes they are "culturally competent." How was that achieved? Is that even possible? What is the definition?

In this context one may argue that *cultural sensitivity* serves as a better term to denote an active process. It is not absolutist, and the term *sensitive* may invoke movement or dynamism to some. The *New Oxford American Dictionary* (2016),[8] defines *sensitive* as "quick to detect or respond to slight changes, signals, or influences; having or displaying a quick and delicate appreciation of others' feelings." Hence it is proposed that cultural sensitivity is a more appropriate term for the lifelong process of learning about others, understanding the myriad facets of culture, and seeking to achieve balance in our professional and personal interactions with others. It ascribes responsibility to our own sense of belonging as a people and as a professional, and it also imparts the realization of the knowledge that must be acquired in efforts to achieve balance and provide the best care to our patients and clients.

Thus far this discussion has centered on the role of the practitioner in the clinician–patient relationship. We must also consider how the patient perceives the practitioner. What influence does the patient's perception have on the relationship and on overall outcomes? Some argue that cultural competence is a bilateral process, whereas others argue it is not. Sánchez[9] presents an argument against the bilaterality of cultural competence. He argues, based on the "difference principle" presented by Rawls,[10,11] that the patient receiving services is not necessarily empowered to expect culturally competent services. This power differential is in line with the concept of cultural humility presented earlier. He further writes, "Cultural expectations, which any member of an alien culture brings with him or her to the doctor–patient relationship, are barriers to proper medical care if and when these expectations are neither understood nor addressed" (p. 5). What patients expect from their health care practitioner will vary by culture. Noting a more comprehensive definition of culture, the patient's perspective, or expectation, will vary by ethnicity, socioeconomic status, prior experience, setting, and any other set of possible factors.

Cultural competence requires an ongoing commitment to identifying our cultural gaps and blind spots and to finding ways to address them.[12]

## 28.4 Guiding Principles for the Speech-Language Pathologist

The American Speech-Language-Hearing Association (ASHA) has a series of documents that serve as guidelines for speech-language pathologists, audiologists, and speech-language-hearing researchers. Among the first in the more recent series is the "Knowledge and Skills Needed by Speech-Language Pathologists and Audiologists to Provide Culturally and Linguistically Appropriate Services," authored by the Multicultural Issues Board.[13] This document outlines the knowledge and skills clinicians should strive to develop in order to provide least-biased and culturally appropriate services to persons with communication, swallowing, and balance disorders. The document also supports the notion of lifelong learning. A list of competencies is provided to achieve further cultural competence, including sensitivity to differences, understanding the influence of culture on service delivery, and the need to advocate for and empower consumers, families, and communities at risk for communication, swallowing, or balance disorders. Later, in 2005, members of the ASHA Multicultural Issues Board authored another related article entitled, "Why Is Yogurt Good for You? Because It Has Live Cultures."[14] The article focuses on the fact that we all present with many cultures, as do our patients. In addition to these two documents, the ASHA Board of Ethics also strongly supported the need to provide culturally appropriate services by developing an Issues in Ethics statement specifically on cultural competence:

> The Code of Ethics requires the provision of competent services to all populations and recognition of the cultural/linguistic or life experiences of both professionals and those they serve. Everyone has a culture. Therefore, cultural competence is as important to successful provision of services as are scientific, technical, and clinical knowledge and skills.[15]

A few years later, members of ASHA produced a policy document entitled, "Cultural Competence in Professional Service Delivery."[16] There is also a set of tools for self-assessment on cultural competence on the ASHA website, within the Practice Portal on Cultural Competence (http://www.asha.org/Practice-Portal/Professional-Issues/Cultural-Competence). The toolbox includes checklists on personal reflection, policies and procedures, and service delivery. In addition, there is a cultural competence awareness tool in an interactive web-based platform. These documents, tools, and many other articles written by respected colleagues in our field serve as a basis for the argument for achieving cultural sensitivity to provide appropriate services to all our stakeholders. Most importantly, these documents and articles also support the notion that culture, multiculturalism, and diversity go beyond race and ethnicity.

# 28.5 Applications to Dysphagia Practice

Very little has been written about how culture and ethics intertwine in the practice of assessment, treatment, and management of dysphagia in adults or children. The myriad of complex challenges and opportunities is similar to that for other health care practice areas, yet some areas of dysphagia practice are quite distinct.

Mutual cultural understanding in the context of health care practice is challenging in part because of the moral meanings of illness, health, and healing systems, which are culturally and religiously grounded.[17] This can render practices such as advanced care planning, disclosure of a terminal illness, or informed consent for research in conflict with local traditions and beliefs. Thus greater sensitivity is required between the practitioner and patient to achieve a balance and mutual understanding that allows for positive outcomes. Marshall and Koenig[17] mention that "moral pluralism and cultural difference have not been central topics of concern in the first decades of American academic bioethics." They further argue bioethics has only recently addressed issues of cultural pluralism, even though the field was founded soon after World War II. In 2002, the World Health Organization (WHO) established an Ethics and Health Unit, which encompasses ethics, trade, human rights, and health law. This initiative by the WHO has sought to foster the development of programs on ethical issues in biomedicine and science in both clinical and research settings worldwide. In the United States, the Fogarty International Center at the National Institutes of Health has developed initiatives focused on bioethics, including a strong program on international research ethics. One such initiative was creating the Global Health Forum on Bioethics, which is a consortium of international agencies, including the Fogarty, WHO, Pan American Health Organization, the Medical Research Council of the United Kingdom, and the Medical Research Council of South Africa. This forum provides an opportunity for scholars and researchers to debate ethical challenges surrounding research and biomedicine practices around the world. Marshall and Koenig argue that, although these are all positive moves toward the globalization of bioethics, it should be understood that many of these initiatives are still based on Western ideology and values.[17]

Of relevance to us, as practitioners in the assessment, treatment, and management of dysphagia, is the fact that we have no standard set of rules or guidelines for being culturally sensitive or for achieving better outcomes in the context of cultural sensitivity. This may be impossible to achieve in the context of individual preferences and perceptions, as well as in the fact that the complexity of challenges increases when there is more than one figure in the dynamic. As is the case in other health care practices, the patient's perception of the practitioner plays a big role in the care provided. How does the patient perceive the role of the practitioner? How does the "first impression" of the practitioner impact their exchange? Does gender play a role? These are all complex areas to explore. In addition, there is the practitioner's perception of the patient. Might the patient's diagnosis be a distractor to the exchange? Are gender or choice of garments influencing the exchange? Does the patient's insurance coverage influence the care to be provided? Again, these are complex factors, all of which cannot be described or analyzed here because they are based on individual responses and perceptions on the part of both the patient and the practitioner.

## 28.5.1 Food Preferences

Specific to dysphagia practice, the first item that usually comes to mind in providing culturally sensitive care is that of food preferences. The menu of food items from which to select is not always culturally relevant, and the practitioner who is making recommendations is not always aware of the diversity of dishes preferred by the patient. Food preference is often an area of practice relayed to our dietitian colleagues. However, in our clinical role of recommending appropriate consistencies that allow for a safer swallow in the context of impaired physiology, we should be informed as to the diet variances each patient presents with and how these vary from our own. For example, when recommending soft or puree consistencies, we often suggest mashed potatoes, and not often do we think of mashed plantains, which is a culinary staple for many in the Caribbean islands. Of course, thanks to globalization and increased awareness of international cooking, many persons who are not of Caribbean origin include plantains in their diet, and persons of Italian descent are not the only ones to eat homemade pasta. The complexity of opportunities to learn from each other continues. In 2002, the American Dietetic Association published the National Dysphagia Diet (NDD)[18] to establish standard terminology and practice applications of diet textures in dysphagia management. The NDD was created through consensus by a panel of dietitians, speech-language pathologists, and a food scientist. The four levels described in the NDD represent classification based on eight textural properties. For more detailed information see the National Dysphagia Diet 2002. A brief overview on the NDD is also provided in McCullough et al.[19]

Most recently, in view of the international use of many different taxonomies for food/diet classifications, the need to agree on terminology both within and across geographic regions has led to the establishment of the International Dysphagia Diet Standardisation Initiative (IDDSI; www.iddsi.org). The goal of this initiative is to develop globally accepted standardized terminology and definitions for texture-modified foods and thickened liquids for individuals with dysphagia of all ages, in all care settings and all cultures. This is clearly stated on the IDDSI website. In a global survey, 54 labels over four to five diet levels were most reported for texture modification.[20] Similar variation was also seen when labeling liquids; 27 different labels were most commonly used over three to four levels of liquid thicknesses. Subsequently, a systematic review was conducted and published in 2015 by Steele et al,[21] which, based on review of 36 articles, found the following for liquids: there is evidence that thickening liquids helps those who aspirate; there is evidence that "too thick" may generate greater residue, which may increase the risk for aspiration. No specific evidence was found to point to particular rheological values that define the boundaries of effective thickening. For texture-modified foods, the systematic review reported there is little evidence at this time, but that solid foods and thicker consistencies require greater effort in oral processing and swallowing. Later in 2015, the IDDSI board of directors, composed of representatives from speech-language pathology, clinical nutrition, gastroenterology, food science, mechanical engineering, nursing, and occupational therapy from around the world, published the IDDSI Framework (**Fig. 28.1**). This framework presents eight levels ranging from 0 for thin liquids to 7 for regular-texture foods. Each level is identified with a color, number, and label. This combination of three identifiers should serve to limit errors in recommending, identifying, preparing, and assembling dysphagia diet orders. Detailed descriptors and testing methods are provided at www.iddsi.org. This may serve as an appropriate multidisciplinary framework for globalizing diet consistency recommendations in the context of food preferences. It is yet to be seen how this will impact compliance with diets recommended to patients with dysphagia.

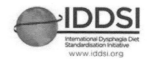

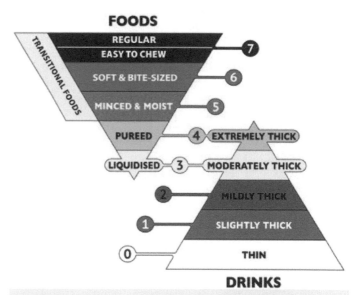

**Fig. 28.1** International Dysphagia Diet Standardisation Initiative

## 28.5.2 Adherence to Treatment

Adherence to treatment is again not often addressed in the context of cultural sensitivity. Clinically, when providing dysphagia services, many practitioners have shifted paradigms from traditional assessment/treatment to management of the person with dysphagia. Another shift in need of attention is that of the use of compensatory, or indirect, treatment strategies employed in concert with direct neuromuscular approaches. This is of relevance to all our patients. In 2005, Colodny[22] published results from a survey conducted with 63 independently feeding adults with dysphagia. Results showed that reasons for nonadherence to treatment recommendations included denial of the swallowing problem, dissatisfaction with food/liquid preparation, assuming a calculated risk, minimizing severity of the problem, projection of blame toward the practitioner, and deflection of nonadherence by referring to an external authority. Also of relevance in the context of compliance with recommendations is the reality of health care disparities.

Specific to health care practices, Beal and Saul[23] reported on the 2004 Commonwealth Fund International Health Policy survey that demonstrated physicians spend less time with "minority" patients (blacks 67%, Hispanics 63%, as compared to whites 87%). Nonwhites also had more unanswered questions after a physician's visit (Hispanics 34%, blacks 31%, as compared to whites 25%). They also presented data suggesting that a strong cultural competency program for medical practitioners improved quality care and overall health care outcomes. This also plays a major role during interactions for informed consent and overall advanced care planning.

To facilitate cultural awareness with all patients, Westby and colleagues[24,25] provide some additional tools. Specifically, Westby introduces the concept of ethnographic interviewing. While originally focused on interviewing parents of children from bilingual homes with possible communication disorders, the overall principles apply to the swallowing specialist and offer ideas on how to present questions in a more open-ended and nonjudgmental manner. Through this process, the practitioner listens to the behaviors and beliefs that the patient or caregiver reports through a systematic and guided dialogue. Ethnographic interviewing conveys empathy/acceptance of the world as defined by the informant, allows the clinician to collect necessary information for generating appropriate support and clinical practice, helps equalize the power differential, provides a means for the professional to discover the culture of the family and their strengths and needs, provides a means for focusing on the perspective of the informant, helps reduce potential bias in assessment and intervention, and allows the clinician to collect data in a more ecologically valid framework.[24] During ethnographic interviewing, the clinician has a general set of questions at the outset, but the flow of questioning is molded by the scope and depth of information obtained as the interview unfolds. The practitioner must also pay attention to how questions are worded, using open-ended rather than closed-ended questions, using presupposition questions effectively, asking one question at a time, and making use of preliminary statements, while maintaining control of the interview.

## 28.6 Questions

1. The word *culture* refers to:

A. Only the skin color of an individual
B. The language a person speaks
C. Integrated patterns of human behavior that include language, thoughts, communications, actions, customs, beliefs, values, and institutions of racial, ethnic, religious, or social groups
D. Religious beliefs and ethnic background only

2. *Cultural humility* refers to:

A. The concept of making cultural awareness a lifelong learning and perspective-taking process
B. Being competent on all aspects of culture, but presenting oneself as humble
C. Accepting that we will never be culturally competent
D. Sensitivity on the part of the patient

3. Some argue that the term *culturally competent* needs improvement because:

A. Knowledge of a culture or language is not absolute or static.
B. It does not sound appropriate in today's politically correct environment.
C. It is too fluid and denotes an active process of accommodation.
D. The multiplicity of culture is not reflected in the terminology.

4. Some argue that the term *culturally sensitive* is more appropriate because:

A. It just sounds better in today's politically correct environment.
B. It appears to be absolute or static.
C. It denotes an active process, possibly invoking dynamism to some.
D. *Sensitive* is nicer and less encompassing.

5. The American Speech-Language-Hearing Association (ASHA) provides guiding principles toward becoming increasingly culturally competent or sensitive in the following documents:

A. Knowledge and Skills Needed by Speech-Language Pathologists and Audiologists to Provide Culturally and Linguistically Appropriate Services
B. Issues in Ethics on Cultural Competence (Board of Ethics, ASHA)
C. Cultural Competence in Professional Service Delivery
D. All of the above

## 28.7 Answers and Explanations

1. **Correct: integrated patterns of human behavior that include language, thoughts, communications, actions, customs, beliefs, values, and institutions of racial, ethnic, religious, or social groups (C).**
*Culture* refers to more than just the color of one's skin or the language an individual speaks. It is a combination a number of factors that ultimately influence human behavior.

2. **Correct: the concept of making cultural awareness a lifelong learning and perspective-taking process (A).**
Clinicians should strive continuously to be culturally aware and realize that the concept of culture is ever-evolving.

3. **Correct: knowledge of a culture or language is not absolute or static (A).**
*Cultural sensitivity* is a more appropriate term than *culturally competent* because cultural concepts are continuously changing.

4. **Correct: it denotes an active process, possibly invoking dynamism to some (C).**
As noted previously, cultural sensitivity is an ever-evolving process.

5. **Correct: all of the above (D).**
ASHA provides a number of resources for clinicians regarding cultural sensitivity, including all those listed

### References

[1] U.S. Department of Health and Human Services, Office of Minority Health. National standards for culturally and linguistically appropriate services in health care: Final report; 2001. http://www.omhrc.gov/clas/
[2] Riquelme LF. The role of cultural competence in providing services to persons with dysphagia. *Top Geriatr Rehabil* 2007;23(3):228–239
[3] Riquelme LF. Cultural competence in dysphagia. *ASHA Lead* 2004;9(7)
[4] Turner L. From the local to the global: bioethics and the concept of culture. *J Med Philos* 2005;30(3):305–320

[5] Riquelme LF. Cultural competence for everyone: a shift in perspectives. *Perspect Gerontol* 2013;*18*(2):42–49

[6] Tervalon M, Murray-García J. Cultural humility versus cultural competence: a critical distinction in defining physician training outcomes in multicultural education. *J Health Care Poor Underserved* 1998;*9*(2):117–125

[7] Crowley CJ, Guest K, Sudler K. Cultural competence needed to distinguish disorder from difference: beyond Kumbaya. *Persp Commun Disord Sci Culturally Linguistically Diverse Pop* 2015;*22*:64–76

[8] New Oxford American Dictionary. Retrieved September 4, 2016

[9] Sánchez CA. Cultural (in) competence, justice and expectations of care: an illustration. *Online J Health Ethics* 2008;*5*(1):1–6

[10] Rawls J. A Theory of Justice. Cambridge, MA: Belknap Press, Harvard University Press, 1971

[11] Rawls J. The Law of Peoples. Cambridge, MA: Harvard University Press, 1999

[12] American Speech-Language-Hearing Association. Professional Issues: Cultural Competence. 2013. http://www.asha.org/Practice-Portal/Professional-Issues/Cultural-Competence

[13] American Speech-Language-Hearing Association. Knowledge and Skills Needed by Speech-Language Pathologists and Audiologists to Provide Culturally and Linguistically Appropriate Services. 2004. https://www.asha.org/policy/ks2004-00215/

[14] Mahendra N, Ribera J, Sevcik R, et al. Why is yogurt good for you? Because it has live cultures. *Persp Neurophysiol Neurogenic Speech Lang* 2005;*15*(1):3–7

[15] American Speech-Language-Hearing Association. Cultural Competence. Issues in Ethics. 2005. https://www.asha.org/policy/et2005-00174/

[16] American Speech-Language-Hearing Association. Cultural Competence in Professional Service Delivery. Professional Issues Statement. 2011. http://www.asha.org/policy/pi2011-00326/

[17] Marshall P, Koenig B. Accounting for culture in a globalized bioethics. *J Law Med Ethics* 2004;*32*(2):252–266, 191

[18] National Dysphagia Diet Task Force. National Dysphagia Diet: Standardization for Optimal Care. Chicago, IL: American Dietetic Association; 2002

[19] McCullough G, Pelletier C, Steele C. National Dysphagia Diet: What to swallow? *ASHA Lead* 2003;*8*:16–27

[20] Cichero JAY, Steele C, Duivestein J, et al. The need for international terminology and definitions for texture modified 6. foods and thickened liquids used in dysphagia management: Foundations of a global initiative. *Curr Phys Med Rehabil Rep* 2013;*1*:280–291

[21] Steele CM, Alsanei WA, Ayanikalath S, et al. The influence of food texture and liquid consistency modification on swallowing physiology and function: a systematic review. *Dysphagia* 2015;*30*(1):2–26 doi: 10.1007/s00455-014-9578-x

[22] Colodny N. Dysphagic independent feeders' justifications for noncompliance with recommendations by a speech-language pathologist. *Am J Speech Lang Pathol* 2005;*14*(1):61–70

[23] Beal A, Saul J. Cultural competency: understanding the present and setting future directions. Paper presented at: Quality of Care for Underserved Populations Conference, The Commonwealth Fund; 2006; New York, NY

[24] Westby C. Ethnographic interviewing: asking the right questions to the right people in the right ways. *J Child Common Dis* 1990;*13*(1):101–111

[25] Westby C, Burda A, Mehta Z. Asking the right questions in the right ways: Strategies for ethnographic interviewing. *ASHA Lead* 2003;*8*:4–17

## Suggested Reading

[1] American Speech-Language-Hearing Association. Practice portal: Cultural Competence. 2015. http://www.asha.org/Practice Portal/Professional-Issues/Cultural-Competence/Cultural-Competence-Content-Development

[2] Crowley C. The ethics of assessment with culturally and linguistically diverse populations. *ASHA Lead* 2004;*9*:6–7. doi: 10.1044/leader.FTR5.09052004.6

# Index

Note: *b* indicates a box; *f*, a figure; and *t*, a table